Behavioral Medicine and Women
A Comprehensive Handbook

Edited by

ELAINE A. BLECHMAN, Ph.D.
KELLY D. BROWNELL, Ph.D.

Forewords by

W. STEWART AGRAS
BONNIE R. STRICKLAND

THE GUILFORD PRESS
New York   London

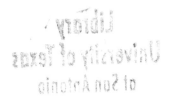

© 1998 The Guilford Press
A Division of Guilford Publications, Inc.
72 Spring Street, New York, NY 10012
www.guilford.com

Printed in the United States of America

This book is printed on acid-free paper.

Last digit is print number: 9 8 7 6 5 4 3 2

Library of Congress Cataloging-in-Publication Data

Behavioral medicine and women: a comprehensive handbook / edited by
  Elaine A. Blechman, Kelly D. Brownell; forewords by W. Stewart
Agras, Bonnie R. Strickland.
     p.   cm.
  Includes bibliographical references and indexes.
  ISBN 1-57230-218-6 (hard.) ISBN 1-57230-522-3 (pbk.)
  1. Women—Health and hygiene—Handbooks, manuals, etc.
2. Women—Psychology—Handbooks, manuals, etc. 3. Medicine and
psychology—Handbooks, manuals, etc. I. Blechman, Elaine A.
II. Brownell, Kelly D.
  [DNLM: 1. Women's Health. 2. Women—psychology. 3. Behavioral
Medicine. WA 309 B419 1998]
RA564.85.B445 1998
610′.82—dc21
DNLM/DLC
for Library of Congress   97–36130
                                                                    CIP

Contributors

BOOK EDITORS

ELAINE A. BLECHMAN, PhD, Department of Psychology, University of Colorado at Boulder, Boulder, Colorado

KELLY D. BROWNELL, PhD, Department of Psychology, Yale University, New Haven, Connecticut

SECTION EDITORS

JEANNE BROOKS-GUNN, PhD, Center for Young Children and Families, Teachers College, Columbia University, New York, New York

LEWAYNE GILCHRIST, PhD, School of Social Work, University of Washington, Seattle, Washington

JULIA A. GRABER, PhD, Senior Research Scientist, Adolescent Study Program, Teachers College, Columbia University, New York, New York

AMY W. HELSTROM, MA, Department of Psychology, University of Colorado at Boulder, Boulder, Colorado

ABBY C. KING, PhD, Department of Health Research and Policy, Stanford Center for Research in Disease Prevention, Stanford University School of Medicine, Stanford, California

BARBARA G. MELAMED, PhD, Ferkauf Graduate School of Psychology, Albert Einstein College of Medicine, Yeshiva University, New York, New York

BETH E. MEYEROWITZ, PhD, Department of Psychology, University of Southern California, Los Angeles, California

GERDI WEIDNER, PhD, Division of Epidemiology and Clinical Applications, National Heart, Lung, and Blood Institute, Bethesda, Maryland

ELIZABETH L. WILLIAMS, MD, MPH, Women's Care, Davies Medical Center, San Francisco, California

CHAPTER AUTHORS

NANCY E. ADLER, PhD, Departments of Psychiatry and Pediatrics, University of California at San Francisco, San Francisco, California

JOHN J. B. ALLEN, PhD, Department of Psychology, University of Arizona, Tucson, Arizona

BARBARA L. ANDERSEN, PhD, Department of Psychology, Ohio State University, Columbus, Ohio

LISA G. ASPINWALL, PhD, Department of Psychology, University of Maryland, College Park, Maryland

AMY K. BACH, MA, Center for the Study of Anxiety and Related Disorders, Boston University, Boston, Massachusetts

DAVID R. BAINES, MD, FAAFP, Association of American Indian Physicians, St. Maries, Idaho

MARY LOU BALASSONE, DSW, School of Social Work, University of Washington, Seattle, Washington

SUSAN A. BALLAGH, MD, Department of Obstetrics/Gynecology, Stanford University Medical Center, Stanford, California

ENRIQUE BARAONA, MD, Department of Alcohol Research and Treatment Center, Department of Veterans Affairs Medical Center, Bronx, New York

DAVID H. BARLOW, PhD, Center for the Study of Anxiety and Related Disorders, Boston University, Boston, Massachusetts

MICHAEL R. BASSO, PhD, Neuropsychology Program, Department of Psychiatry, Ohio State University, Columbus, Ohio

STEVEN R. H. BEACH, PhD, Department of Psychology, University of Georgia, Athens, Georgia

KLEA D. BERTAKIS, MD, MPH, Center for Health Services Research in Primary Care, Department of Family Practice, University of California at Davis, Davis, California

DAVID R. BLACK, PhD, MPH, CHES, FASHA, Department of Health Promotion and Health Kinesiology and Leisure Studies, Purdue University, West Lafayette, Indiana

EDWARD B. BLANCHARD, PhD, Center for Stress and Anxiety Disorders, Department of Psychology, State University of New York at Albany, Albany, New York

RICHARD J. BODNAR, PhD, Neuropsychology Doctoral Program, Department of Psychology, Queens College, The City University of New York, New York, New York

JULIENNE E. BOWER, MA, Department of Psychology, University of California at Los Angeles, Los Angeles, California

SARAH S. BROWN, MPH, Institute of Medicine, National Academy of Sciences, Washington, D.C.

ROBERT L. BRUNNER, PhD, Nutrition Education and Research Program, School of Medicine, University of Nevada, Reno, Nevada

CHARLES S. CARVER, PhD, Department of Psychology, University of Miami, Coral Gables, Florida

THOMAS F. CASH, PhD, Department of Psychology, Old Dominion University, Norfolk, Virginia

HENRY N. CLAMAN, MD, School of Medicine, University of Colorado at Denver, Denver, Colorado

CLAIRE COESHOTT, PhD, Group Leader for Immunology, Cortech, Inc., Denver, Colorado

COLLEEN COFFEY, MA, Department of Psychology, University of Colorado at Boulder, Boulder, Colorado

B. JANE CORNMAN, RN, CS, PhD, School of Nursing, University of Washington, Seattle, WA

W. EDWARD CRAIGHEAD, PhD, Department of Psychology, University of Colorado at Boulder, Boulder, Colorado

VICKI L. DOUTHITT, PhD, Experimental and Applied Sciences, Golden, Colorado.

PATRICIA M. DUBBERT, PhD, Psychological Services, Veterans Affairs Medical Center, Jackson, Mississippi; School of Medicine, University of Mississippi, Jackson, Mississippi

CHRISTINE DUNKEL-SCHETTER, PhD, Department of Psychology, University of California at Los Angeles, Los Angeles, California

MARGARET EDMUNDS, PhD, Institute of Medicine, National Academy of Sciences, Washington, D.C.

ROBERT C. EKLUND, PhD, Department of Health, Physical Education, and Recreation, University of North Dakota, Grand Forks, North Dakota

H. J. EYSENCK, DSc, (deceased), Department of Psychology, Institute of Psychiatry, London, England, United Kingdom

TIFFANY FIELD, PhD, Department of Pediatrics, Touch Research Institute, School of Medicine, University of Miami, Coral Gables, Florida

FRANK D. FINCHAM, PhD, School of Psychology, University of Wales, Cardiff, Wales, United Kingdom

EDNA B. FOA, PhD, Center for the Treatment and Study of Anxiety, Department of Psychiatry, Medical College of Pennsylvania, Philadelphia, Pennsylvania

FREDERICK W. FOLEY, PhD, Ferkauf Graduate School of Psychology, Albert Einstein College of Medicine, Yeshiva University, New York, New York

ROBERT R. FREEDMAN, PhD, Departments of Psychiatry, and of Obstetrics/Gynecology, Wayne State University, Detroit, Michigan

PATRICIA A. GANZ, MD, Division of Cancer Prevention and Control Research, School of Medicine and Public Health, Johnson Comprehensive Cancer Center, University of California at Los Angeles, Los Angeles, California

LINDA C. GIUDICE, MD, PhD, Reproductive Endocrinology Laboratory, Division of Reproductive Endocrinology and Infertility; Stanford University Medical Center, Stanford, California, Children's Hospital at Stanford, Stanford, California,

KAREN GLANZ, PhD, MPH, Cancer Research Center of Hawaii, University of Hawaii, Honolulu, Hawaii

IAN H. GOTLIB, PhD, Department of Psychology, Stanford University, Stanford, California

NICOLA S. GRAY, BS, School of Medicine, University of Pittsburgh, Pittsburgh, Pennsylvania

MARY BANKS JASNOSKI GREGERSON, PhD, Family Therapy Institute, George Washington University, Washington, D.C.

SIGRID B. GUSTAFSON, PhD, Department of Psychology, Virginia Polytechnic Institute and State University, Blacksburg, Virginia

WILLIAM E. HALEY, PhD, Department of Gerontology, University of South Florida, Tampa, Florida

SHARON HALL, PhD, Department of Psychiatry, University of California at San Francisco, San Francisco, California, Psychiatry Service, Department of Veterans Affairs Medical Center, San Francisco, California

BONNIE L. HALPERN-FELSHER, PhD, Department of Pediatrics, University of California at San Francisco, San Francisco, California

JANET B. HARDY, MDCM, Department of Pediatrics, School of Medicine, Johns Hopkins University, Population Center, School of Hygiene and Public Health, Johns Hopkins University, Baltimore, Maryland

KAREN HEFFERNAN, MS, Payne Whitney Clinic, New York, New York

MARK H. HERMANOFF, MD, Department of Immunology, Division of Allergy and Clinical Immunology, National Jewish Center for Immunology and Respiratory Diseases, University of Colorado Health Sciences Center, Denver, Colorado, Denver, Colorado

CORINNE G. HUSTEN, MD, MPH, Office on Smoking and Health, Centers for Disease Control and Prevention, Atlanta, Georgia

C. DAVID JENKINS, PhD, The Highlands, Chapel Hill, North Carolina

PRIYA JORGANNATHAN, National Asian Women's Health, San Francisco, California

ROBERT M. KAPLAN, PhD, Department of Family and Preventive Medicine, Division of Health Care Sciences, University of California at San Diego, San Diego, California

JOEL D. KILLEN, PhD, Department of Medicine, Stanford University School of Medicine, Stanford, California

MIRIAM H. LABBOK, MD, MPH, Institute for Reproductive Health, Department of Obstetrics and Gynecology, Georgetown University, Washington, D.C.

MARK L. LAUDENSLAGER, PhD, Departments of Psychiatry, University of Colorado Health Sciences Center, Denver, Colorado

RUTH A. LAWRENCE, MD, Departments of Pediatrics and of Obstetrics/Gynecology, University of Rochester Medical Center, Rochester, New York

AMI LAWS, MD, Stanford Medical Group, Palo Alto, California

LINDA LERESCHE, ScD, Department of Oral Medicine, School of Dentistry, University of Washington, Seattle, Washington

RONA L. LEVY, PhD, MSW, MPH, School of Social Work, University of Washington, Seattle, Washington

RICHARD R. J. LEWINE, PhD, Schizophrenic Disorders Program, Department of Psychiatry and Behavioral Sciences, Emory University School of Medicine, Atlanta, Georgia

MARCI LOBEL, PhD, Department of Psychology, State University of New York at Stony Brook, Stony Brook, New York

SALVATORE R. MADDI, PhD, Department of Psychology, School of Social Ecology, University of California at Irvine, Irvine, California

MARLENE M. MAHEU, PhD, Nicotine Recovery Institute, San Diego, California

JOANNE E. MANTELL, PhD, MSPH, MSSW, HIV Center for Clinical and Behavioral Studies, Psychosocial Core, New York State Psychiatric Institute, Columbia University, New York, New York

JONI A. MAYER, PhD, Graduate School of Public Health, San Diego State University, San Diego, California

MARY E. McCAUL, PhD, Comprehensive Women's Center and Program for Alcohol and Other Drug Dependencies, Johns Hopkins University School of Medicine, Baltimore, Maryland

PETER McLEAN, PhD, Department of Psychiatry, The University of British Columbia, Vancouver, British Columbia, Canada

LILY D. McNAIR, PhD, Department of Psychology, University of Georgia, Athens, GA

JESSICA MOTHERWELL McFARLANE, PhD, Counselor, Women, Children, and Families, Vancouver, British Columbia, Canada

TRACI L. McFARLANE, MA, Department of Psychology, Erindale College, University of Toronto, Mississauga, Ontario, Canada

DAVID J. MIKLOWITZ, PhD, Department of Psychology, University of Colorado at Boulder, Boulder, Colorado

SUSAN G. MILLSTEIN, PhD, Department of Pediatrics, University of California at San Francisco, San Francisco, California

PHYLLIS MOEN, PhD, Bronfenbrenner Life Course Center, Cornell University, Ithaca, New York

PATRICIA J. MOROKOFF, PhD, Department of Psychology, University of Rhode Island, Kingston, Rhode Island

HEIDI D. NELSON, MD, MPH, Co-Director, Women's Health Fellowship, Oregon Health Sciences University, Portland, Oregon

M. KAREN NEWELL, PhD, Division of Rheumatology and Immunobiology, College of Medicine, University of Vermont, Burlington, Vermont

MARILYN NEWSOM, MD, Department of Neurology, Boulder Medical Center, Boulder, Colorado

DAVID O. NORRIS, PhD, Department of Environmental, Population, and Organismic Biology, University of Colorado at Boulder, Boulder, Colorado

KATHERINE A. O'HANLAN, MD, Division of Gynecologic Oncology, Department of Obstetrics/Gynecology, Stanford University Medical Center, Stanford, California

K. DANIEL O'LEARY, PhD, Department of Psychology, State University of New York at Stony Brook, Stony Brook, New York

HEATHER CARMICHAEL OLSON, PhD, Fetal Alcohol and Drug Unit, Children's Mental Health and Substance Abuse Program, University of Washington, Seattle, Washington

JOHN W. OSBORNE, DDS, MSD, University of Colorado School of Dentistry, Denver, Colorado

MELISSA J. PERRY, ScD, Center for AIDS Intervention Research, Medical College of Wisconsin, Milwaukee, Wisconsin

ANNE C. PETERSEN, PhD, W.K. Kellogg Foundation, Battle Creek, Michigan

THOMAS G. PICKERING, MD, DPhil, Hypertension Center, Department of Medicine, New York Hospital, Cornell University Medical Center, New York, New York

PENNY F. PIERCE, PhD, RN, School of Nursing, and Institute of Social Research, University of Michigan, Ann Arbor, Michigan

JANET POLIVY, PhD, Department of Psychology and Psychiatry, Erindale College, University of Toronto, Mississauga, Ontario, Canada

THOMAS PRUZINSKY, PhD, Department of Psychology, Quinnipiac College, Hamden, Connecticut; Institute of Reconstructive Plastic Surgery; New York University Medical School, New York, New York; Division of Plastic Surgery, Yale University Medical School, New Haven, Connecticut

RENA L. REPETTI, PhD, Department of Psychology, University of California at Los Angeles, Los Angeles, California.

JEAN L. RICHARDSON, DrPH, Department of Preventive Medicine, University of Southern California School of Medicine, Los Angeles, California

GEORGE W. ROBERTS, PhD, Senior Behavioral Scientist, Centers for Disease Control and Prevention, National Center for Injury Prevention and Control, Atlanta, Georgia

JUDITH G. ROGERS, OTR, Through the Looking Glass, Berkeley, California

DAMARIS J. ROHSENOW, PhD, Department of Veterans Affairs Medical Center, Providence, Rhode Island, Center for Alcohol and Addiction Studies, Brown University, Providence, Rhode Island

JAMES C. ROSEN, PhD, Department of Psychology, University of Vermont, Burlington, Vermont

LESLIE D. ROSENSTEIN, PhD, Olin E. Teague Veterans Center, Temple, Texas

SANFORD H. ROTH, MD, Arthritis Center, Ltd., Phoenix, Arizona

JULIA H. ROWLAND, PhD, Psycho-Oncology Program; Department of Psychiatry and Lombardi Cancer Center, Georgetown University School of Medicine, Washington, D.C.

DIANE N. RUBLE, PhD, Department of Psychology, New York University, New York, New York

LAURIE RUGGIERO, PhD, Department of Psychology and Cancer Preventive Research Center, University of Rhode Island, Kingston, Rhode Island

CAROL D. RYFF, PhD, Department of Psychology, University of Wisconsin, Madison, Madison, Wisconsin

WILLIAM C. SANDERSON, PhD, Cognitive Behavior Therapy Program, Department of Psychiatry, Montefiore Medical Center, Albert Einstein College of Medicine, New York, New York

KAREN B. SCHMALING, PhD, Department of Psychiatry and Behavioral Sciences, University of Washington, Seattle, Washington

ULRIKE SCHMIDT, MRC, Paterson Centre for Mental Health, London, England, United Kingdom

ROSA N. SCHNYER, DiplAc, Department of Psychology, University of Arizona, Tuscon, Arizona

LISA A. SCOTT, BA, Health Kinesiology and Leisure Studies, Department of Health Promotion, Purdue University, West Lafayette, Indiana

MARSHA MAILICK SELTZER, PhD, Waisman Center, University of Wisconsin, Madison, Wisconsin

PHYLISS D. SHOLINSKY, MSPH, Epidemiology and Biometry Program, Division of Epidemiology and Clinical Applications, National Heart, Lung, and Blood Institute, Bethesda, Maryland

ILENE C. SIEGLER, PhD, MPH, Duke University Medical Center, Durham, North Carolina

KATHLEEN J. SIKKEMA, PhD, Medical College of Wisconsin, Milwaukee, Wisconsin

LAUREN B. SMITH, BA, University of California at San Francisco, San Francisco, California

TIMOTHY W. SMITH, PhD, Department of Psychology, University of Utah, Salt Lake City, Utah

MAE S. SOKOL, MD, Department of Psychiatry, University of Pittsburgh School of Medicine, Pittsburgh, Pennsylvania; Center for Overcoming Problem Eating, Western Psychiatric Institute and Clinic, Pittsburgh, Pennsylvania

ARNELI A. SOLIDUM, MD, Department of Obstetrics and Gynecology, College of Physicians and Surgeons, Columbia University, New York, New York

SACHIKO T. ST. JEOR, PhD, RD, Nutrition Education and Research Program, University of Nevada School of Medicine, Reno, Nevada

ANNETTE L. STANTON, PhD, Department of Psychology, University of Kansas, Lawrence, Kansas

CATHERINE M. STONEY, PhD, Department of Psychology, Ohio State University, Columbus, Ohio; Department of Psychiatry, Brown University School of Medicine, Providence, Rhode Island

EZRA S. SUSSER, MD, DPH, Division of Epidemiology and Community Psychiatry; Associate Director, HIV Center for Clinical Behavioral Studies, New York, New York

HELEN SWEETING, PhD, Medical Research Council, Medical Sociology Unit, Glasgow, Scotland, United Kingdom

JOEL SZKRYBALO, BA, Department of Psychology, New York University, New York, New York

EVELYN B. THOMAN, PhD, Sleep Studies Laboratory, Department of Biobehavioral Science, University of Connecticut, Storrs, Connecticut

SANDRA P. THOMAS, PhD, RN, University of Tennessee, Knoxville, Tennessee

NICHOLAS TROOP, BSc, Eating Disorder Research Group, Institute of Psychiatry, London, England, United Kingdom

JALIE A. TUCKER, PhD, Department of Psychology, Auburn University, Auburn, Alabama

FIONA C. VAJK, BA, Department of Psychology, University of Colorado at Boulder, Boulder, Colorado

AMY W. WAGNER, PhD, Department of Psychology, University of Wyoming, Laramie, Wyoming

JACQUELINE WALLEN, PhD, MSW, Department of Family Studies, University of Maryland, College Park, Maryland

LILA A. WALLIS, MD, MACP, Clinical Professor of Medicine, Cornell University Medical College, New York, NY; Former President, the American Medical Women's Association (AMWA); Chair, AMWA's Task Force on Women's Health Curriculum;

Co-Chair, the National Academy on Women's Health Medical Education (NAWHME); and Founding President, the National Council on Women's Health (NCWH).

MICHELLE P. WARREN, MD, Department of Obstetrics and Gynecology, College of Physicians and Surgeons, Columbia University, New York, New York

SYLVIA WASSERTHEIL-SMOLLER, PhD, Albert Einstein College of Medicine, Yeshiva University, New York, New York

RISA B. WEISBERG, BA, The Center for the Study of Anxiety and Related Disorders, Boston University, Boston, Massachusetts

MARCIA WESTKOTT, PhD, Department of Women's Studies, University of Colorado at Boulder, Boulder, Colorado

WILLIAM E. WHITEHEAD, PhD, Division of Digestive Diseases, Departments of Medicine and Psychology, University of North Carolina at Chapel Hill, Chapel Hill, North Carolina

ALCUIN WILKIE, MRCPsych, Department of Psychiatry, St. Charles Hospital, London, England, United Kingdom

THOMAS ASHBY WILLS, PhD, Ferkauf Graduate School of Psychology and Department of Epidemiology and Social Medicine, Albert Einstein College of Medicine, Yeshiva University, New York, New York

RENA R. WING, PhD, Department of Psychiatry, University of Pittsburgh School of Medicine, Pittsburgh, Pennsylvania

PATRICIA A. WISOCKI, PhD, Professor of Psychology, University of Massachusetts at Amherst, Amherst, Massachusetts

BRYAN T. WOODS, MD, Olin E. Teague Veterans Center, Department of Medicine, Temple, Texas

ALBERT M. WOODWARD, PhD, MBA, Office of Applied Studies, Substance Abuse and Mental Health Services Administration, Rockville, Maryland

SUZANNE L. WOODWARD, PhD, Department of Psychiatry, Wayne State University School of Medicine, Detroit, Michigan

SHEILA WOODY, PhD, Department of Psychology, Yale University, New Haven, Connecticut

MARGARET O'DOUGHERTY WRIGHT, PhD, Department of Psychology, Miami University, Oxford, Ohio

JUDITH WYLIE-ROSETT, EdD, RD, Department of Epidemiology and Social Medicine, Albert Einstein College of Medicine, Yeshiva University, New York, New York

ALEX J. ZAUTRA, PhD, Department of Psychology, Arizona State University, Tempe, Arizona

ANTONETTE M. ZEISS, PhD, Department of Veterans Affairs, Palo Alto Health Care System, Palo Alto, California

Foreword

Not so long ago, the entire compass of behavioral medicine could be contained within a single and relatively slim volume, and much of the field could be contained within a single head. No special emphasis upon the disorders of women was then apparent. Research during the past 20 years has dramatically altered that situation: The linkages between behavior and disease have been studied at various levels of organization, and in terms of treatment and prevention. No longer can one researcher or clinician be familiar with the entire field. More recently still, the singular aspects of women's health and disease have been intensively studied; this research has been catalyzed in part by a greater emphasis on this important area by funding agencies.

A comparison between the first volume specifically addressing this topic, Blechman and Brownell's 1988 *Handbook of Behavioral Medicine for Women,* and the present book demonstrates the expanded range of interests and findings in the area of women's health. If the format of the first handbook had been followed, the present book would have run to three or four very heavy volumes, straining both muscles and mind.

Instead, the editors have decided to limit the length of individual contributions to under 10 pages, to dispense with the voluminous references found in most texts, and to divide the field into nine sections that are logically chosen and sequenced. This organization has led to chapters that are easy for the reader to find, and also easy to read and to abstract critical information from in a very short time.

The enormous popular interest in the content areas covered by this handbook is reflected in the number of paperbacks devoted to many of these topics. Some of these are of dubious quality, departing from the scientific findings underpinning the field. Hence there is much misinformation in the public domain— misinformation that affects patients' attitudes toward their treatment. This handbook offers an excellent corrective to this situation, allowing clinicians treating women to obtain authoritative information quickly on topics with which they may have only a passing familiarity, and allowing them to convey such information to their patients in a balanced manner. This should result in better care for that half of humanity to whose care this book is addressed.

W. Stewart Agras, MD
School of Medicine
Stanford University

Foreword

*T*en years ago, the *Handbook of Behavioral Medicine for Women* was published to enthusiastic reviews. For the first time, a comprehensive, empirically supported consideration of behavioral approaches to women's health was available. According to a reviewer for the *American Scientist*, Blechman and Brownell had prepared "an excellent starting point for anyone interested in women's issues . . . informative, provocative, stimulating. I hope this is the first of many editions."

The hope of this reviewer has been more than realized with this new book, *Behavioral Medicine and Women*. Indeed, all of us are indebted to Blechman and Brownell. In the earlier volume, they did the difficult work of first identifying health issues specific to women, and then finding science-based experts who could describe these needs and discuss appropriate treatments. Spurred by the emerging interests in women's health (no doubt inspired in part by the first book) and by the considerable advances in understanding and treating women's health needs, their preparation of the present book is up to date and even more comprehensive than the first.

Over 150 of the very best-known people in women's health and medicine cover an exhaustive compendium of topics. Older areas of disease and dysfunction, such as arthritis, anxiety, and diabetes, are covered; so are more recent concerns, such as occupational disorders, HIV, and Alzheimer's disease. Traditional areas of treatment for the medical problems of women are simply and yet thoroughly described, as are alternative treatments (e.g., acupuncture). Populations of women extending from the white middle class to the homeless are included. Perhaps, most importantly, the present volume brings new information about social and behavioral coping processes that are a major part of women's lives in regard to health, prevention, illness, and health care utilization.

As new areas of interests emerge, scientists and clinicians depend heavily on an encyclopedic knowledge base that encompasses both theoretical understandings and practical applications. Usually such information is not available. Blechman and Brownell have done us all a service by incorporating women's health needs and treatments within a comprehensive behavioral model that covers the important aspects of individual well-being and public health across both psychological and physical disorders.

BONNIE R. STRICKLAND, PHD, ABPP
Department of Psychology
University of Massachusetts at Amherst

Preface and Acknowledgments

*I*n 1984, The Guilford Press brought out Elaine Blechman's first edited volume, *Behavior Modification with Women*. This was arguably the first edited book to integrate knowledge about women's mental health in a social–environmental context. In 1988, the two of us edited the *Handbook of Behavioral Medicine for Women*— a volume focusing on linkages between women's mental and physical health, once again in a social–environmental context. Our purpose was to promote awareness of the scarcity of knowledge about topics important to at least half the people on this planet. Our current book, *Behavioral Medicine and Women: A Comprehensive Handbook,* aims to help promote new knowledge about women's health, including numerous contradictory findings.

Along with an increase in information about intersections between women's physical and mental health has come growing bewilderment among women about which behavioral, dietary, pharmacological, and surgical practices are beneficial and which are harmful, and about what constitutes a healthy lifestyle. Some women are so perplexed that they either have given up any attempt to maintain a healthy lifestyle, or have adopted prescientific, superstitious beliefs and strategies to cope with disease. Thus our aim in this volume is to provide a rational integration of what is known about women's health in a format that will prove useful, intellectually stimulating, and even emotionally reassuring to consumers, practitioners, scientists, and students. The extensive and intensive chapter coverage of topics, the scholarly section introductions, and the annotated "Further Reading" lists (which take the place of extensive in-text citations and lengthy, conventional reference lists) should allow this volume to serve as a textbook for some readers and as a general or specialized reference book for others. Some readers will consult this book to learn what to do about a specific condition or disorder; others will consult it to identify topics in need of future inquiry.

When we edited the 1988 volume, we identified a number of topics pertinent to women's health for which there was no research evidence and about which no experts were willing to speculate. When we solicited chapters for that book, a substantial number of eminent scientists challenged us to explain the need for a book devoted to women's health. Many presumed, wrongly, that gender differences in the prevalence of disorders would be the sole (and to them trivial) focus of the book. They seemed genuinely baffled by the notion that women's behavior and health are shaped by distinctive social and environmental forces, and thus that equally distinctive prevention and intervention measures are needed. Most of the chapters in the 1988 book were written by brave souls who argued against mind–body dualism; pointed out gaps in our knowledge about women's health; lobbied for basic research, clinical trials, and prevention programs; and made the most of relevant, though often sparse, research findings.

Not even a decade later, we find ourselves editing a book under quite different constraints. Educated women no longer need to be convinced that psychological disorders have physiological antecedents, components, and consequences, just as physical disorders have psychological antecedents, components, and consequences. Just about every day, we read research reports in top-echelon psychological and medical journals about issues pertinent to women's health. In the current handbook, chapter authors covering topics that at first seemed overly narrow have found it difficult to review recent empirical advances and methodological developments within their page limits. Areas about which nothing could have been said less than a decade ago have spawned far more subtopics, data, and chapters than we or our associate editors ever anticipated. As a result, we have in some cases included multiple chapters on the same topic from differing perspectives. Had we the space, we could have covered most topics in this book with chapters written from the vantage points of epidemiology, prevention, and intervention, and from psychological and medical perspectives.

We attribute the growth in research on women's behavioral medicine not to ephemeral concerns about political correctness, but to what we hope are lasting changes in the politics of North American behavioral science. In the past decade, a numerically small but disproportionately influential group of women who were graduate students and medical students in the 1970s entered the senior ranks in their universities, medical schools, and professions; they thus gained the power and safety to influence decision making about research funding and journal publication, and to investigate topics long considered "career breakers." The disciplinary boundaries that once obstructed investigation of the health of women as whole people (with somas and psyches) are vanishing. The celebrity of both female and male contributors to this book indicates that women's health is no longer a marginal or incendiary topic in scientific circles. Sophisticated treatments of gender differences (and their absence) are paving the way for an understanding of fundamental health-related mechanisms that operate in the same way across genders, while yielding to the unique social environments inhabited by each gender.

Self-congratulation is not yet in order, for much more remains to be learned. In their section introductions, each of our section editors has identified gaps in knowledge and neglected areas of research; widely accepted yet flawed research methods; and trendy diagnoses and interventions that are uncritically accepted one year and forgotten the next. The next version of this book will certainly require two volumes and must include data-based chapters on topics that include antisocial personality disorder, hormone replacement therapy, chronic yeast infection, nutritional supplements, and consumer treatment preferences. We hope that much more will be known by then about the impact on women's mental and physical health of normative developmental transitions (e.g., the change from being married to being divorced or widowed) and of exceptional life choices (e.g., single parenting with and without a male or female partner). Assuming that the "new age" of the 1990s will persist into the next century, we expect to see data-based chapters on every aspect of what is now considered alternative medicine, including massage, meditation, and yoga. At the top of our wish list for the next version are chapters reporting definitive findings about the developmental mechanisms that account for diverse disorders, and about the causal mechanisms that promote successful prevention and intervention strategies.

This book could not have been completed without the painstaking, thoughtful, persistent, and cheerful efforts of Amy W. Helstrom, our editorial assistant and an editor of Section IX. Our other section editors—Jeanne Brooks-Gunn, Julia A. Graber, Abby C. King, Lewayne Gilchrist, Elizabeth L. Williams, Beth E. Meyerowitz, Gerdi Weidner, and Barbara G. Melamed—labored long and hard to recommend and recruit contributors, bore with us through an unanticipated reorganization of this book, and produced, each in her or his own way, section introductions that make this book much more than an unrelated jumble of chapters. Seymour Weingarten, Editor-in-Chief of The Guilford Press, encouraged and supported our efforts despite unanticipated delays.

Jerry Frank, of Pergamon Press, editor of our previous volume, is no longer with us. We mourn the loss of this jolly bon vivant and recall that without his enthusiasm, neither the 1988 book nor this one would have seen the light of day.

Finally, our joy at the publication of this book was tempered by news of the death of one of the contributors to this volume, Dr. H. J. Eysenck, who was great in scholarship, intellectual courage, and gentility. At this point, we can only begin to contemplate the enormity of Dr. Eysenck's contributions to our understanding of the intersection of stress, coping, and health.

ELAINE A. BLECHMAN,
Boulder, Colorado

KELLY D. BROWNELL,
New Haven, Connecticut

SUGGESTED READING

Eysenck, H. J. (1994). The outcome problem in psychotherapy: What have we learned? *Behavior Research and Therapy, 32,* 447–495.

Contents

IV HEALTH CARE PARADIGMS, POLICIES, AND SETTINGS

Addresses the question "What do we know about innovations in health care policies, paradigms, and settings that affects women's health?"

V BODY IMAGE AND SUBSTANCE USE

Addresses the question "What do we know about linkages between body image and substance use on the one hand, and women's physical and mental health on the other?"

VI SEXUALITY AND REPRODUCTION

Addresses the question "What do we know about linkages between sexuality, reproduction, and women's physical and mental health?"

VII PHYSIOLOGICAL DISORDERS WITH BEHAVIORAL AND PSYCHOSOCIAL COMPONENTS

Addresses the question "What do we know about physiological disorders among women that should be known by any mental health or health care provider or educated woman?"

VIII LINKAGES BETWEEN BEHAVIORAL, PSYCHOSOCIAL, AND PHYSICAL DISORDERS

Addresses the question "What do we know about behavior disorders among women that should be known by any mental health or health care provider or educated woman?"

Section I

LIFE COURSE
PERSPECTIVES

1

Section Editors' Overview

Jeanne Brooks-Gunn
Julia A. Graber

*I*n this section, "Life Course Perspectives," chapter authors have written about various epochs or transitions in individuals' lives that have consequences for the health of girls and women. Although developmental transitions and their link to health are the specific foci of this section, it is notable that the entire volume is dedicated to understanding women's health across the life course. As such, the editors have carefully selected topics with an eye toward the causes and consequences of health status and how it changes over time, as well as how the definition of health itself is altered as the individual develops. Indeed, the question of who becomes sick and who does not (or, more precisely, how and when individuals move in and out of health) could be framed in terms of life epochs; this approach contrasts with the more traditional discussions of causes and consequences or outcome-based approaches.

The topics covered in this section are broad, in order to encompass the "flavor" of this approach. Chapters are presented on prenatal development, infancy, childhood, early adolescence (puberty), late adolescence (sexuality and teenage childbearing), young adulthood (specifically issues related to parenting), midlife, and later life. These are most, if not all, of the life stages of women. More specific chapters relevant to the topics discussed in this section and linked to life epochs are found throughout the book (e.g., menopause, osteoporosis, access to prenatal care, health care in public high schools, and postpartum depression, to name just a few).

LIFE PHASES OR LIFE STAGES

What do we mean by a "life course perspective"? Moen's chapter on aging opens with the statement that changes in biological, social, emotional, and cognitive realms occur over the life course and interact in complex ways. Life course scholars attempt to understand the timing and sequencing of these changes, as well as the differential effects that such changes have on individuals and groups at different points in their lives. In addition to discontinuities, continuities over life phases are of interest, as are phase-specific behaviors that "set the stage" for health in subsequent life phases. As Moen emphasizes in her chapter, the point of such a framework is to see the life course as more than just a series of snapshots. Unfortunately, given the costliness and length of time needed to conduct long-term longitudinal studies, the bulk of the work to date has examined lives within life phases, rather than in terms of trajectories across life phases. At the same time, a life course perspective may be used to examine a particular life phase more intensively and extensively, since each life phase is itself made up of a series of biological and social events. Often researchers have focused on the movement into and/or out of a particular life phase (e.g., adolescence), in order to capture the breadth of possibilities that arise as individuals make important transitions.

How do we define a life phase or epoch? We have deliberately avoided the use of the term "stage," since theorists from Sigmund Freud to Erik Erikson and beyond have used this word to denote a particular view of development. Stage theories hold, among other tenets, that challenges and intrapsychic issues are unique to each stage; that reorganization occurs as a result of successful negotiation of each stage; and that development is stymied if the issues of a previous stage were not resolved. Along these lines, some stage theories propose critical periods for development. According to these theories, not only is development compromised by continuing issues, but resolution or advancement cannot occur once a critical period is past. These assumptions do not underlie the notion of life phases or epochs, even though such assumptions certainly could be tested.

Life phases are usually defined in terms of biological and social events that occur from conception to death. Although different cutoff points and distinctions have been made, the following groupings are fairly standard, at least in Western societies: the prenatal period, infancy, early childhood, late childhood, early adolescence, late adolescence, early adulthood, middle age (middle adulthood), and old age (late adulthood). These groupings are based on a mix of biological, social-cognitive, and role changes. In cultures with formal and extended schooling, the timing of changes in school type and environment is a primary defining feature of childhood and adolescence (e.g., the entry into elementary school marks the beginning of late childhood; the entry into middle or junior high school marks the beginning of early adolescence). Role changes are paramount in late adolescence and adulthood (e.g., getting a job, becoming a parent). At the same time, biological changes (over and above the general aging process) are implicated in defining the prenatal period, infancy, early and late adolescence, and early and middle adulthood. The salience of reproductive changes is the defining feature of three of these phases—puberty in early adolescence, pregnancy in late adolescence/early adulthood, and menopause in middle adulthood. Reproductive changes are also part of the prenatal period, in that the fetus "becomes" a female or a male through differences in brain organization and in internal and external sex characteristics. The critical nature of reproduction in women's lives is illustrated time and again in this volume. Almost half of the chapters in the book address aspects of reproduction (broadly defined).

REPRODUCTIVE TRANSITIONS

We believe that reproductive transitions provide a useful frame for studying many (but not all) aspects of women's health. Such transitions are critical landmarks in women's lives, from the prenatal development of a female through menopause. In addition, if social aspects of reproduction are considered as well as biological substrates, we might add parenthood as a reproductive transition, in that becoming a mother or a father is gender-specific (even if both parents exhibit parenting behavior). Some might even add early childhood to this list, since this is the life phase when children acquire gender constancy. However, we are more concerned with those transitions that involve biological change, in addition to role and social-cognitive changes.

It is important to note that life phase transitions are usually made up of a series of events or markers. For example, pubertal change encompasses a series of events—breast development, fat accumulation, height spurt, menarche, hormonal increases. Pubertal changes co-occur with a number of social and school changes, including the move to middle school (in Western societies), increased independence from the family, and the beginning of dating relationships, to name a few. Hence the combination of these biological, social, and psychological changes characterizes the life phase of early adolescence, but it will also predict health in later adolescence and potentially across the life course. Like puberty, the other reproductive transitions are linked to social and psychological changes. As such, reproductive transitions are embedded in a life course that must be considered in all of its contextual features. The rich interaction between biology and context is especially important to consider when studying reproductive transitions. The facile explanation of behavioral changes at puberty, pregnancy, or menopause is that behavior is "caused" by biological processes. However, the picture of behavioral change is much more complex.

The context of a life phase is also defined by intergenerational influences, in that the life experiences of generations, particularly within families, are interconnected and interactive. That is, we and others such as Rossi and Rossi have suggested that a woman's experience of menopause may be quite different if her daughter is experiencing puberty, is sexually active, or is a pregnant young woman. Moreover, a girl's experience of puberty is no doubt influenced by her mother's reproductive life phase, just as the daughter's phase influences the mother's menopausal experience. (See further readings for examples of such reciprocal influences on mothers' and daughters' dieting behavior and depressed affect by us and members of our group.)

The timing of reproductive events is also an important consideration in understanding their link to health outcomes. For example, effects of mothers' menopausal status on daughters' eating behavior are only found for early-maturing girls. Becoming a grandmother early (i.e., in young to middle adulthood), as is the case when one's daughter is a teenager or when one was a teenage mother herself, has a different meaning than becoming a grandmother in middle to late adulthood.

Studies looking across reproductive transitions should allow for comparisons of the factors contributing to successful negotiation of the different transitions. Similar factors (or at least a similar model) may be applicable to puberty, pregnancy, and menopause, for example. Regrettably, little work on reproductive transitions to date has been comparative. Several lines of comparative research could be considered. One focus has to do with the social, biological, and psychological correlates of reproductive transitions more generally. The following discussion is a brief overview of a specific model for linking reproductive transitions and health outcomes via the experience of stress during these transitions.

STRESS AND WOMEN'S REPRODUCTIVE TRANSITIONS

A wealth of research has been amassed on the effects of different types of stressors on health at both the physiological and psychological levels as has been indicated in recent reviews. Reproductive transitions may be periods in the life course when more stressors occur, and/or reproductive transitions may increase the physiological and psychological vulnerability to stress. From the perspective of women's health, the ultimate question is whether or not increased numbers of stresses, increased physiological or psychological responsiveness to stresses, or both lead to heightened risk for morbidity or mortality. In the case of pubertal development, the risk for morbidity is more common, although potential lifelong effects that influence mortality are possible.

In our research on the pubertal transition, we have been asked the following sets of questions: What are the factors occurring during puberty that lead to stress during this time? That is, do more stresses occur during the pubertal transition than at other periods of development (excluding other reproductive transitions)? In contrast, do the stresses that occur during the pubertal years have more of an impact on health outcomes than if the same stresses occurred prior to or after the transition? Evidence exists for both situations during the pubertal transition. (Research on pregnancy and menopause has not typically taken this approach.)

First, in research examining whether or not more potentially stressful life events occur during puberty than at other life phases (excluding other reproductive transitions), preliminary evidence indicates that adolescents do in fact experience an increased number of such life events coinciding with the peak pubertal years. In two longitudinal studies of adolescents (by our group and by Ge and his colleagues), the number of stressful life events has been shown to increase during the early adolescent years. The number of events experienced peaked between ages 12 and 14 for girls in the Early Adolescent Study by Brooks-Gunn, and by age 15 for girls in the Iowa Youth and Families Project as reported by Ge and his colleagues. The peak in events noted in the Early Adolescent Study occurred simultaneously with the period of middle to late pubertal development for most girls in this sample. In both studies, subsequent declines were seen in the reported number of events after these peak ages.

Second, research by others has also demonstrated that the experience of so-called stressful events has a greater impact on adjustment when events occur simultaneously with pubertal development. In the work of Petersen and her colleagues, the experience of pubertal changes at the same time as a school change (e.g., moving from an elementary to a junior high school) led to poorer adjustment in the junior high school years, as well as to longer-term influences on depressive affect in late adolescence.

As indicated in the examples noted above, much of the research examining the outcome of stress during pubertal development has focused on affective outcomes—specifically, depressive affect and depression. Comparable research on stress during puberty has also examined such health-related outcomes as changes in bone density, fat deposition, and obesity. Parallel work has been done on menopause. The development of bone density at puberty, and changes in lipid levels at menopause, provide interesting examples of this work.

During the adolescent decade, 48% of bone mass is accrued. The accrual of bone mass begins with the onset of puberty, but continues for several years after puberty into young adulthood. Although bone density is typically subject to fluctuation (often in relation to estrogen levels), stressors also affect the accrual of bone mass during puberty in ways that may have lasting effects throughout the life course. As yet, little research has addressed whether disruptions in bone mass accrual in adolescence lead in fact to longer-term structural deficits, or whether such deficits are ameliorated in adulthood if the stressor is discontinued.

Research on changes in bone density during puberty and adolescence has demonstrated the strong effects of estrogen on bone density during this time. However, lower levels of circulating estrogen, and resultant amenorrhea or delaying of pubertal development, have been caused by behavioral stressors such as high levels of exercise and disturbed eating behaviors as demonstrated in work by Warren and others—that is, subclinical and clinical eating disorders. Even though these studies have included adolescents of a broad age range (e.g., 13–20 years in Dhuper et al., 1990), the exercise and dieting stresses are occurring during puberty for many of these girls. In addition to affecting processes such as normal bone development, these same activities affect several aspects of pubertal development, in some cases elongating the pubertal development period by delaying puberty. Puberty is not, however, completely delayed by exercise. Warren (1980) reports that changes in exercise behavior were related to progressions in breast development and menstruation but not to pubic hair development, which progressed during periods of delayed breast development. Hence, these stressors are likely to be affecting health outcomes via gonadal estrogen production rather than via adrenal systems.

Another example is the work of Matthews and colleagues. This team has shown that lipid levels in blood during the menopausal transition are strongly influenced by the occurrence of stressful life events. Women who experience stress just before the menopausal transition begins exhibit an increase in low-density lipoproteins and a decrease in high-density lipoproteins, compared to women who do not report stressful experiences in the premenopausal phase.

Finally, is it possible that the nature of reproductive transitions means that stressful events at these times has specific or stronger effects on women's health than stress experienced at other times in the life cycle? Few data exist to support, or to refute, this premise. Perhaps experiences of stress during periods of physiological change may be qualitatively different and may have different effects on girls' and women's health than during times of hormonal stability. As indicated in our examples, estrogen influences have been found on many physiological systems of the body, including cardiovascular, lipids, bone accretion, and fat deposition, as well as affective function across the lifespan. Hence estrogen influences on health may be especially likely to occur during reproductive transitions. In addition, because of the interactive nature of the endocrine system, bidirectional effects are also likely to exist among stress and reproductive hormones; that is, stress affects the production of reproductive hormones, as seen in the elongation of the follicular phase of the menstrual cycle in response to psychological stressors. Reproductive hormones affect the magnitude of cardiovascular and neuroendocrine responses to stress, as evidenced by Matthews's work on blood pressure responses to stress in men and women in middle age (e.g., postmenopausal women had higher blood pressure than same-age premenopausal women). Further comparative considerations of reproductive transitions are needed to address these questions, but perhaps the most intriguing questions require examinations of the transitional experiences within individuals across the life course.

FURTHER READING

Adler, N., & Matthews, K. A. (1994). Health psychology: Why do some people get sick and some stay well? *Annual Review of Psychology, 45,* 229–259.
The authors provide a comprehensive overview of current issues in health psychology.

Brooks-Gunn, J. (1992). Growing up female: Stressful events and the transition to adolescence. In T. Field, P. McCabe, & N. Schneiderman (Eds.), *Stress and coping in infancy and childhood* (pp. 119–145). Hillsdale, NJ: Erlbaum.
This chapter reviews several studies of girls' development at adolescence and highlights data on the experience of stressful life events in early adolescence.

Brooks-Gunn, J., & Chase-Lansdale, P. L. (1995). Adolescent parenthood. In M. Bornstein (Ed.), *Handbook of parenting: Vol. 3. Status and social conditions of parenting* (pp. 113–149). Mahwah, NJ: Erlbaum.
This chapter reviews the literature on teenagers as parents highlighting innovative research on multigenerational parenting practices and situations.

Brooks-Gunn, J., & Ruble, D. N. (1982). The development of menstrual-related beliefs and behaviors during early adolescence. *Child Development, 53,* 1567–1577.
Findings on the experience of menarche and menstruation are reported from a large multimethod two-study project.

Deutsch, F. M., Ruble, D. N., Fleming, A., Brooks-Gunn, J., & Stangor, C. (1988). Information-seeking and self-definition during the transition to motherhood. *Journal of Personality and Social Psychology, 55*(3), 420–431.
In a large cross-sectional study of the transition to motherhood, self-socialization processes are examined in connection with the construction of identity.

Dhuper, S., Warren, M. P., Brooks-Gunn, J., & Fox, R. (1990). Effects of hormonal status on bone density at maturity in adolescent girls. *Journal of Clinical Endocrinology and Metabolism, 71*(5), 1083–1087.
Findings are reported on a study of estrogen effects on bone density in a sample of adolescent girls and young adult women.

Elder, G. H., Jr. (1985). Perspectives on the life course. In G. H. Elder, Jr. (Ed.), *Life course dynamics: Trajectories and transitions, 1968–1980* (pp. 23–49). Ithaca, NY: Cornell University Press.
The author explains a model for understanding development across the life course.

Ge, X., Lorenz, F. O., Conger, R. D., Elder, G. H., Jr., & Simons, R. L. (1994). Trajectories of stressful life events and depressive symptoms during adolescence. *Developmental Psychology, 30,* 467–483.
Findings on the experience of stressful life events during adolescence are reported for a sample of European-American adolescents residing in rural communities.

Graber, J. A., & Brooks-Gunn, J. (1996). Reproductive transitions: The experience of mothers and daughters. In C. D. Ryff & M. M. Seltzer (Eds.), *The parental experience in midlife* (pp. 255–299). Chicago: University of Chicago Press.
This chapter examines models for intergenerational influences on the lives of mothers and daughters at times of reproductive transition and reviews findings from a series of studies conducted by the authors and their colleagues.

Graber, J. A., & Brooks-Gunn, J. (1996). Transitions and turning points: Navigating the passage from childhood through adolescence. *Developmental Psychology, 32*(4), 768–776.
This article reviews and develops models for understanding behavioral change at developmental transitions focusing on adolescent development.

Maier, S. F., Watkins, L. R., & Fleshner, M. (1994). Psychoneuroimmunology: The interface between behavior, brain, and immunity. *American Psychologist, 49,* 1004–1017.
A synthesis of potential mechanisms linking stress and health is provided.

Marshall, W. A., & Tanner, J. M. (1986). Puberty. In F. Falkner & J. M. Tanner (Eds.), *Human growth: Vol. 2. Postnatal growth neurobiology* (pp. 171–209). New York: Plenum Press.
This chapter is a comprehensive review of the literature on pubertal development drawing upon the voluminous collaborative work of the coauthors.

Matthews, K. A. (1989). Interactive effects of behavior and reproductive hormones on sex differences in risk for coronary heart disease. *Health Psychology, 8,* 373–387.
A synthesis of findings linking reproductive hormones and health in women is presented with the development of a model for subsequent research.

Paikoff, R. L., Brooks-Gunn, J., & Carlton-Ford, S. (1991). Effect of reproductive status changes upon family functioning and well-being of mothers and daughters. *Journal of Early Adolescence, 11*(2), 201–220.
This study is one of the few to examine empirically the simultaneous effects of reproductive transitions on mothers and daughters.

Parlee, M. B. (1984). Reproductive issues, including menopause. In G. Baruch & J. Brooks-Gunn (Eds.), *Women in midlife* (pp. 303–313). New York: Plenum Press.
This groundbreaking chapter argued for the development of biopsychosocial models for studying menopause, setting the course for subsequent research.

Petersen, A. C., Sarigiani, P. A., & Kennedy, R. E. (1991). Adolescent depression: Why more girls? *Journal of Youth and Adolescence, 20,* 247–271.
One of the few studies to test a simultaneous change model finding prediction from early adolescence to subsequent depression.

Rossi, A. S., & Rossi, P. H. (1990). *Of human bonding.* New York: Aldine de Gruyter.
This volume documents the reciprocal nature of influences that parents and children have on one another.

Rodin, J., & Kupfer, D. (1992). *In and out of health.* Unpublished manuscript, Yale University.
This paper was developed as part of the guidelines for the John D. and Catherine T. MacArthur Foundation Research Network on Health-Promoting and Disease-Preventing Behaviors.

Simmons, R. G., & Blyth, D. A. (1987). *Moving into adolescence: The impact of pubertal change and school context.* New York: Aldine.
This book reports on a seminal study of development during adolescence with comprehensive examination of the influence of school context on adjustment and behavior.

Smith, S. (1995). Two generation programs: A new intervention strategy and directions for the future. In P. L. Chase-Lansdale & J. Brooks-Gunn (Eds.), *Escape from poverty: What makes a difference for children?* (pp. 299–314). New York: Cambridge University Press.
The author argues for further development of two-generation intervention programs to meet the needs not only of young parents as they enter the work force but also of their young children.

Warren, M. P. (1980). The effects of exercise on pubertal progression and reproductive function in girls. *Journal of Clinical Endocrinology and Metabolism, 51,* 1150–1157.
How exercise delays puberty separate from changes in weight is investigated in a sample of adolescent athletes.

Warren, M. P., & Brooks-Gunn, J. (1989). Delayed menarche in athletes: The role of low energy intake and eating disorders and their relation to bone density. In C. Laron & A. D. Rogol (Eds.), *Serono Symposia publications: Vol. 55. Hormones and sport* (pp. 41–54). New York: Raven Press.
Findings are reported on the unique contributions of hereditary factors, exercise, and other behaviors on bone density during the pubertal years.

2

Brain and Behavior Development

Bryan T. Woods
Leslie D. Rosenstein

*I*t has been less than a decade since the topic of brain and behavior development was reviewed for the 1988 *Handbook of Behavioral Medicine for Women,* and yet the information available on the subject has undergone the same exponential growth as so much of neurobiology has. Therefore,we have made an effort to describe what is known now about the major issues, rather than to review in detail the earlier history of the field—however fascinating the evolution of ideas may have been. The chapter is divided into the following sections: (1) the neurobiology of sexual differentiation in the central nervous system (CNS) in humans, and in animal models where these are relevant to humans; (2) the nature of male–female brain differences not directly linked to reproduction; (3) normal and pathological male–female differences in cognition; and (4) the interaction of sex differences in brain anatomy with cognitive function and dysfunction.

THE BASIC NEUROBIOLOGY OF SEXUAL DIFFERENTIATION

Reproduction in higher organisms is under a significant degree of neural control, such that fundamental differences in the reproductive roles and behaviors of the sexes are believed to be determined by differences in the male and female nervous systems. Until recently, anatomical evidence for sexually dimorphic brain structures was limited to birds and small mammals, but there are now both pathological and *in vivo* brain imaging studies demonstrating such dimorphism in humans.

Sexual differentiation in vertebrates is determined by a single chromosome of a single pair. In mammals one chromosome of the pair is always an X chromosome, but the other one may be a second X (in which case the organism will be female) or a Y (in which case a male will result). It is of fundamental importance to note that in mammals the "default" condition is female; that is, a single X and no Y (X,O) leads to female development, while the presence of a single Y, even in the presence of up to four X's, results in male development. (In birds the opposite relationship prevails.) It has also been clear for some time that the Y chromosome exerts its determining effect on genital sexual differentiation by way of testis development, rather than by directly exerting a general effect on somatic cells.

The responsible gene on the Y chromosome, known as the *sry* gene, was isolated in 1990 and its protein product sequence determined. Since then the basic molecular biological basis for this stimulatory effect on testis development has been emerging rapidly. It has now been shown that SRY (the *sry* gene's protein) has a DNA binding region that is critical for its function, which suggests that SRY acts either directly to activate other genes that bring about testis growth, or indirectly to suppress a gene that inhibits testicular growth. The testis in turn synthesizes testosterone and other hormonal factors that result in differentiation of the fetus into a phenotypic male. Of interest is the fact that the gene controlling synthesis of the cellular receptors for testosterone and its active metabolite, dihydrotestosterone, is located on the X chromosome; a mutation of this androgen receptor gene can block the effects of testosterone and cause a genotypic male (X,Y) to develop as a phenotypic female.

Understanding of the sexual differentiation of those areas of the CNS that directly relate to sexual and reproductive behavior is much further advanced in laboratory animals than in humans. For example, there is clear evidence in the rat (1) that certain hypothalamic nuclei are sexually dimorphic (i.e., they differ in size and/or shape); (2) that this sexual dimorphism is determined by differences in exposure to circulating testosterone at a critical period in development; and (3) that these dimorphic nuclei exert control on adult reproductive behavior. In humans, however, (1) the observations of sexually dimorphic hypothalamic nuclei are recent, and the specifics are still controversial; (2) the data *directly* linking the differential development of these nuclei to fetal androgen levels are lacking; and, finally, (3) the relationship of these dimorphic nuclei to adult sexual behavior (including sexual orientation) is still tenuous.

BRAIN DIFFERENCES NOT DIRECTLY RELATED TO REPRODUCTIVE BEHAVIOR

By contrast, understanding of sexual differences in anatomy and function of the much larger portions of the CNS that are *not* directly involved in sexual and reproductive behavior is largely based on human data, and with the rapid recent development of *in vivo* brain imaging techniques, knowledge in this area is expanding dramatically. Here, too, these questions arise: What parts of the brain are sexually dimorphic, how and when do the differences arise, and how do such differences make themselves manifest functionally?

Systematic observations indicating that on average adult men have larger brains than adult women were first reported in the 19th century, and in spite of the controversy that has surrounded the *interpretation* of this observation, the existence of a mean brain volume difference of about 10% is not disputed. What are disputed are the basis of the difference and its functional significance, if any. A currently widely held view is that sex differences in whole-brain volume simply parallel (and reflect) similar sex differences in body size, and are thus in a functional sense trivial. This view has recently been disputed on the basis that the previously utilized methods of correcting for body size are statistically inappropriate, and that if appropriate corrections for body size are made, the male–female differences in brain size persist.

These differing conclusions are largely based on analysis and reanalysis of data from adult autopsy series, but it is instructive to look at data on childhood growth norms. In this case brain size must be inferred from head size (expressed as head circumference), but since brain growth drives head growth during development, the two are closely correlated in normal children. In Figure 2.1 we have taken standard growth chart tables used in pediatrics and plotted the median (50th-percentile) male and female values for head circumference and height from birth to age 18.

Several points should be noted. First, male and female median head circumferences diverge in the first 2 years of life, and then male circumference remains proportionally larger over the whole age range of the graph. (It should be noted that since the head is roughly spheroid, circumference is related to brain volume by a cubic function, and the differences in circumference of 1.5–2.0 cm equate to volume differences of 50–80 cc.) Second, male and female median heights (and weights) closely overlap until age 14, and between the ages of 10 and 13 the female values are slightly larger than the male values. Third, head growth continues for *both* males and females up through age 18, even though female height starts to plateau several years earlier than male height.

What are the implications of these observed trends? First, sexual divergence in brain growth appears to be complete by age 2, whereas significant divergence in body size is

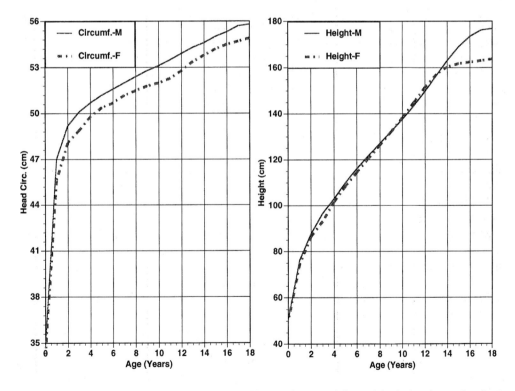

FIGURE 2.1. Median male anad female head circumference (left) and body height (right) from birth to age 18. The data are from Behrman (1992).

delayed until adolescence. Second, in females brain growth *persists* for several years after body growth plateaus. Third, the relative ratios of brain size to body size for males and females are markedly age-dependent, such that from birth until age 14 the male ratio is higher, but by age 18 the female ratio is higher. These divergent trends strongly suggest that brain and body growth patterns within the human species are separately pro-grammed and lack any strong causal relationship in either direction, and that this holds for sensual dimorphism as well. In other words, differences between human male and female brains are almost independent of differences in human male and female body size.

SEX DIFFERENCES IN COGNITIVE FUNCTION

In contrast to these sex differences in brain size, there are negligible sex differences in median overall scores on general measures of intellectual functioning, such as the Wechsler tests. There are, however, sex differences in measures of more narrowly defined functions, variously described as differences in means, variances, distribution, or quality of performance. The most consistent findings of female superiority come with tests that emphasize perceptual and psychomotor abilities and processing speed. The most consis-tent demonstrations of male superiority are in tests emphasizing visual–spatial functions (e.g., mental rotation of objects in space), mechanical reasoning, and mathematical skills.

Not all performance differences have been stable over time. For example, a previous female superiority on the Verbal portion of the Scholastic Aptitude Test has dissipated recently, possibly because of changing sex patterns among the students who take the test. That is, there has been a recent shift in the sex ratio of high school dropouts, with an increase in male dropouts, and thus a presumed elimination of the potentially lowest scorers in the male population taking the test. Similarly, there has been an expansion in the numbers of students characterized as learning-disabled and thus not taking the standard test; since most learning-disabled individuals are male, this too would have the effect of eliminating low scorers disproportionately from the male test population.

A second important aspect of sex difference in measured abilities is variance, and this tends to be greater in male populations. This becomes important at the upper extremes of score distributions, because if variance differs there may be only a small difference in mean scores and yet a four- or fivefold difference in numbers of males and females in the top 0.5%.

When it comes to addressing the issue of the development of sex differences in cognitive functions, one has not only to ask whether the level of a function differs but whether the timetable of development of the function differs. In spite of the methodo-logical difficulties, however, the patterns of relative functional strengths and weaknesses appear to parallel adult findings even as early as first grade.

The greatest problem with interpretation of cognitive tests is determining what functions are actually being tested. On some tests, cognitive "style" may interact with test requirements to favor one sex over the other. For example, males have been found to be more impulsive in their test-taking behavior than females, favoring speed over accuracy; a test that heavily penalizes guessing may favor the more careful and accurate approach of females, whereas one that rewards guessing can have the opposite effect. Nevertheless, it is still true that the mean male–female differences in cognitive abilities appear to be much smaller than the mean difference in brain size.

THE RELATIONSHIP OF ANATOMICAL DIFFERENCES TO COGNITIVE DIFFERENCES

If body size differences aren't the answer to the paradox of unequal brain size but equal cognitive functioning, what is? Several answers have been proposed. First, specific functions that show male superiority (e.g., mental rotation of objects) may require relatively large volumes of brain tissue, whereas functions that show female superiority (psychomotor processing speed) may be independent of tissue volume but critically dependent on circuit organization. Second, neuronal density may be normally greater in certain critical areas of the female brain, reducing volume without reducing efficacy. Third, the greater hemispheric lateralization thought to be characteristic of males may confer certain functional advantages but result in male intrahemispheric brain tissue redundancy for other functions. Finally, it should be noted that even though the sex difference in median brain size is about one standard deviation, the within-sex range of brain sizes of normal adults is much larger. Since by most reports the within-sex correlations of head size with standard cognitive test performance are quite low (accounting for less than 5% of test score variance), and the within-sex correlation of head size to body size is also quite low, the problem of accounting for differences in brain size is actually more general than the sexual dimorphism issue. Nevertheless, the problem may be methodologically more tractable if efforts are first directed to looking for the basis of the difference in brain size between the sexes.

In order for researchers to begin to address the question, means of determining whether brain functions are related to brain structure in different ways in males and females are needed. This problem has been approached in a number of ways. First, various behavioral tasks that are known from brain lesion studies to reflect functional lateralization (e.g., dichotic listening ear preference tasks) have been applied to normal subjects. Second, there has been a search in normal brains for quantitative sex differences in size or cell density of localized anatomical regions that are known to be related to certain functions (e.g., the speech areas of the left hemisphere, the splenium of the corpus callosum). Third, observers have studied the effects of static brain lesions (e.g., localized strokes) on functional performance, looking for sex differences in the impairments produced by anatomically comparable lesions. Finally, studies in normal subjects have begun to utilize the recent rapid advances in functional brain imaging that allow fairly precise quantitation of localized changes in brain blood flow/metabolism in response to well-defined cognitive tasks.

Behavioral Findings and Anatomical Differences in Specific Regions

A number of behavioral studies (reviewed in the chapter by Woods and Hebben in the 1988 *Handbook*) have looked at sex differences in hemispheric lateralization on behavioral tasks in both normal adults and children, and have tended to conclude that the lateralization of verbal functions to the left hemisphere and visual–spatial functions to the right hemisphere (of right-handed individuals) is more pronounced in males, with the difference beginning in childhood and continuing into adult life. These studies have provided one of the major lines of evidence for the theory that hemispheric functional specialization in general is greater in males.

Although there does not appear to be any significant sex difference in relative hemispheric size, one likely requirement of less hemispheric lateralization of function is greater interhemispheric communication. For this reason, a number of investigators have looked for sex differences in the size of the major interhemispheric communication channels—the corpus callosum and the anterior commissure. Earlier pathological studies failed to agree on whether a significant sex difference in callosal size exists or not. Several recent studies that have utilized magnetic resonance imaging (MRI) to look at callosal area found that callosal area varied directly and significantly with intracranial area, and inversely and significantly with age; however, it has been argued that once the effects of these variables are eliminated, there is no significant gender effect. There is a single neuropathological study indicating that the anterior commissure is larger in females.

There are various reports of sex differences in brain areas that are critical for language functions (e.g., observations that the usual male pattern of the left planum temporale's being larger than the right is seen less frequently in females), but a number of other studies looking at the frontal operculum or the angulation of the sylvian fissure have not found significant sex differences in patterns of asymmetry. There is, however, a very recent neuropathological study by Witelson and colleagues indicating that neuronal density in the auditory cortex is 11% greater in females than in males.

Differential Effects of Focal Brain Lesions

There are several readily reproducible consequences of lateralized brain lesions in adult male patients, and these have been used for the study of sex differences in degree of hemispheric specialization. The first such consequence is aphasia after left-hemisphere strokes. McGlone noted in 1980 that the incidence of aphasia after left-hemisphere stokes in women is only one-third what it is in men. Later, however, Kimura pointed out that there is a greater tendency for aphasia after anterior than after posterior left-hemisphere strokes in women, whereas the converse tends to be true in men. She noted furthermore that since anterior strokes are much less frequent than posterior strokes, it follows that the sex difference in incidence of aphasia after left-hemisphere strokes of unspecified location can be explained not by assuming that language is less hemispherically lateralized in women than men, but by assuming that it is more compactly organized *within* the left hemisphere in women than in men.

Another such approach is to look at sex differences in deficits in verbal memory after left temporal lobectomy. A study by Trenerry and colleagues used this paradigm and reported that males showed a greater impairment in verbal memory after left temporal lobectomy for complex partial (temporal lobe) seizures than did females after the same surgery. They did not find a sex difference in the effect of right temporal lobectomy on verbal memory (which improved postoperatively in both sexes)—contrary to what one would expect if verbal memory were lateralized to the left hemisphere in males but bilaterally represented in females. Therefore, they interpreted their results as evidence of greater functional plasticity after brain insults in females than in males. Unfortunately for this theory, the females in the study were much younger at age of seizure onset (and presumably lesion onset) than males (mean age was 8.7 years for females vs. 15.1 years for males). Because loss of functional plasticity for at least language is essentially complete by puberty, if not earlier, the authors' use of analysis of covariance to eliminate age-of-onset effects does not solve the problem of the age-of-onset difference; their result may be an age effect, not a sex effect.

A third brain lesion consequence that has been reported to show sex differences is a greater impairment in males than females of Verbal IQ scores relative to Performance IQ scores with left-hemisphere lesions, and the converse with right-hemisphere lesions. However, this effect may be test-dependent: It was reported to be present when the older Wechsler–Bellevue test was used, but not when the data were from the Wechsler Adult Intelligence Scale (WAIS). Kimura reported the results of WAIS subtests, and her data show a complex picture of sex differences varying by subtest. On several Verbal subtests females were more adversely affected than males by right-hemisphere lesions, but on the Performance subtests only Picture Arrangement showed greater male than female sensitivity to right-hemisphere lesions. On two other Performance subtests, Picture Completion and Object Assembly, there was a sex difference not in hemispheric laterality effects, but in sensitivity to anterior versus posterior lesions.

Functional Imaging Results

There are two major methods currently available for functional imaging: positron emission tomography (PET) scanning, and functional MRI (fMRI). Both measure changes in blood flow induced by neuronal activity rather than the electrical activity of brain cells, and both have certain limitations as to anatomical and temporal resolution, such that activity changes can only be detected if they involve tissue volumes measured in cubic centimeters and if they persist for minutes. Moreover, getting significant results may require averaging across individuals, and since brains vary in size and shape, spatial corrections tend to degrade spatial resolution further.

One commonly utilized functional imaging paradigm consists of a series of tasks that are cumulative, in the sense that each new element incorporates the previous elements and adds to them. For example, the first task might be to look at a random pattern on a screen; the second task, to look at a picture of the same size, shape, and light–dark contrast; and the third to try to select an appropriate one-word title for the picture. Images of brain activation induced by the first task are then subtracted from the images induced by the second task, and similarly the images from the second task are subtracted from those obtained during the final task. The differences are assumed to be task-specific.

A recent fMRI study by Shaywitz and colleagues used a subtraction paradigm to look for sex differences in young adults in localized increases in brain activity induced by a reading task. The first element of the task required judgment of orientation of slanted lines (e.g., | | | | vs. \ \ \ \); the next element required recognition of a pattern of equivalence of orthographic letter case alternation (e.g., kTGh = fLPd); the third element was discrimination between rhyming and nonrhyming nonsense words; and the last task component was deciding whether two words came from the same semantic category. The study found that in male subjects activation specific to the phonological (rhyming) component of the task was more focal and limited to the left hemisphere, whereas in females the activation was less focal and bihemispheric.

In another recent study, Gur and colleagues used PET scanning to examine resting cerebral metabolism; they found that in both hemispheres men showed higher metabolic rates in the lateral and ventromedial temporal lobes, while women had higher rates in the middle and posterior cingulate gyri. In this study the sex differences were intrahemispheric, not interhemispheric. (It should, however, be noted that resting studies are problematical for interpretation because they cannot control for mental activity during the resting state, and thus cannot exclude systematic differences.)

CONCLUSIONS

Evidence for sex differences in brain organization comes from behavioral studies in normal individuals, quantitative radiographic or neuropathological comparisons of presumably intact male and female brains, analysis of localized brain lesion effects on specific functions, and functional imaging studies. It seems clear from the data that significant sex differences in brain organization exist, but that they are more subtle and complex in both their origins and their manifestations than early theories envisioned.

Progress in science depends on developments in methodology, but it also depends on broader social forces that help determine which scientific questions are "legitimate" or "interesting." Because anthropometric data on differences in male and female brain size were misused in the past by being linked to "intelligence," and then employed as biological justifications for educational and occupational discrimination, the study of anatomical and functional sex differences in the brain came for a time to be regarded as somewhat suspect as a proper topic for mainline research. However, with the increasing appreciation that the brain is characterized to a significant degree by hard-wired functional modularity (so that one should speak not of a unitary "intelligence" but rather of a number of different "intelligences"), and with the number of female neuroscientists who have taken the lead in reporting clinical and anatomical data confirming sex differences in brain structure, it would seem that the topic is now widely viewed as "legitimate." This sea change in attitude, coming just as the new brain imaging methodologies offer unique possibilities for studying quantitative differences in the functional neuroanatomy of normal individuals, suggests that further progress in this field will now come very rapidly.

FURTHER READING

Behrman, R. E. (Ed.). (1992). *Nelson's textbook of pediatrics* (8th ed.). Philadelphia: W. B. Saunders.
This is a standard text providing tables and nomograms for head and body growth from birth to age 18.

Byne, W., & Parsons, B. (1995). Human sexual orientation: The biologic theories reappraised. *Archives of General Psychiatry, 50,* 228–239.
A critical review of the expanding literature relating anatomical brain differences to sexual orientation.

Gur, R. C., Mozley, L. H., Mozley, P. D., Resnick, S. M., Karp, J. S., Alavi, A., Arnold, S. E., & Gur, R. R. (1995). Sex differences in regional cerebral glucose metabolism during a resting state. *Science, 267,* 528–531.
Describes results from positron emission tomography (one of the two major current methods of functional brain imaging) suggesting that there are sex differences in resting brain activity, but that they are bilaterally symmetrical.

Hedges, L. V., & Nowell, A. (1995). Sex differences in mental test scores, variability, and numbers of high-scoring individuals. *Science, 269,* 41–49.
A review demonstrating that the practical consequences of sex difference in test performance variance may be great even if mean differences are small.

Kimura, D. (1987). Are men's and women's brains really different? *Canadian Psychology/Psychologie Canadienne, 28,* 133–147.

An analysis of gender variation in interaction of lesion localization with WAIS subtest scores.

McGlone, J. (1980). Sex differences in human brain symmetry: A critical review. *The Behavioral and Brain Sciences, 3,* 215–263.
A thoughtful and critical review of the human brain lesion evidence for sex differences in the localization of anatomical substrates for cognition.

Parashos, I. A., Wilkinson, W. E., & Coffey, C. E. (1995). Magnetic resonance imaging of the corpus callosum: Predictors of size in normal adults. *Journal of Neuropsychiatry and Clinical Neurosciences, 7,* 35–41.
A summary of recent brain imaging studies of sex differences in the size and morphology of the corpus collosum.

Peters, M. (1991). Sex differences in human brain size and the general meaning of differences in brain size. *Canadian Journal of Psychology, 45,* 507–522.
A reasoned and balanced discussion of the neurobiological implications of various theories of sexual dimorphism of the human brain.

Shaywitz, B. A., Shaywitz, S. E., Pugh, K. R., Constable, R. T., Skudlarski, P., Fulbright, R. K., Bronen, R. A., Fletcher, J. M., Shankweiler, D. P., Katz, I., & Gore, J. C. (1995). Sex differences in the functional organization of the brain for language. *Nature, 373,* 607–609.
An important recent documentation of the use of the newest functional imaging methodology to confirm old suppositions about sex differences in the localization of language.

Swaab, D. F., & Hofman, M. A. (1995) Sexual differentiation of the human hypothalamus in relation to gender and sexual orientation. *Trends in Neuroscience, 18,* 264–270.
A recent update of the complex literature on sexual dimorphism of hypothalamic nuclei in animal models and human brains as it relates to reproductive behavior.

Trenerry, M. R., Jack, C. R., Cascino, G. D., Sharbrough, F. W., & Ivnik, R. J. (1995). Gender differences in post-temporal lobectomy verbal memory and relationships between MRI hippocamal volumes and preoperative verbal memory. *Epilepsy Research, 20,* 69–76.

Witelson, S. F., Glezer, I. I., & Kigar, D. L. (1995). Women have greater density of neurons in posterior temporal cortex. *Journal of Neuroscience, 15,* 3418–3428.

3

Infancy

Evelyn B. Thoman

W ith the birth of an infant, a mother's horizon expands to include learning and feelings that go with caring for a new and very dependent person. In her new role, she accepts sometimes extraordinary demands on her physical, emotional, and logistical energies. At the same time, the new baby is adapting to an extrauterine world of people and things, and to experiences of met and unmet needs.

From birth, the baby is in many ways optimally designed for this adaptation because of sensory and affective sensitivities and responsiveness, biological rhythms, and a capability for learning from what is perceived and experienced. A major function of these capabilities early in life is to establish a synchrony with the mother, who assures the baby's survival and is the baby's major source of stimulation, affection, challenge, and ongoing partnership.

THE ROLE OF LEARNING DURING INFANCY

The learning capabilities of infants continue to be uncovered by scientists using creative and carefully designed studies. As examples, newborns can modify their pattern of sucking (the number of sucks and the duration of pauses between bouts of sucks) in order to hear their mothers' voices, to receive a small amount of sweetened water, or to see a visual pattern that they "like."

The visual system and attentiveness are indications of the infant's preparation for being an active member of the mother–infant system. As a newborn, the infant's focal distance is about 10 inches—just the right distance to perceive the mother's face when she is holding and talking to her baby. And putting the baby in the upright position, which the mother may use during this interaction, is the optimal physical stimulation to cause a baby to be highly alert. When alert, the baby has a preference for the characteristics that are inherent in a face, especially the round pattern of eyes (note that a round, bull's-eye pattern is also present on the mother's breasts). From such alert attentiveness comes much learning about the baby's closest social partner. This learning can continue at greater physical distances as the infant's focal distance increases over the early weeks.

Learning about the mother actually begins prenatally. A baby is exposed repeatedly to the mother's voice throughout gestation. Very shortly after birth, the baby prefers to hear the mother's voice rather than that of a strange woman. Likewise, the newborn exhibits a preference for the mother's odor. From the early months, infants can learn contingent behaviors to achieve pleasing consequences. For example, babies are great imitators, and they learn to repeat behaviors that elicit pleasurable responses from their parents. In the early months, they will learn to make specific movements of the head in order to cause a mobile to move. Even preterm infants can organize their random-appearing movements to achieve contact and cuddle with a "breathing" teddy bear that has the same breathing rate as the babies. The teddy bear findings highlight the importance of rhythmic stimulation (which even the most immature infants find attractive), as well as the appeal of opportunities for entraining to appropriate biological rhythms (which are later available from the mother).

By 6 months of age, infants can show rudimentary abilities to count. Also at this age, once having looked at an object attentively, infants will prefer to pay more attention to a novel object—something new to learn about. In fact, tests of such attentiveness at 6 months reliably predict children's mental developmental status at school age. Early opportunities for learning can have lasting consequences. For example, exposure to music at a very early age facilitates later acquisition of aspects of musical and linguistic perception. Likewise, negative experiences may or may not have enhancing consequences for development, depending on whether the experience constitutes a challenge or a stress. Obviously, not all experiences can be "positive," and tumbles and minor "hurts" are a necessary way of becoming acquainted with the world and learning to cope with its challenges.

Most parents feel that their infants are terribly smart from the beginning, and growing evidence says that they are generally right. However, it is not necessary, or even beneficial, to use intensive "training" procedures to enhance an infant's intelligence (flash cards, etc.). Social interaction with the mother has great variability and subtlety, as well as biological significance for the infant, which is not to be found in specific kinds of skill training at a very early age. For instance, even the experience of breastfeeding offers opportunities for the baby to learn to adjust to changes in the feel of the nipple and breast, as well as to changes in sucking pressure and size of swallows required throughout a feeding. Likewise, bottle feeding offers varied views for the baby, with different positions for feeding and even the possibility for the father's face to provide the view.

It is also not necessary to provide an overabundance of brightly colored toys that can quickly fill the rooms of a home. Each toy may be of special interest to the parents and, initially, to the baby; however, an infant's visual system can be overstimulated and an already high arousal level can be exacerbated by excessive numbers of brightly colored toys and sound-making objects in the environment. One way to titrate the toy experience is to rotate toys from the closet to the toybox, so that the baby can find pleasure in the "new" toys brought out or even take pleasure in reconnecting with "old friend" toys. Also, there are numerous toys that allow more freedom of action and elicit creative interaction. For example, the timeless kindergarten blocks are made of natural wood and offer endless possibilities for imaginative arrangements, with appeal and benefits from infancy through later ages. Legos are in this category as well. An additional benefit of the blocks (not one that the baby is aware of, naturally) is practice with mathematical logic, because the blocks are cut in multiples of a basic unit.

With age and increased capacity for action, locomotion, and communication, infants learn what things are manipulable and how they can be manipulated, what things are harmful, what things are edible, what things can be put together with other things or put inside other things, and so forth. They also learn which objects can be used for desired purposes, and especially how to make people provide what is desired. But each baby learns these "lessons" at his or her own pace. Even in their motor development, some may learn to use fine motor movements more readily than gross motor skills, or the reverse. Gentle (i.e., optional) activities, rather than overly structured play, allow a baby's interests and mental development to proceed along his or her own unique path.

THE SLEEP–WAKE STATES

Among the very basic characteristics that an infant brings to the mother–infant system are biological and behavioral rhythms. A mother has a day–night rhythm of sleep and wakefulness, as well as shorter rhythms throughout the day. One goal of the developing mother–infant interaction is to synchronize these rhythms, with the result of more positive feelings for both partners. It has even been argued that the function of a baby's sleep is to give the parents a respite and rest.

On the average, during the earliest weeks, babies sleep about 16½ hours a day; by 1 month, 15½ hours; and by 3 months, 15 hours. The amount continues to decrease gradually to almost 14 hours at 1 year, and to 13 hours at 2 years. Until about 4 years, some sleep occurs in daytime naps. But more important to parents is when the baby will sleep through the night. This is highly variable: Some babies will sleep for a 6-hour stretch at night within the first few weeks; others may not do so until after they are a year old.

Some babies wake up during the night and "self-soothe," then go back to sleep. (In such cases, parents may not know they have awakened. We only know this because researchers have recorded those periods.) Other babies sleep erratically during the night and cry whenever they awaken. Some are consolable, but others may cry inconsolably, especially during the evening or at night (these are considered to be the "colicky" babies). Others may be irritable day or night, but they can be consoled by being held and carried, so that their mothers may find themselves carrying their babies about for many hours during the day and then, at times of exhaustion, just letting the babies cry. The constant carrying leads some mothers to sleep with their babies at night (this is called "co-sleeping" by infant researchers). Suggestions for relieving the strain on the relationship that can unquestionably result from these efforts are included in the appendix to this chapter. These suggestions have been found to help mothers (and fathers) and babies organize their day in a way that leads to more synchrony in their mutual expectations. They can be useful by way of helping parents to help babies learn when to expect playful attention, as well as when and how to go to sleep and to self-soothe.

Co-sleeping is encouraged by some researchers as a way of facilitating the baby's development, while other experts remain skeptical and are concerned for the possibility of "laying over" (the mother's rolling over onto the infant), which is known to occur (although the incidence is unknown). The almost passionate views on this issue can be highlighted by a quote from one woman speaking about the pleasures of a mother's sleeping with her baby and letting the baby nurse: "How can you expect to hold onto them later in life if you begin their lives by pushing them away? I don't care what the doctors say. I believe it best for the mother and child to be together." On the other hand,

Brazelton and many other infant experts advise not allowing the baby to sleep with the parents or even to go to sleep in a parent's arms, because the baby will not learn to self-soothe and go to sleep on his or her own. A transitional object in the crib at sleep time (pacifier, blanket, mother's undershirt, or soft toy) is recommended as a way of facilitating the acquisition of sleeping independence.

The arguments against co-sleeping also include findings that this practice is associated with more frequent awakenings in the night, and that sleeping practices interfering with continuous nighttime sleep are predictive of sleep disturbances at a later age. By contrast, babies who learn to sleep alone by going to bed awake and self-soothing, possibly with a sleep aid, are more likely to be good sleepers at a later age. However, as with many decisions regarding the welfare of babies, parents have options because the decisions are primarily based on cultural goals. In North American culture, independence is valued as a goal for children from the earliest age. Also, such independence may be necessary when both parents are working, and a good night's sleep for each of them is essential for their health and ability to cope with the roles of work and baby caregiver.

In a less ambiguous category, the current recommendation of the American Pediatrics Association is that babies should be put in their cribs on their backs or propped on their sides rather than in a prone position. This recommendation for infants' sleep position stems from evidence that the prone position places infants at a higher risk for sudden infant death syndrome (SIDS). However, the supine position is not appropriate for babies who are susceptible to frequent regurgitation. By the time babies are able to roll over and determine their own sleep position, the peak of SIDS incidence (3 months) has fortunately passed. It is also important to note that soft quilts or bedding materials are to be avoided in all circumstances, as they offer the possibility of a baby's rebreathing a pocket of an increasing level of carbon dioxide.

It may be of interest to parents to know that all normal babies have frequent, brief apneas (periods of nonbreathing) during sleep. These episodes typically last from 2 to 5 seconds, and they occur 40 or 50 times in an hour's sleep. An occasional apnea as long as 10 seconds may occur, and this is also normal. However, since such occurrences are extremely rare, they are not events to watch for or worry about.

Not only do babies develop a circadian rhythm of day–night sleep, but there are within-sleep rhythms as well. A most important ultradian biobehavioral rhythm is the cycle of active (rapid-eye-movement or REM) and quiet (non-REM) sleep. This cycle is about 60 minutes in the early weeks; then, with development, babies are able to establish more rhythmic and more prolonged active–quiet sleep cycles (reaching 90 minutes in adulthood). These two sleep states are readily observable: During active sleep, one can clearly see REM (fluttering of the eyelids or slow, rolling movement of the eyeballs under the lids), and small twitches of the fingers or toes; during quiet sleep, breathing is very regular, and the baby is very quiescent. (This is the state when the baby is so still that many of us as parents admit to having given a baby a gentle poke to make the baby stir, just to be reassured that he or she was still really breathing!)

The sleep states are important, and not only as a basic biological rhythm. Active sleep is the prelude to the dreaming state of the older child and adult. Do babies dream? It is assumed that they do, but within the limits of their brains' stores of memories and experiences. Thus, at the very early ages, babies' dreams cannot consist of specific images, as is the case with young children and adults.

Sleep serves other demonstrated functions as well. First, sleep is considered to be a modulator of the immune system, and in turn the immune system plays a role in sleep.

Quiet sleep is thought to be most intimately involved in this. Second, the release of growth hormone occurs primarily during periods of quiet sleep. Third, much evidence indicates that consolidation of learning occurs during active (dream) sleep. Finally, the states of sleep and wakefulness serve the baby more generally (but very importantly) by mediating all incoming stimulation and by modulating the baby's responses to all that he or she perceives.

INFANTS' AFFECTS

Most important for the baby and the developing mother–infant relationship are the baby's affects. Babies are "feelers," and they are designed to elicit the most primitively positive feelings in parents. Because babies are not capable of specific emotions (jealousy, envy, resentment, etc.), their feelings are generally referred to as "affects." The negative emotions just listed are fortunately not yet learned in infancy; experience will be the teacher of each of these and other more complex emotions. However, from the time of birth, a baby has a wide range of affective expressions, and many researchers accept these expressions at "face value"—that is, as indicating the baby's feelings. Interestingly, these are most richly observed (and presumably experienced, or dreamed) during the state of active sleep; they include smiles, frowns, grimaces, looks of puzzlement, sighs and sighing sobs, vocalizations including coo sounds and brief cries, and various movement patterns with the limbs and whole body. Over the early months, these expressions are less often observed in sleep and more often seen in wakefulness, especially in the course of social exchanges, but sometimes in response to toys (e.g., a mobile). In addition, wakefulness permits active interest and curiosity, which are expressed by attentiveness and exploration, both visually and motorically.

A baby's interest is especially piqued by the mother's conversation when she talks to him or her using "mothereze," the high-frequency, musical "baby talk" adults find very comfortable when speaking with babies. (The only other circumstances noted for this mode of speaking are conversations between young lovers, and pet owners' talking to their pets.) Such talk often elicits soft vocalizations from the baby, and the conversation facilitates imitation of the mother's joyful, affective tone. The two can be said to "sing" together while the baby is learning and entraining to the mother's rhythms.

CONCLUSION

From the earliest age, learning, the sleep–wake rhythms, and affect are intimately linked processes, both in the baby's central nervous system and in the baby's behaviors. The states are the gate for experience. Whereas sleep is fundamental for rest and a determinant for mood when awake, wakefulness permits attention. And affect is associated with the reinforcements received from seeking, social enticement, and satisfaction during wakefulness. Thus, the baby's expression of these processes, including a range of facial, vocal, and movement behaviors, are integral to the development of synchrony in the mother–infant exchange. They provide cues to the mother as to the baby's interests, needs, and feelings and how to respond to them; at the same time, they provide her with an understanding of her baby and her ability to satisfy the baby's needs. Her pleasure and that of her baby are fuel for their relationship and for the infant's development.

APPENDIX FOR MOTHERS (AND FATHERS): THINGS THAT HELP MAKE BABIES HAPPY

The following suggestions are meant to help you provide cues for your infant. A regular routine will help to teach your baby what to expect at certain times during the day and night (e.g., when to sleep and when to play).

  1. Try to feed the baby as regularly as possible. Most important is giving the evening feeding at the same time every night. It is suggested that a baby can even be awakened for this feeding, called the "anchor feeding." Giving an anchor feeding can also help the baby lengthen the time between feeds during the night.
  2. If you can anticipate the time when the baby most often has a crying spell (usually in the evening when you are most weary!), you may be able to "fool the rule" by using a period of time before the usual unhappy hour to keep the baby as comfortable and calm as possible, with minimal stimulation.
  3. Maximize light exposure during the daytime, with (ideally) some sun exposure; provide some light even during daytime naps. Minimize light levels during the nighttime, especially during periods when the baby wakes up and is fed during the night. A very dim light (e.g., a small red light) is better than a lamp or room light.
  4. If possible, have a few minutes during each day for a regular playtime, when your attention is exclusively devoted to the baby. This should be at a time of day when you are not too tired and the baby is most likely to be awake and alert. The attention can be gentle, such as singing to the baby, or however you want to enjoy your baby. Of course, you will play with the baby at other times of the day. But if you can have one time that you consistently give the baby attention, this will be another cue that helps the baby to learn expectations.
  5. If the baby cries at night and has been fed within a short time, the suggested routine is to stroke the baby's back or head gently to try to calm the baby; then pick the baby up if crying continues (before you both get overwrought). If the baby is picked up, handling should be very gentle, and any talking or singing should be very low-voiced.

FURTHER READING

Ferber, R. (1985). *Solve your child's sleep problems.* New York: Simon & Schuster.
This book, by a noted clinician and researcher, gives much-needed information for parents whose infants sleep erratically and cry excessively.

Ferber, R., & Kryger, M. (Eds.). (1995). *Principles and practice of sleep medicine in the child.* Philadelphia: W. B. Saunders.
This volume includes chapters describing the normal development of sleep in infants and children, and the nature and typical ages for sleep problems to occur.

Seligman, M. E. P., Reivich, K., Jaycox, L., & Gillham, J. (1995). *The optimistic child.* Boston: Houghton Mifflin.
Although the stated objective of this book is to provide a parenting approach that "safeguards children against depression and builds lifelong resilience," Seligman and colleagues clearly support the view that the issues of emotional development are critical from earliest infancy.

Thoman, E. B., & Acebo, C. (1984). The first affections of infancy. In R. W. Bell, J. Elias, R. L. Greene, & J. H. Harvey (Eds.), *Interfaces in psychology: Vol. 1. Developmental psychobiology and neuropsychology* (pp. 17–56). Lubbock: Texas Tech University Press.

This chapter reviews the ontogenetic and biological evidence for the "wholeness" of infants as persons from the time of birth, including not only the ability to learn, but the ability to sense emotions in others and to respond with a range of emotions (or affects).

Thoman, E. B., & Browder, S. (1988). *Born dancing: How intuitive parents understand their baby's unspoken language and natural rhythms.* New York: Harper & Row.

This book depicts infants as unique, complete, competent, and feeling beings from the time of birth, and proposes that a major form of adaptation of mothers and infants is the achievement of synchrony of their individual rhythms—in sleeping, feeding, and other activities.

Thoman, E. B., & Ingersoll, E. W. (1993). Learning in premature infants. *Developmental Psychology, 29,* 692–700.

A study of premature infants with a surrogate companion (a "breathing" teddy bear) indicates that these immature infants can show an approach response to the bear; that they smile in their sleep more than infants with a nonbreathing bear; and that their respiration pattern appears to become entrained by the bear's very regular "breathing."

4

Maternal Cocaine Use and Fetal Development

Tiffany Field

Cocaine is reported to be used by as many as 10–15% of pregnant women. Cocaine exposure has been associated with a greater rate of prenatal and perinatal complications, including spontaneous abortion, placenta previa, intrauterine growth retardation, intraventricular hemorrhage, cardiac anomalies, low birthweight, low head circumference, and prematurity. In addition, behavioral studies have noted a tendency for cocaine-exposed newborns to show more stress behaviors than nonexposed infants, including restlessness, irritability, hypertonia, tremors/clonus, and abnormal reflexes. However, other investigators have reported minimal effects. In the case of preterm cocaine-exposed newborns, neither the contribution of prematurity itself nor the effects of cocaine exposure on top of prematurity have been studied in prior research. Two recent studies—one on full-term cocaine-exposed newborns, and one on preterm cocaine-exposed infants—are reviewed below.

FULL-TERM COCAINE-EXPOSED INFANTS

In our study on full-term infants (Eisen and colleagues), 26 neonates with a positive urine screen for cocaine were compared to 26 neonates with negative urine screens for cocaine and marijuana. The infants had an average gestational age of 38 weeks, an average birthweight of 2,400 grams, and an average chronological age of 4 days. The two groups of primarily inner-city, African-American, low-socioeconomic-status mothers did not differ on demographic factors. However, more cocaine-using mothers were single (23 vs. 14), smoked cigarettes (18 vs. 3), and drank alcohol (17 vs. 2). Marijuana use was reported by 39% of the cocaine-using mothers, and use of cigarettes and alcohol combined by 27%. Only 15% of the mothers used cocaine alone, suggesting that 85% of the cocaine-using sample were polydrug users.

The cocaine-exposed newborn group did not differ from the nonexposed group in sex distribution, gestational age, chronological age, birthweight, birth length, or postnatal complications. However, the cocaine-exposed neonates had smaller head circumferences and more obstetric complications. The cocaine-exposed neonates also tended to show more stress behaviors, particularly abnormal reflex behavior and autonomic instability. It is interesting that on the scale measuring these behaviors, maternal alcohol use contributed more to the variance than cocaine use. The only variables that entered a stepwise regression were obstetric complications and maternal alcohol use, which together contributed to 24% of the variance. On the Brazelton Neonatal Behavior Assessment Scale, the cocaine-exposed neonates received inferior scores on the habituation cluster, suggesting that they required more trials to habituate to stimuli than did the nonexposed neonates.

In the stepwise regression on the habituation score, cocaine use was the only variable accounting for a significant amount of the variance. Another study, by Coles and colleagues, also reported inferior performance on the habituation items of the Brazelton by cocaine-exposed neonates. This finding is perhaps not surprising, inasmuch as habituation is related to dopaminergic function, and cocaine has been implicated in dopamine dysfunction. Given that habituation has been related to central nervous system dysfunction and inferior intellectual development in alcohol-exposed infants, these findings highlight the need for intervention.

PRETERM COCAINE-EXPOSED NEONATES

Because many cocaine-exposed infants are born prematurely, the purpose of comparing cocaine-exposed preterm infants with nonexposed preterm infants in the study described here was to determine the combined effects of cocaine exposure and prematurity. For this study, we (Scafidi and colleagues) recruited 30 preterm newborns (15 females) with a positive urine toxicology for cocaine (mean gestational age = 30 weeks, mean birthweight = 1,239 grams) and 30 preterm neonates (18 females) with a negative toxicology (mean gestational age = 30 weeks, mean birthweight = 1,212 grams), following random stratification on demographic variables. The groups did not differ in socioeconomic status or ethnic composition (68% African-American, 18% European-American, 7% Hispanic).

The cocaine-using mothers were more often single (as they were in our study on cocaine-exposed full-term infants) and averaged a higher number of previous pregnancies (four vs. two), although the groups did not differ on maternal age or ethnicity. Although the cocaine-exposed infants did not differ from nonexposed infants on the traditional birth measures, including gestational age, birthweight, birth length, Apgar scores, or postnatal complications, the cocaine-exposed infants had more obstetric complications (lower scores) and smaller head circumferences, like the cocaine-exposed full-term infants we studied. They were also in the neonatal intensive care unit for longer periods of time, which may explain their greater daily weight gain while in the unit. In addition, they were on more medications (typically caffeine) and had a greater incidence of intraventricular hemorrhage. The intraventricular hemorrhage rating for the cocaine-exposed group was most frequently a grade 1. The fact that the cocaine-using mothers visited their infants less frequently and touched, held, and fed them less frequently when they visited them could have been related to the mothers' drug-using behavior and lifestyle, and/or to the more fragile condition of their immature infants.

On the Brazelton Neonatal Behavior Assessment Scale, the cocaine-exposed infants did surprisingly better on the habituation cluster than the nonexposed infants—possibly because of accelerated development related to intrauterine stress, or possibly because they were "shutting down" sooner because of their stress condition. In contrast, their performance was inferior on the range of state and regulation-of-state factors, and they received more depressed scores on the Lester depression cluster. On the supplemental items, they received lower scores on cost of attention, regulatory capacity, and regulation of state.

During the 45-minute sleep–wake behavior recordings (scored second by second on a laptop computer from time lapse videotapes), the cocaine-exposed infants showed different sleep patterns. First, they spent less time in quiet sleep (40% vs. 63%) and more time in indeterminate sleep (31% vs. 14%). In addition, they showed significantly more multiple limb movements (30% vs. 13% of the time), more mouthing behaviors (9% vs. 5%), and more tremulousness (11% vs. less than 1%). These sleep behavior differences suggested not only that the cocaine-exposed preterm infants were showing less mature sleep behavior than the nonexposed preterms (i.e., they were spending less time in quiet sleep), but also that their sleep was more disorganized, as suggested by the high levels of indeterminate sleep. The last finding is disturbing, given that indeterminate sleep was the one neonatal variable that was inversely related to 12-year-old's IQ scores in a longitudinal follow-up study by Sigman and Parmelee.

Finally, the cocaine-exposed preterm infants had higher levels of urinary norepinephrine, dopamine, and cortisol. These results were surprising, given that the infants' urines were sampled long after acute drug effects would be apparent (at 1 month after birth). In an earlier study, Hertzel and colleagues reported elevated catecholamines, which could simply have been related to the residual effects of cocaine. However, the elevated catecholamines, and cortisol in our study may have derived from chronic sympathetic and adrenocortical activity. Enhanced norepinephrine levels could relate to enhanced maturity of the sympathetic nervous system, as has been reported earlier for preterm infants receiving supplemental stimulation. This enhanced development may relate to excessive stress in the perinatal period.

As we noted in our conclusions to the Scafidi et al. study, there is reason to be concerned. That is, many of the findings (e.g., inferior state regulation, indeterminate sleep, intraventricular hemorrhage) are known to contribute to developmental delay, suggesting the need for early intervention for cocaine-exposed preterm neonates.

FURTHER READING

Cole, B. J., & Robbins, T. W. (1989). Effects of 6-hydroxydopamine lesions of the nucleus accumbens septi on performance of a 5-choice serial reaction time task in rats: Implications for theories of selective attention and arousal. *Behavioral Brain Research, 33,* 165–179.
In this study, cocaine exposure was shown to affect habituation and dopaminergic function.

Coles, C., Platzman, K., Smith, I., James, M., & Falek, A. (1991). Effects of cocaine, alcohol, and other drugs used in pregnancy in neonatal growth and neurobehavioral status. *Neurotoxicology and Tetralogy, 13*(4), 1–11.
In this study, cocaine-exposed infants showed inferior performance on habituation items.

Eisen, L., Field, T., Bandstra, E., Roberts, J., Morrow, C., Larson, S., & Steele, B. (1991). Perinatal cocaine effects in neonatal stress behavior and performance on the Brazelton scale. *Pediatrics, 88,* 477–480.

Hertzel, J., Christensen, N. J., Pedersen, D. A., & Kuhl, C. (1982). Plasma noradrenaline and adrenaline in infants of diabetic mothers at birth and at two hours of age. *Acta Paediatrica Scandinavia, 71,* 941–945.

Infants in this study showed elevated catecholamines (stress hormones).

Kuhn, C., Schanberg, S., Field, T., Symanski, R., Zimmerman, E., Scafidi, F., & Roberts, J. (1991). Tactile/kinesthetic stimulation effects on sympathetic and adrenocortical function in preterm infants. *Journal of Pediatrics, 119,* 434–440.

This study showed that supplemental stimulation led to enhanced maturity of the sympathetic nervous system.

Scafidi, F. A., Field, T., Wheeden, A., Schanberg, S., Kuhn, C., Symanski, R., Zimmerman, E., & Bandstra, E. (in press). Cocaine-exposed preterm neonates show behavioral and hormonal differences. *Pediatrics, 97,* 851–855.

In this study, cocaine-exposed newborns showed inferior performance in many ways.

Sigman, M., & Parmelee, A. (1989, January). *Longitudinal predictors of cognitive development.* Paper presented at the meeting of the American Association for the Advancement of Science in San Francisco.

This study showed that newborns who showed more disorganized sleep had lower childhood IQs.

Singer, L. T., Garber, R., & Kliegman, R. (1991). Neurobehavioral sequelae of fetal cocaine exposure. *Journal of Pediatrics, 119,* 667–672.

This is a review of the literature on cocaine exposure's effects on young infants.

Streissguth, A. P., Barr, H. M., & Martin, D. C. (1983). Maternal alcohol use and neonatal habituation assessed with the Brazelton scale. *Child Development, 54,* 1109–1118.

This study found inferior intellectual development in alcohol-exposed infants.

5

Maternal Alcohol Use and Fetal Development

Heather Carmichael Olson

*I*t has long been recognized that alcohol use during pregnancy is a concern both for a woman's health and for the health of her child. Now it is known that alcohol is a teratogen that can cause abnormal fetal development, given over 20 years of thorough human studies and experimental animal research. A full spectrum of alcohol-related birth defects (ARBDs) and alcohol-related neurodevelopmental disorder (ARND) have been identified among the offspring of some women who drink while pregnant. Alcohol effects have come to be seen as a public health concern and economic burden to society; moreover, the prevention and treatment of risk drinking and ARBD/ARND have become priorities in health promotion for women and children.

ALCOHOL-RELATED BIRTH DEFECTS AND ALCOHOL-RELATED NEURODEVELOPMENTAL DISORDER

Prenatal alcohol exposure can produce a continuum of effects, ranging from subtle functional deficits to the distinct medical diagnosis and lifelong developmental disability of fetal alcohol syndrome (FAS). As defined so far by the Institute of Medicine, the minimal criteria for diagnosing FAS are prenatal and/or postnatal growth retardation, a cluster of characteristic craniofacial anomalies, and variable central nervous system (CNS) involvement that can include neurological abnormalities, developmental delays, behavioral dysfunction, intellectual impairment, and skull or brain malformations. Offspring prenatally exposed to alcohol who do not have the full FAS can still show associated conditions. Among these individuals, the specific physical characteristics that define the full syndrome are reported with a higher frequency; there is a greater risk for growth problems; and there is an increased risk for behavioral deficits similar in type and extent to those seen in patients with the complete FAS.

ARBDs and ARND are often subtle and hard to evaluate, and there are reasons for both under- and overdiagnosis of the problems. The influence of racial and familial traits, similarities to other disorders, and nonspecific abnormalities must be taken into account. Unless the full spectrum of FAS features is present, it is generally not possible to establish with certainty whether abnormalities are actually caused by alcohol; in these cases a descriptive diagnosis is recommended. Diagnostic criteria for ARBDs and ARND are being refined as additional data are collected and as clinicians gain more experience with the problem; a diagnostic manual has recently been developed (see Astley & Clarren, 1997). At this point, no prenatal diagnostic test has been developed; the effects of gestational alcohol exposure cannot always be recognized in newborns; and the full syndrome is most accurately identified between the ages of 8 months and puberty. Yet the diagnosis is often not made soon enough for early intervention to be provided, because a child's emerging cognitive and behavioral problems have not yet become a concern. Diagnosis requires solid information about prenatal exposure, as well as the services of a team of health professionals trained in neurodevelopmental assessment and the specific features of alcohol effects. Efforts are now being made to train more diagnosticians and to develop diagnostic aids (in the form of checklists, laboratory and imaging studies, computer analysis of facial photographs, psychological profiles, and screening tests).

It is difficult to estimate the incidence and prevalence of FAS, because of diagnostic issues, underreporting, and the limitations of available data, though the syndrome has been found in every population that uses alcohol. One widely accepted worldwide estimate is 1.9 cases of FAS per 1,000 live births, and the incidence of other ARBDs and ARND is undoubtedly higher. There is no solid evidence that specific demographic groups are at greater risk for alcohol effects in general, or for the full syndrome, given the lack of population-based prevalence studies.

Exploratory studies of the behavioral characteristics of fetal alcohol-affected individuals have been conducted across the lifespan. Findings have focused both on the "primary" cognitive and behavioral disabilities resulting from CNS dysfunction, and more recently on "secondary" disabilities in lifestyle and daily functioning. Over the next few years, research will more completely describe the diverse profile of fetal alcohol effects, with a broader range of patients and comparison groups studied, more data on patients' deficits and strengths, and more information on risk and protective factors.

FAS has been called the leading known cause of mental retardation in the Western world. But this syndrome cannot simply be viewed as another type of mental retardation, since many individuals with FAS have IQ scores falling in the borderline or average range. A research summary by two American Academy of Pediatrics committees states that about three-quarters of babies with FAS show irritability during infancy, including signs of tremulousness or jitteriness. Many show difficulties with sucking and muscle tone, and some may be labeled as "failure to thrive." Problems become more evident as the child grows. In early childhood, about three-quarters of those diagnosed with FAS reported in this research summary show mild to moderate mental retardation, though a range of IQs exists (and new data appears to show higher functioning). About half of young children with FAS show poor coordination, decreased muscle tone, hyperactivity, and/or attention deficits, and they may also have language problems. For a small number of children with FAS, autistic-like behavior may occur.

As they grow, according to clinical observations and existing research, children with FAS often have memory and learning deficits; even when accounting for their age and IQ level, they frequently show special difficulties in relating cause and effect, making social judgments, understanding another's point of view, and planning. There are emerging discrepancies between apparent ability level and actual level of achievement and daily functioning. For example, there may be a discrepancy between relatively better verbal fluency and vocabulary, and relatively poor ability to communicate and function effectively in social situations. These cognitive and linguistic deficits seem related to the frequent troubles these children have in handling the complexities of peer interaction and conforming to social norms, and to the varied behavior problems they can present (e.g., persistent temper tantrums, poor peer relations and social skills, and apparent lying and stealing).

In adolescence and adulthood, facial dysmorphology changes and becomes less distinctive, as do growth deficiencies. Yet there can be continuing and serious problems in CNS dysfunction among fetal alcohol-affected individuals, with complex and long-term life problems. Data from Streissguth and colleagues on a group of 61 adolescents and adults with FAS, or a partial expression of the syndrome then called "possible fetal alcohol effects (FAE)," showed average IQ in the range of mild mental retardation; however, almost half of the group were not technically mentally retarded. More recent data on 415 alcohol-affected individuals documented average IQ in the borderline range of intelligence for those with FAS, and in the average range for those with FAE. Streissguth and her coworkers have described these and other patients as often showing special difficulties in arithmetic skills, which seem related to difficulties they have with abstractions such as time and space, cause and effect, and generalizing from one situation to another. Streissguth has commented that these patients typically show superficially good verbal skills, but have difficulties with independent living, poor judgment, and generally dysfunctional lives. Adolescents and adults with FAS also commonly have problems establishing and maintaining lasting interpersonal relationships. All this suggests that individuals with significant fetal alcohol effects may run a higher risk of problems that are not easily accounted for by deficits in either their intellectual ability or their rearing environment. These "secondary disabilities" may include mental health problems, school disruption, legal and correctional involvement, substance abuse, inappropriate sexual behavior, and difficulties with independent living. In addition, if a woman who is fetal alcohol-affected engages in risk drinking during pregnancy, there is the chance that her child will also show alcohol effects, and so alcohol-related secondary disabilities may emerge again in the next generation.

Given these potential problems, it is essential to retain a balanced view of fetal alcohol effects, since affected individuals can also show characteristics that are quite positive. Yet the best outcomes among alcohol-affected individuals have not been adequately documented, because such individuals may not receive research attention. At this point, there are anecdotal reports of a wide range of positive outcomes, even among patients with the full FAS—including those in one useful and interesting 1992 book entitled *Fantastic Antone Succeeds!: Experiences in Educating Children with Fetal Alcohol Syndrome*. Very recent research has revealed protective factors important in the lives of alcohol-affected individuals, such as early diagnosis, high-quality and stable home environment, and eligibility for social services from the Division of Developmental Disabilities. Effective intervention can be set up to promote these protective influences.

IMPACT OF DOSE, PATTERN, AND TIMING OF ALCOHOL EXPOSURE

The impact of alcohol, like that of other teratogens, depends on the quantity, frequency, and gestational timing of prenatal exposure. A number of prospective longitudinal studies have examined the relationship between the full range of drinking patterns during pregnancy and offspring development. Group research findings have generally shown a positive association between the degree of prenatal alcohol exposure and the extent of physical, cognitive, and behavioral deficits. Greater levels of exposure have been associated with more serious impairment, and group data show that even moderate doses of alcohol (in the "social drinking" range) can have subtle developmental consequences.

There are marked differences between individuals in vulnerability to any given level of exposure. Some researchers have tried to define "safe" or especially detrimental levels of alcohol consumption, but such thresholds have not yet been established. The U.S. Surgeon General has advised that all pregnant women abstain from drinking throughout pregnancy, because there is no way to determine clearly which babies may be at risk for damage from very low levels of prenatal exposure. Children with the full FAS are usually (though not always) born to women who clearly abused alcohol during pregnancy; the risk of having a child with FAS has been estimated at approximately 6% among alcoholic women.

Animal research has shown that a high peak blood alcohol level (resulting from much drinking in a short time) is one critical factor in subsequent offspring effects. Animal data also document that the specific types of birth defect produced depend on the system(s) in the fetus undergoing development at the time of exposure. Heavy and consistent drinking throughout pregnancy risks the entire constellation of structural defects, whereas "binge-like" (heavy and occasional) drinking may damage particular systems. Organ systems are most vulnerable during their embryonic period of most dynamic development. Thus there may be critical periods for alcohol damage during embryonic development, and there may be different profiles of ARBDs depending on when the exposure occurred. Limited data suggest that drinking early in pregnancy appears related to physical anomalies (and may be most damaging to brain structure), and that drinking in the third trimester seems to affect body size more directly. But because the brain is sensitive to the effects of alcohol throughout gestation, the brain damage that underlies later behavioral effects may occur at any time. Yet stopping alcohol use at any time during pregnancy is likely to be beneficial, even for functions affected by earlier drinking.

IMPACT OF MEDIATING FACTORS

Although excessive drinking increases the overall risk for FAS, not all women who drink heavily during pregnancy give birth to children with ARBDs or ARND. Characteristics of mothers and children may explain why some infants are spared and others not, and researchers are pursuing this question intensively. Twin studies are examining genetic variables in children, and one special group of women now under investigation consists of those who have already produced a child with FAS. Maternal characteristics of particular interest are older age and higher number of previous pregnancies. Also of interest are nutrition, metabolic characteristics, disease, smoking, overall state of physical and mental health, lifestyle characteristics, and genetic background; deficits in many of these are associated with chronic alcohol use by women. A mother's use of other drugs is another mediating variable under study, since women who use one substance are also likely to use others, especially if they are heavy users. There may be interactions between combinations of substances; the combination of tobacco and alcohol, for example, produces smaller offspring than the separate use of either substance. Note there is also some evidence that fathers' alcohol consumption may directly induce deficits in their progeny.

MECHANISMS OF FETAL ALCOHOL DAMAGE

Alcohol has a myriad of structural and functional effects on the sensory–motor, neuroanatomical, neurochemical, neurohormonal, and immunological systems of the developing fetus. There may be several mechanisms responsible for these deleterious effects, so that the varied features of ARBDs and ARND may arise from different causes. There are probably both direct and indirect effects of alcohol and/or its metabolites on the developing fetus, and an impact at both the molecular and cellular levels. Prenatal alcohol exposure may affect fetal development by damaging or killing developing fetal cells, thus decreasing cell size and number in several organ systems, and may interfere with the processes of cell migration and adhesion. Alcohol may also affect placental function in the mother, and influence many of the numerous biochemical steps involved in the process of fetal development.

The most common brain abnormalities in FAS are a decrease in the overall size of the brain and, because the total number of cells is reduced, diminished thickness of the outer layers of the brain (the cortex), as well as reductions in the volume of deep cerebral white matter. The brain regions of the hippocampus and cerebellum have been found to be vulnerable to alcohol, and recent studies using magnetic resonance imaging show diverse defects in these and other regions of the brain, such as the basal ganglia and the corpus callosum. In some children with FAS, nerve cells fail to migrate to appropriate sites; this leads to clumps of misplaced cells, which are assumed not to be fulfilling their normal roles within the brain. Now under study are the relationships between abnormal behavior and the disturbed structure and function of brain systems induced by alcohol.

CURRENT PREVENTION AND TREATMENT STRATEGIES

Prevention and Treatment of Drinking during Pregnancy

Nationwide, and even internationally, there are a growing number of community-based and culturally appropriate efforts to prevent drinking during pregnancy, and thus to prevent ARBDs. Warning signs at points of liquor purchase, warning labels on alcoholic beverages, educational campaigns in the electronic and print media, hotlines to provide alcohol and drug use information, training of health care providers and teachers, preconception counseling, and prenatal clinic programs have been initiated across the United States. In response to these varied efforts, U.S. women's knowledge of the risks of heavy drinking during pregnancy, their awareness of FAS, and their ability to correctly describe FAS increased between 1985 and 1990. But still needed are more prevention and education efforts, focusing on behavior rather than attitudes. Target groups especially in need of prevention may be drinkers who are young (< 30 years), black, or Hispanic, or who have limited years of education.

Recent prevention research has focused on developing brief but accurate checklists to assess risky drinking during pregnancy. Such checklists can also serve as openings for healthcare providers to present hazards and advice about drinking during pregnancy. These checklists inquire about such topics as tolerance to alcohol, whether people have annoyed the woman by criticizing her drinking, or whether she ever has a drink first thing in the morning as an "eye-opener." Prevention efforts have focused on training physicians and other health care professionals about alcohol abuse, assessment of at-risk drinking during pregnancy (and after), what to do if a woman is not ready for treatment, complications of chronic alcohol use (e.g., poor nutrition) and how to handle them, and treatment approaches and availability. These training efforts must continue.

Once a pregnant woman is identified as an at-risk drinker, she will be eligible for high-risk follow-up and should be referred for substance abuse assessment and possible treatment. There has recently been a major drive to create specialized, woman-oriented chemical dependency treatment. This approach focuses on issues important to women struggling with addiction. Woman-oriented services also focus on removing obstacles to treatment by providing such services as specialized case management, detoxification for pregnant women, on-site or readily available child care, family support services, and easily accessible prenatal care.

Treatment of Alcohol-Related Birth Defects

As I have described elsewhere, treatment of ARBDs and ARND can be seen as a four-step process. The first step involves reframing an affected individual's developmental and behavioral problems as organically based and long-term, and reframing the treatment process and goals accordingly. The second step requires creation of flexible, individualized intervention strategies, tailored to the needs of the affected individual as revealed in appropriate assessment, and easily changeable when they are no longer effective or the problems have changed. The third step involves building a protective environment for the affected individual. Because some of the patient's problems will be resistant to change, the best strategy is to provide an environment that limits harmful consequences and makes the most of the patient's skills. The fourth and final step focuses on building a partnership of services; this is necessary, given the complexity and long-term nature of the patient's problems and the fact that he or she may be involved in multiple intervention systems (e.g., special education, counseling, the correctional system, etc.).

Growing numbers of resources are helpful in creating the flexible and individualized intervention strategies needed for individuals with ARBDs and ARND. Self-help books and videotapes are becoming available. A growing number of health and education professionals are beginning to understand fetal alcohol effects. Researchers are starting to develop and test specific intervention strategies aimed at the population of individuals with fetal alcohol effects. Services appropriate to the complex and ongoing needs of alcohol-affected individuals (and their families) are developing, although much more work remains to be done. Such services include grassroots parent support groups and informational newsletters; specialized diagnostic and referral clinics; adoption support services; referral for Supplemental Security Income funding; specialized group homes; specialized treatment in schools, as well as in substance abuse, public health, mental health, and correctional facilities; and advocacy programs tailored to the needs of families involved in substance abuse and raising children with fetal alcohol effects. A major focus in future research will be on the effectiveness of these programs and intervention techniques developed specifically for this population.

FURTHER READING

Aase, J. M. (Ed.). (1994). Special focus: Alcohol-related birth defects [Special issue]. *Alcohol Health and Research World, 18*(1), 5–9.
Recent monograph containing state-of-the-art research reports on important topics in the field of alcohol-related birth defects by such authors as Aase, Abel, Becker, Burgess, Cicero, Coles, Cordero, Day, Dufour, Jacobson and Jacobson, Mattson, Morse and Weiner, Randall, Riley, Russell, Sokol, and Streissguth.

Astley, S. J., & Clarren, S. K. (1996). A case definition and photographic screening tool for the facial phenotype of fetal alcohol syndrome. *Journal of Pediatrics, 129,* 33–41.
Presentation of a highly accurate method useful for case definition through screening of facial photographs to find individuals with the critical features of FAS.

Astley, S. J., & Clarren, S. K. (1997). *Diagnostic guide for fetal alcohol syndrome and related conditions.* Seattle: University of Washington Press.
Presentation of a descriptive, easily usable diagnostic system for FAS and related conditions. This diagnostic approach is designed to increase diagnostic precision and accuracy, and better characterize the disabilities of alcohol-exposed individuals who do not have FAS.

Carmichael Olson, H. (1994). The effects of prenatal alcohol exposure on child development. *Infants and Young Children, 6*(3), 10–25.
Clinically oriented article giving brief case reports of children with FAS, and outlining a useful intervention framework for caregivers and professionals.

Committee on Substance Abuse & Committee on Children with Disabilities. (1993). Fetal alcohol syndrome and fetal alcohol effects. *Pediatrics, 91*(5), 1004–1006.
Research summary on "fetal alcohol effects" and clinical recommendations for the pediatric community.

Comprehensive Health Education Foundation. (1995). *The Washington State fetal alcohol resource guide.* Olympia: Washington State Department of Social and Health Services.
Compilation of videos, slides, books, and other resources useful for public and professional education, and for developing individual and community strategies of prevention and treatment for ARBDs.

Connor, P. D., & Streissguth, A. P. (1996). Effects of prenatal exposure to alcohol across the lifespan. *Alcohol Health and Research World, 20*(3), 170–174.
Straightforward, brief, and easily understood presentation of nomenclature and diagnostic criteria, the structural damage to the brain that alcohol can cause, alcohol-related neuropsychological deficits, treatment strategies, and prevention issues.

Kleinfeld, J., & Westcott, S. (Eds.). (1992). *Fantastic Antone succeeds!: Experiences in educating children with fetal alcohol syndrome.* Anchorage: University of Alaska Press.
Practical, easy-to-read book including chapters written by parents, professionals (e.g., teachers, art therapists, and counselors), and researchers; offers a wide variety of intervention ideas for individuals with FAS and "possible fetal alcohol effects."

National Institute for Alcoholism and Alcohol Abuse (NIAAA). (1994). *Eighth special report to the U.S. Congress on alcohol and health* (DHHS Publication No. NIH 94-3699). Washington, DC: U.S. Government Printing Office.
Thorough compendium of research on the full range of ABBDs, including data from animal research, information on alcohol-induced brain damage, data on the effects of social drinking from epidemiological research, and clinical studies of FAS.

Stratton, K. R., Howe, C. J., & Battaglia, F. C. (Eds.). (1996). *Fetal alcohol syndrome: Diagnosis, epidemiology, prevention, and treatment.* Washington, DC: National Academy Press.
Comprehensive discussion of nomenclature, prevalence, diagnostic issues, approaches to prevention, and the available information about treatment of FAS and other alcohol-related birth defects. This resource sets the latest guidelines for the study of fetal alcohol effects.

Streissguth, A. P. (1994). A long-term perspective of FAS. *Alcohol Health and Research World, 18*(1), 74–81.
Reflections and data on the longterm behavioral outcome of individuals with fetal alcohol effects, presented in an easy-to-understand article.

Streissguth, A. P., Aase, J. M., Clarren, S. K., LaDue, R. A., Randels, S. P., & Smith, D. F. (1991). Fetal alcohol syndrome in adolescents and adults. *Journal of the American Medical Association, 265*(15), 1961–1967.
Ground-breaking study presenting data on adolescents and adults with FAS or FAE, and documenting the lifespan effects of prenatal alcohol exposure on cognition and adaptive behavior, as well as the "secondary disabilities" seen in this clinical population (such as mental health, legal, job, and academic problems).

Streissguth, A. P., Barr, H. M., Kogan, K., & Bookstein, F. L. (1996). *Understanding the occurrence of secondary disabilities in clients with fetal alcohol syndrome (FAS) and fetal alcohol effects (FAE).* Seattle: University of Washington Press.
This report, funded by the Centers for Disease Control and Prevention, documents findings from caregiver interviews of a very large clinical sample of fetal alcohol-affected individuals. Patients ranged in age from infancy to middle age, and the sample included both patients with diagnosed FAS and those with the clinical label of FAE. Results show a strikingly high prevalence of "secondary disabilities" among individuals with FAS or FAE. Such disabilities include mental health problems, school disruption, difficulties with the law, parenting problems, substance abuse, and other deficits. Risk and protective factors are identified in this correlational data set, and recommendations made to meet the challenge of overcoming these secondary disabilities.

6

Childhood: Gender Role Development

Joel Szkrybalo
Diane N. Ruble

A growing body of research suggests that women's vulnerability to such health problems as eating disorders and depression may be rooted in childhood development. In particular, childhood is a crucial period in the formation of gender roles. It is a time when girls become cognizant of their gender identity; when they learn about the positive and negative stereotypes commonly associated with their gender group; when they become aware of status and power differences between the sexes; and when they face socialization pressures from parents, teachers, peers, and the mass media to adhere to the prevailing gender role norms of their culture. This chapter examines the implications of female gender role development for women's health, highlighting the potential links among early gender stereotyping, gender role socialization, and the greater incidence of eating disorders and depression in women.

THE DEVELOPMENT OF GENDER ROLE KNOWLEDGE

Most studies find that boys and girls show the same general pattern of gender role development. At about age 2½, they are both able to correctly identify their own gender and the gender of other children. From the ages of 3–5, they show dramatic increases in their knowledge of gender stereotypes. They know, for instance, that dresses and dolls are "for girls" whereas ties and toy trucks are "for boys," and that nursing is a "woman's job" whereas carpentry is a "man's job." Their preferences for same-sex friends and gender-stereotypic toys also become well established. At slightly older ages, children start to develop more abstract and internal notions about gender. They show an awareness of gender-typed personality traits (e.g., boys are "angry," girls are "fearful") and can grasp the gender-typed connotations of TV commercials. Finally, in the early elementary school years, children have a tendency to apply gender stereotypes in a dogmatic fashion, arguing that boys and girls should not deviate from their prescribed gender roles. They may even ignore attempts by their parents or teachers to modify their rigid, sexist thinking. With age, however, children become more aware of exceptions to the rule and more accepting of gender role flexibility.

There are a few noteworthy exceptions to this pattern of gender role development. First, children of both sexes tend to view the male role as more rigidly defined than the female role. Boys who cross gender role boundaries are usually treated with greater peer disapproval and derision than girls who do so are. Second, girls are often found to be more egalitarian in their views than boys, stating that traditionally male-typed or female-typed activities should be open to both sexes. What might account for the greater flexibility of females and the female gender role? In part, children may be responding to recent cultural changes that have granted opportunities for women to pursue nontraditional occupations and familial roles. The loosening of the male gender role has proceeded at a slower pace. It is also likely that these differences reflect children's growing awareness of the lower social status and power attributed to women in North American culture (and, indeed, in most cultures). Girls may argue for flexibility in gender stereotypes, or engage in traditionally male-typed activities such as baseball, because they want to experience the greater power and prestige associated with the male role.

Some evidence supports this second interpretation of gender role flexibility in girls. Studies of gender role attitudes report that both boys and girls show an "in-group bias" at about age 5, in which they proclaim that their own gender group is better than the other one. This bias seems to reflect a type of basic identity validation: "I value my own attributes over the attributes of others who differ from me." By the time children reach age 7, however, the influence of masculine domination becomes apparent. Both sexes are more likely to evaluate males and the masculine role more positively, and girls are more likely to say that they would prefer to be the other sex. At age 10, children show an awareness of gender prejudice toward women.

This growing knowledge about cultural sex differences in power and status may have a negative impact upon girls' self-perceptions. One possible consequence is that girls may be more willing to accept negative gender stereotypes about their capabilities. For instance, a girl who does poorly on a math test at school may be likely to accept the stereotype that "boys are better in math than girls," rather than to attribute her poor performance to the fact that she did not study enough. Not surprisingly, studies that find childhood sex differences in self-confidence and expectations for success in achievement domains, such as school performance, almost always favor boys. This finding emerges despite the fact that *actual* sex differences in scholastic abilities are quite small; indeed, in many cases (e.g., verbal skills), they favor girls.

Another way in which gender stereotypes affect girls' self-image is by fostering certain coping styles. One fairly common stereotype about females is that they are inherently more emotional, empathic, and dependent upon other people's support than males are. In research parlance, males are presumed to be more "instrumental," while females are stereotypically viewed as more "expressive." Does the research evidence support this distinction between the sexes?

Studies of toddler-age children report few consistent sex differences in emotional expression. At best, boys show up as slightly more irritable, and girls as slightly more fearful. In early elementary school—the time of rigid gender stereotyping in children—sex differences become more pronounced. Boys hide their painful emotions more often and exhibit more anger, whereas girls are more likely to hide emotions that hurt other people's feelings. Finally, by adolescence, girls report more sadness, shame, and guilt than boys, and claim that they experience emotions more intensely. They also describe themselves as more empathic than their male counterparts, even though physiological measures and unobtrusive observations do not bear out this conclusion.

These findings suggest that gender-stereotypic beliefs about scholastic abilities, physical skills, and emotional expressiveness may influence girls' self-perceptions, coping styles, and attributions of success or failure. Young children show relatively few sex differences in abilities and emotional behavior, prior to their knowledge of stereotypes. When sex differences do emerge, they tend to be small and dependent upon age. With the growth of knowledge about gender stereotypes, girls begin to realize that their traditional role in adult society is devalued. They may judge their poor performance in masculine domains as a validation of cultural stereotypes, or may attribute their successes to luck or effort rather than natural ability. They may cope with distress through emotional or interpersonal outlets, reporting greater sadness or dependency needs. Given the central role of negative beliefs and attributions in current theories of depression, childhood may thus set the stage for women to show greater vulnerability to depression.

THE IMPACT OF GENDER ROLE SOCIALIZATION

Any description of gender development cannot be considered complete without acknowledging the role of parents, teachers, peers, and the mass media in shaping children's beliefs and behaviors. These "socializing agents," as they are sometimes called, are intimately involved in teaching girls what it means to be female in a given culture and time period. To the extent that they serve as custodians of gender norms or role models of flexibility and personal choice, they influence girls' ideas about the physical activities, personality traits, and future occupations that are appropriate for their gender group. Peers and the media also maintain standards of acceptable clothing, appearances, and conduct, determining what is "in style" for girls. The health and well-being of women may be tied as much to these external influences as to their early gender-stereotypic beliefs and attributions.

The primary socializing agents in the lives of most young girls are the parents. Parents can exercise influence over gender role development in a number of ways, either deliberately or unwittingly. They can encourage gender role compliance through direct praise and punishment. For instance, a mother can foster dependency in her daughter by encouraging proximity-seeking behaviors and deploring acts of assertiveness and autonomy. Parents can also structure the home environment in a manner that creates different kinds of experiences and challenges for sons and daughters. For instance, providing dolls, dollhouses, and tea sets for daughters can cultivate their social skills; limiting their access to toy trucks, construction tools, and building blocks can impede the development of visual–spatial and mechanical skills. Finally, parents can serve as important models of gender role behaviors and attitudes for their children. Studies of maternal employment have found that girls develop more egalitarian beliefs when their mothers are in the work force, particularly if the mothers' job status and work satisfaction are high.

The consequences of parental socialization for women most likely depend upon a number of factors, including parental attitudes and beliefs about the female role, the degree to which parents communicate these beliefs to their daughters, and the quality of parent–daughter relationships. Research findings suggest some possible links. According to one recent study, parents who hold more stereotypic beliefs about sex differences in English, math, and sports abilities are more apt to expect these differences in their children, even when there is no legitimate basis for them. Moreover, their children tend to fulfill their expectations eventually, rather than to perform at levels congruent with actual abilities. Since girls are stereotypically viewed as being less competent in math and "masculine" sports, they may be discouraged from engaging in certain athletic activities or entering math-related fields (e.g., engineering), in which they would otherwise excel. The consequences may be especially poignant for females whose abilities or aspirations come into conflict with the expectations of their parents. In such cases, a young woman's decision to pursue her own ambitions may entail a loss of parental support, thereby increasing her vulnerability to depression.

Parents are certainly not alone in guiding children's gender development. As a testing ground for gender roles outside the family, schools can also have a lasting impact on children's attitudes and beliefs about their gender group. One way that schools accomplish this is through the socializing influence of teachers. Although nowadays many teachers try to foster gender equality in the classroom, studies suggest that boys and girls continue to receive subtle forms of differential treatment. For instance, teachers have been found to discourage high activity levels and masculine behavior in preschool girls. In later grades, teachers are more attentive to boys and allow them more time to speak in class. They are also more likely to accept answers from boys who call out in class, whereas they may tell girls to raise their hands first. Such cues may reinforce stereotypes that girls are more sedentary, compliant, and less confident in their intellectual skills than boys. Conversely, they support the view of boys as more active and aggressive.

Another way in which gender role differences are made salient in school is through the influence of peers. Peers can serve as models of appropriate gender roles, as well as fierce advocates of gender-stereotypic norms. Any boy who has been called a "sissy" for playing with dolls knows that a violation of gender norms can be met with swift disapproval from peers. Although parents and teachers probably exert greater influence during the early elementary school years, peers may become increasingly important as children approach adolescence. The preadolescent peer group is often involved in creating and projecting images of what is "cool" and what leads to popularity among one's peers. They respond to idealized images in the mass media of how young boys and girls should look, how they should act, and what they should strive to become.

Unfortunately, many of these images have gender-stereotypic connotations that bode poorly for women. Within the peer group, popularity for preadolescent boys is frequently based upon athletic ability and toughness. Popularity for girls is more closely related to physical appearance, social skills, and parents' socioeconomic status. Hence, the tacit message that girls must strive to be attractive, soft, dependent, and emotionally attuned to others is reinforced within the school setting. In particular, the greater emphasis on physical appearance for girls may set the stage for later concerns with body image and dieting, both of which figure prominently in the etiology of eating disorders.

The popular media certainly have a hand in perpetuating stereotypic images of male and female roles. On TV, women are more often portrayed as young, thin, beautiful, and provocatively dressed. Magazines directed at young women place greater emphasis on appearances and dieting than do male-oriented magazines, though the trends are slowly changing. Gender stereotyping in children's television programs is also quite conspicuous: Male cartoon characters are more likely to be problem solvers, whereas female characters are more likely to be sweet, childlike, and dependent. Shows written for boys contain more action, loud music, and quick scene changes; shows for girls employ more soft music, female narration, and fading scene changes. Again, the message conveyed by the media is that males are more competent, independent, powerful, and heroic than females. To get ahead in the world, females are supposed to rely on external measures of self-worth rather than their internal resources and problem-solving abilities.

Since children are watching more television today than in past years, the role of the media in shaping stereotypic beliefs is likely to increase. Several studies have already demonstrated that high levels of TV viewing in children correlate with stronger gender stereotyping. However, the direction of influence remains unclear. Children who hold stereotypic beliefs may simply be more inclined to watch TV programs than other children. On the positive side, other studies report that nontraditional portrayals of men and women may help counter gender stereotypes about domestic roles and occupations in children. The media may thus be a promising venue for challenging traditional roles instead of merely perpetuating them.

Taken together, the influence of socializing agents upon children's gender role beliefs and behaviors are pervasive. Girls encounter subtle and not-so-subtle messages about their accepted role in society from many different sources. When these messages are stereotypic and traditional, they impose restrictions on the kinds of behaviors, personality traits, and aspirations that girls can exhibit. They also offer idealized images of what girls should strive to become, which can lead to an unhealthy focus on external appearance and body weight. Women's greater vulnerability to depression and eating disorders probably has some links to these early socialization experiences.

A few cautionary notes should be added here. Our presentation of gender role knowledge and socialization influences under separate headings is consistent with the way these issues have been examined in the developmental literature. Most researchers tend to focus on one area or the other for the sake of clarity and convenience. Nevertheless, it is widely acknowledged that this dichotomy is artificial; knowledge development and socialization probably interact in complex ways. Girls are not passive recipients of gender role socialization. Their maturing cognitive capacities determine the kinds of information that they can absorb and how this information is evaluated.

Some research also suggests that socializing agents do not simply impose stereotypic expectations upon children. In some cases, they may respond to actual differences exhibited by boys and girls. These differences may be rooted in biology or in children's unique beliefs about gender roles. The direction of effects between socialization and biological/cognitive factors thus needs to be clarified in future research. Finally, socialization effects are often dependent upon context. Studies of school-based interventions report moderate success in promoting egalitarian beliefs in children, but changes seldom generalize beyond the classroom.

SUMMARY

There is growing evidence that women's vulnerability to depression and eating disorders may be linked to early gender role development. As young girls acquire a firm sense of gender identity and learn the stereotypes associated with their gender group, they become increasingly aware of power and status differences between men and women. Their self-image, attributions of success or failure, and styles of coping may be influenced by negative gender stereotypes, potentially increasing their vulnerability to depression. The socialization influences of parents, teachers, peers, and the mass media may also serve to perpetuate gender stereotypes. In particular, idealized images of gender roles in the media and peer subculture may adversely affect preadolescent girls by emphasizing the importance of appearance, body weight, and dependency in females. Though children's gender-typed beliefs and gender role socialization are often examined separately in the literature, they probably exercise a mutual influence over female role development. Biological sex differences and contextual factors also appear to contribute to differential socialization of boys and girls.

FURTHER READING

Basow, S. A. (1992). *Gender stereotypes and roles.* Pacific Grove, CA: Brooks/Cole.
Chapter 8 of this textbook examines the impact of gender stereotypes and roles on the physical and mental health of both men and women.

Eccles, J. S., Jacobs, J. E., Harold, R. D., Yoon, K. S., Arbreton, A., & Freedman-Doan, C. (1993). Parents and gender role socialization during middle childhood and adolescent years. In S. Oskamp & M. Costanzo (Eds.), *Gender issues in contemporary society* (pp. 59–83). Newbury Park, CA: Sage.
Summarizes research findings by Eccles and others on the effect of parental socialization on children's performance in academic and sports domains.

Lutz, S. E., & Ruble, D. N. (1995). Children and gender prejudice: Context, motivation, and the development of gender conceptions. *Annals of Child Development, 10,* 131–166.
A theoretical paper describing the links between children's gender role knowledge and the development of gender prejudice toward females.

Ruble, D. N., Greulich, F., Pomerantz, E. M., & Gochberg, B. (1993). The role of gender-related processes in the development of sex differences in self-evaluation and depression. *Journal of Affective Disorders, 29,* 97–128.
A scholarly review of the literature on childhood sex differences in self-evaluation. Original data are also presented to explore the hypothesis that girls exhibit more depressive symptomatology than boys during childhood.

Ruble, D. N., & Martin, C. L. (in press). Gender development. In W. Damon (Series Ed.) & N. Eisenberg (Vol. Ed.), *Handbook of child psychology* (5th ed.): *Vol. 3. Social, emotional, and personality development.* New York: Wiley.
A thorough review of the literature on gender development from the early 1980s to the present. Different theoretical perspectives of gender development are also summarized.

Signorella, M. L., Bigler, R. S., & Liben, L. S. (1993). Developmental differences in children's gender schemata about others: A meta-analytic review. *Developmental Review, 13,* 147–183.
An analysis of developmental trends in children's gender stereotype knowledge across a large collection of studies. The effects of TV viewing and maternal employment on gender stereotyping are also examined.

7

Adolescence

Anne C. Petersen

Adolescence is a fascinating phase of life to examine in relation to society. Except for the biological transition of puberty, adolescence is rooted in society. As many have noted, such a period only emerged with the Industrial Revolution and did not take a contemporary form until after World War II. Even today, there are many cultures around the world and subgroups in the United States in which the only aspect of adolescence that youngsters experience is the biological transition through puberty. The existence of a phase between childhood and adulthood is only possible when there is a period of time in which the young person looks like an adult but does not yet take on adult roles.

In agrarian societies, historically and now, children begin working with adults in the fields (and, for girls, in the home) from an early age. They may even accompany parents as infants, beginning to observe the work life of their parents—the life the children will move into. In these societies and families there is little age segregation, and learning about adult roles is relatively easy for a child. These societies tend to have rites of passage from childhood to adulthood, usually occurring when a young person manifests biological readiness for adult reproductive roles. Such rites signal clearly to children that they are expected to begin to function as adults in the society.

Contrast the agrarian developmental progression with that of current U.S. society. There is typically a 10- to 15-year gap between biological maturity and entry into adult work roles. Entry to adult family roles, at least as measured by becoming a parent, is currently much more variable in U.S. society: Some girls become mothers in early adolescence, and others delay motherhood until their late 20s or 30s. Although significant knowledge and experience are required to become an effective parent, no knowledge is required to procreate, making this a less salient index of adult status in current times. Adult work roles, in contrast, are extremely difficult to learn, with very few young people having much opportunity to observe even their parents as workers. Because many positions require a college education, and many employers for positions not requiring this education have a bias about hiring young people for responsible roles until they are into their 20s, most young people are not able to enter meaningful adult work roles until their early to middle 20s. Even more complex are societal expectations for the kinds of persons youths are expected to be. It is not surprising, then, that the United States has high morbidity and mortality for youths.

DEFINING ADOLESCENCE

The linkage of adolescence to societal issues makes it difficult to define uniformly and simply. Many scholars now use the second decade of life as a uniform definition for all young people. In a more precise definition, adolescence begins with the biological changes of puberty and ends with the assumption of adult work and family roles, yielding different developmental ages for each young person.

However we define the period of adolescence, it is now typically a long period with distinct phases. Early adolescence is characterized by puberty and related changes, and is usually considered as the ages of 10–13 years. Middle adolescence, characterized by the behavior and appearance of the adolescent stereotype, includes the ages of 14–16 years. Late adolescence is characterized by the transition into adulthood and related changes, and is thought of as the ages of 17–20 years.

Adolescence overall is a period of life in which there is change in every aspect of individual development and in every important social context. This developmental change is stressful, or at least challenging, in and of itself. When it is combined with life events that might occur at any age, such as death, disease, or difficult life circumstances, a young person can become overwhelmed and unable to progress developmentally. Most young people, however, are able to cope effectively with change. Indeed, the need to deal with such challenges may stimulate significant personal growth.

INDIVIDUAL CHANGE IN ADOLESCENCE

Biological Development

The biological changes of puberty are the most rapid and dramatic in life, with the exception of infancy. Notably, infants do not experience their changes or the reactions of others to them in the way that adolescents do. With puberty, children take on adult size, shape, and reproductive capacity. The period takes 4–5 years on average, with tremendous variations. The timing of puberty is about 2 years earlier in girls than in boys. For both boys and girls, pubertal timing is the most influential aspect of biological change for behavior and responses of others. Early-developing girls are at increased risk for depression, body image disturbances, and eating disorders, as well as early pregnancy and other problem behaviors (e.g., drug and alcohol abuse).

Cognitive Development

Cognitive capacity increases throughout childhood and continues to develop into adolescence. In general, young people develop increased capacity to think abstractly during early adolescence. This improves their ability to think hypothetically (e.g., about the future), to think logically, and to make more effective decisions. Among adolescents (as with adults), emotions may interfere with these cognitions and impair judgment.

Psychosocial Development

Adolescents increasingly develop a sense of self in all aspects of functioning. Interestingly, overall self-esteem increases during adolescence, but body image becomes more negative for a time—especially for girls. Moral development and ego development increase over adolescence, reaching adult levels (which are not typically at the highest levels) by midadolescence and manifesting gender differences in level and nature. A sense of oneself relative to others increases over childhood and adolescence; this is probably linked to the increasingly large and diverse groups of others one interacts with. Social development over adolescence moves increasingly in the direction of intimacy with peers (including romantic partners), with decreasing time spent with parents—again with gender differences.

Summary

In contrast to the stereotype of adolescence as a time of problems and frequently of disintegration, developmental research demonstrates that adolescents move toward adult, mature status in all aspects of individual development. They have increasing capacity to behave responsibly and competently as adults. The development of boys and girls diverges in most aspects, varying in patterns similar to those seen in adults.

CHANGES IN SOCIAL CONTEXTS

Peer Group

As youngsters develop through childhood and adolescence, their peer groups become larger and more complex. In childhood, peer groups are typically small and convenient; in adolescence, peer groups are increasingly linked to interests (e.g., classes, teams, clubs, etc.). Moreover, romantic relationships play an increasing role in peer interactions, developing from distant crushes in early adolescence to more adult-like intimate relationships later in adolescence.

Family

Parent–adolescent relationships change over the course of adolescence. The family's response to a young adolescent may depend on birth order; the oldest sibling typically encounters more rules and more resistance to developing autonomy. This difference influences family dynamics, but the stereotype of inevitably conflictual relationships is typical only of early adolescence, and then only focused on mundane conflicts. Research demonstrates that in general, an authoritative parenting style is related to more positive adolescent behaviors, but large variations by ethnic group have been found.

Schools

Schools for young adolescents in the United States are larger, more complex, and more distant from home than are elementary schools. These settings are experienced by young adolescents as more anonymous, as limiting autonomous behavior in the classroom, and perhaps as unsafe outside the classroom. Schools change little in nature by middle adolescence, but most of these older youngsters are able to deal with the challenges of large, anonymous schools. Many have argued that schools for young adolescents are developmentally damaging.

Society

Societal expectations are different for younger versus older adolescents. In the United States, cartoons and other popular media suggest that adults expect trouble from youngsters when they become pubertal, perhaps creating a self-fulfilling prophecy. By later adolescence, young people are expected to have a sense of direction and be prepared to enter adult work roles. It is not clear that any societal institutions take responsibility for preparing all adolescents to meet these expectations.

Summary

All important social contexts are different for adolescents than for children. Although change is surely appropriate, insufficient thought has been given to the nature of change and whether it is developmentally appropriate. Evidence is accumulating that many of these settings are causing difficulties rather than enhancing development.

SOCIAL IMPLICATIONS OF ADOLESCENCE

Young people are the future of any nation. Therefore, it seems essential to nurture youngsters thoughtfully in order to prepare them for adult roles. Too many youths in the United States fail to reach adulthood at all, becoming casualties of murder, suicide, or accidents. Girls are more likely to fall prey to depression and eating disorders, and increasingly are victims of violence. It has been estimated that half of all youths reach adulthood damaged by their experiences. Many assume that these casualties result from the nature of adolescence; nothing could be further from the truth. In fact, the development that ought to take place in adolescence involves accumulating potential to achieve and perform responsibly. Why does this fail to happen in too many cases?

Youngsters today are confronted with many challenges, on a much broader scale than previous generations. In the United States, youths have higher death rates than in any other developed nation. Today, sex in adolescence may lead not only to pregnancy, but to illness and death through AIDS and other sexually transmitted diseases. The prevalence of guns makes it possible for unprecedented numbers of teens to die from gunshot wounds. And affluence in the United States puts many youngsters behind the wheels of cars; this, together with the availability of alcohol and other judgment-impairing drugs, also produces significant morbidity and mortality among youths in the United States compared to other developed countries.

The powerful and largely unprincipled mass media bombard youths with messages about hedonistic pursuits, without similar attention to the importance of developing responsibility for others and for pursuing productive roles in the society. Although some social institutions provide opportunities for young people to learn how to become effective adults and citizens, these opportunities are not available for all, and frequently need to be sought out when they do exist. Conversely, powerful constraints operate on young people to keep them out of the work force, especially if they are not college-bound, and even more powerfully if they are poor. Adolescents look to the society for messages about the types of adults they are to become. What they generally hear is not encouraging.

Much can be done to change this situation. The Carnegie Council on Adolescent Development has provided a great deal of information about how schools can improve, and more is also being learned about what families can do. Much work is yet needed to persuade the mass media and businesses that they should play a more positive role in youth development. But change is possible and extremely important.

FURTHER READING

Carnegie Council on Adolescent Development. (1995). *Great transitions: Preparing adolescents for a new century.* New York: Carnegie Corporation of New York.
This volume represents the final report of the Carnegie Council on Adolescent Development, documenting the risks encountered in traversing adolescence today, especially early adolescence, while also highlighting the tremendous opportunities of this developmental period when young people are supported to reach adulthood. Essential requirements for healthy adolescent development are specified, with recommendations for how to help them reach it.

Feldman, S. S., & Elliott, G. R. (Eds.). (1990). *At the threshold: The developing adolescent.* Cambridge, MA: Harvard University Press.
This Carnegie Corporation of New York edited volume provides a comprehensive overview of current research on normal development in early adolescence. The 19 chapters review interdisciplinary knowledge about biopsychosocial development in all the key contexts during early adolescence.

Millstein, S. G., Petersen, A. C., & Nightingale, E. O. (Eds.). (1993). *Promoting the health of adolescents: New directions for the twenty-first century.* New York: Oxford University Press.
This edited volume pursues the pathways to healthy development in various areas during adolescence, including consideration of special issues such as economics, social processes, and lifestyles. The 16 chapters by experts in adolescent health and development are supplemented by commentaries on health care considerations by physicians and nurses.

Petersen, A. C. (1988). Adolescent development. *Annual Review of Psychology, 39,* 583–607.
This first Annual Review article on adolescent development reviewed the dramatically increasing body of research on the second decade of life, noted its multidisciplinary nature, and highlighted key findings. Dramatic advances have occurred in knowledge about adolescent mental health, effects of puberty, and effects of family processes, among many other areas.

Petersen, A. C., Leffert, N., Graham, B., Ding, S., & Overbey, T. (1994). Depression and body image disorders in adolescence. *Women's Health Issues, 4*(2), 98–108.
This article reviews findings from Petersen's research on the pubertal and social development processes that lead to depression and body image disorders in adolescents, especially producing more problems among girls.

Piper, M. (1994). *Reviving Ophelia: Saving the selves of adolescent girls.* New York: Ballantine Books.
This popular volume on adolescent girls draws accurately on the research on adolescence, as well as the author's clinical experience to paint a vivid picture of the risks of adolescence in U.S. society for girls.

Rutter, M. (Ed.). (1995). *Psychosocial disturbances in young people: Challenges for prevention.* Cambridge, UK: Cambridge University Press.
This edited volume considers why psychosocial disorders have increased among young people at the same time that health and living conditions have improved. The 11 chapters review time trends in various problems and consider preventive approaches at the individual, school, and community levels.

Rutter, M., & Smith, D. (Eds.). (1995). *Psychosocial disorders of young people: Time trends and their causes.* New York: Wiley.
This edited volume represents the report of a study group of Academia Europaea to consider whether psychosocial disorders had become more or less frequent over the past 50 years, to review casual explanations, and establish priorities for future research. The study concluded that psychosocial disorders have increased since the end of World War II. Several factors are implicated in this rise, with some others ruled out by the research.

Simmons, R. G., & Blyth, D. A. (1987). *Moving into adolescence: The impact of pubertal and school context.* Hawthorne, NY: Aldine.
This volume culminates several years of research by the authors on the roles of pubertal change and school transition on adolescent self-image, academic achievement, and extracurricular participation. Differences between boys and girls in changes and effects on behavior are especially emphasized.

Takanishi, R. (Ed.). (1993). *Adolescence in the 1990s: Risk and opportunity.* New York: Teachers College Press.
This volume includes chapters by experts studying and working with adolescents with an emphasis on schools.

8

Puberty

Julia A. Graber
Jeanne Brooks-Gunn

*T*he changes of puberty result in the attainment of reproductive functioning and adult-like physical form, and define the developmental transition from child to adolescent. As such, pubertal development directly influences not only girls' biological systems and functioning, but also their social and emotional development. In addition to the physical, emotional, and social changes experienced by girls themselves at puberty, their experiences influence their social context as family, friends, and teachers respond to their changing appearance. Even girls' feelings about themselves are subject to the satisfaction or anxiety they experience about their changing appearance in a social context. Internal rather than external pubertal processes have also been proposed as the cause for behavioral change at adolescence. For example, brain development at puberty has been hypothesized to cause changes in cognitive skills and abilities, and increases in hormones have been hypothesized to cause moodiness and irritability. The following is a brief description of pubertal development in girls and the psychosocial correlates of puberty.

PUBERTAL PROCESSES

Marshall and Tanner have identified five primary areas of growth and development during the pubertal process: (1) alterations in the nervous system and development of the reproductive endocrine system, regulating the other pubertal developmental processes; (2) the development of secondary sexual characteristics, along with maturation of the reproductive organs; (3) the growth spurt in height and weight; (4) changes in the distribution of fat and muscle tissue and their ratio in the body; and (5) circulatory and respiratory system development. The reproductive endocrine system consists primarily of the hypothalamus, the pituitary gland, and the gonads. Whereas the hormonal pathways that ultimately regulate puberty and reproduction are organized prenatally, resulting in the development of the external genitalia, the system remains relatively dormant from the postnatal period until the middle childhood years. The activation of this system begins with "adrenarche," the maturation of the adrenal gland, which produces androgens; this is followed about 2 years later by "gonadarche," the maturation of the gonads and the hypothalamus–pituitary–gonadal (HPG) system. (These processes have been described in detail by Reiter and Grumbach and are reviewed briefly here.) As yet, the mechanisms that control when the system will be activated are undetermined. Maturation of the reproductive system results in the production of gonadotropin-releasing hormone (GnRH) by the medial basal hypothalamus. The pituitary responds to stimulation by GnRH by releasing pulsatile bursts of gonadotropins, luteinizing hormone (LH) and follicle-stimulating hormone (FSH). Even though LH and FSH are secreted at low levels by the pituitary throughout childhood, it is only when episodic nocturnal bursts of LH are seen that the hormonal activity can be defined as indicating early stages of puberty. Levels of FSH rise steadily until adult levels of production are reached, whereas LH is only released throughout the day in adult-like patterns in the later stages of puberty. Estradiol is released by the ovaries in response to LH and FSH levels, completing the basic feedback loop of the HPG system. In order for the menstrual cycle to be functional, each facet of the loop must be sufficiently mature to stimulate the ovulatory LH surge.

Most girls experience the development of secondary sexual characteristics at about 10.5 years of age with the beginning of breast development, followed closely by the appearance of pubic hair; however, individual variations are common in pubertal development, such that pubic hair appears prior to breast budding in one-fifth of all girls. Variations in onset can probably be attributed to differences in hormonal control of breast and pubic hair development. Breast growth is predominantly related to estrogen, secreted by the ovaries, whereas hair growth is stimulated by androgen secretions, some of which come from the hypothalamus–pituitary–adrenal axis. Girls take about 4.5 years to progress through the stages of breast development, which encompass most of the pubertal process. Mature patterns of pubic hair growth are attained before breast development is complete for most girls. Acceleration in growth in height, or the growth spurt, begins 6–12 months before breast development and peaks at about the middle of breast and pubic hair development. Just after the peak in the growth spurt is passed, and in the middle of the weight spurt, "menarche" (first menstruation) occurs at approximately 12.5 years of age in the United States. Final adult stature is reached by age 18 in nearly all girls.

The age norms for activation of the hormonal system and subsequent development of secondary sexual characteristics vary considerably within each gender. This variation is observed in both the timing of the onset of development and the rates at which individuals progress through puberty. In fact, recent investigations have focused on individual differences in the age norms associated with pubertal development. Large-scale studies of both African-American and European-American girls, such as that done by the National Heart, Lung, and Blood Institute (NHLBI) Research Group, have demonstrated earlier ages of pubertal development in African-American girls. In particular, the NHLBI Growth and Health Study examined the physical development of over 2,300 girls aged 9 and 10 years. Comparisons indicated that twice as many 9-year-old African-American as European-American girls had begun breast development (36% vs. 16.5%). African-American girls were also significantly taller and heavier, and had a higher percentage of body fat, than European-American girls. The meaning of these group differences to girls themselves is only just beginning to be studied.

LINKS BETWEEN PUBERTY AND PSYCHOSOCIAL DEVELOPMENT

Because pubertal development encompasses multiple processes, links between pubertal and psychosocial development have been examined in connection with specific processes. The most commonly studied aspects of pubertal development are (1) the hormonal changes of puberty; (2) changes in secondary sexual characteristics (i.e., movement from Tanner 1 to Tanner 2 stages of breast development and the acceleration of growth in height); and (3) the timing of pubertal development, as compared to the average age of development of one's peers. Each aspect of development has demonstrated effects on psychosocial development. Pubertal processes have usually been investigated in terms of how specific processes are experienced by adolescents and as antecedents to behavioral change, although bidirectional associations between puberty and behavior have begun to be tested.

Behavioral Correlates of Hormonal Changes

It has long been assumed that behavioral changes at puberty, or at least the negative changes, are results of the increases in hormones occurring during puberty. Despite the belief in this assertion for nearly a century, formal tests of hormone effects on behavior at puberty have been limited to the past 10–15 years. Several review articles have delineated the associations between pubertal hormones and changes in mood, affect, and behavior at adolescence, with most studies examining aggressive behavior, depressive affect, or sexual arousal.

In studies of aggressive behaviors and feelings, both global hormonal functioning (as indexed by estradiol) and adrenal androgens have demonstrated small negative associations with aggression in girls. Such associations have more often been studied in boys; this research has found direct effects of testosterone on provoked aggressive behavior in boys, along with indirect effects (via impatience and irritability) on other aggressive behaviors. Results across studies are mixed, with different hormones relating to aggressive behaviors and feelings, depending on gender, the hormones being assessed, and the aspect of aggression under study. Increases in a single hormone probably do not lead to aggression; it is more likely that increased hormones lead to arousal, which stimulates an emotional response.

Associations between pubertal hormones and changes in depressive affect have also been documented. In work by members of our group, it was hypothesized that hormone levels are most likely to be associated with behavior when the hormonal systems are being activated, such that links should be seen in the early stages of puberty but not later. In testing this hypothesis in a sample of 100 girls, Warren and Brooks-Gunn found a curvilinear association between estradiol category and depressive affect. Because the hormones linking the HPG system are highly correlated, it was feasible to base categories of hormonal and reproductive functioning on estradiol levels. Specifically, depressive affect was found to be highest for girls with rapidly increasing but subadult hormonal levels.

Other researchers, such as Buchanan and colleagues, have emphasized that only some girls demonstrate alterations in mood in association with hormonal levels; thus, girls may have different sensitivities to physiological substrates. Such interpretations have also been made about arousal effects, as arousal may be interpreted differently among adolescents and therefore may be expressed as aggression, anxiety, depressive affect, or another emotion. For example, even though boys experience greater increases in testosterone during puberty, girls may be more emotionally or biologically responsive to small increases in testosterone.

The investigations conducted to date indicate that increases in pubertal hormones do affect behavior, at least in children who are already well into the pubertal transition. Most important is the lack of information on larger samples of girls, especially non-European-American samples, and limited information on the earlier hormonal changes. Indications that changes in affect may be strongest with the initial rise in hormones need to be investigated more fully in younger samples, which should be followed longitudinally as each child experiences these changes.

Psychological Response to Changes in Secondary Sexual Characteristics

In addition to potential physiological effects on behavior via arousal or direct effects of hormones on mood, pubertal development is also experienced as a psychological and social event. The psychological meaning or significance of different pubertal processes varies greatly, depending on the aspect of puberty being studied. Most research attention has been focused on the significance of the menarcheal experience. Cross-cultural studies have frequently identified menarche as a time of transition and particular significance in girls' development. Theoretical perspectives make disparate hypotheses, including the suggestion that menarche may be anxiety-provoking and/or a traumatic event, as well as the idea that it may elicit positive social cues as an indicator of maturity. Research with adolescent girls during the pubertal years supports both types of responses, noting that individual differences exist among girls in how they experience menarche: Girls who experience menarche earlier than their peers and girls who report being unprepared for it have more negative experiences than other girls. Even though menarche may signal reproductive capacity and may take on special meaning in the transition from child to adult, it is not an externally apparent transition; that is, others are only aware that it has occurred if girls choose to tell them about it. Girls usually only tell their mothers and closest friends.

In contrast, other aspects of development are more noticeable to the external world and may also have psychological significance for girls. The meaning and significance of other aspects of pubertal development have been much less studied in girls; even less attention has been given to the significance of pubertal development in boys. Girls' responses to breast development have been examined in a few studies, such as one by Brooks-Gunn and colleagues. Whereas girls with more advanced breast development reported more positive feelings on measures of adjustment and relations with peers, about 50% of these girls also reported being teased about this development. Subsequent research using projective measures to assess feelings about breast development indicated again that even though development was viewed positively, negative feelings did arise in the context of interactions with others, especially embarrassment with fathers.

The literature to date thus suggests that advancing through the stages of pubertal development is not a particularly negative experience for most adolescent girls. Responses to puberty tend to be neutral or positive, although individual differences clearly exist among girls. Explaining individual differences requires examining the contexts that are associated with negative experiences (e.g., lack of preparation or experience of teasing) that may ultimately lead to poorer adjustment.

The Significance of the Timing of Puberty

How girls cope with puberty and how they are influenced by it depend upon their emotional and cognitive skills at the time when pubertal transitions occur. The timing of the onset or experience of a particular pubertal event varies greatly across girls. For example, even though the average age of menarche is 12.5 years, girls may reach menarche at any time between the ages of 9.5 and 15.5 and still be within the range of normal development. Hence, girls are at different levels of emotional and cognitive development when they experience different pubertal events. Girls who experience puberty earlier than most other girls are more likely to be unprepared emotionally and cognitively for such changes. In addition, the timing of development has meaning in the social context; that is, girls come in contact with other girls and adults who may place particular values on "normative" versus "non-normative" development. Such considerations suggest that girls who do not mature at the same time as their peers will be at increased risk for negative developmental outcomes, with the earliest-maturing girls being at the highest risk, as they are likely to be less psychologically and socially prepared for the changes of puberty.

Indeed, research has begun to demonstrate that girls who mature earlier than their peers have poorer adjustment along several dimensions than do other girls or boys. In several studies, girls who matured earlier than their peers had poorer body image than other girls. Girls with chronically disturbed eating behaviors across adolescence were also more likely to be earlier maturers than girls with healthy eating attitudes and behavior. Research on depression in both girls and boys found that earlier maturation, together with other stressful adolescent transitions at school and in the family during the middle school years, led to increased depressive affect into late adolescence in both girls and boys. Thus, at least in this depression research, the synchrony of changes rather than gender per se predicted poor outcome. However, in view of the age when most girls reach menarche and when most school systems institute a school transition between grades, it is much more likely that girls will experience these two changes simultaneously. Recent findings exemplify the complexity of the relationship of pubertal timing and adjustment. Caspi and Moffitt found that not all early-maturing girls experienced adjustment problems, and not all girls with a history of adjustment problems were early maturers. Yet those girls with a history of problems who matured early had the worst adjustment outcomes by midadolescence. How and why such combinations result in negative outcomes are questions that have not been fully addressed.

Many of these studies were restricted to samples of girls; the nature of associations between timing and adjustment merits further studies allowing for comparison of these hypotheses in girls and boys. Earlier maturers of both genders have been found to initiate problem behaviors (e.g., alcohol use) at earlier ages. Earlier onset of risky behaviors in general has been linked to negative outcomes later in adolescence. This work suggests that timing effects may exist for boys but have been studied less often than for girls. In summary, the existing literature suggests that adjustment, coping skills, and prepubertal biological predispositions combine with different types of pubertal transitions to influence longer-term developmental outcomes.

Bidirectional Links between Puberty and Social Context

More complex models delineating the interrelationship among hormones, behavior, and environmental factors are also important in explaining how pubertal development is experienced, and ultimately in predicting who is at risk for longer-term problems. Specifically, environment and context not only change in response to girls' pubertal development, but may also shape and alter the nature of that development. For example, pubertal development is affected by such behaviors as nutritional intake, exercise, and dieting; that is, increased exercise and dieting, and/or lowered nutritional intake, will delay pubertal development. Whereas it has long been accepted that hormones are receptive to environmental stressors (e.g., dieting and exercise), the importance and influence of behavioral stressors on the developing hormonal system have only recently been considered.

Research on family conflict and family structure has documented interesting effects of family environment on the timing of pubertal development. Earlier ages of menarche were reported for girls living in households in which no father was residing in the home during the childhood years. Earlier ages of menarche were also reported by girls who lived with both biological parents if family conflict was also reported. Socioeconomic or weight differences among the girls did not account for these findings.

In our own research, we have also found that earlier maturation was predicted by conflict and lack of approval in families with both parents residing in the home. In addition, controlling for body fat and hereditary factors did not diminish the effects. These effects were also not attributable to family responses to pubertal development; that is, early pubertal development did not increase conflict in the family. Controlling for level of breast development (a visible cue of development) did not diminish the amount of variance explained by family relations. In combination, these results indicate that psychological stressors, at least those experienced in the family environment, affect the timing of pubertal development. These findings represent the beginnings of research that seeks to identify the depth and breadth of interaction between the social environment and the physiological underpinnings of puberty.

FURTHER READING

Brooks-Gunn, J., Graber, J. A., & Paikoff, R. L. (1994). Studying links between hormones and negative affect: Models and measures. *Journal of Research on Adolescence, 4*(4), 469–486.
Key models are reviewed, with highlights of innovative studies conducted within the domain of each.

Brooks-Gunn, J., Newman, D., Holderness, C., & Warren, M. P. (1994). The experience of breast development and girls: Stories about the purchase of a bra. *Journal of Youth and Adolescence, 23*(5), 539–565.
A unique study of the impact of breast development on girls' psychosocial development, which combined projective techniques with questionnaire measures.

Brooks-Gunn, J., & Petersen, A. C. (Eds.). (1983). *Girls at puberty: Biological and psychosocial perspectives.* New York: Plenum Press.
This edited volume is a landmark compilation of the conceptual and empirical work on girls and puberty up to the early 1980s.

Brooks-Gunn, J., & Reiter, E. O. (1990). The role of pubertal processes in the early adolescent transition. In S. Feldman & G. Elliott (Eds.), *At the threshold: The developing adolescent* (pp. 16–53). Cambridge, MA: Harvard University Press.
The authors provide a comprehensive review of the biological, psychological, and social processes that occur at puberty.

Buchanan, C. M., Eccles, J. S., & Becker, J. B. (1992). Are adolescents the victims of raging hormones?: Evidence for activational effects of hormones on moods and behavior at adolescence. *Psychological Bulletin, 111,* 62–107.
This paper provides an in-depth review of the studies that have examined pubertal hormonal activity in association with changes in mood and behavior at adolescence.

Caspi, A., & Moffitt, T. E. (1991). Individual differences are accentuated during periods of social change: The sample case of girls at puberty. *Journal of Personality and Social Psychology, 61,* 157–168.
This study tests the accentuation principle, using a longitudinal sample of girls in New Zealand studied from early childhood through adolescence.

Graber, J. A., Brooks-Gunn, J., & Warren, M. P. (1995). The antecedents of menarcheal age: Heredity, family environment, and stressful life events. *Child Development, 66,* 346–359.
A bidirectional model linking puberty and family relationships is explored in a study of early adolescence.

Graber, J. A., Petersen, A. C., & Brooks-Gunn, J. (1996). Transition to puberty: Methods, measures, and models. In J. A. Graber, J. Brooks-Gunn, & A. C. Petersen (Eds.), *Transitions through adolescence: Interpersonal domains and context.* Mahwah, NJ: Erlbaum.
The authors explore the measurement of pubertal development and how measurement affects findings on puberty and adjustment; psychosocial correlates of pubertal timing are explored in depth.

Jessor, R. (1993). Successful adolescent development among youth in high-risk settings. *American Psychologist, 48*(2), 117–126.
The author delineates a model for understanding adolescent risk behavior that incorporates protective factors to predict adjustment.

Marshall, W. A., & Tanner, J. M. (1986). Puberty. In F. Falkner & J. M. Tanner (Eds.), *Human growth: Vol. 2. Postnatal growth. Neurobiology* (pp. 171–209). New York: Plenum Press.
This chapter is a comprehensive review of the literature on pubertal development, drawing upon the voluminous collaborative work of the coauthors.

Moffitt, T. E., Caspi, A., Belsky, J., & Silva, P. A. (1992). Childhood experience and the onset of menarche: A test of a sociobiological model. *Child Development, 63,* 47–58.
A sociobiological model for predicting age at menarche is tested in a sample of girls studied from early childhood through adolescence in New Zealand.

National Heart, Lung, and Blood Institute [NHLBI] Growth and Health Study Research Group. (1992). Obesity and cardiovascular disease risk factors in black and white girls: The NHLBI Growth and Health Study. *American Journal of Public Health, 82,* 1613–1620.
The NHLBI reports on a large, multisite study of girls' health and physical development beginning with girls ages 9 and 10.

Petersen, A. C., Sarigiani, P. A., & Kennedy, R. E. (1991). Adolescent depression: Why more girls? *Journal of Youth and Adolescence, 20,* 247–271.
One of the few studies to test a simultaneous change model finding prediction from early adolescence to subsequent depression.

Petersen, A. C., & Taylor, B. (1980). The biological approach to adolescence: Biological change and psychological adaptation. In J. Adelson (Ed.), *Handbook of adolescent psychology* (pp. 117–155). New York: Wiley.
The authors identify models for understanding behavioral change at puberty.

Reiter, E. O., & Grumbach, M. M. (1982). Neuroendocrine control mechanisms and the onset of puberty. *Annual Review of Physiology, 44,* 595–613.
This paper provides an excellent review of the hormonal changes at puberty.

Stattin, H., & Magnusson, D. (1990). *Paths through life: Vol. 2. Pubertal maturation in female development*. Hillsdale, NJ: Erlbaum.
The book is a compilation of findings from the authors' longitudinal study of girls from early adolescence into adulthood.

Warren, M. P., & Brooks-Gunn, J. (1989). Mood and behavior at adolescence: Evidence for hormonal factors. *Journal of Clinical Endocrinology and Metabolism, 69,* 77–83.
Changes in aggressive and depressive affect are linked with rapidly increasing hormones at puberty in girls; the sample is one of the largest collected for studying hormones at puberty.

9

Adolescent Sexuality

Susan G. Millstein
Bonnie L. Halpern-Felsher

Adolescence is a period marked by rapid and extreme biological, social, and cognitive changes. Pubertal changes typically begin the life stage we call adolescence, as described in Graber and Brooks-Gunn's chapter on puberty; and hormonal changes drive the somatic changes, such as breast and pubic hair development. The age of onset and duration of biological changes have broad and different ranges in males and females, vary among individuals, and are associated with differences in psychosocial functioning. Pubertal onset for females ranges from 8 to 13 years of age, with completion at 13 to 18 years. For males, onset is from 9.5 to 13.5 years of age, with completion at 13.5 to 17.5 years.

Certain aspects of pubertal change (e.g., menarche) are often viewed positively by girls, as signifying a desired transition to adulthood. However, other aspects are not viewed positively. For example, girls often become unhappy with their newly forming bodies as they begin to heed messages that the slimmer prepubescent body is more appealing in Western society. Many postpubertal females develop a negative body image and begin dieting, attempting to maintain a preadolescent figure. A small percentage of girls develop more serious eating disorders, such as anorexia nervosa or bulimia nervosa. During this time there is also much comparison among peers in terms of their physical maturation, with early-maturing girls often feeling abnormal and isolated.

SEXUAL BEHAVIOR

Adolescent sexual behavior generally does not begin with intercourse, nor does it necessarily begin in adolescence. During late childhood and early adolescence, for example, autoerotic sexual behaviors include fantasies and masturbation. Later, sexual behaviors are extended to involve another person. For many but not all adolescents, the course of these new sexual behaviors follows a pattern beginning with embracing and kissing, then leading to petting, and finally more intimate behaviors, including oral sex and vaginal and anal intercourse. The timing and pattern of when these behaviors emerge vary as a function of cultural background. For example, African-American adolescents are more likely to proceed directly from kissing to sexual intercourse, and to do so at earlier ages.

Data from the 1995 Youth Risk Behavior Survey indicate that 53.5% of Hispanic, 49% of European-American, and 67% of African-American high school girls have experienced coitus at least once. Overall, the median age of onset of sexual intercourse for females is 17.4 years. Males engage in sexual intercourse earlier than females, with 48.9% of European-American males to 81% of African-American males sexually active by age 19 years. However, the difference in the age of onset between males and females has been narrowing since the 1960s. The frequency of sexual activity among adolescents is typically sporadic; it rarely occurs more than once a week. The frequency of intercourse between a couple typically increases as the relationship becomes more intimate. Most sexually active adolescents have engaged in coitus with multiple partners, with the number of partners related to the number of years an adolescent has been sexually active.

Much research has examined factors associated with the onset of sexual activity during adolescence. Risk factors include early physical maturation, low educational goals, poor academic performance, living in single-parent families, and poverty. Cultural norms and religious beliefs regarding sexuality also play a role.

CONCERNS ABOUT ADOLESCENT FEMALE SEXUALITY

Adults generally express concerns about adolescent sexuality for a number of different reasons. Among these are beliefs that premarital sex is wrong, that adolescent sexuality is developmentally inappropriate, and that adolescent sexuality has undesirable consequences. Moral, religious, and social constraints against "uncontrolled" female sexuality have also been dominant forces in U.S. society. These forces continue to exert their influence on adolescent females today.

The extensive changes that take place during the adolescent years call for different expectations about what constitutes appropriate sexual behavior. Many adults consider sexual activity in a 14-year-old girl troubling, but fewer may feel this way about an 18-year-old. For some older adolescents, mutually consensual sexual activity can be an expression of true intimacy and healthy sexual development. But for younger adolescents, sexual activity can have negative consequences.

For all adolescents, the primary negative consequences of adolescent sexual behavior are sexually transmitted diseases (STDs) and pregnancy. Among the more serious consequences of STDs for females are pelvic inflammatory disease and its sequelae: chronic pelvic pain, infertility, and ectopic pregnancy. Prevalence rates for most STD agents peak during adolescence and young adulthood, because of a combination of biological and behavioral vulnerabilities. Females who begin sexual activity early are at particular biological risk for STDs. Current statistics underestimate the burden of sexually transmitted disease in this age group, because the two most frequently occurring STDs among adolescents (chlamydia and human papilloma viral infection) are not routinely reported to the Centers for Disease Control. Furthermore, although adolescents currently represent a minority of AIDS cases, many of the AIDS cases reported in the 20- to 25-year-old age group are the result of HIV infection that occurred during adolescence.

Pregnancy rates among adolescents are lower than at other points in history, but they are still distressingly high, with 12% of adolescents becoming pregnant each year.

Approximately 50% of pregnancies among adolescents end in live births. Roughly one-fifth of all births in the United States are to adolescents. The negative social and economic outcomes associated with adolescent parenting have been well documented; they include leaving school prior to high school graduation, increased reliance on public assistance, higher divorce rates, and fewer economic opportunities. There are also negative consequences for the children born to adolescents, such as low birthweight.

Although pregnancies and STDs are preventable, adolescents' use of contraception in general and condoms in particular is inconsistent and less than optimal. Thirty-five percent of 15- to 19-year-old girls do not use any form of contraception at first intercourse. The younger an adolescent girl is at her sexual debut, the less likely she is to use contraception at first intercourse and later in her sexual career. Less than half of sexually active adolescents use condoms consistently, with variations by race and ethnicity. Fifty-two percent of girls do not use condoms at first intercourse. In addition, adolescents are less likely to use condoms in established sexual relationships than they are with casual partners. This may be due to feelings of increased trust and commitment, or to the less sporadic nature of sex in these relationships. Other reasons postulated for adolescents' poor contraceptive use is the often unplanned and sporadic nature of adolescent sex; adolescents may also not like using available methods.

GENDER STEREOTYPES AND ADOLESCENT SEXUALITY

Most adolescents engage in premarital sexual intercourse, making adolescent sexuality a normative event in adolescent development for both boys and girls. However, gender stereotypes still prevail, with gender-disparate messages the norm rather than the exception. Males are expected to surrender to their sexual desires, and adolescence for males is considered a time of sexual exploration and self-definition. In contrast, female adolescents' sexual desires are constrained, and the expression of their sexuality is viewed as wrong, immoral, and fraught with danger.

However, females are presented with conflicting messages. While being exposed to messages admonishing them to avoid sexual activity, they are simultaneously bombarded with mass media images that encourage them to enhance their sexual attractiveness, exposed to social programs designed to teach them how to use contraception, and pressured by boyfriends to prove their love sexually. The conflict between the deep-seated gender stereotypes and the other messages delivered by the social environment leaves female adolescents in a precarious position. For adolescent females who wish to remain virgins, the supportive function once provided by socially consistent messages, which offered them a socially sanctioned way to refuse males' sexual advances, no longer exists. For adolescent females who are mature and ready to engage in sexual activity, the message that sex is wrong and should somehow be hidden undermines their own acceptance of their behavior, thwarting healthy sexual development.

MEANING OF SEXUALITY TO ADOLESCENT FEMALES

The first experience with sexual intercourse is typically viewed more negatively by females than by males. Females often express feelings of regret about the experience, which may reflect the inherent conflicts discussed above. Throughout adolescence, sexual behavior appears to have different meanings for males and females. Although the range of meaning is great within both genders, females typically associate sexual activity with a committed, intimate, and loving relationship; by contrast, males view sex as a way of satisfying their sexual needs and desires, as a learning experience, and as a self-defining act, rather than as a demonstration of love and commitment. These differences between males' and females' attributions for sex probably explain, at least in part, why males are more likely to engage in casual sex (including one-night stands) than are female adolescents.

These different patterns can be problematic for adolescent females who believe that a sexual relationship should be based on love, intimacy, and commitment. Adolescent males are aware of such beliefs. Thus, they may be able to convince girls that they are in love; may state that if the girls were really in love, they would have sex; or may say that sex is needed to maintain a relationship. Therefore, girls may be misled into having unwanted sexual intercourse.

SEXUAL COERCION, RAPE, AND SEXUAL ABUSE

It is estimated that from 15% to 25% of U.S. women will be forced to have sex against their will during their lifetimes. Rates of sexual coercion vary dramatically, depending on the type of coercion measured. Sexual coercion can be emotional or physical, and it can range from subtle manipulation to verbal threats to rape. Most coercive acts involve someone known by the victim, such as an acquaintance, boyfriend, or family member.

The incidence of rape in female adolescents is believed to be higher than for any other age group, and rape is probably underreported because of fear of stigmatization, feelings of shame, and recognition that females who come forth are often considered responsible for being raped. Sexually abused females have a host of personality, psychological, and behavioral problems, including posttraumatic stress disorder, recurrent nightmares, depression, withdrawal, and school difficulties. We know less about the long-term effects of more subtle forms of coercion.

Gender stereotypes may also help explain why sexual coercion is so common. Males are often portrayed as being the aggressors, and females as their submissive and gentle counterparts. Consequently, a male often feels that he has the right to be sexually forceful with a woman, especially one he is dating. Many adolescent males believe they have the right to expect sexual intimacies if, for example, they take girls out to dinner. In contrast, females, who are not supposed to express their sexual desires, are expected by males to resist sexual advances. Therefore, their indications that they are not interested in sex are often taken as permission for males to proceed. Changes in the socialization of adolescent males and females are important and necessary.

ACKNOWLEDGMENT

This research was supported in part by the Maternal and Child Health Bureau (MCJ000978).

FURTHER READING

Brooks-Gunn, J., & Paikoff, R. L. (1993). "Sex is a gamble, kissing is a game": Adolescent sexuality and health promotion. In S. G. Millstein, A. C. Petersen, & E. O. Nightingale (Eds.),

Promoting the health of adolescents: New directions for the twenty-first century (pp. 180–208). New York: Oxford University Press.
Excellent chapter focusing on (1) adolescent sexual well-being, including feelings about puberty and sexual arousal, sexual behavior, and safe sex; (2) factors related to sexual well-being, such as culture, family, and peers; and (3) interventions designed to increase adolescents' sexual well-being.

Cates, W., Jr. (1990). The epidemiology and control of sexually transmitted diseases in adolescents. *Adolescent Medicine: State of the Art Reviews, 1,* 409–428.
State-of-the-art review of trends in and control of STDs among adolescents.

Forrest, J. D., & Singh, S. (1990). The sexual and reproduction behavior of American women, 1982–1988. *Family Planning Perspectives, 22,* 206–214.
Study using data from the 1992 National Survey of Family Growth to describe the sexual, contraceptive, and reproductive behavior of women aged 15–44.

Gullotta, T. P., Adams, G. R., & Montemayor, R. (Eds.). (1993). *Adolescent sexuality.* Newbury Park, CA: Sage.
Excellent edited book with chapters describing a variety of aspects of adolescent sexual behavior, including biological development, sexual well-being, aberrant sexual experiences, gay and lesbian youth, STDs, and pregnancy.

Hayes, C. D. (1987). *Risking the future: Vol. 1. Adolescent sexuality, pregnancy and childbearing.* Washington, DC: National Academy Press.
Report from the National Research Council, National Academy of Sciences, on adolescent sexuality, pregnancy, and childbearing.

Moore, S., & Rosenthal, D. (1993). *Sexuality in adolescence.* New York: Routledge.
Excellent book with chapters on the biological and social determinants of adolescent sexuality and sexual risk.

Nathanson, C. A. (1991). *Dangerous passage: The social control of sexuality in women's adolescence.* Philadelphia: Temple University Press.
Outstanding book discussing the historical, social, and cultural contexts surrounding adolescent sexuality.

Udry, J. R., Talbert, L. M., & Morris, N. M. (1986). Biosocial foundations for adolescent female sexuality. *Demography, 23,* 217–227.
Cross-sectional study examining how and the extent to which hormones play a role in adolescents' sexual debut at puberty.

10

Teenage and Adolescent Pregnancy

Janet B. Hardy

THE SCOPE OF THE PROBLEM

The long-standing problems of teenage pregnancy and childbearing are of social concern and controversy in the United States. The high risk of adverse long-term consequences, particularly among those childbearing adolescents (i.e., below age 18), and those 18- and 19-year-olds who are having a second or higher-order birth, is associated with high societal costs.

In 1992, approximately 1 million high school teenagers were pregnant. Over ½ million delivered a live infant; 363,550 elective abortions were reported and an estimated 132,178 miscarriages and fetal deaths occurred. In 1994, the most recent year for which national statistics are available, 518,389 teenagers had a live birth, accounting for 13% of all births. Among the teenagers, 298,219 (57.4%) of births were to older teens, aged 18–19, 208,070 (40.1%) were to adolescents, aged 15–17, and almost 13,000 (2.5%) were to even younger girls, 10–14 years old. Among the infants born to preteen and teenage mothers, 402,444 (78%) were first born and 115,945 were second or higher-order births.

Live birth rates per 1,000 U.S. teenagers, which had risen steadily to 62.1 in 1991, appeared to have peaked in that year. In 1993, the rate was 59.6, and in 1994, it was 58.9. However, the rate for the youngest girls, aged 10–14, remained at 1.4 per 1,000 between 1990 and 1994. Abortion rates showed comparable decreases.

The figures cited above do not reflect the considerable disparity in teenage pregnancy rates by ethnic background and place of residence within the United States. In 1992, the national birth rate of 61 per 1,000 females aged 15–19, masks rates of 52 for white and 112 for black teenagers. The rates in the poor areas of large cities and in some pockets of rural areas are far higher than those of more affluent suburban areas.

The U.S. teenage live birth rate of 62.1 in 1991 was by far the highest among Westernized countries. It was almost twice that of the United Kingdom, the country with the next highest rate, and 12 times that of Japan, the country with the lowest rate. Because many European countries provide more generous public support for women and children than is the case in the U.S., it seems unlikely that eligibility for welfare is a significant incentive for U.S. girls to become pregnant.

Recent estimates of public costs of teenage childbearing include direct, single-year costs of about $22 billion for Aid to Families with Dependent Children, Medicaid, and food stamps and their administration. It should be noted that these costs do not include the costs for the Supplemental Nutrition Program for Women, Infants and Children (WIC) and relevant special educational programs, or of those born by other public and private agencies or by families, or the opportunity costs related to unrealized human capital.

DIFFERENCES BETWEEN TEENAGE AND ADOLESCENT PREGNANCY

As a girl's level of cognitive, social and emotional development strongly influences her behavior, and as immature physical development may have an adverse effect on her pregnancy, the interchangeable use of the two designations "teenage" and "adolescent" is counterproductive and should be discouraged. The period between puberty, which may occur as early as 9 or 10 years or as late as 16 years of age, and young adulthood is a time of great physical, cognitive, social, and emotional change. Because a girl's developmental level in these domains strongly influences the effectiveness of strategies for both pregnancy management and prevention, let us consider some of the differences between pregnancy in "older teens," aged 18 and 19 years, and "adolescents," aged up to 18 years.

Although a birth to an older teenager may carry increased social risk, particularly if the young woman is not married or is having a second or higher-order birth, it is very different from a birth to a true adolescent. An older teenager has usually completed her physical growth; she is socially and emotionally more mature. She is more likely to have completed high school and to be employed; she may be married or have a stable partner. Furthermore, her obstetrical risks are low. Pregnancy in this age group appears to reflect current social norms and the permissive attitudes toward adult sexual behavior brought about by the "sexual revolution" of the past 30 years. In this age group, high rates of sexual activity and pregnancy are prevalent at all levels of society.

Pregnancy for a true adolescent, on the other hand, tends to be associated with increased health and social risks for both mother and infant. In general, a pregnant adolescent will not (1) have completed her psychological and social developmental tasks; (2) have finished high school (even more problematic, pregnancy in this age group is associated with academic problems, truancy, and dropout); (3) be married to the child's father; (4) have been employed or had any training for employment; (5) have the knowledge and role models necessary for effective parenting; or (6) have attained legal majority (age 18 in most states), which would allow her full participation in important decisions regarding her own and her baby's future. Furthermore, pregnant adolescents generally face higher obstetrical risks than older teens. They are more likely to have a delayed onset of, or no, prenatal care; they are also at greater risk of pregnancy complications, such as anemia, toxemia, and preterm delivery. Many are depressed, which has an adverse impact on self-care and infant care. Their infants are at high risk for low birthweight and infant mortality. Finally, these young mothers are at risk for early, repeated conception and for having larger families than they desire.

A colleague, L. S. Zabin, and I have found that adolescent pregnancy tends to be intergenerational: 80% of the mothers we studied had their first births as teenagers, and 51% as adolescents. Childbearing among girls aged under 18 is associated with poverty and social disadvantage. Girls in more affluent areas begin their sexual careers at older ages and are much less likely to become pregnant. If pregnancy does occur, they are far more likely to have abortions than are inner-city adolescents. The cost of abortion is a significant barrier for poor families; because of the severe restrictions on public funding for abortion, there is little choice but for a poor adolescent to continue her pregnancy (and to keep the baby, since adoption is not an acceptable option for most adolescents). Finally, the exact contribution of sexual abuse of adolescent girls to the frequency of pregnancy in this age group is unknown, but evidence is accumulating to suggest that it is not negligible and must be considered in both pregnancy prevention and the care of pregnant girls.

CONSEQUENCES OF ADOLESCENT CHILDBEARING

The consequences of adolescent childbearing may be severe for the young mother, her child (or children), her family of origin, and the young father, particularly if his education is truncated by marriage and efforts to support his family. The young mother's lack of education, immaturity, and lack of resources are likely to have adverse effects on her ability to be an effective parent, and therefore on the development of her child. Her poor education and lack of readily available child care are serious barriers to continued education and employment. Welfare support was used for all or part of the first 18 months after delivery by 91% of a random sample of adolescents we studied in the city of Baltimore. Health problems were of frequent occurrence among both mothers and babies, particularly white mothers and infants. During the first 18 months, 18% of babies were hospitalized, 18% required outpatient treatment for injuries, and 13% had chronic health problems; in each category, the proportion of white infants significantly exceeded that of black infants. Among blacks, 88% had Medicaid coverage and 10% were enrolled in health maintenance organizations, as opposed to 68% and 4%, respectively, among the whites. In this sample, black adolescents had significantly higher educational attainment than the whites, but very few of the blacks were married as compared with 25% of the whites. In a recently reported longitudinal study of inner-city children and their mothers, my colleagues and I found that the children of inner-city adolescent mothers were less likely to have graduated from high school or have a Graduate Equivalency Degree, at age 27 to 33, than children of older mothers in the same population.

The social consequences for a young mother, her partner, and her child (or children) are inextricably intertwined with those of poverty and social disadvantage: inadequate housing and nutrition; living in high-crime areas; family instability; and general lack of resources, including lack of information for making informed choices about lifestyle (e.g., use of cigarettes, alcohol, and illicit drugs) and reproductive health (e.g., those risks attributable to the early initiation of sexual activity, lack of contraception, multiple partners, sexually transmitted infections, and AIDS). Because of the conditions under which many inner-city adolescents live, and the imperatives for survival in a hostile environment, choice may seem irrelevant as they face a future without hope of improvement. In our random sample, 11% had difficulty obtaining adequate food during pregnancy, and 16% had such difficulty in the 18 months after delivery; 9% were refused medical care because of lack of health insurance and inability to pay for care.

The fathers in our random sample of births to adolescent mothers in Baltimore spanned a wide age range. They were on average 2–4 years older than the mothers; white fathers tended to be older than black ones. In the majority of couples, the partners had known each other for 2 years or longer prior to conception. It was the rare father who was not told about the birth of his child. Like the mothers, the fathers on average had substantial educational and occupational deficits, which made it very difficult (if not impossible) for them to establish homes and support their families. Eighteen months after their children's births, the majority of these fathers were still living with their own parents, who were usually single mothers. Seven percent were in jail. Contact between a father and a child became less frequent during the child's first 18 months; by 15 months, 16% of fathers had no contact, and 26% had contact only once a month or less often. Finally, 20% of the fathers were reported by the mothers to have one or more children by other women. Among fathers aged 20 or more at the study children's births, 29% of the white and 36% of the black had children by other women. This is a bleak picture, but one must not lose sight of the fact that 10% of these inner-city fathers were able to obtain adequate employment and make independent homes for their families; other couples lived together with parents.

Diverse outcomes 7 and 12 years after delivery (in the early 1960s) were seen among a large sample of adolescent mothers and their children followed in the Johns Hopkins Collaborative Perinatal Study. However, continued problems for most young mothers and children were frequent, as compared with older mothers and their children. The adolescents in general failed to catch up educationally; they also had unstable marriages and partnerships. Moreover, a higher proportion required welfare support, and their children had less adequate cognitive and academic development at age 7 than those of older women. Another Baltimore study found considerable diversity among black adolescent mothers followed over a 17-year period. Many had supportive families and continued their education. Those with additional education were more likely to obtain steady employment, and that or stable marriages enabled them to do well. Their children, however, generally fared less well, with many educational and social problems.

MANAGEMENT OF TEENAGE AND ADOLESCENT PREGNANCY

The 18- or 19-year-old with a first pregnancy requires the level of prenatal care appropriate for a low-risk woman in her 20s—that is, early diagnosis, pregnancy option counseling, and adequate prenatal and delivery care (including education in nutrition, family planning, and parenting, as well as follow-up). An older teen with a higher-order pregnancy may need additional services, as she may continue to face the risks similar to those of a first pregnancy in adolescence.

Socially disadvantaged adolescents are a medically underserved group with many health problems, which often originate in poor nutrition, the early onset of sexual activity, cigarette smoking, illicit drug or alcohol use, and depression. When such adolescents become pregnant, they too need the early pregnancy diagnosis, option counseling, and referral required by older women. Because of their multiple problems, their needs for pregnancy care are best met in a comprehensive program appropriate for their level of physical, cognitive, and social development. Such a program, using a case management approach, should provide first-rate medical care backed up by (1) nutrition, health, and pregnancy-related education; (2) counseling and psychosocial support; and (3) referral to community agencies for financial help, crisis management, and continued schooling. A pregnant girl's parents and the baby's father should participate in the planning and should be helped to understand the girl's need for support and for ongoing education. Successful comprehensive programs help adolescents understand their pregnancies and motivate them to participate in their own care. Although such programs are more costly than traditional prenatal care because of labor intensiveness, they are cost-effective in terms of averted costs for the management of pregnancy complications, low birthweight, and early, repeated conception and both maternal and child health problems in the early years after birth.

Comprehensive follow-up care for both a young mother and an infant, continuing for 2 to 3 years after the birth, is essential to ensure good health for mother and child and to prevent the early recurrence of unintended conception.

FURTHER READING

Bolin, F. S. (1990). *Growing up caring: Exploring values and decision making.* Mission Hills, CA: Glencoe/McGraw-Hill.
Sponsored by the J. P. Kennedy, Jr., Foundation's Community of Caring Program in Washington, D.C., this volume presents a values-based curriculum for use in schools to enhance students' life chances and to prevent substance abuse, adolescent pregnancy, AIDS, and other behavioral problems.

Child Trends. (1996, January). *Facts at a glance: Trends in teenage birth rates, 1960–1993; abortion rates, 1973–1991; and age at first sex and non-marital births to teens, 1950–1993.* Washington, DC: Author.

Furstenberg, F. F., Jr., & Brooks-Gunn, J. (1986). Adolescent mothers and their children in later life. *Developmental Reviews, 6,* 224–251.
This paper describes the children of adolescents and their high frequency of developmental problems during childhood and adolescence.

Furstenberg, F. F., Jr., Brooks-Gunn, J., & Morgan, S. P. (1987). *Adolescent mothers in later life.* Cambridge, UK: Cambridge University Press.
This volume describes a follow-up study of urban adolescent mothers, which documents the great diversity of long-term outcomes experienced by this high-risk group of young mothers.

Hardy, J. B., Shapiro, S., Mellits, E. D., Skinner, E. A., Astone, N. M., Ensminger, M. E., LaVeist, T., Baumgardner, R. A., & Starfield, B. H. (1997). Self-sufficiency at ages 27 to 33 years: Factors present between birth and 18 years that predict educational attainment among children born to inner-city families. *Pediatrics, 99,* 80–87.
This paper describes the frequency of self-sufficient adult outcomes among 1,758 inner-city children followed from birth to ages 27 to 33 with emphasis on the prediction of educational attainment. The children of adolescent mothers were less likely to graduate from high school or have a graduate equivalency degree (GED) than those of older women in the same population.

Hardy, J. B., & Zabin, L. S. (1991). *Adolescent pregnancy in an urban environment: Issues, programs, and evaluation.* Washington, DC: The Urban Institute Press.
This volume presents a comprehensive picture of adolescent pregnancy and related problems, and describes the content and evaluation of a university hospital-based urban program for maternal and infant care and for school-based pregnancy prevention.

Hayes, C. D. (Ed.). (1987). *Risking the future: Adolescent sexuality, pregnancy, and childbearing.* Washington, DC: National Academy Press.
This volume presents a comprehensive review of the antecedents, consequences, and costs of teenage sexuality and pregnancy.

National Center for Health Statistics. (1994). Advance report of final natality statistics, 1992. *Monthly vital statistics report, 43*(5, Suppl.).
National Center for Health Statistics. (1996). Advance report of final natality statistics, 1992. *Monthly vital statistics report, 45*(11, Suppl.).
These government publications provide annual vital statistics for births in the United States by maternal age, race, marital status, and ordinal position and birthweight of children for 1992, and 1994 with discussion of important trends during the past 10–20 years. Note that the specific dates on the supplement publications are important for identification.

11

Parenting

Amy W. Helstrom
Elaine A. Blechman

Women enter new social roles and acquire new perceptions of themselves and others as they begin biological and foster parenthood and caregiving to grandchildren and elderly parents. The transition to parenting is a normative biological task for women and for men. But women, unlike men, typically spend the majority of their lives involved in caregiving and parenting. Unlike men, women's views of themselves, and others' views of them, are organized around the parenting and caretaking process. "Outcomes" of the parenting process (such as children's behavior problems) are, more often than not, attributed to mothers' rather than fathers' efforts. At work, women are often expected by themselves and by others, to act more "caring" than their male colleagues even when such behavior is detrimental to their own productivity and peace of mind and to their ability to juggle family and work responsibilities. While parenthood is an experience that most women treasure, few women reckon with parenthood's lifelong impact on their physical and psychological well-being. The scientific community seems to know as little as women themselves about how women are shaped by parenting. While parents' effects on children's adjustment is a topic that has yielded countless research reports, fingers and toes suffice to count data-based publications concerned with children's effects on parents.

Parenting, like other normative developmental tasks such as marriage and work, involves a behavioral component (e.g., How warmly and skillfully does 22-year-old Mary toilet train her 2-year-old son, John?), a cognitive component (e.g., What does Mary believe is the right way to toilet train a 2-year-old?), and an emotional component (e.g., How much does Mary enjoy being with John?). Like other developmental tasks, parenting requires continuous behavioral, cognitive, and emotional responses to unexpected challenges, problems, and stressors.

Mary is a single mother; her son John looks a lot like the abusive husband who deserted her during pregnancy. It is not unreasonable to expect (although the research literature is relatively silent on this point), that Mary will cope with the challenge of raising John much as she copes with challenges at work, in her extended family, and with friends. Mary's parents and her five siblings are all very supportive of Mary's efforts to raise John. Mary is a skilled manager and has earned merit raises at each of her job performance reviews. It is not unreasonable to expect (although again relevant data are hard to find) that family social support and Mary's verbal intelligence and interpersonal skills will improve Mary's capacity to cope prosocially with the parenting challenge in ways that will benefit her, her son John, and the rest of society.

In sum, what we do know about parenting (although we don't know why) is that the health consequences of parenting depend upon a vast array of factors including perceived social support from friends and family, marital satisfaction, socioeconomic status, number of children, and children's physical and psychological health. In the remainder of this chapter, we summarize particularly interesting and statistically significant reports about the correlates, concurrent and longitudinal, of parenting. We do our best to differentiate between speculation about mechanisms and data-based findings.

THE TRANSITION TO PARENTING

Common physical problems associated with the postpartum period include anemia, breast engorgement, constipation, discomfort during sexual intercourse, fatigue, hemorrhoids, postsurgical discomfort (following a cesarean section or episiotomy), sleep disturbance, and uterine cramps. The stress of pregnancy and childbirth may exacerbate preexisting chronic physical conditions and diseases, contributing to lasting physical impairment. In addition, the stress of pregnancy and childbirth may exacerbate preexisting psychological vulnerabilities impeding physical recovery from childbirth and paving the way for lasting psychological impairment. For a detailed consideration of the antecedents and consequences of postpartum depression, see Gotlib's chapter in this volume.

The ease of transition to first-time parenting depends upon numerous factors. (What we don't know is which of these factors have greater impact on adjustment and which have less.) Women and men may benefit if they can afford to maintain pleasurable aspects of the pre-pregnancy lifestyle after the first child is born. For most parents, abrupt changes in lifestyle coincident with pregnancy and childbirth (e.g., fewer contacts with coworkers and friends) are both stressful and inevitable.

Alexander and Higgins compared parents' prebirth and postbirth scores on measures of self-perception and well-being to learn more about why parenting sometimes reduces distress and sometimes increases distress ($n = 29$ couples). The authors found that self-discrepancies (between one's actual self-concept and one's ideal self-concept) were correlated with the amount of post-birth distress. Parents for whom there was a large discrepancy between how they saw themselves and their ideal selves suffered an increase in dejection post-birth than parents low in actual–ideal discrepancy.

PARENTING CHILDREN OF DIFFERENT AGES

In the child's first few years of life, parents' physical and psychological vulnerability continues although not at the same level as in the postpartum period. At day care and at school, young children are exposed to hepatitis A, meningitis, diarrhea, otitis media, and upper respiratory diseases. In turn, young children expose their parents to these diseases.

In respect to psychological adjustment, the Cowans are engaged in a longitudinal study of the impact of parenting on parents. In 1992, Leventhal-Belfer, Cowan, and Cowan described new parents' adjustment to parenting in the early-childhood period (until the first child was 42 months of age). They found that fathers' satisfaction with day-care arrangements predicted mothers' satisfaction with the parenting role.

Most parents would agree that the psychological stress associated with parenting adolescents is as great (or greater than) what they experienced during the postpartum period. While all parents of adolescents have some common experiences, the impact of this process on parents may well depend upon the same variables that influenced well-being in the postpartum period. In addition, variables such as gender of child and age of parent take on a new significance during adolescence for children and for their parents. Ge and colleagues reported stronger cross-gender associations in self-rated distress (mother with teen son, teen daughter with father) than same-gender associations (mother with daughter, father with son).

PARENTING AND MARRIAGE

Is marriage, even an unhappy marriage, better for mothers than no marriage at all? Is single motherhood more beneficial than married motherhood for women who are autonomous and self-sufficient and more detrimental for women who depend upon others for direction and support?

Koski and Steinberg studied mothers of 10- to 15-year-old adolescents ($n = 129$ families). Satisfaction with parenting was moderated by mothers' marital satisfaction and overall psychological well being. The women most satisfied with parenting rated themselves low on mid-life crisis and high on marital satisfaction. Compas and Williams, in 1990, found that single mothers reported more total psychological symptoms than married mothers of adolescents ($n = 216$). However, single mothers used different coping strategies than married mothers, including accepting more responsibility, problem solving, and positive appraisal. Duffy reported that single mothers with higher levels of education and income reported better mental health.

PARENTING AND WORK

Is work a source of additional stress for mothers or a source of respite, support, and distraction? Is it work per se or the coping strategies employed by women who choose to work while raising children that makes the difference? The answer is (as Repetti's chapter in this volume suggests), "It depends."

Sogaard and colleagues, in a 1994 survey of over 3,000 women, found that, after adjusting for age, education, marital status, and place of residence, homemakers with young children reported the highest levels of coping problems, dissatisfaction with life, and depression compared to women who were employed. Homemakers reported more psychological health problems than employed women except for unmarried employed women. Rosalind Barnett, in a 1992 publication, reported that the combination of work and parenting protects women from the negative effects of relationships with their children. Fong and Amatea, in a study of women with academic jobs, found that women who were married and parents reported less stress than single women. In contrast to Compas's findings reported above, Fong and Amatea reported that single women were most likely to report the use of passive coping styles.

PROXY VARIABLES AND PSYCHOLOGICAL MECHANISMS

Research concerned with the impact of parenting on women's health has implicated a good number of proxy variables such as child's gender, parent's age, parent's employment, and parent's marital status. What this research has generally failed to do is to scratch beneath the surface for underlying psychological processes, to measure psychological processes by more than just self-report, and to pit rival causal models against each other. Absent such research, we know what our grandmothers knew about the centrality of parenting to women's well-being, but not much more.

FURTHER READING

Alexander, M. J., & Higgins, E. T. (1993). Emotional trade-offs of becoming a parent: How social roles influence self-discrepancy effects. *Journal of Personality and Social Psychology, 65*, 1259–1269.
A study that examines the reasons that some people suffer more distress after becoming a parent while other people suffer less distress.

Barnett, R. C, Marshall, N. L., & Sayer, A. (1992). Positive-spillover effects from job to home: A closer look. *Women and Health, 19*, 13–41.
Examines types of employment that are associated with levels of psychological distress for mothers.

Compas, B. E., & Williams, R. A. (1990). Stress, coping, and adjustment in mothers and young adolescents in single- and two-parent families. *American Journal of Community Psychology, 18*, 525–545.
A look at the differences and difficulties associated with being a single parent of an adolescent.

Duffy, M. E. (1989). Mental well-being and primary prevention practices in women heads of one-parent families. *Journal of Divorce, 13*, 45–64.
Asks questions concerning primary prevention strategies for women who are single parents and looks at possible mediators of independent variables such as education.

Fong, M. L., & Amatea, E. S. (1992). Stress and single professional women: An exploration of causal factors. *Journal of Mental Health Counseling, 14*, 20–29.
An investigation of the coping strategies of single and married women and women who are parents.

Koski, K. J., & Steinberg, L. (1990). Parenting satisfaction of mothers during midlife. *Journal of Youth and Adolescence, 19*, 465–474.
Examines the relationship between marital satisfaction, and psychological symptoms for mothers in midlife.

Ge, X., Conger, R. D., Lorenz, F. O., Shanahan, M., & Elder, G. J. (1995). Mutual influences in parent and adolescent psychological distress, *Developmental Psychology, 31*, 406–419.
A study examining the mutual influences of parent and adolescent psychological distress.

Leventhal-Belfer, L., Cowan, P. A., & Cowan, C. P. (1992). Satisfaction with child care arrangements: Effects on adaptation to parenthood. *American Journal of Orthopsychiatry, 62*, 165–177.
Examines the parents' mental health as it is related to their decisions about child care.

Sogaard, A. J., Kritz-Silverstein, D., & Wingard, D. L. (1994). Finnmark heart study: Employment status and parenthood as predictors of psychological health in women, 20–49 years. *International Journal of Epidemiology, 23*, 82–90.

A study examining the differences between working women and nonworking parents compared to women who are not parents in relationship to problems of coping, dissatisfaction with life, depression, and loneliness.

Telleen, S., Herzog, A., & Kilbane, T. (1989). Impact of a family support program on mothers' social support and parenting stress. *American Journal of Orthopsychiatry, 59*, 410–419.

An evaluation of support programs for parents.

Terry, D. J., Mayocchi, L., & Hynes, G. J. (1996). Depressive symptomatology in new mothers: A stress and coping perspective. *Journal of Abnormal Psychology, 105*, 220–231.

A study examining the relationship between levels of stress and postpartum depression.

12

Parenting of Adults with Mental Retardation

Marsha Mailick Seltzer

A UNIQUE GROUP OF PARENTS

This chapter describes a unique group of older women—aging mothers who care for adult children with mental retardation. These mothers face an atypical and poorly understood dual challenge—namely, the continuing caregiving responsibility for these adult children, and the personal challenge of adjusting to their own aging. These women have had different experiences from those of mothers who have nonhandicapped children, including unusually prolonged periods of active parenting, a distinct tempo of family life, and added emotional challenges and demands for coping.

Mental retardation affects 7.2 million people in the United States. The "ripple effects" of this disability are of much greater magnitude, as their parents and siblings are affected as well. Fully 80% of persons with mental retardation live with their families, often throughout their lives.

Although family caregiving is not an unusual role for women, the experiences of aging mothers who care for adult children with mental retardation are distinctive, for several reasons. First, whereas the provision of direct care by a parent for a child is normative when the family is young, this arrangement is not normative when a mother is approaching or has reached old age and a son or daughter has reached adulthood.

Another unique aspect of the caregiving experiences of this group aging mothers is the duration of their direct caregiving responsibility. Parenthood is an irrevocable role for all who have reared children. However, there is a substantial difference between normative parenting in old age, which is generally a "hands-off" role, and parenting an adult with disabilities, which involves a prolonged process of direct caregiving. In normative parenting, the direct care responsibilities last about two decades. In contrast, the duration of direct caregiving for a son or daughter with mental retardation can be five or six decades, or even longer.

Finally, aging mothers of adults with mental retardation are unique because they have had sustained interaction with professionals throughout their years of parenting. This pattern of relatively frequent contact with health and human service professionals throughout the parenting years is distinct from the essentially private parenting experience that is characteristic of most mothers of children without disabilities.

Health professionals are currently taking a great deal of interest in aging women who have provided long-term care to adult children with lifelong developmental disabilities. This interest is the result of the increased longevity of persons with mental retardation, who previously had a shorter lifespan than the general population. Because they now receive better services and health care, persons with developmental disabilities are now living well into adulthood and even into old age. Thus, the period of active parenting often extends throughout the mother's life.

Older mothers of adults with mental retardation constitute one example of the more general phenomenon of the provision of care by elderly persons to younger family members with disabilities or chronic illness. Other examples include aging mothers of adults with mental illness, cerebral palsy, and head injury. Even AIDS can be considered within this paradigm, in some cases in which parents rather than peers become the primary caregivers.

OUR RESEARCH PROGRAM

Until recently, little was known about the effects of this type of parenting on the health, psychological well-being, and social role participation of aging women. Since 1988, however, Marty Krauss and I have been studying 461 aging mothers (mean age = 66, range = 55–85) of sons and daughters with mental retardation (mean age = 35, range = 15–66) who live at home with them. When the study began, over three-fourths of the mothers were in good or excellent health. About two-thirds were married, and most of the others were widows. Over 80% had at least a high school education. About three-fourths of their adult sons and daughters had mild or moderate retardation and were in good or excellent health. About one-third had Down syndrome, which is associated with earlier onset of Alzheimer's disease and higher rates of mortality than are other types of mental retardation.

During the course of this study we have learned a great deal about these women, including how they have coped with their additional caregiving responsibilities, the nature of their plans for the future care of their sons or daughters after they are no longer able to be the primary caregivers, and the extent to which their other children expect to become the next generation of caregivers. In addition, we have attempted to gauge the impact of long-term parenting on these women's health, psychological well-being, and social participation.

THE WEAR-AND-TEAR HYPOTHESIS
VERSUS THE ADAPTATIONAL HYPOTHESIS

In our investigation of the impact of long-term parenting, we have examined two competing hypotheses. The first is the "wear-and-tear" hypothesis, which predicts that family caregiving will have a negative effect on the caregiver's mental and physical health.

The other hypothesis is the "adaptational" hypothesis, which predicts that new adaptive capacities will emerge during the course of caregiving.

Most research on caregiving for the elderly provides support for the wear-and-tear hypothesis; caregiving women have been found to be at risk for depression, poor health, and social isolation. However, there is also some evidence in support of the adaptational hypothesis. For example, Townsend and his colleagues studied adult children who provided care to impaired elderly parents, and found that many of these adult children exhibited stability or improvements, rather than decrements, in their mental health during the time that they were providing care.

In order to examine the wear-and-tear hypothesis versus the adaptational hypothesis in the case of aging mothers of adults with mental retardation, we compared the aging mothers in our sample with several contrast groups. First, we compared the mothers with older women who were not caregivers. Second, we compared them with women who were caregivers for the elderly. Third, we compared them with mothers of young children with disabilities. We expected that the wear-and-tear hypothesis would be more descriptive of the well-being of our aging caregivers than the adaptational hypothesis would be, because the very long years of active parenting would have taken a physical and emotional toll.

We found, to our surprise, that the mothers in our sample were functioning as well as or better than these contrast groups. For example, fully 71% of the mothers in our sample rated themselves as being in good or excellent health, whereas only 60% of a national probability sample of women the same age considered themselves to be in equally good health. Similarly, the women in our sample were substantially more satisfied with their lives in general and were less depressed than a comparison sample of women caring for elderly relatives; they were comparable on these dimensions with older noncaregiving women. Furthermore, the mothers in our sample were no more burdened or stressed than comparison groups of family caregivers for the elderly or mothers of young children with disabilities, even though they had been caregivers for so many more years than those in these comparison groups. Finally, the women in our sample had social support networks that were nearly as large as those of their noncaregiving generational peers. (These results are described more fully in my 1993 paper with Krauss.)

Why should these aging mothers—whom we expected would be at greater risk for poor physical health, depression, dissatisfaction with life, feelings of burden and stress, and social isolation—appear to be just the opposite? At least three factors may come into play here. First, there is a self-selection process regarding which families elect to rear sons or daughters with mental retardation at home, even after the children have reached adulthood. However, as noted earlier, it is the rule rather than the exception for a child with retardation to be reared at home and to continue to live at home in adulthood. Thus, self-selection is not fully explanatory of the favorable well-being of our aging mothers of adults with mental retardation.

A second explanation for the unexpectedly positive profile is that after so many years of caregiving, these women have adjusted to their children's disability and accommodated to their responsibilities as long-term family caregivers. Many mothers have told us that earlier in life, they experienced more burden and distress associated with having children with retardation. However, with the passage of time, it has become easier to accept the children's limitations and to develop an appreciation of their strengths.

A third explanation for the favorable health and well-being of these women is that they are often deriving benefit directly from the adult children. For example, many of the adults in our sample do chores for their mothers around the house. In some situations in which the mothers are becoming physically frail, the adult children are essential for the maintenance of their households. In addition, many mothers have described the importance of the companionship provided by these sons or daughters, and of the strong bonds of affection between them.

It also appears that some of these mothers have maintained their health and emotional fortitude in part *because* of the caregiving role, which honed their coping skills early in adulthood, and now gives them an added sense of purpose in life. Many of these mothers have responded to the challenge of rearing children with retardation by developing new adaptive capacities, reaching into previously untapped personal reserves, and envisioning new opportunities for personal growth and development.

For any one or a combination of these reasons, the women we have studied are currently, on balance, a well-functioning group of aging women. Few deny that they have experienced grief, frustrations, and many disappointments, especially during the early years when they were thrust into the rocky territory of parenting children with a disability. However, most now report more gratification than frustration in the role of long-term active mothers to their sons or daughters with mental retardation.

PARENTING OF ADULTS WITH RETARDATION VERSUS ADULTS WITH MENTAL ILLNESS

In order to gain an understanding of the generality of our findings across different types of disabilities, we compared the mothers in our sample with another group of aging mothers—mothers of adult children with serious and persistent mental illness. In this work, we are collaborating with our colleague Jan Greenberg. We sought to compare these two groups because their challenges are in many respects very similar. Both groups of older women provide care to their adult children in the areas of personal hygiene, transportation, and money and medication management. Also, both experience feelings of loss and grief associated with the realization that their children have not experienced a normal life. In addition, both groups express pervasive worry about the future, when they will no longer be able to be the primary caregivers for their children.

However, despite these similarities, we found the favorable health and well-being of aging mothers of adults with mental retardation to contrast sharply with that of aging mothers of adults with mental illness. Aging mothers of adults with mental illness feel substantially more burdened by their long years of active parenting than their counter-parts whose adult children have mental retardation, experience less closeness in their relationship with their adult children, and have higher levels of depressive symptoms. We hypothesized that the coping strategies used by these two groups of mothers might be an important factor in accounting for these differences.

To this end, we compared the coping strategies of a sample of aging mothers of adults with mental illness with the strategies used by the sample of aging mothers of adults with mental retardation described above. The two samples were recruited by means of similar strategies, and the criteria for inclusion in the study and the measures we used were identical.

We found that the two groups of mothers reported using problem-focused coping strategies with equal frequency. These included strategies such as active coping, planning, positive reinterpretation and growth, and suppression of competing activities. However, mothers of adults with mental illness were significantly more likely than mothers of adults with mental retardation to report using emotion-focused coping strategies, including focus on and venting emotions, denial, behavioral disengagement, and mental disengagement. This use of emotion-focused coping strategies was found to be associated with higher levels of depressive symptoms. Thus, part of the explanation for the disparity between the two groups of aging mothers in psychological well-being seems to be that the mothers of adults with mental illness are more likely to use emotion-focused coping strategies.

In addition, we found that when mothers of adults with mental retardation used problem-focused coping strategies, they benefited more than when mothers of adults with mental illness used the very same strategies. When faced with the stress of children with a disability, aging mothers of adults with retardation who used the coping strategies of planning and positive reinterpretation and growth were able to reduce their depressive symptoms. However, mothers of adults with mental illness had high levels of depressive symptoms even when they used these coping strategies.

What might account for the differential effects of coping that we observed? One possibility is that aging mothers of adults with mental illness are faced with a caregiving context over which they can exert only limited control. Hence, even though they are likely to use strategies such as planning and positive reinterpretation/growth, their adult children's behavior is likely to be unpredictable. These children often disrupt plans that the mothers have made, and this makes it difficult to reframe or reinterpret the caregiving responsibility as a meaningful role in later life.

In contrast, mothers of adults with mental retardation can rely on the relative stability of their children's functioning and the relative receptivity of the formal service system to their involvement. Thus, their planning efforts are more likely to pay off and engender feelings of efficacy, which in turn may make it easier for them to reinterpret the caregiving role in a positive light. Over the course of decades, the differential effects of the coping efforts of mothers of adults with mental retardation and those of adults with mental illness may result in the differences in levels of depressive symptoms, subjective burden, and relationship closeness that we have observed. (These findings are described more fully in my 1993 study with Greenberg and Greenley, and my 1995 study with Greenberg and Krauss.)

What can be concluded? First, we should not generalize from studies of aging mothers of children with one type of disability to other situations. The nature of the caregiving challenge is experienced differently by the two samples we studied, even though in many respects the "facts" of their caregiving responsibilities are similar. In particular, when the caregiving challenge gives an older woman a sense of control, her coping efforts are more likely to be effective, and she is more able to preserve her sense of well-being. Thus, although there is evidence that the early years of parenting a child with retardation have an assaultive quality, this period is replaced by adaptation and increased personal well-being.

With respect to self-reported health status, depressive symptoms, life satisfaction, and social support, aging mothers of adults with mental retardation are more similar to their generational peers who do not have continuing parenting responsibilities; they are different in these respects from aging mothers of adults with mental illness, who share a similar caregiving challenge. Over time, the caregiving challenge experienced by mothers of adults with retardation becomes increasingly predictable, and their relationships with their sons or daughters are characterized by growing companionship and mutual interdependence. Thus, their role as active parents in old age is non-normative, but nevertheless can be conducive to pleasant, healthy, and productive lives.

FURTHER READING

Greenberg, J. S., Seltzer, M. M., & Greenley, J. R. (1993). Aging parents of adults with disabilities: The gratifications and frustrations of later life caregiving. *The Gerontologist, 33,* 542–550.
Aging mothers caring for adults with mental retardation report more gratification with caregiving and less burden than aging mothers caring for adults with mental illness.

Krauss, M. W., & Seltzer, M. M. (1993). Current well-being and future plans of older caregiving mothers. *Irish Journal of Psychology, 14,* 47–64.
Aging mothers of adults with mental retardation have surprisingly favorable psychological well-being while still caregivers, but vary in the extent of their future planning.

Seltzer, M. M., Greenberg, J. S., & Krauss, M. W. (1995). A comparison of coping strategies of aging mothers of adults with mental illness or mental retardation. *Psychology and Aging, 10,* 64–75.
Aging mothers of adults with mental retardation use problem-focused coping strategies when faced with caregiving stress more effectively than aging mothers of adults with mental illness do.

Seltzer, M. M., & Ryff, C. D. (1994). Parenting across the lifespan: The normative and nonnormative cases. In D. L. Featherman, L. Lerner, & M. Perlmutter (Eds.), *Life-span development and behavior* (Vol. 12, pp. 2–40). Hillsdale, NJ: Erlbaum.
Although most studies of parenting examine how parents influence child development, the experience of parenting also affects the adult development of the parents, in both normative and non-normative cases.

Townsend, A., Noelker, L., Deimling, G., & Bass, D. (1989). Longitudinal impact of inner-household caregiving stressors. *Psychology and Aging, 4,* 393–401.
Although in some instances caregiving has a "wear-and-tear" effect on the caregiver, there is also evidence of adaptational processes.

13

Midlife

Sandra P. Thomas

*R*apid changes in the ideology of women's roles; shifting sociocultural and economic forces; and a confluence of remarkable historical events have produced a cohort of midlife women unlike any previous generations. We are not even sure how to define "midlife" any more. Although it was often defined in the literature of the 1970s and 1980s as the age period from 35 to 55 years (after which people were called "elderly"), the upper boundary is 65 or 70 years of age in newer studies. Today's vigorous, active 55-year-old woman would surely bristle at being called "elderly," and she looks forward to 25 more years of living. Because physiological and mental ages are seldom synchronous with chronological age, and because hereditary and lifestyle factors result in such wide variation among individuals, the age parameters of middle adulthood should be considered rough estimates.

Although the likelihood of developing a chronic condition such as arthritis, diabetes, or heart disease is increasing during the middle years, only a minority of women are significantly debilitated. In fact, most midlife women report good physical health. Despite the portrayal of menopause in medical literature as the major health issue for midlife women, studies show that it is a rather benign, minor event for most. Studies also show that midlifers are more interested in health-promoting activities than are younger adults, and they tend to have the financial resources to purchase needed health services.

Good mental health also characterizes most midlife women. Sometime between the ages of 30 and 40, they complete their separation–individuation from their mothers. Later in the midlife period, most complete their own child-rearing obligations. Despite the love they have for their children, they usually express relief when the last one leaves home (refuting the myth of the "empty nest" syndrome). The "refilled nest" syndrome is actually more problematic for this cohort of midlife women, when adult children return to the parental home because of job loss or divorce. Contrary to another popular myth, midlife women do not experience a reduction in sexual interest or satisfaction. Likewise, the majority continue to feel positive about their appearance, despite the gradual changes caused by aging. Although depression occurs all too frequently in women throughout the lifespan, its incidence is not higher in midlife. There is no significant decline in intelligence or cognitive functioning. Therefore, it is time for health professionals to adopt a more positive and realistic view of midlife women.

Nevertheless, middle adulthood presents women with a number of stressful challenges. To the extent that they cope effectively with these, their personal development will be enhanced, and their health will not be adversely affected. However, health professionals must have a good grasp of normal midlife development and the savvy to initiate health-promoting interventions when ineffective coping is observed.

MIDLIFE DEVELOPMENT

Carl Jung was the first to propose that midlife is a time of psychological upheaval. He wrote of the necessity for both men and women to incorporate the contrasexual aspects of themselves. For men, this involves owning their suppressed nurturant, tender qualities; for women, it involves allowing expression of their aggressive impulses. Jung also viewed middle age as a time for redirection of psychic energy toward spiritual values. Erikson defined the developmental task of midlife as "generativity versus stagnation." He contrasted generativity, which includes the nurturance and guidance of one's children (or social contributions by childless individuals), with regression to an obsessive need for pseudointimacy accompanied by a pervading sense of stagnation. The task for the ego is to arrive at a favorable balance of generativity over stagnation, by accepting responsibilities toward the larger society and mentoring the next generation.

The ideas of these seminal early thinkers have been challenged. Sheehy has asserted, "Generativity is a fine concept as far as it goes. . . . Overlooked is the fact that serving others is what most women have been doing all along. . . . It is not through more care-giving that a woman looks for a replenishment of purpose in the second half of her life. " Gilligan has alleged that life cycle theories fail to account properly for women's experience, because they are based on the lives of men. Jung's proposed sex role identity "crossover," in which midlife men become more "feminine" and women become more "masculine," has been refuted by several newer studies. In recent years, some theorists have disputed the notion of any universal kinds of experiences during midlife.

DO WOMEN HAVE A MIDLIFE CRISIS?

Debate continues as to whether there really is a "midlife crisis" for women, or whether the term "transition" is more appropriate. Some studies do support a period of turmoil, which for women is more likely to occur in their 40s than in their 50s. Apter reports that all 80 of her study participants had a crisis. There is evidence that the death of a parent or friend can shatter a comfortable existence and precipitate a confrontation with one's own mortality. Women's reactions to losses in midlife are dependent in part on their history of previous losses and the extent of unfinished grieving versus acceptance and resolution. It has been argued that the mourning process can actually promote personal development, because incorporating aspects of lost loved ones transforms individuals.

Whether or not women report a "midlife crisis," most acknowledge a time of reassessment and coming to terms with the future as well as the past. Goals are revised or replaced with new ones. There is less emphasis on material possessions, and more reflection about the brevity and meaning of life. Unresolved and unsettled issues of childhood and adolescence may be revived, and one researcher found that for her informants, the rediscovery of the girls they had been from ages 8 to 10 provided direction for conscious development of adult identity in midlife.

Hulbert and Schuster contend that women may arrive at midlife with a stronger and more integrated sense of self than men do, because they have dealt more actively with conflicting expectations, options, values, and role commitments throughout young adulthood. Their life "scripts" are not as simple as men's straightforward career trajectories. Whereas men may stop short in middle adulthood and ruefully deplore their neglect of relationships during years of intense career involvement, women have blended intimacy and achievement all along. The consensus of a dozen longitudinal studies is that most midlife women report a strong sense of their own competence and high levels of life satisfaction. Some refer to this period as "women's prime of life."

PSYCHOSOCIAL FACTORS AFFECTING MIDLIFE WOMEN'S HEALTH

Psychosocial factors known to affect midlife women's health include a sense of control or mastery; self-esteem; optimism; a sense of purpose in life; level of perceived stress; level of social support; and quality of experience in major roles, such as wife, mother, and worker (and particular combinations of roles that may produce role conflict or role overload). Research shows that it is not *occupancy* of multiple roles that affects health, but rather a woman's subjective evaluation of the costs and benefits of her role commitments. In studies of midlife women, the role of paid worker is usually correlated with better health, with some scholars suggesting that work minimizes the stress of the midlife transition. Many women are at the peak of their career productivity during the middle years, although some are just gearing up for intensive job involvement. Several studies have documented the increased *joie de vivre* exhibited by "late bloomers" who revive their long-postponed career goals in midlife, switching from household work to outside employment (or from part-time to full-time career commitment). However, work is more likely to be beneficial to women whose jobs confer greater status, autonomy, and control than it is to women in service, clerical, or factory work, which is less prestigious and rewarding.

Quality of experience in the roles of wife and mother is also highly salient to midlife health. Distressing aspects of these roles are more strongly linked to health than the rewards are. Stress resulting from interactions with spouse or children markedly increased the rates of negative health outcomes in a 5-year study of middle-aged women conducted by the McKinlays and their colleagues. Midlife women are particularly vulnerable to stress because of the simultaneous demands of younger and older generations.

THE NATURE OF MIDLIFE STRESS

We now know that stress is fundamentally a perceptual construct, because life events seen as catastrophic by some individuals are energizing challenges to others. To the extent that individuals have anticipated certain midlife events (e.g., death of a parent, retirement) and prepared for them, these events may be less disruptive. However, unexpected events (e.g., accidents, job loss, or discovery of a mate's infidelity) are predictably very distressful. In addition to such episodic major stressors, middle-aged individuals have heavy ongoing daily responsibilities. In one of my studies, 66% of the sample reported severe daily hassles, and most of these women were also experiencing major life changes. The midlife woman still struggles with society's gender-based mandate to be the primary nurturer of the sick. Jolene, mother of three, told us:

> In the past year I've had to start taking care of my dad and my grandmother. My dad developed dementia. . . . I feel like I'm losing control of myself. I'm somebody's mom. I'm somebody's wife. I'm somebody's daughter. I'm somebody's granddaughter. And I help to take care of all these people. . . . You can't slow down. You're always on the clock . . . you're trying to take care of somebody else and trying to get ready to go to work. Some days it's really made me cry. I just lose my emotional stability.

As if this were not enough, many women do a lot of "worry work" for others including their spouses, children, and friends. In fact, vicarious stress topped the list in a subsequent study, where we asked women to describe their greatest current stressor. Typical responses included worries about a husband's unemployment, a grandson's bad grades, a daughter-in-law's mother's illness, and a son's divorce. This perpetual caring for others can exact heavy costs, not only in terms of time and energy, but also in neglect of a woman's own health-promoting activities (e.g., aerobic exercise and relaxation). Women must be encouraged to know their limits and take time to care for themselves. Medicating their midlife worry and stress via alcohol, drugs, and other chemical "fixes"—including excessive eating—must be discouraged.

MIDLIFE COPING

There is some evidence that as people age, and as they handle ever more complex problems, they become more adept at coping. One team of researchers found that middle-aged people use more confrontive coping and support seeking than older people. A number of our own study participants have found their anger during their midlife years and used it to liberate themselves from overly demanding roles and relationships. Roberta said:

> I'm about tired. I guess it took 40 years to get tired. I can't do it. I just can't keep up with all their needs. I mean, if I'm not pulled in that direction, I'm pulled in the other, and they're going to pull me apart one of these days.

Dale told us:

> I'm not sure if it's because I turned 40, but this past year has been the climax of my anger. . . . It was like I woke up and I said, "*No*, I'm not going to be silent anymore!"

Midlife women also receive valuable empathy and support from their female friends. One recent study showed that friendships were the strongest correlate of well-being for midlife women.

CONCLUSION

Research on midlife women is still scant, although several important studies have been completed and others recently initiated. Less is known about the midlife experience of impoverished women, because many of the major studies have examined middle- or upper-class samples. There is also a dearth of research about the middle adulthood of ethnic/racial minorities and of women who have never married or are living with same-sex partners. Therefore, generalizations about "women" as a group should be avoided. By the year 2000, the number of midlife women between the ages of 35 and 64 will have increased to slightly more than 50 million, approximately 42% of the female population. Clearly, the physical and mental health of women in this age group will continue to be a vital concern to both care providers and policy makers.

FURTHER READING

Apter, T. (1995). *Secret paths: Women in the new midlife.* New York: Norton.
Interview study of 80 U.S. and British midlife women, documenting developmental crisis and personal growth.

Baruch, G., Barnett, R., & Rivers, C. (1983). *Lifeprints: New patterns of love and work for today's women.* New York: McGraw-Hill.
Important study of 238 women in Brookline, Massachusetts, examining midlife role quality and well-being.

Erikson, E. (1968). Generativity and ego integrity. In B. Neugarten (Ed.), *Middle age and aging.* Chicago: The University of Chicago Press.
Classic theory outlining the internal psychic issues of midlife, with emphasis on development of a sense of generativity.

Gilligan, C. (1979). Woman's place in man's life cycle. *Harvard Educational Review, 49,* 431–446.
Essay proposing that extant life cycle theories fail to account for women's experience; women reach midlife with a different perspective than men on the importance of relationships.

Hulbert, K. D., & Schuster, D. T. (Eds.). (1993). *Women's lives through time: Educated American women of the twentieth century.* San Francisco: Jossey-Bass.
Of the 15 longitudinal studies summarized in this book, 12 followed women into midlife and beyond. The studies illuminate not only human development, but also the influence of historical events and societal forces on the various cohorts of women.

Hunter, S., & Sundel, M. (Eds.). (1989). *Midlife myths: Issues, findings, and practice implications.* Newbury Park, CA: Sage.
Excellent edited book with chapters on physical status, cognition, mental health and personality development, family relationships, and social responsibility.

Jung, C. G. (1954). *The development of personality. Collected works, vol. 17.* New York: Pantheon Books.
Earliest formulation of the shift in ego energies during midlife, with emphasis on reclaiming repressed aspects of the self.

Matthews, K., Wing, R., Kuller, L., Meilahn, E., Kelsey, S., Costello, E., & Caggiula, A. (1990). Influences of natural menopause on psychological characteristics and symptoms of middle-aged healthy women. *Journal of Consulting and Clinical Psychology, 58,* 345–351.
One of several journal articles reporting on a longitudinal study of 541 initially premenopausal healthy women.

McKinlay, S. M., Triant, R. S., McKinlay, J., Brambilla, D., & Ferdock, M. (1990). Multiple roles for middle-aged women and their impact on health. In M. Ory & H. Warner (Eds.), *Gender, health, and longevity: Multidisciplinary perspectives* (pp. 119–136). New York: Springer.
One of several reports on a longitudinal study of over 2,000 midlife Massachusetts women, examining multiple roles, stress, and health variables.

Sheehy, G. (1976). *Passages: Predictable crises of adult life.* New York: Dutton.
Synthesis of developmental theories for the lay audience; useful in helping clients understand life transitions.

Thomas, S. P. (1990). Predictors of health status for mid-life women: Implications for later adulthood. *Journal of Women and Aging, 2,* 49–77.
Study examining psychological, behavioral, environmental, and sociodemographic predictors of health status of midlife women; 59% of the variance in health status was explained by the predictors.

Thomas, S. P. (1995). Psychosocial correlates of women's health in middle adulthood. *Issues in Mental Health Nursing, 16,* 285–314.
Secondary analysis of Baruch and Barnett's data set, with emphasis on prediction of midlife health status rather than psychological well-being.

Thomas, S. P., & Donnellan, M. (1993). Stress, role responsibilities, social support, and anger. In S. P. Thomas (Ed.), *Women and anger* (pp. 112–128). New York: Springer.
Study illuminating vicarious stress in women's lives and its correlation with their anger.

Thomas, S. P., & Jefferson, C. (1996). *Use your anger: A woman's guide to empowerment.* New York: Pocket Books.
Summary of strategies for healthy anger management, based on the Women's Anger Study findings; useful for female clients with high levels of stress and anger.

Woods, N. F. (1993). Midlife women's health: There's more to it than menopause. In B. J. McElmurry & R. S. Parker (Eds.), *Annual review of women's health* (pp. 163–196). New York: National League for Nursing.
Excellent annotated bibliography, along with an overview of midlife women's health issues by the author.

14

Aging and Women's Life Course

Phyllis Moen

*T*he process of aging is frequently depicted as synonymous with the onset of poor health and disability. But women as well as men move through adulthood and old age in complex ways, which include social and psychological processes as much as biological ones. Reduced activity levels and sickness may often be concomitant with aging, but the relationship between growing older and poor health is not immutable. Considerable numbers of women age successfully, with few health problems or disabilities, whereas others face such difficulties quite early in life. Most studies of women's health either include women of all ages or look specifically at a particular life stage, such as the teenage years or midlife. A life course view of successful, healthful aging highlights the dynamic processes of development and change over the lifespan, as well as the importance of the social contexts of lives. The focus is on the multiple meanings of age: as a biological aging process, as a social life stage, and as representing each cohort's unique historical context.

A LIFE COURSE PERSPECTIVE ON AGING

A life course perspective challenges traditional ways of investigating the interplay between gender and health. Instead of considering snapshots of individual lives at one point in time, a life course approach focuses on life pathways, considering role transitions, trajectories, and turning points in lives over time. In fact, one useful way of depicting the life course is as a series of movements in and out of various roles. Women's life course reflects the interweave of work, family, and community role trajectories, which change in conjunction with age as well as with changing circumstances and options. For example, an individual life can be characterized as a series of interrelated trajectories through occupation, marriage, parenthood, and caregiving, as well as volunteer and community participation. An important theoretical and practical implication of this approach is that occupying particular roles (e.g., wife, widow, or worker) at any one point in time may matter less in terms of health and psychological adjustment than may the duration of roles (e.g., wife, widow, or worker), the number and predictability of role entries and exits throughout adulthood, and their timing in relation to age as well as other life events. In turn, role continuities and changes are tied to developmental trajectories in physical health and emotional well-being throughout women's life course. Three life course themes are crucial in seeking to understand women's lives, women's health, and the link between the two: "timing," "process," and "context."

Timing relates to the incidence, direction, and sequence of roles throughout the life course. For example, the employment role has been positively related to women's health. But knowing whether or not a woman is employed at any one point in time may be less useful than knowing the duration and patterning of her labor force participation throughout adulthood.

Process focuses on aging as a series of role transitions, rather than as a single event. Some roles (e.g., that of wife or worker) are left, and others (e.g., that of widow or retiree) are entered. Process, like timing, also draws attention to role trajectories, or the way roles are played out over the life course.

Context can be seen on two levels: personal and historical. The personal circumstances of women's lives—their education, income, social network, marital status, and family size, as well as their age—may have important repercussions for their social integration and health in the later years of adulthood. But historical shifts may matter as well affecting the options and opportunities of women at different ages. Women from different cohorts were born into vastly different worlds, with changing expectations regarding women's roles and lives. Women from different cohorts will be of different ages at any one point in time; hence any historical variations may well be obfuscated by differences in age. Focusing on the context of women's lives draws attention to potential differences by age cohort, as well as differences by educational background, prior health, household composition, and economic situation.

THE IMPORTANCE OF PATHWAYS

The study of aging and health from a life course perspective becomes an investigation of *pathways*—of the connections between different phases of life, and of ways in which circumstances in early adulthood may affect health and social integration later in life. One promising corollary, and possible precursor, of women's health in later adulthood is social integration, in the form of involvement in multiple roles. Occupying multiple roles (e.g., those of worker, club member, volunteer, and churchgoer) has been positively linked to health and to longevity. Such multiple role occupancy may be especially important in later adulthood—a time when role reduction, rather than role accumulation, becomes increasingly common.

However, cross-sectional research linking health with social connectedness is problematic because the direction of effects is unclear. A key issue is one of "social causation" versus "social selection." Social causation assumes that social integration (occupying multiple roles) influences health. By contrast, social selection assumes that healthy women are the ones most likely to take on and maintain multiple social roles. But the issue of social causation versus social selection is less crucial than is an understanding of the pathways to *both* health and social integration in later adulthood. Studies suggest that successful aging encompasses both social integration (multiple roles) and health in the later years of life.

A focus on social integration is especially important when looking at women's lives, since women's public participation in the larger society tends to be circumscribed by the primacy of their private family obligations. Women are also more likely than men to spend their later adulthood alone, without the presence (and support) of a spouse. Aging women are particularly susceptible to social isolation as they leave or lose employment, their children grow up and lead their own lives, and as many lose the wife role through divorce or widowhood. The primary issue is not whether multiple role involvement affects health or vice versa, but how various pathways lead to social integration and health in women's later years.

THE IMPORTANCE OF PREVIOUS EXPERIENCES

A key life course proposition is that early experiences matter—in other words, knowing something about women's life experiences should help to explain their health in later adulthood. Thus, a life course approach to women's roles and health suggests the following questions. What is the relationship between social integration (multiple roles) in early adulthood and how well women age? Is it current roles or women's role biography (roles over their life course) that most affects their health? If social involvement promotes health, what factors promote social connectedness (integration) as women age?

Social integration (defined as multiple role involvements) at one life phase may or may not be conducive to social integration and health in the later years of adulthood. For example, family responsibilities often constrain women's involvement in employment or community activities for a number of years; however, experiences during this child-rearing phase may have little effect on women's social integration or health in later adulthood. On the other hand, active community participation during early adulthood, despite heavy family demands, may signal an active involvement in society that persists into old age. Research evidence drawing on a life course approach documents that women's role involvements during the prime adult years appear to promote both social integration and health in the later years of their lives. But is it multiple role occupancy generally, or the duration or timing of particular roles, that is most conducive to health?

WOMEN'S ROLE BIOGRAPHIES

Both current and past role involvement can be important for women's health. Women's lives and lifestyles are defined by their private family roles as well as their public activities in society.

Family Roles

Marriage has been positively linked to health, whereas divorce and widowhood typically have negative health effects. A life course focus draws attention to the timing of a marital dissolution. It is not clear from existing research whether the state of nonmarriage is the critical factor in inhibiting health, or whether it is the recency of the transition from marriage to nonmarriage. Moreover, since widowhood becomes increasingly common in the later years of women's lives, being nonmarried may have fewer negative health impacts for older women than for women whose marriages ended in earlier adulthood.

Motherhood is also a common role for women, and, unlike marriage, it is one from which women rarely exit. (Women who have children are mothers for life, no matter how old their children.) Little is known about the impact of motherhood on social integration and health in later life. Still, the number of children raised or the amount of one's life spent in raising children could have long-term health consequences. Having children in the home may promote health-enhancing regimens as women attempt to establish good examples for their children; on the other hand, parenting obligations may result in women's spending less time and effort on self-care. My own research has shown that number of children was positively related to longevity among women who were wives and mothers in the 1950s, and other research has found that the presence of children in the home deters women from engaging in negative health behaviors.

But family roles carry obligations as well as benefits. One potentially costly role, in terms of women's health and social integration, is that of caregiver to adult relatives. Whereas the care involved in the raising of young children is anticipated, frequently welcomed, and circumscribed in the lifespan, caring for an infirm parent (or spouse) or for a handicapped adult child can become an unexpected but absorptive role that may restrict women's participation in other activities and produce debilitating strains in their lives. (However, this need not always be the case, as Seltzer points out in her chapter on the parenting of adults with mental retardation.)

Work and Community Roles

Two nonfamily roles—as an employee in paid work or a volunteer in unpaid work—provide mechanisms for women's active participation in the larger society. Recent research has examined the positive effects of employment for women's health, but the long-term significance of the duration, number of spells, or timing of employment throughout adulthood for health in later life is not clear.

Volunteer work can also produce positive health consequences. Indeed, the existing evidence suggests that engaging in social participation at any point in the life course has positive health outcomes. My colleagues and I found that membership in clubs or organizations was positively related to women's longevity. In our research following women over a 30-year period, we also found that volunteering at various times throughout adulthood was positively associated with functional ability and occupying multiple roles in later adulthood; in addition, being a club or organizational member in earlier adulthood was positively related to functional ability and subjective health 30 years later, as well as to the duration of health. It may be the degree of choice involved in social participation in community activities that is beneficial. Social participation may also provide gratifying social involvement and recognition, reductions in anxiety and in self-preoccupation, and many forms of socioemotional support. Given these beneficial side effects, participation in formal, organized volunteer activities throughout adulthood appears to promote health. It also contributes to activity in old age, and consequently to multiple roles later in life.

OBJECTIVE SOCIAL CONDITIONS

Health in childhood and early adulthood, as well as high socioeconomic status, are resources that should promote women's health throughout their life course. Education matters for health in later adulthood, precisely because it shapes women's economic status, lifestyle, and social connectedness. Educated women are more likely than those with fewer years of schooling to adopt behavior conducive to health throughout the life course; they are also more apt to have the economic means for optimal health care. Educational achievement, occupational prestige and income have been shown to be highly correlated with women's health. Moreover, lifestyles incorporating risk factors such as smoking have been linked to social class, with older educated (or those with higher socioeconomic status) women less likely to smoke and more likely to exercise than those women with less education.

CONCLUSIONS

The life course perspective offers no simple interpretation of the relationship between social integration earlier in life and health in women's later years of adulthood. Rather, it suggests that the connection should be viewed as a dynamic and possibly cumulative process, wherein the roles women occupy in early adulthood play out in patterns of involvement over the life course, which in turn sustain health.

The life course perspective also places women's social integration and health within the context of a changing society. For example, younger cohorts of women may be more healthy than older cohorts precisely because they are more socially integrated. Because health has been shown to be linked to multiple roles, it is important to assess factors affecting the number of roles women occupy at all stages of the life course.

One role in particular—being a member of a club or organization that is involved in volunteer work—appears to be positively related to women's health. On the other hand, the evidence suggests that the duration of time spent caring for infirm or aged parents, spouses, or other relatives may be negatively related to a caregiver's own health.

A life course approach suggests first a cumulative accentuation process, in which the least healthy are the most vulnerable later in life, whereas those who are most healthy and most socially connected (in terms of multiple roles) in the prime of adulthood are the most resilient as they age. Women who are actively connected to the larger society throughout their adult years are apt to be the most healthy and actively involved later in life. Second, social participation in paid or unpaid work is important. Volunteer work in service clubs or organizations seems especially conducive to subsequent health and integration. Whether this reflects women's active choices; a personality characteristic related to "joiners"; the social contacts, support, and other psychosocial payoffs of social participation; or some other, unmeasured construct remains to be investigated.

"Successful aging" can be depicted as living both a healthy and an active, involved life. Both social integration and health in women's later years may reflect choices and experiences throughout adulthood. Research suggests that the aging process may vary widely as a result of women's social roles in the prime of life, with multiple role involvements having long-term benefits for women's health. Moreover, social participation, in terms of volunteering and club membership at any time during adulthood, appears to be an especially important influence on the ways in which women grow old.

ACKNOWLEDGMENT

Support for the preparation of this chapter was provided by a grant from the National Institute on Aging (IT50 AG11711-01).

FURTHER READING

Elder, G. H., Jr. (1995). The life course paradigm: Social change and individual development. In P. Moen, G. H. Elder, Jr., & K. Luscher (Eds.), *Examining lives in context* (pp. 101–139). Washington, DC: American Psychological Association.
A nice overview of this theoretical perspective.

Gove, W. R., & Hughes, M. (1979). Possible causes of the apparent sex differences in physical health: An empirical investigation. *American Sociological Review, 44,* 126–146.
An early and important analysis of why men and women differ in terms of their health.

House, J. S., Landis, K. R., & Umberson, D. (1988). Social relationships and health. *Science, 241,* 550–545.
A review of the evidence (to the mid-1980s) on the positive health effects of social connections.

Moen, P., Dempster-McClain, D., & Williams, R. M., Jr. (1989). Social integration and longevity: An event history analysis of women's roles and resilience. *American Sociological Review, 54,* 635–647.
A study of women over a 30-year period, demonstrating that multiple roles in earlier adulthood promote longevity.

Moen, P., Dempster-McClain, D., & Williams, R. M., Jr. (1992). Successful aging: A life course perspective on women's roles and health. *American Journal of Sociology, 97*(6), 1612–1638.
A study of women over a 30-year period providing evidence of the links between multiple roles on subjective assessments of health in the later years.

Moen, P., Robison, J., & Dempster-McClain, D. (1995). Caregiving and women's well being: A life course approach. *Journal of Health and Social Behavior, 36,* 259–273.
Shows that the impacts of caregiving on health depends on the contexts and resources that women bring to the caregiving role.

Thoits, P. A. (1986). Multiple identities: Examining gender and marital status differences in distress. *American Sociological Review, 51,* 259–272.
A nice theoretical overview, as well as an empirical study of gender differences in stress.

Umberson, D. (1987). Family status and health behaviors: Social control as a dimension of social integration. *Journal of Health and Social Behavior, 28,* 306–319.
Study suggesting that family members help promote preventive behaviors in individuals, accounting for the positive relationship between marriage and family on the one hand and health on the other.

Section II

STRESS AND COPING

15

Section Editor's Overview

Elaine A. Blechman

*H*ow much control does any woman have over her physical and mental health? Are all women passive victims of risk factors such as genetic endowment that, regardless of their actions, predestine the length and quality of their lives? Or can women assume total control of their destinies through effective coping strategies? Common sense and empirical evidence suggest a middle ground, which I call "coping–competence theory" and illustrate in Table 15.1. Coping–competence theory asserts that how a woman copes with current stress is the most direct, substantial influence on her future physical and mental health.

The way a woman currently copes with stress mediates the indirect influences on her health: the influences of personal attributes that are either invariable (e.g., ethnicity) or hard to alter (e.g., temperament), of close relationship characteristics (e.g., marital conflict), and of personal style (e.g., humor). Current stressors are known contributors to ill health and include features of the physical environment (e.g., prevalent infectious diseases, environmental contaminants) and of the social environment (e.g., cultural norms, neighborhood disorganization). Current stressors influence and are influenced by health outcomes (e.g., when a woman succumbs to a chronic illness, she may assume a more financially dependent and more stressful social role in her family). Current coping strategies include a long list of methods believed to be beneficial to health. Each woman's approach to a particular stressor is jointly determined by the nature of that stressor itself (e.g., humor is a good way to cope with some stressors but not with others) and by her typical personal style (e.g., the extent to which she generally makes use of humor). Current coping strategies directly influence future health outcomes, and indirectly influence future status in regard to coping and to other risk protection factors. Thus a woman with multiple sclerosis who uses social support to confront her illness increases her future chances of social support and of popularity with her friends and neighbors.

Coping–competence theory provides a heuristic device for integrating chapters in this section of the book. All these chapters consider how various coping processes influence women's health and women's competence. By competence, I mean a woman's satisfaction with her regulation of emotions, interpersonal relationships, and academic and occupa-

TABLE 15.1. Coping and Women's Health

Relationships	Self attributes	Stressors	Coping strategies	Health outcomes
Bonding	Age	Chronic illness	Acceptance	Resistance
Marital satisfaction	Education	Cultural norms	Achievement	Onset
Parenting satisfaction	Ethnicity	Daily hassles	Aggression	Severity
Parenting skill	Gender	Developmental transitions	Attachment	Recovery
Parent warmth	Genetic endowment	Disease vectors	Avoidance	Relapse from mental and physical
Peer acceptance	Lifestyle	Disabilities	Blaming	disorders and
Peer network size	Income	Environmental contaminants	Commitment	diseases
Perceived peer support	Occupation	Neighborhood organization	Compliance	
Peer popularity	Physical attractiveness	Normative challenges	Creativity	
	Religion	Physiological reactivity	Denial	
	Self-esteem	Social roles	Distraction	
	Temperament		Exercise	
	Verbal intelligence		Hardiness	
			Hostility	
			Humor	
			Impatience	
			Optimism	
			Perseverance	
			Power	
			Problem solving	
			Recreation	
			Resilience	
			Rest	
			Self-disclosure	
			Self-regulation	
			Social comparison	
			Social support	
			Substance use	

tional achievement. Since these chapters overlap somewhat in their consideration of key variables (such as social support or attachment) while assigning to these variables different operational definitions (as a quality of close relationships, a personal style, or a coping strategy), Table 15.1 places some variables within more than one construct. Variables that have been found elsewhere to predict mental and physical health outcomes are included in Table 15.1 even if they are not the topics of chapters in this section.

CLOSE RELATIONSHIPS

Beach, Fincham, O'Leary, and Wills consider how various characteristics of close relationships with families and friends influence women's health outcomes.

Attachment

According to Beach, attachment in adults reflects their "internal working models"—cognitive schemas dating from infancy that represent how the individuals characteristically cope with the emotional and social frustrations inherent in close relationships. Women's attachment styles have been shown to predict their future chances of marital satisfaction and social support. Securely attached adult women cope relatively more successfully with the frustrations inherent in marriage, providing them with more perceived support from others and more satisfaction with that support. In contrast, ambivalently attached and avoidantly attached women may lack social resources because of their excessive preoccupation with autonomy and mistrust, and may be particularly vulnerable to depression when confronted with less than satisfactory marriages.

Marital Quality

Fincham argues that a bad marriage not only deprives partners of the benefits of social support and intimacy, but imposes special costs. A pessimistic coping style may predispose women both to marital distress and to depression. Marital distress may contribute to poor physical health via repeated arguments that cause unrelieved physiological reactivity and impaired immune system functioning. A husband's protective and supportive attitudes may contribute to marital satisfaction and sustain a woman's recovery from affective disorders, whereas his hostile attitudes and criticism of negative symptoms may obstruct marital satisfaction and recovery.

Marital Conflict

O'Leary points out that although marital conflict is inevitable and divorce rates are high, many women prefer being married to being separated or divorced, and feel good unless the quality of their relationships is poor or they are abused by their husbands. For women whose depression is the product of severe but remediable marital conflict and abuse, the answer lies not in individual therapy aimed at improving these wives' coping strategies, but in conjoint therapy aimed at raising relationship quality and in individual or group therapy aimed at reducing husbands' aggression. Training in improved coping strategies seems in order either when marital conflict is irremediable or when chronic dysthymia has preceded marital conflict. O'Leary leaves us with tantalizing questions about how unhappy women in bad marriages can be matched beforehand with the optimal treatment approach.

Social Support

Wills reports that women with more social support have less depression, a lower risk of mortality, and a better chance of recovery from illness. For Wills, "social support" is either the sheer number of social relationships (structural support) or the perceived quality of social support (emotional support) available in those relationships. Wills suggests that social support functions in a number of ways to avert bad health outcomes: by reducing the risk associated with current stressors, by promoting more effective coping and a healthier lifestyle, and by moderating personal attributes (e.g., self-esteem and physiological reactivity) in ways that increase the range and appropriateness of coping strategies. Anticipating the need for research that delineates causal mechanisms, Wills hypothesizes that structural support may influence health by reducing stress while emotional support may influence health by improving coping strategies.

PERSONAL STYLE

Eysenck, Basso, Smith, Gustafson, Carver, Maddi, and Wright consider how a woman's characteristic style of responding to stress (what some, such as Eysenck, call her "personality") influences health outcomes.

Self-Regulation

Eysenck equates unhealthy coping with neurotic emotional responses and excessive dependence upon other people; he equates healthy coping with self-regulation. In support of his view about the healthy impact of self-regulated coping, he presents mortality data from a 15-year follow-up of 2,608 women, in which self-regulation was negatively correlated with death from cancer, coronary heart disease (CHD) and all other causes after controlling for smoking, drinking, and other risky behaviors. According to Eysenck, three health-relevant personality types are the classic Type A personality, who is vulnerable to CHD and prone to anger, hostility, and aggression; the Type B personality, who is physically healthy and adept at emotional self-regulation; and the Type C personality, who is vulnerable to depression and relies on neurotic defense mechanisms.

Type A Behavior Pattern

Basso defines the Type A behavior pattern (TABP) as "a relatively stable disposition to respond to achievement- or control-related challenges in an intensely aggressive, competitive, impatient, and ambitious manner" that may promote chronic, health-eroding physiological reactivity. Basso suggests that women who are vulnerable to CHD because they consistently rely on a TABP coping strategy may be inclined to perceive a broad range of events as stressful, may be preoccupied with achievement, or may have very low self-esteem. Regardless of why a woman uses a TABP coping style, persistent TABP is widely believed to influence CHD pathogenesis through a cascade of physiological events beginning with excessive and frequent sympathetic activation and concluding with myocardial infarction.

Hostility

For Smith, hostility is the cognitive manifestation of a phenomenon that often includes anger (an emotional response) and aggression (a behavioral response). Smith describes a longitudinal study finding that in both men and women, hostility predicted increased risk of myocardial infarction and all-cause mortality after lifestyle risk factors were controlled. Three possibly interdependent mechanisms may be responsible: greater physiological reactivity to daily stressors, fewer psychosocial resources (e.g., social support), and more unhealthy lifestyle behaviors (e.g., drug use).

Achievement

Gustafson focuses on the way in which families influence women's strategies for coping with academic challenges. Gustafson's findings suggest that characteristics of close family relationships distinguish young women who cope successfully with academic demands from those who cope unsuccessfully. Parents of academically successful females are particularly warm and encouraging, expressing high aspirations for their daughters and strong beliefs in their daughters' capabilities.

Optimism

Carver distinguishes between optimistic and pessimistic styles of coping with stress. Optimistic coping, in which a woman attempts to resolve controllable challenges while accepting uncontrollable challenges, may lead to better recovery from cancer surgery, better adaptation to infertility and other problems, less morbidity, and later mortality. Pessimistic coping may have adverse effects on health because it involves a fatalistic expectation of bad outcomes regardless of personal efforts, and a generally unhealthy and reckless lifestyle. Coping style may have its greatest impact on health from youth to midlife, whereas genetic endowment may have its greatest impact in later adulthood and old age.

Hardiness

Maddi defines "hardiness" as a characteristic cognitive style that includes beliefs in commitment (to active involvement), control (over event outcomes), and challenge (to grow in wisdom through positive and negative experiences). Maddi argues that hardiness protects against stress-related physical and mental illness by altering the way women cope with stress; it promotes transformational (active, decisive) coping and beneficial health practices.

Resilience

Wright defines "resilience" as the capacity for successful coping despite high-risk status, chronic adversity, and exposure to major stressors. She illustrates the research on resilience by describing studies focusing on the risk factors of childhood poverty, teen pregnancy, and sexual victimization. Direct and indirect protection against high risk and severe stress may come from personal attributes (e.g., positive temperament, self-esteem); from close relationship characteristics (e.g., responsive parents, social support); and from strategies for coping with stress that are optimistic, self-directed, realistic, socially and morally mature, and problem-focused.

CURRENT STRESSORS

Repetti and Sweeting consider how levels and types of current stressors influence women's health outcomes.

Multiple Roles

Repetti considers how women's physical and mental health is directly affected by their need to cope with multiple roles, including those of worker, spouse, mother, and (eventually) daughter of aged parents who is indirectly affected by their coping strategies. The role enhancement hypothesis suggests that multiple role involvement should benefit women's health—for example, by conferring additional social and economic resources. The role strain hypothesis suggests that multiple role involvement should injure women's health—for example, by requiring superhuman investments of energy, patience, and flexibility. Seemingly confirming the role enhancement hypothesis, healthier women are more likely to enter the work force and remain employed (and to do well in their multiple roles, perhaps because of self-selection). Also in apparent support of the role enhancement hypothesis, married women report better health (particularly if they are satisfied with their marriages), perhaps because unhealthy women never get married or are divorced. In apparent support of the role strain hypothesis, parenthood has negative consequences for marital satisfaction and for health, particularly if a mother has young children or is unemployed.

Life Events

Sweeting writes about the linkage between stressful life events and women's physical and mental health, as well as the impact of dominant coping strategies on life event experiences. She points out that only undesirable events (not all life changes) are potentially damaging, and that prediction of health is not aided by differential weighting of events. The correlations between life events and health are often significant, but are usually too low to be of much explanatory usefulness. Furthermore, such correlations at best indicate bidirectional relationships between stress and life outcomes, such that family fights may cause or be caused by depressive symptoms, or some third variable may cause both. Dominant coping strategies may influence not only the acute and chronic stressors a woman confronts, but the future consequences of stressor confrontation. Women's greater susceptibility to depression and anxiety may result from their more frequent exposure either to stressful life events or to more stressors related to close relationships, although results are inconclusive. Women and men may experience similar levels of life events, but women may react more strongly to any life event or to identity-relevant family-related events. Women may have more social support resources on average then men; however, because of their multiple roles (as workers, wives, and mothers), they may become distressed about a broader range of identity-relevant events (e.g., their own difficulties at work and their husbands' problems on the job).

CURRENT COPING STRATEGIES

Although many other authors in this section consider characteristic personal styles of coping, only Aspinwall focuses on a coping strategy (*social comparison*) that is a fractional component of numerous coping styles. According to Aspinwall, a woman's method of coping with stress (including acute and chronic illness) and her perceived satisfaction with her physical and mental health may depend upon information she derives by comparing herself with others. Information derived from social comparison helps women reduce uncertainty about their health, gauge the appropriateness of their reactions, regulate their emotions, and problem solve. Through downward social comparison, women may regulate negative emotions associated with life-threatening and chronic illnesses, although at times downward comparison may increase fear and depression. Through upward comparison, women may learn expert problem-solving strategies, although at times upward comparisons may induce feelings of inferiority.

HEALTH OUTCOMES

Ryff, the only author in this section to focus on the outcome of successful coping, argues that *positive mental health* results from adaptive coping with stress via autonomy, environmental mastery, personal growth, positive relations with others, purpose in life, and self-acceptance. Although adaptive coping strategies and chances for positive mental health may vary with age, gender, ethnicity, and social class, supportive relationships and positive interpretations of chronic stressors may be prime vehicles for adaptive coping among women.

CONCLUSIONS

There is universal agreement that the way a woman copes with stress influences her future health. Distinctions between emotion-focused coping as bad and problem-focused coping as good are gradually giving way to an appreciation of the subtlety of the coping process. Many stressors cannot be "solved," There is not enough time in the day to wrestle with all the potentially solvable problems that face us. Sometimes just venting about a stressor to a good friend and listener puts the situation in perspective and reduces concern about the problem situation. While denial is potentially harmful, particularly when it takes the form of substance abuse or violence against self or others, there are times when the best strategy is to get on with things and engage in distracting activities that reduce concern about insurmountable problems. For these reasons, I focus in my research on the virtues of prosocial coping. In prosocial coping, a woman confronts stress in diverse ways that share only one common element: her strategy is intentionally chosen (from all reasonable alternatives) to benefit her and others in the short-run and in the long-run. This is my operational definition of "effective" coping.

Hunches abound about the core characteristics (listed in Table 15.1) of effective coping with stress and about the necessary and sufficient antecedents of effective coping (listed in Table 15.1 in the "relationship" and "self" attributes columns). We need research that will investigate these hunches so that we can delineate health-promoting causal mechanisms and design theory-driven, health-promoting prevention and intervention programs. In particular, we must determine if relationship and self attributes (e.g., bonding, age) have direct effects on health outcomes irrespective of coping strategy and stress. Emerging, optimistic evidence suggests that a woman's current coping strategies directly influence her future health outcomes while mediating or moderating the indirect effects of past relationships, immutable personal qualities, and current stress. If coping matters little, then prevention efforts must identify malleable relationship, self, and stress attributes and attempt to alter them. If coping matters a lot, then prevention efforts must focus on teaching prosocial coping strategies such as self-disclosure that allow a woman to benefit herself without harming others despite any bad cards fate has dealt her.

FURTHER READING

Blechman, E. A. (1996). Coping, competence, and aggression prevention: Part 2. Universal, school-based prevention. *Applied and Preventive Psychology, 5,* 19–35.
Considers the practical implications of coping–competence theory for school-based prevention of violence and delinquency.

Blechman, E. A., & Culhane, S. E. (1993). Early adolescence and the development of aggression, depression, coping, and competence. *Journal of Early Adolescence, 13,* 361—382.
Presents coping–competence theory as a potential common pathway for the development of aggression and depression in childhood.

Blechman, E. A., Dumas, J. E., & Prinz, R. J. (1994). Prosocial coping by youth exposed to violence. *Journal of Child and Adolescent Group Therapy, 4,* 205–227.
Describes the successful results of a program that trained aggressive elementary school students to communicate prosocially with peers and authority figures.

Blechman, E. A., Prinz, R. J., & Dumas, J. E. (1995). Coping, competence, and aggression prevention: Part 1. Developmental model. *Applied and Preventive Psychology, 4,* 211—232.
Links the literature on risk-protection factors to coping–competence theory.

16

Attachment

Steven R. H. Beach

*B*owlby's theory of attachment and consequent developments in infant attachment research were first applied to the study of adult intimate relationships in the seminal work of Hazan and Shaver. Hazan and Shaver proposed that adults may show the same types of attachment patterns that are displayed by very young children in the experimental paradigm called the "Strange Situation." Hence, "securely" attached adults were described by Hazan and Shaver as those for whom closeness and trust are comfortable. Two types of "insecurely" or "anxiously" attached adults were identified: "Ambivalently" attached adults were described as worrying about abandonment and wanting to get closer, whereas "avoidantly" attached adults were described as being uncomfortable in relationships because they do not trust or feel they can depend on close others. Subsequently, Bartholomew and Horowitz further divided the avoidant group into two types of avoidantly attached persons: (1) a "fearful" group, composed of individuals who desire social contact and intimacy, but experience a pervasive fear of rejection and therefore actively avoid situations and relationships in which they perceive themselves as vulnerable to rejection; and (2) a "dismissing" group, consisting of individuals who develop models of the self as fully adequate and capable, but who view social contact and intimacy as unnecessary.

Like the earlier work on attachment styles among children, our current understanding of attachment in adults appears to be largely compatible with a cognitive perspective. Adults' attachment styles are hypothesized to reflect "internal working models," mental models that strongly resemble cognitive schemas, with affective as well as propositional information represented; these models appear to include representations of the self, important others, and the nature of relationships in general. Internal working models guide expectations about the self and others, as well as interpretations of social interactions. Internal working models are presumed to derive from individuals' relationships with their primary caregivers and from other social experiences in the past. Thus, persons enter new relationships with sets of expectations about themselves and others as partners. Despite the obstacles to changing fundamental expectations about the self and others, current relationships may often provide an opportunity for the revision of internal working models.

Since its introduction, attachment theory has been found to be a useful framework for explaining and understanding adult interactions and socioemotional reactions. In addition to predicting the quality of close relationships in adulthood, attachment style appears to have important implications for individual well-being and coping with interpersonal or major life stressors. It is currently believed that attachment styles reflect highly organized individual differences in cognition and affect, which may play a central role in the way individuals deal with stressful or challenging life events. Because of the large empirical literature suggesting the beneficial effects of socially supportive interactions on emotional response to stress (see the chapter by Wills on social support in this volume), an area of particular interest is the effect of attachment styles on the utilization of social resources. Also of interest is the relationship of attachment style to "perceived support" in relationships, as well as cognitive factors and personality factors that may be related to health. Finally, because of the potential health consequences of both marital discord (see O'Leary's chapter on marital conflict) and depression, the extent to which persons with different attachment styles may be differentially vulnerable to the development of marital discord and depression is of importance.

DOES ATTACHMENT STYLE INFLUENCE UTILIZATION OF SOCIAL RESOURCES?

Several studies suggest that attachment style does indeed influence the extent to which individuals make use of available social resources. In one study, Simpson, Rholes, and Nelligan examined the role of attachment in predicting both support seeking and support giving among romantic partners faced with an anxiety-provoking situation. To control for the degree of stress, all women participants were told that they were to be exposed to a procedure that would arouse considerable anxiety and distress in most people, but that the experimenter could not give them any further information until after the experiment. After each female subject was shown a room normally used for physiological assessment, she was led back to the waiting room, and her male partner was brought to the waiting room as well. A small video camera then unobtrusively recorded the couple's interaction for the next 5 minutes. Women who earlier had reported secure attachment engaged in more support seeking in the anxiety-provoking situation. Conversely, avoidant women engaged in less support-seeking behavior in the anxiety-provoking situation. It appears, then, that the anxiety cues associated with the experimental situation led securely attached women to react differently from avoidantly attached women. Because seeking support in this situation was an adaptive response, it would also appear that securely attached women made better use of social resources than did their avoidant counterparts.

In a nonexperimental replication of Simpson and colleagues' results, another group of researchers found that attachment style could predict utilization of social resources in response to real-world stressful events as well. Mikulincer, Florian, and Weller examined the response of a group of Israeli college students to the threat of Iraqi Scud missile attack during the Gulf War. As in the earlier experimental study, secure students, relative to ambivalent or avoidant students, were found to make greater use of social support as a way of coping with the anxiety caused by the bombardment. Conversely, among students living in the most dangerous areas, it was found that the avoidantly attached actually showed greater use of distancing strategies than other students did. Again, it appears that attachment style may influence utilization of social resources in response to stress, in ways that may carry long-term implications for health. In addition, it appears that behaviors reflective of self-reported attachment styles may be most likely during conditions of high stress.

IS ATTACHMENT STYLE RELATED TO "PERCEIVED SUPPORT" IN RELATIONSHIPS AND GENERAL INTERPERSONAL ORIENTATION?

Attachment theory suggests that some individuals have a "head start" in feeling supported by partners, and that this should positively influence their feelings of well-being and their health. Because they expect their needs to be met, securely attached adults report less neuroticism than their insecure counterparts do, and securely attached women report higher levels of support from their husbands. In contrast, ambivalent individuals report feeling more anxious and more jealous in their relationships than securely attached subjects, but tend to idealize their partners (at least early in relationships). Ambivalent individuals therefore are more prone to high-intensity negative affect in response to their partner's behavior. At the other extreme, persons with both types of avoidant attachment (fearful and dismissing) tend to display low emotional intensity in describing their romantic partners; they are often characterized by low levels of agreeableness and openness to feelings, and by high neuroticism. Overall, then, particular attachment styles appear to be associated with characteristic sets of expectations, and thus with characteristic modes of relating to the social environment.

Attachment styles also predict individuals' perceived support and satisfaction with the support being provided by their partners. Securely attached adults perceive that more social support is available, as well as reporting high levels of satisfaction with available support; insecurely attached adults report the reverse. Securely attached adults are less likely than insecurely attached adults to report expectations that seeking help from others will be risky, costly, and futile. Among the insecure attachment groups, the avoidantly attached are more likely to focus on needs for autonomy and independence, while the ambivalently attached report greater mistrust of others. To the extent that attachment style continues to emerge as a coherent way of organizing individual differences in orientation toward close relationships, these initial findings suggest that early attachment experiences may be an important influence on later beliefs that shape support seeking and support provision.

IS ATTACHMENT STYLE RELATED TO MARITAL DISCORD AND DEPRESSION?

How do attachment styles, which are identifiable in spouses before they are even married, exert an influence on later marital functioning? Recent research indicates a tendency toward assortative pairing with regard to attachment style. Accordingly, spouses with secure attachment styles will often be paired with spouses who also have secure attachment styles. Such couples report significantly more intimacy than couples in which one or both spouses are insecurely attached. Unfortunately, the mechanism that leads to assortative mating for attachment style is not well understood. Of particular interest, from the standpoint of the development of depression, is whether women with insecure attachment styles are at greater risk of depression in response to marital discord than are the securely attached. Currently, the answer to this question is not known. However, securely attached married couples report less withdrawal during conflictual discussions, and also report less verbal aggression, than couples containing at least one insecure spouse. This strongly suggests that attachment style may predict change in marital satisfaction, because withdrawal has been found to predict later deterioration in marital adjustment, and conflict is a strong concurrent correlate of dissatisfaction. Accordingly, the attachment styles couples bring to marriage may influence the quality of the marriage over time. Given the importance of the marital relationship for depression, it seems clear that attachment style may play an important role in the development of depression.

CONCLUSION

The explosion of research on attachment has found attachment style in adulthood to be related to a wide range of health-related perceptions, personality styles, and behaviors. This underscores the importance of future research that will examine the development of relationships in light of the attachment styles partners bring to relationships. If attachment style is found to be an important predictor of both marital discord and the development of depression, it will suggest potentially useful strategies for prevention of both interpersonal stress and emotional disorder.

FURTHER READING

Baldwin, M. W. (1992). Relational schemas and the processing of social information. *Psychological Bulletin, 112,* 461–484.
For those interested in a more "cognitive" account.

Bartholomew, K., & Horowitz, L. M. (1991). Attachment styles among young adults: A test of a four category model. *Journal of Personality and Social Psychology, 61,* 226–244.
This paper puts forward the proposal that attachment can be viewed in terms of two dimensions, yielding four rather than three attachment styles.

Beach, S. R. H., Smith, D. A., & Fincham, F. D. (1994). Marital interventions for depression: Empirical foundation and future prospects. *Applied and Preventive Psychology, 3,* 233–250.
This paper provides numerous citations regarding the effect of marital satisfaction on mood and depression.

Bowlby, J. (1980). *Attachment and loss: Vol. III.* New York: Basic Books.
A classic in attachment literature.

Hazan, C., & Shaver, P. (1987). Romantic love conceptualized as an attachment process. *Journal of Personality and Social Psychology, 52,* 511–524.
This is the classic paper on the application of attachment to adult romantic relationships.

Kobak, R., & Hazan, C. (1991). Attachment in marriage: The effects of security and accuracy of working models. *Journal of Personality and Social Psychology, 60,* 861–869.
A very nice discussion of the effect of attachment models on marital behavior.

Mikulincer, M., Florian, V., & Weller, A. (1993). Attachment styles, coping strategies, and posttraumatic psychological distress: The impact of the Gulf War in Israel. *Journal of Personality and Social Psychology, 64,* 817–826.
A good field study of attachment and coping.

Shaver, P. R., & Brennan, K. A. (1992). Attachment styles and the "Big Five" personality traits: Their connections with each other and with romantic relationship outcomes. *Personality and Social Psychology Bulletin, 18*(5), 536–545.
A good source of information about the possible overlap of attachment and personality.

Simpson, J. A., Rholes, W. S., & Nelligan, J. S. (1992). Support seeking and support giving within couples in an anxiety-provoking situation: The role of attachment styles. *Journal of Personality and Social Psychology, 62,* 434–446.
A very nice experimental study of attachment and coping.

17

Marital Quality

Frank D. Fincham

Approximately 40% of the problems for which people seek professional help in the United States concern their spouses or marriages—a proportion that is twice the size of any other problem area. Because women (especially those with a high school education) are more likely than men to define a problem in mental health terms, marital quality may be particularly important for understanding women's mental health. In a similar vein, the recent emergence of the biopsychosocial perspective on physical health has stimulated investigation of family relationships and health problems, and suggests that marital quality may also be relevant for understanding women's physical well-being. This chapter examines whether marital quality is associated with the onset of women's mental and physical health problems, is relevant to their course, and has implications for their treatment.

MARITAL QUALITY AND PROBLEM ONSET

Epidemiological and survey studies have consistently shown a relationship between being married and positive mental health, physical well-being, and mortality. Where gender differences have been found, they usually show that marriage is less of a protective factor for women than for men. Even so, marriage is assumed to protect both men and women because of the social support and intimacy it affords. With the vast majority of the general population reporting happy marriages, this finding may simply reflect the benefits of a satisfactory marriage. But does lowered marital quality result only in the loss of potential benefits, or are there costs associated with being in a distressed marriage? The more complete picture that emerges from the investigation of marital quality suggests that unsatisfactory marriages are a risk factor for health.

Mental Health

Marriages in which one spouse exhibits a mental health disorder (e.g., depression, anxiety, schizophrenia, or alcoholism) are characterized by, among other things, lower marital satisfaction. This association is best documented for depression—a disorder that is experienced by large numbers of women (it is estimated that up to 26% of women experience major depressive disorder in their lifetimes), and is exhibited about twice as often by women than by men.

Although the link between marital distress and depression does not differ across gender, marital distress significantly increases the risk of depression, with findings varying from a 10-fold increase in newlyweds to a 25-fold increase in the general population. This association does not show that marital distress causes depression. However, both retrospective reports and data from prospective longitudinal studies are consistent with the view that marital distress is implicated in the etiology of depression, particularly in the presence of a severely stressful event that involves loss or that is likely to result in humiliation or feelings of entrapment. The finding that marital distress may cause depression does not preclude depression from influencing marital satisfaction. Evidence for both processes exists.

Why are marital distress and depression linked? We have not yet determined why there are sex differences in depression, and speculation about the association between marital distress and depression is even more rudimentary. Some hypotheses offered to explain sex differences in depression suggest that coping style may be involved. For example, a pessimistic way of explaining events has been linked to a number of poor outcomes, including marital distress and depression, and is a factor that might account for their association. This possibility is particularly appealing, in light of some evidence that girls are more likely than boys to be socialized into using a pessimistic explanatory style. At present, the mechanisms linking marital distress and depression have received little attention.

Physical Health

Much of the evidence relating to physical health focuses on the protective role of social relationships such as marriage, rather than on the health costs of being in an unsatisfactory relationship. Being married is typically used as an index of social support and intimacy, and is correlated with a health outcome. The evidence showing that being unmarried (assumed lack of social relationship) is a major risk factor for health is thought to rival that available to establish such factors as smoking, high blood pressure, and physical inactivity as health risks. However, lifestyle, selection into marriage, stress versus support, and combinations of such factors can be used to explain differential risk across marital status groups. It is quite possible that the purported protective effect of marriage may simply reflect the increased risks faced by those who are not married.

Much stronger evidence linking marriage to health would exist if marital quality were shown to be related to physical well-being. Only a handful of studies have attempted to do this, and they have not focused specifically on women's health. One possible exception is research on pregnancy, which has shown that marital dissatisfaction is associated with more somatic symptoms, depression, and diffuse anxiety. Not surprisingly, texts on women's health rarely mention marital variables.

Interesting preliminary evidence involving the immune system points to a possible association between marital quality and women's health. Specifically, it has been shown that lower marital quality predicts poorer immune system functioning, and that greater frequency of behaviors characteristic of marital distress (e.g., criticism, interruption) during a discussion of marital problems is associated with larger decrements in immune functioning over a 24-hour period. Such findings are consistent with research showing that marital satisfaction is linked to physiological reactivity (e.g., heart rate) during discussion of a marital difficulty.

Such findings raise intriguing possibilities. For example, marital distress may be a stressor that changes health-related behaviors (e.g., sleeping habits); such changes may influence the immune system and thereby lead to poorer health. Alternatively, marital distress may result in negative marital interactions that increase physiological arousal, thereby impairing immune system functioning and lowering resistance. Indeed, prolonged physiological arousal resulting from enduring negative interaction could lead directly to poor health outcomes. If such speculations are supported by future research findings, improving marital quality will be a means of preventing health problems.

MARITAL QUALITY AND PROBLEM COURSE

Mental Health

Marital distress has been implicated both in recovery from mental health problems and in relapse. Again the most robust evidence, and perhaps that most relevant to women's mental health, concerns depression. Marital problems are the topics most frequently raised by depressed patients, and failure to achieve resolution of marital problems predicts poor outcome. In fact, wives' ratings of the marital relationship predict recovery 6 months after hospitalization. The feelings of nondepressed spouses (usually husbands) toward the depressed partners also predict the speed of recovery. When spouses' responses are more positive toward the depressed persons (e.g., more protective and supportive), episodes are briefer. Finally, the effects of both medication and psychotherapy for depression appear to be attenuated when administered in the context of a distressed marriage as compared to a happy marriage. Thus, marital satisfaction is important in predicting the course and resolution of depressive episodes.

Marital distress also appears to produce relapse. Wives whose depression has remitted are particularly vulnerable to family tension and to hostile statements made by family members (often their spouses). High rates of criticism by their spouses predict relapse. Interestingly, spouses' reports that their partners are critical also predict relapse, and do so more efficiently than observer counts of the number of critical comments made by the partners. Thus, both self-reported marital distress and observer-rated marital problems predict relapse.

Interestingly, family members are less tolerant of negative symptoms (e.g., lack of volition, withdrawal) of mental disorders than they are of positive symptoms, possibly because they view such symptoms as lack of motivation or laziness. However, several disorders that occur more frequently in women (e.g., depression, agoraphobia) tend to be characterized by such negative symptoms, and hence husbands' hostility and criticism of afflicted wives is particularly important in understanding the course of these disorders.

Physical Health

Relatively few studies have investigated whether marital distress influences the course of physical health problems, especially among women. Most available studies focus on cardiac problems, with wives playing the nonpatient role. These studies have not yet established a convincing link between marital quality and the course of physical health problems, though there is some evidence that a partner's illness puts a nonpatient spouse at risk for physical and psychological problems. It appears that the degree of risk depends on features of the illness (e.g., chronicity, degree of impairment), level of marital satisfaction, changes in family functioning (e.g., finances, sex), and the characteristics of each spouse (e.g., age, coping style).

Further research is necessary before we can draw conclusions about any link between marital quality and the course of physical problems. Intuitively, however, one would expect that a satisfactory marriage would facilitate recovery from illness, and that a distressing marriage might worsen symptoms or impede recovery.

MARITAL QUALITY AND TREATMENT

Although available research on many of the issues addressed earlier remains rather rudimentary, it has some important implications for treatment. Perhaps the most important of these involve prevention. Both prevention of marital distress and alleviation of marital problems can be viewed as preventive health measures. Behaviorally oriented interventions have been shown to be most effective in both preventing and alleviating marital distress.

A further important implication is that nonpatient spouses may need to be included in the treatment of mental and physical health problems. To draw once again on depression research as an example, it has been shown that marital therapy is as effective as individual therapy in the treatment of depressed spouses. Although both marital and individual treatments are effective in alleviating depression, relative to no treatment, only marital therapy improves marital satisfaction.

Merely including a patient's partner in treatment is, however, unlikely to be sufficient. Spouse's behavior has been shown to have an impact on patients' behavior; therefore, an important factor in treatment effectiveness is likely to be change on the part of nonpatient spouses. Particular attention should be given to changing hostile and critical behaviors, as such behaviors appear to be important for psychological and physical disorders. Thus, interventions must actively involve nonpatient spouses and, where appropriate, produce change in these spouses. Notwithstanding the value of including nonpatient spouses in treatment, careful evaluation is required to determine their role in treatment and the issues that need to be addressed.

FURTHER READING

Beach, S. R. H., Sandeen, E. E., & O'Leary, K. D. (1990). *Depression in marriage*. New York: Guilford Press.
An impressive description of how to treat co-occurring depression and marital discord that includes an overview of depression, theories of depression, and a marital discord model of depression.

Brown, G. W., Harris, T. O., & Hepworth, C. (1995). Loss, humiliation and entrapment among women developing depression: A patient and non-patient comparison. *Psychological Medicine, 25,* 7–21.

This empirical paper is one of several by the first author that identifies the absence of a close, confiding relationship and difficulties in such relationships (often marriage) as risk factors for the onset of depression among women in the general population.

Burman, B., & Margolin, G. (1992). Analysis of the association between marital relationships and health problems: An interactional perspective. *Psychological Bulletin, 112,* 39–63.

A comprehensive review of the relation between marriage (marital status, marital adjustment, and marital interaction) and the etiology and course/treatment of health problems.

Cutrona, C. E. (1996). *Social support in couples: Marriage as a resource in times of stress.* Thousand Oaks, CA: Sage.

An excellent overview of social support in marriage that pays close attention to gender differences and reviews the role of social support when one partner is seriously ill.

Gotlib, I. H., & McCabe, S. B. (1990). Marriage and psychopathology. In F. D. Fincham & T. N. Bradbury (Eds.), *The psychology of marriage: Basic issues and applications.* New York: Guilford Press.

A concise, valuable review of the association between marriage (marriage status, marriage distress) and marital therapy and several psychopathologies (anxiety disorders, depression, alcoholism and schizophrenia).

18

Marital Conflict

K. Daniel O'Leary

PREVALENCE OF MARITAL CONFLICT

Conflict in marriage seems inevitable. Even among engaged couples about to be married, psychologically denigrating comments (e.g., insulting or swearing at partners) occur in at least 75%. The actual divorce rate in the United States is often debated, but estimates of the likelihood of being divorced range from 40% to 50%. Even for those who are not divorced and who would call themselves happily married, we can surmise that conflict is sometimes marked. In large nonclinical samples, the percentages of couples who are discordant vary, depending upon which populations are studied and how marital discord is measured. Overall, however, 15–20% of individuals call themselves discordant or have scores that fall into some discordant classification.

On the other hand, marriage has very positive aspects, and despite the divorce rates in the United States, approximately 95% of all men and women marry. Even among those who divorce, from 38% to 63% remarry, depending upon the age cohort. Moreover, in the United States, approximately 3–5% of the population engages in what is called "serial marriage" (i.e., at least three marriages). Thus, despite its negative aspects, marriage is a highly sought-after institution.

IMPACT OF MARITAL CONFLICT ON WOMEN

In the 1970s, sociologists such as Jesse Bernard (1972) depicted marriage as good for men and bad for women; in contrast, recent data indicate that marriage has positive physical and psychological benefits for both men and women. However, it is not the marital state per se that is most at issue when the psychological assets and liabilities of marriage are considered. Instead, it is the quality of marriage that is most likely to be predictive of the mental health of the partners. Consider the roles of marital discord and physical abuse in women's psychological states.

As Fincham notes in his chapter on marital quality, and as my colleagues and I have found, marital discord has been repeatedly associated with women's depressive symptomatology (and, incidentally, men's as well). The magnitude of the association in the general population ranges from approximately .35 to .50. Furthermore, our longitudinal research in a large sample of newly married couples indicates that marital discord is predictive of later depressive symptomatology whereas depressive symptomatology, is not predictive of later marital discord. Finally, in our own research, we found that when women who have never had a depressive episode were assessed within 3 weeks after a significant negative marital event, 38% of the women met criteria for a major depressive episode. Of interest, given my earlier description of marriage as a sought-after institution, is the finding that the events having the most negative impacts involved perceived or actual loss of the partner through affairs and/or separation.

As one might expect, physical abuse of women is also associated with depressive symptomatology. The magnitude of the association varies with the type of population studied, but the strongest associations appear in women seeking assistance from agencies for abused women. For example, we found a correlation of .54 between depressive symptomatology and both frequency and severity of violence in such a population. More startling, however, was the fact that 52% of the women had scores over 20 on the Beck Depression Inventory. For women seeking marital treatment in bidirectionally violent relationships, researchers in our clinic found a correlation of .32 between the level of physical abuse and depressive symptomatology. Furthermore, physical abuse has been found to be an immediate precipitant of women's suicide attempts, especially by African-American women seen in a large urban hospital. In summary, there is certainly a relation between physical aggression in marriage and depressive symptomatology.

Over the past 5 years, research on marital problems has shown that discord is also associated with reduced immune system functioning. In turn, it is hypothesized that this reduced immune functioning places such individuals at risk for developing varied illnesses. It does not seem far-fetched to believe that long-standing marital stress may lead to anxiety and depression, and that the physical symptomatology of anxiety or depression alone (e.g., hypervigilance and lack of sleep) could lead a person to develop various illnesses.

COPING WITH MARITAL CONFLICT

Coping with marital conflict can be accomplished in may ways. Indeed, the topics of several of the chapters in this section on coping processes reflect many of the important ways in which women can cope with marital conflict—for example, optimism; personality styles, such as repression; and social comparison ("My marriage is not that bad, compared to Jane's and Susan's"). Of course, a woman may realistically come to believe that her husband is so negative and abusive, either psychologically or physically, that the only clear alternative available to her is separation and/or divorce. Clinical judgment indicates that in many of these cases, a woman's psychological health improves following her separation from the abusive partner. None of the chapters in this section, however, cover an individual coping strategy that has been used by partners for centuries and discussed more commonly by different mental health professionals—namely, acceptance.

It is important to address the issue of coping with marital conflict as a couple's problem, because there is no consistent evidence that helping an individual will increase marital satisfaction. On the other hand, there is evidence from over a dozen studies that conjoint marital therapy leads to increases in marital satisfaction. Most recently, Shadish, Ragsdale, Glaser, and Montgomery found that in 27 studies marital therapy effect sizes were significant (d = .60) and, according to the authors, larger than one finds typically in pharmaceutical trials. In the case of physical and psychological abuse, my colleagues and I found to our surprise that helping women cope with the abuse by decreasing their self-blame, looking at alternatives to marriage, and recognizing the cycle of violence so that they could help decrease escalation of disagreements led to increases in marital satisfaction and decreases in depressive symptomatology. However, it is important to note that we had the husbands simultaneously enrolled in a treatment program that was designed to reduce their physical and psychological aggression; according to the wives' reports of the husbands' behavior, it did. In short, although the women were not in conjoint treatment, they knew that their husbands were also in treatment to address the physical and psychological abuse, and in turn the marital problems.

A recent study by Tutty, Bidgood, and Rothery showed that women in physically abusive relationships who were in group treatment also improved, in that their marital satisfaction increased and their depression decreased—even though their husbands were not in a parallel treatment program. The mechanisms of successful change in this latter program are unclear, as the husbands were not explicitly in any treatment, and their behavior may not have changed at all. Being in a group with others with whom the women could identify, having members of the group to call for support, decreasing self-blame, developing an understanding for their husbands' behavior, and perhaps recognizing some of the ways in which they themselves contributed to marital problems may have facilitated both the individual and marital improvements reported by these women.

Many programs for psychologically and physically abused women place strong emphasis on understanding the misuse of power by men and the role of the patriarchy in shaping men's domination over women. Although this depiction of certain marriages makes excellent sense, I do not know of any treatment programs using this approach that have been systematically evaluated with data from both men and women. In the program Neidig, Heyman, and I developed for women, core concepts of control and patriarchy were clearly part of the program; as mentioned above, however, the husbands were also in a program to reduce physical and psychological aggression. In any case, there is an urgent need for evaluation of treatment programs for abused women.

Both individual and marital treatment have been evaluated for women who are both depressed and maritally discordant. Beach and I compared cognitive-behavioral marital therapy for depressed, maritally discordant women and their husbands with Beck's individual cognitive therapy for the depressed, maritally discordant women. Basically, the women met criteria for major depressive disorder in the *Diagnostic and Statistical Manual of Mental Disorders,* third edition, revised; they also met a clinical cutoff on the Dyadic Adjustment Scale of marital discord. The treatment sessions were weekly and lasted for approximately 4 months. When compared to a waiting list control group, the women receiving individual cognitive therapy experienced decreases in depressive symptomatology, but not increases in marital satisfaction. On the other hand, the women receiving marital therapy experienced increases in marital satisfaction *and* reductions in depressive symptomatology. These results were replicated by Jacobson and colleagues at the University of Washington, and marital/couple therapy has been recognized in the

American Psychiatric Association's practice guidelines as a treatment for depressed individuals with significant relationship problems.

There are certain cases where the individual problems of women would seem to be best addressed individually, rather than in a marital context. For example, if a woman is coping with chronic anxiety that may be unrelated to the marriage, or if the woman has chronic low levels of depression (i.e., dysthymia), individual therapy may be the best coping mechanism—even if the marriage is distressed. In longitudinal research with newly married couples, Beach and I found that women who had symptoms of dysthymia had marriages that quickly became discordant. Women with dysthymia may be best treated with individual psychological therapy or with antidepressant medication. A multisite study sponsored by Squibb is currently being conducted to compare these two treatments for individuals with chronic depression. Finally, individual treatment is usually the treatment of choice for women coping with severe physical abuse.

Individual coping through reading and religious study or involvement may also help many women to cope with marital problems. A visit to any major bookstore reveals over 50 books on ways to understand and cope with marital/sexual problems. Although very serious marital problems may not be helped by reading material about marriage, women with lesser problems may be helped. Furthermore, a method that has been neglected by most mental health professionals as a coping strategy with family problems is prayer or meditation. Prayer was one of the two most frequently used coping mechanisms among African-American women in Washington, D.C., who were exposed to violence in the streets and in their neighborhoods. Given this finding, one would expect that prayer may be a coping method frequently used by many women dealing with marital conflict.

CONCLUSIONS

Coping with marital conflict can take many forms. Individual strategies for coping with marital conflict have not been well catalogued to assess their relative frequency but initial findings indicate that catharsis, distraction, taking action, and thinking about solutions are the four most commonly used coping strategies for dealing with daily marital stressors (personal communication, Drs. Christine Marco and Arthur Stone, The University at Stony Brook, November 21, 1995). Research is needed to evaluate the relative effects of these and other coping strategies on individual mental health indices as well as marital satisfaction. Coping with marital problems by seeking professional help has proven efficacious for many, as conjoint marital therapy has proven effective in numerous individual studies and in meta-analyses. Generally, individual therapy for marital problems has been less effective than conjoint therapy, but for certain individual problems (e.g., coping with physical abuse) it is often a preferred treatment.

FURTHER READING

Beach, S. R. H., & O'Leary, K. D. (1993). Marital discord and dysphoria: For whom does the relationship predict depressive symptoms? *Journal of Social and Personal Relationships, 10,* 405–420.
Empirical evaluation of the role of marital discord as a predictor of depressive symptomatology in a sample of 272 newlywed couples

Bernard, J. (1972). *The future of marriage.* New Haven, CT: Yale University Press.
Review of reasons why marriage is good for men and bad for women.

Christensen, A., Jacobson, N. S., & Babcock, J. (1995). Integrative behavioral couple therapy. In N. S. Jacobson & A. S. Gurman (Eds.), *Clinical handbook of couple therapy* (pp. 31–64). New York: Guilford Press.
Although acceptance has been a central part of many therapies for decades, this chapter is the first to place critical emphasis on acceptance in behavioral couple therapy.

Kiecolt-Glaser, J. K., & Glaser, R. (1992). Psychoneuroimmunology: Can psychological interventions modulate immunity? *Journal of Consulting and Clinical Psychology, 60,* 569–575.
Review of peer-reviewed studies of psychoneuroimmunology interventions. Distress and poorer personal relationships appear to be associated with down-regulation of immunity across a number of studies.

Lilliard, L. A., & Waite, L. J. (1995). Till death do us part: Marital disruption and mortality. *American Journal of Sociology, 100,* 1131–1156.
Data are provided from a sample of 5,053 men and 6,059 women to document the role that marriage plays in reducing mortality rates.

O'Leary, K. D., & Beach, S. R. H. (1990). Marital therapy: A viable treatment for depression and marital discord. *American Journal of Psychiatry, 147,* 183–186.
In this study, marital therapy was compared to Beck's cognitive therapy for depressed, maritally discordant women. Both led to reductions in depression but only marital therapy led to reduction in depressive symptomatology *and* increases in marital satisfaction.

O'Leary, K. D., Neidig, P. N., & Heyman, R. E. (1995). Assessment and treatment of partner abuse: A synopsis for the legal profession. *Albany Law Review, 58,* 1215–1234.
Review of the literature on prevalence, assessment, and treatment of partner abuse, with special emphasis for attorneys.

Shadish, W. R., Ragsdale, K., Glaser, R. R., & Montgomery, L. M. (1995). The efficacy and effectiveness of marital and family therapy. *Journal of Marital and Family Therapy, 4,* 345–360.
Reviews major findings from a multiproject metaanalysis of the effects of marital and family therapy. Effects were moderate, statistically significant, and often clinically significant.

Stark, E., & Flitcraft, A. (1995). Killing the beast within: Women battering and female suicidality. *International Journal of Health Services, 25,* 43–64.
Documents the role of wife abuse in suicide attempts in a large metropolitan hospital, and provides concrete documentation of the role of battering in suicide attempts of African-American women.

Tutty, L. M., Bidgood, B. A., & Rothery, M. A. (1993). Support groups for battered women: Research on their efficacy. *Journal of Family Violence, 8,* 325–343.
An evaluation of 12 support groups for women victims of domestic assault. Significant improvements were found on a number of measures, including self-esteem, perceived stress, marital functioning, and decreases in psychological and physical aggression.

19

Social Support

Thomas Ashby Wills

*T*his chapter considers how social support is related to health in women. "Social support" is defined broadly as (1) the number of social relationships a person has, and (2) the quality of the supportive functions that these relationships provide. It should be noted that qualitative and quantitative measures have different meanings for research on social support. With regard to health status, the chapter discusses measures of mental health and measures of physical health, indexed by disease morbidity and mortality. Research has consistently shown that social support indices are related both to better mental health and to better physical health status. The issue emphasized in this chapter is *how* social support produces better health outcomes—that is, what the mechanisms of the observed effects are.

STRUCTURAL VERSUS FUNCTIONAL MEASURES

Research has involved a distinction between two different approaches to conceptualizing and measuring social support. "Structural" measures tap the number of social relationships that exist and the structure of interconnections among these relationships. For example, a typical structural measure will ask whether the respondent is married; has close friends; has children in the household or living nearby; visits with neighbors or relatives; is employed; belongs to a community organization; or belongs to a church, temple, or other formal religious group. The intent is to obtain a count of the total number of social connections a person has, and this index, termed "network size," taps the extent of regular social relationships in which an individual participates.

"Functional" measures ask whether the respondent knows one or more persons who can provide particular functions if the respondent has a problem. The functions typically include emotional support (availability of someone who can provide confiding, reassurance, and sympathetic listening), instrumental support (someone who can provide help with instrumental needs, such as financial assistance, housework, transportation, or child care), informational support (someone who can provide useful information or advice about a problem), and social companionship (someone who can participate in leisure or recreation activities). The intent is to obtain a score for the perceived availability of these functions from a person's social relationships, thus indexing the ability of network members to be useful in helping a person to deal with problem situations.

The reason for the distinction between structural and functional measures is that research shows they are not strongly correlated. Both types of measures have been shown to be related to better health status, but structural and functional measures clearly index different aspects of social support, and their effects may occur through different mechanisms.

POSSIBLE MECHANISMS FOR SOCIAL SUPPORT'S EFFECTS ON HEALTH

When one considers the issue of how social support is related to health status, several different mechanisms are theoretically possible. The major possibilities examined in the literature are as follows:

1. *Self-esteem.* The existence of normative social connections provides status in the community, thereby producing higher self-esteem.

2. *Appraisal.* The knowledge that adequate support is available may alter the subjective appraisal of negative events, and thereby may enable persons to be less anxious or depressed in times of adversity.

3. *Coping.* Support may provide assistance with information gathering, problem solving, and implementation of solutions, thereby enabling persons to cope better with problematic situations.

4. *Help-seeking.* Social connections or social support may increase the likelihood that persons will be aware of and utilize relevant community resources (e.g., cancer screening), and thus may decrease risk for health problems.

5. *Physiological.* Support may have a direct calming effect on physiological systems involved in stress reactions, thereby producing better affective states and (potentially) better immune system functioning.

6. *Behavioral.* Support may reduce the likelihood of risk-promoting behaviors (e.g., cigarette smoking), and reduce the likelihood of relapse among persons who are trying to improve their health (e.g., quitting smoking), thereby decreasing risk for development of risk factors for physical illness.

These six mechanisms, of course, are not mutually exclusive.

SOCIAL SUPPORT AND MENTAL HEALTH

A large number of studies have found social support to be related to lower levels of anxiety or depressive symptomatology, and prospective studies have shown that high support is antecedent in time to a lower level of depression. A prominent issue concerns whether social support is primarily useful to persons currently experiencing many negative life events (termed "stress buffering"), or whether support is related to mental health independent of a person's current stress level. Research indicates that functional measures, such as emotional support or instrumental support, are consistently involved in stress-buffering effects: They are related to lower depression primarily among persons experiencing a great deal of life stress. In contrast, structural measures are generally related to mental health independent of stress level. The prevailing interpretation is that functional support is relevant for mental health because it helps a person cope with problems, whereas structural support is related to mental health because it provides regular interaction and acceptance in the community.

Research has not shown strong gender differences in the effects of support on depression. Structural and functional measures are found to be related to lower levels of depressive symptomatology for both men and women. Some research has indicated that women's mental health is more closely related to emotional support and the availability of a confidant to share concerns and feelings with; in contrast, there is evidence that men benefit from a more diffuse network of cooperative relationships and community involvements. However, the similarities appear more important than the differences, and the evidence is strong that social support is relevant to mental health for both genders.

With respect to the mechanisms of social support's effects on mental health, research is surprisingly sparse. Some studies have shown emotional support to be related to higher self-esteem, but there have been few direct tests of whether self-esteem is the sole mediator of relationships to mental health status. Mediation analyses with children have shown that social support is related to more adaptive coping and better competence, which would be consistent with a coping mechanism for support effects, but there are few such analyses from studies with adults. Thus the available evidence is consistent with self-esteem and coping mechanisms, but further research is needed to establish more definitive conclusions about how the effect of social support on mental health outcomes is mediated.

SOCIAL SUPPORT AND MORTALITY

A number of epidemiological studies based on large, representative samples have shown that persons with higher structural support scores have lower rates of mortality. These studies have employed prospective designs, using structural measures from a baseline measurement to predict mortality rates over 5- to 10-year time spans. Studies have been conducted within the United States in a metropolitan area in California, and in rural areas in Michigan and Georgia. European studies have been conducted in urban and rural areas in Sweden and Finland. Though results for men and women have varied somewhat across studies, the general finding is that persons with a lower number of social connections show a two- to threefold increase in risk of mortality over the follow-up period. The prospective design rules out the possibility that lower social connections are a consequence (not a cause) of physical illness, and statistical adjustments for age, socioeconomic status, and other important risk factors indicate that the effect of social connections is not attributable to possible confounding variables. The effect of structural support indices has been found for mortality from a variety of causes, and does not seem to be concentrated in any particular disease entity.

Research with mortality as the outcome has primarily involved structural measures. The findings indicate that the total number of a person's social connections with family, neighborhood, and community is an important protective factor with regard to physical health status. Recent Swedish studies have shown functional (emotional) support to be related to lower mortality rates, but this research is based on male samples, and its applicability to women's health remains to be determined.

A number of separate studies have suggested aspects of the mechanisms through which social connections may be related to physical health status. Persons with more social connections are less likely to be cigarette smokers or heavy drinkers, and less likely to relapse after cessation or treatment, thus providing evidence for a behavioral mechanism. In addition, several studies have shown that persons with larger social networks are more likely to utilize preventive services (e.g., mammography screening), so there is suggestive evidence that social connections are related to health through a help-seeking mechanism. The suggestion that the effect of social support operates through a direct physiological mechanism, reducing reactivity to stressors and consequent release of stress hormones, is plausible on the basis of animal research. Available evidence on humans is generally consistent with this formulation, and includes some studies showing social support to be related to lower reactivity and enhanced immune system functioning; however, the diversity of the evidence precludes definitive conclusions at this time.

SOCIAL SUPPORT, MORBIDITY, AND RECOVERY

A limitation for evidence from mortality studies is that it is difficult to determine where in the disease process support acts to produce a beneficial effect. From findings showing that support reduces the risk of mortality, it is unclear whether support operates to avert the development of risk factors in the first place (i.e., to decrease risk), or to reduce the severity of disease symptomatology among persons who have existing risk factors (i.e., to decrease morbidity) and to lessen the lethality of disease among persons who have suffered an episode of clinical illness (i.e., to promote recovery). This has been addressed in studies of morbidity and recovery from illness.

Research conducted under the general rubric of disease incidence has been tantalizing but inconsistent. Several studies have been conducted about the onset of coronary heart disease (CHD) symptoms (usually angina or myocardial infarction) among subjects who were free of any signs of disease at baseline. Although some studies of angiography samples have found social support to be related to less severe artery occlusion, incidence studies have generally failed to find a consistent predictive effect of social support with regard to onset of disease symptomatology. However, these studies are not conclusive; the follow-up intervals have been short, and the symptomatology measures have been of relatively low reliability. This research is tantalizing, because social support has been related both to behavioral indices (e.g., cigarette smoking) and to neuroendocrine indices (e.g., epinephrine and cortisol) that have known relationships to symptom onset. Yet at present there is not a compelling body of evidence relating social support to the onset of disease symptomatology.

In contrast, notable consistency has been found in studies examining the relationship of social support to recovery versus mortality from CHD. Studies with large samples of patients followed over long time periods have shown that persons with higher support levels at the time of hospitalization are more likely to recover. These studies have used representative samples and have found effects of support on recovery, even after statistical control for demographic variables, disease severity, and other risk factors. Two samples of older adults have included females, and the results have shown that social support is related to recovery among both men and women. This research provides a strong conclusion regarding a beneficial effect of social support in enhancing recovery from illness.

The way in which social support improves recovery from illness has not been clarified at the present time. Because protective effects are observed with statistical control for illness severity, it is not simply the case that persons with better support have less severe symptomatology. It is probable that both structural and functional mechanisms are involved. Persons with social connections are more likely to have someone nearby in case of a medical emergency; emotional support may reduce emotional distress among persons who are hospitalized and can motivate persistence in efforts at recovery; and instrumental support may enhance the ability of ill persons to comply with medical regimens and make lifestyle modifications that will lead to more complete recovery.

CONCLUSIONS AND IMPLICATIONS

Research has shown that persons with more social support have lower levels of depression, a lower risk of mortality, and a greater likelihood of recovery from clinical illness. The magnitude of effect for mortality outcomes is comparable to that of known biomedical risk factors for CHD. The beneficial effect of social support has been established in population-based, prospective studies that employed statistical control for relevant confounders. Though different modes of action are suggested for structural and functional measures, beneficial effects are observed for both aspects of support. Thus, the scientific evidence on social support as a protective factor is compelling. Research on the mechanisms through which social support acts as a protective factor indicates some evidence for self-esteem, help-seeking, coping, and behavioral (i.e., substance use) mechanisms as involved in the contribution of social support to better health status. Where in the disease process social support acts to produce better health outcomes has not been clarified at this time. There is moderate (but not conclusive) evidence that support may act to avert development of CHD risk factors, and there is strong evidence that support acts to enhance recovery from illness. Research to determine the point(s) at which social support acts in the disease process is a high priority for understanding how social relationships contribute to health.

The evidence on social support and health has a number of implications for practitioners who are concerned with women's health. Social support is clearly beneficial for women, so attention to a woman's social network and available support is important from the standpoint of assessment. It is clear that involving family members in a woman's treatment program will have a beneficial effect, and this should be done to the maximum extent possible. Interventions may be designed that would educate persons about how to seek help more effectively from family members and community resources, and thereby increase the ability of persons to utilize all the supportive resources that are potentially available to them. It is also evident that persons who are married, have close relationships with family members, and are socially integrated in the community have better health status. Thus it can be expected that social or policy factors that act to degrade the quality of family relationships will be reflected in higher costs for health care.

FURTHER READING

Berkman, L. F., Leo-Summers, L., & Horwitz, R. I. (1992). Emotional support and survival after myocardial infarction: A prospective, population-based study of the elderly. *Annals of Internal Medicine, 117*, 1003–1009.
This empirical article reports a study of 165 elderly persons who were followed after being hospitalized for a heart attack. Emotional support was related to longer survival time.

Berkman, L. F., Vaccarino, V., & Seeman, T. (1993). Gender differences in cardiovascular morbidity and mortality: The contribution of social networks and social support. *Annals of Behavioral Medicine, 15,* 112–118.

This review article considers evidence on how social support is related to heart disease, and discusses hypotheses about how social support processes may differ for women and men. The authors note that effects of social support are generally found to be similar for men and women.

Cohen, S., & Herbert, T. B. (1996). Health psychology: Psychological factors and physical disease from the perspective of human psychoneuroimmunology. *Annual Review of Psychology, 47,* 113–142.

The authors address evidence about psychological effects on immune system functioning. They outline how the immune system works, discuss studies on how psychological factors such as stress or depression affect immune system parameters, and consider how these may be related to infectious illness or chronic disease.

House, J. S., Landis, K. R., & Umberson, D. (1988). Social relationships and health. *Science, 241,* 540-545.

This paper discusses studies of social networks and mortality rates, conducted in several different regions and countries, which show that persons with greater social integration have lower mortality rates (after adjustment for age and a number of other control variables). The authors note that effects tend to be larger for men than for women.

Seeman, T. E., Berkman, L. F., Blazer, D., & Rowe, J. W. (1994). Social support and neuroendocrine function. *Annals of Behavioral Medicine, 16,* 95–106.

This paper considers how social support may be related to levels of stress-related hormones that have been linked to heart disease. They report findings from a study of community-dwelling elderly. Women with greater social integration had lower levels of epinephrine, norepinephrine, and cortisol.

Turk, D. C., & Kerns, R. D. (Eds.). (1985). *Health, illness, and families.* New York: Wiley.

This book includes several chapters discussing how family interaction may be linked to health status. Linkages to health behavior are discussed with reference to family systems theory, and processes linking support from family members to compliance with medical regimens are outlined. Examples from the areas of blood pressure and obesity are discussed.

Williams, R. B., Barefoot, J. C., Califf, R. M., Haney, T. L., Saunders, W. B., Pryor, D. B., Hlatky, M. A., Siegler, I. C., & Mark, D. B. (1992). Prognostic importance of social resources among patients with CAD. *Journal of the American Medical Association, 267,* 520-524.

The authors studied a large sample of patients with diagnosed coronary artery disease, following the sample for an average of 9 years after diagnosis. They found that persons with higher emotional support (married and able to confide in their spouses) had significantly lower rates of mortality, even after demographic characteristics and medical risk factors were controlled for.

Wills, T. A. (1991). Social support and interpersonal relationships. In M. S. Clark (Ed.), *Review of personality and social psychology* (Vol. 12, pp. 265-289). Newbury Park, CA: Sage.

This review article considers different types of supportive functions, including emotional, instrumental, and informational support. Availability of these functions has been related to lower levels of anxiety and depression, as well as to more favorable health status. The article notes that emotional support is most consistently indicated as beneficial for adjustment, and that this effect has been observed for persons in different stages of the life cycle.

Wills, T. A., Blechman, E. A., & McNamara, G. (1996). Family support, coping and competence. In E. M. Hetherington & E. A. Blechman (Eds.), *Stress, coping, and resiliency in children and families* (pp. 107–133). Mahwah, NJ: Erlbaum.

The authors consider how support from parents is beneficial for children and adolescents. They report findings showing that emotional and instrumental support from parents are related to better coping and greater competence for children; in turn, these effects are related to lower likelihood of adolescents' substance use.

20

Personality

H. J. Eysenck

*H*ealth, stress, and personality are much more closely interrelated than orthodox medicine is ready to acknowledge. In 1906, Sir William Osler, often called the father of British medicine, said: "It is very often much more important what person has the disease, than what disease the person has." Stress has important health consequences, but cannot be defined or understood other than in relation to personality. The same objective situation (e.g., having to address a large audience, getting divorced, being in an accident) may be traumatic for one person, leave another unmoved, and prove exciting for a third. Coping behaviors and efficiency differ from person to person and strongly influence a person's reactions and health consequences. When we talk about the health consequences of "stress," we mean the damage done by a stressor for which the victim has no appropriate coping behavior, and which leads to strong autonomic and immune system innervation. Strong emotional reactions and absence of coping behaviors characterize a person likely to suffer bad health consequences; weak emotional reactions and presence of appropriate coping behaviors characterize a person likely to remain healthy.

THE RELATIONSHIP BETWEEN PERSONALITY TYPES AND HEALTH

There are many different concepts subsumed under the heading of the psychologically healthy person. Qualities frequently named are self-directedness, low sympathetic arousal, hardiness, optimism, fighting spirit, self-efficacy, autonomy, and self-regulation. Common to most theories are the absence of neurotic emotional responses, the absence of emotional coping mechanisms, and the lack of excessive emotional dependence on other people. As an example of the relationship between personality and health, consider Figure 20.1, which shows the results of a 15-year follow-up study of 2,608 women with a mean age of about 50 at the beginning of the experiment. Each subject was interviewed and given a 105-item questionnaire designed to measure self-regulation. After 15 years,

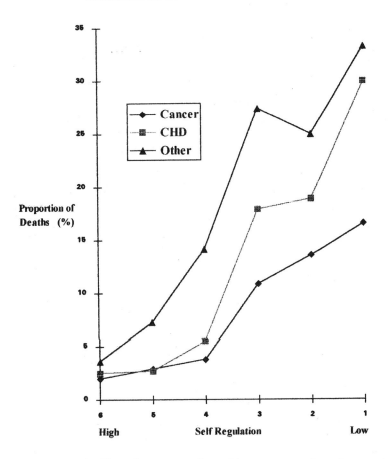

Prospective 1973-1988 Study: Females (N=2,608)

FIGURE 20.1. Degree of self-regulation (as indicated by mean questionnaire score) as a factor in mortality from cancer, coronary heart disease (CHD), and other causes. From Grossarth-Maticek and Eysenck (1995).

mortality was ascertained. Scores on the questionnaire were divided into six bands, from a high score of 6 to a low score of 1.

The results show a clear tendency for high scores to go with survival and low scores to go with mortality. This is true for death from cancer, coronary heart disease (CHD), and all other causes. It is noteworthy that women obtained significantly higher scores than men on the test; 26.6% of women were in the two highest categories, compared with 13.2% of men. As for the two bottom groups, 21.2% of men and 17.8% of women were in these categories. It is tempting to say that this difference may be relevant to the well-known tendency of women to live longer, but such a causal interpretation would be premature. (Note that these figures are independent of smoking, drinking, and other risk factors also investigated in this study.) Many other studies have shown similar health-related effects of an autonomous, self-regulated personality; however, these studies usually have disease rather than mortality as the criterion, and also have shorter follow-up periods.

If the healthy, autonomous personality constitutes one "type," disease-prone person-alities constitute the opposite end of the continuum. Over the centuries physicians have claimed that their observations have established the existence of a cancer-prone type, characterized by a strong tendency to repress emotions and show a bland exterior, in spite of strong emotional reactions inside. Such a person would also have problems in coping with depression. Such a person might be said to belong to "Type C," a personality type quite different from the CHD-prone "Type A," characterized by strong feelings of anger, hostility, and aggression. (The original hypothesis of a CHD-prone Type A was much broader, but most of the other features belonging to it have been shown to be irrelevant. For a further discussion of Type A behavior, see Basso's chapter.) Following this alphabetical description, we might follow the originators of the "Type A" notion by calling the healthy type "Type B."

There is now a great deal of evidence that Type A and Type C do exist, can be diagnosed in healthy men and women, and can be used to predict later CHD and cancer, respectively. A good example is the work of Carolyne Thomas, who studied 1,300 young medical students at Johns Hopkins University in Baltimore and then followed them up for over 40 years. She found that those students whose personalities resembled Type C were 16 times more likely to die of cancer than were those of other personality types. Temoshok and Dreher have given a good popular summary of all the available evidence, and have also included numerous case studies of women who died of cancer, with corresponding personality descriptions. My 1991 study, including similar data for CHD, also surveyed the literature; here also, the evidence shows that some Type A features in healthy men and women are considerably useful in predicting future CHD mortality.

Of course, a healthy personality does not guarantee freedom from cancer and CHD; Type A and Type C personalities are potent risk factors, but there are other risk factors largely independent from personality, such as heredity. Table 20.1 shows results for a subsample of my 1991 study. Two groups of women were chosen—namely, 33 who had died of breast cancer, and 606 who were healthy and living; the rest of the total sample of 1,085 women had died of other causes. The women in each group were divided into those with no close relative who had died of breast cancer, and those with one, two, or three such relatives. The greater the number of such relatives, the greater the genetic risk factor. It will be seen that self-regulation scores (S-R in the table) were independent of group membership; genetic risk was not correlated with personality. (There was of course a marked difference in self-regulation between healthy women and the victims of breast cancer.) CHD, personality type, and stress must always be seen in the context of all these risk factors.

TABLE 20.1. Personality (as Indicated by Mean Self-Regulation [S-R] Score) and Heredity (as Indicated by Number of Relatives Who Died of Breast Cancer) as Risk Factors for Death from Breast Cancer

Group (no. of relatives)	n	S-R	Died of breast cancer	n	%	S-R	Healthy and living	n
0	544	3.6	1	0.2	3.1	316	58.1	4.6
1	349	3.5	9	2.5	3.0	205	58.7	4.7
2	138	3.6	9	6.5	2.9	64	46.4	4.9
3	54	3.9	14	25.9	3.1	21	38.9	5.0
Totals	1,085		33	3.0		606	55.6	

INTERVENTIONS

Knowing that one is at risk for cancer or CHD, or even disease in general, is not much good to anyone unless there is some form of intervention that can help to reduce the risks. Fortunately, the evidence suggests that behavior therapy or cognitive-behavioral therapy can drastically alter the probability of contracting cancer or CHD. Several follow-up studies, in which some subjects were randomly assigned to therapy and others to control conditions, have been done on cancer-prone and CHD-prone people. In some studies therapy was individual, extending over 30 hours in all; in others group therapy was used, again running to between 20 and 30 hours in all. In one typical study using individual therapy, 50 cancer-prone persons receiving the therapy were compared with 50 no-treatment controls 10 years after therapy was concluded. Of those in the therapy group, none died of cancer; sixteen of those in the control group died. In my similar experiment with Grossarth-Maticek, 16 of 92 CHD-prone persons died of CHD in the control group, whereas only 3 died in the therapy group. Results with group therapy were similar.

To return to our self-regulation study, two groups of low scorers were formed on a random basis; one received a mixture of individual and group therapy, and the other received no therapy. There were 341 persons in each group. Nineteen years later mortality was ascertained. In the therapy group, 94 had died; in the control group, 152 had died—a very significant difference. In the therapy group, 210 were living and healthy, compared with 128 in the control group (61.7% vs. 37.6%). Thirty-seven in the therapy group, as opposed to 61 in the control group, were living but ill. Clearly therapy was effective, almost halving the number of victims in this prospective study.

Even patients suffering from cancer or CHD can be helped very significantly by behavior therapy. Thus, Spiegel and colleagues more than doubled survival time for treated women with terminal breast cancer. Other studies have obtained similar results. One of these used 100 women with terminal breast cancer, half of whom had chosen to have chemotherapy and half of whom had rejected it. In each of these groups, half received behavior therapy and half did not. Those who received chemotherapy alone, or behavior therapy alone, survived significantly longer than those receiving neither; there was no significant difference between the effects of the two types of therapy. But the effects of these two types of treatment combined synergistically: The women who received both survived significantly longer than would have been expected just from adding the effects of the two methods of therapy. Positive effects have also been found for patients suffering from CHD.

CONCLUSIONS

The evidence is now very strong in favor of the proposition that some people are psychologically predisposed to succumb to stress and develop physical diseases of various kinds (cancer, CHD, etc.), with the disease in question also partly depending on personality. There are now good theories linking personality and stress on the one hand, and disease on the other. Thus, failure to cope leads to feelings of helplessness, hopelessness, and finally depression; depression is closely linked with high cortisol levels, and cortisol is known to inhibit the activity of the immune system. Reduced activity of the immune system allows the ever-present cancer cells to grow and develop into life-threatening full-blown cancers. The demonstration that personality and stress can be changed through psychological intervention that promotes healthy coping, and thus greatly reduces the risk of illness, is a major discovery. Prevention is clearly better than cure, particularly when "cures" are hard to come by. In spite of the expenditure of $25 billion over the past 20 years by U.S. cancer groups, the incidence of cancer has *increased* by 7%, while survival time has only risen by a very small amount. Psychological treatment holds the key to prevention; *jointly with medical treatment,* it holds out great promise to increase survival time significantly. Undoubtedly, future research will greatly improve on our present methods of treatment, but already these hold considerable promise.

FURTHER READING

Eysenck, H. J. (1991). *Smoking, personality and stress: Psychosocial factors in the prevention of cancer and coronary heart disease.* New York: Springer-Verlag.
General survey of the relationship between stress and personality with cancer and CHD.

Eysenck, H. J., & Grossarth-Maticek, R. (1991). Creative novation behaviour therapy as a prophylactic treatment for cancer and coronary heart disease: Part II. Effects of treatment. *Behaviour Research and Therapy, 29,* 17–31.
Method and effect of psychological treatments for the prevention of cancer and CHD, and for prolonging life in cases of incurable cancer.

Grossarth-Maticek, R., & Eysenck, H. J. (1995). Self-regulation and mortality from cancer, coronary heart disease, and other causes: A prospective study. *Personality and Individual Differences, 19*(6), 786.
Study of the healthy personality, and the relationship between personality and mortality.

Osler, W. (1906). *Aequanimitas.* New York: McGraw-Hill.

Spiegel, D., Bloom, J. R., Kraemer, H. C., & Gottlieb, E. (1989, November 14). Effect of psychosocial treatment on survival of patients with metastatic breast cancer. *Lancet,* 888–891.
A demonstration of how psychological treatment can double the length of survival in cases of inoperable breast cancer.

Temoshok, L., & Dreher, H. (1992). *The Type C connection.* New York: Random House.
Nontechnical survey of the literature on personality and cancer.

Thomas, C. B., Duszynski, R., & Shaffer, J. W. (1979). Family attitudes reported in youth as potential predictors of cancer. *Psychosomatic Medicine, 41,* 287–302.

21

Type A Behavior Pattern

Michael R. Basso

*T*he Type A behavior pattern (TABP) is a relatively stable disposition to respond to achievement- or control-related challenges in an intensely aggressive, competitive, impatient, and ambitious manner. Characteristically, Type A individuals have an intrusive and emphatic speech style, accelerated rate of activity, intensified sense of time urgency, and heightened physiological reactivity. They also tend to have an increased propensity toward angry and irritable emotional responses.

Although much of the early research defining the TABP concerned white middle-class men, these characteristics tend to be equally applicable to women classified as Type A. As has also been found in research with men, Type A women are usually of higher socioeconomic status, have higher levels of education, and are employed in higher-status occupations than non-Type A women. When socioeconomic status is taken into account, prevalence rates of the TABP do not differ between men and women. It is estimated that at least 25% of women may be classified as Type A. Type A behavior is most prominent in middle adulthood and least so in old age. White women tend to show more Type A characteristics than black women, and salaried workers are more likely to show TABP behaviors than nonsalaried workers.

The importance of the TABP arises from its demonstrated association with the leading cause of death in men and women older than 40, coronary heart disease (CHD). In a number of studies, individuals classified as Type A were more likely to develop CHD or other vascular-related illnesses than non-Type A people. For instance, in one prospective study, employed Type A women were four times as likely as their non-Type A counterparts to develop CHD during an 8-year period. The increased incidence related to TABP was independent of other suspected risk factors, such as smoking, exercise, or family history of CHD.

In addition to CHD, other health problems seem to be associated with the TABP. Type A individuals have a greater incidence of stress-related illnesses, such as respiratory infections, ulcers, allergies, and headaches.

THEORY AND PROPOSED MECHANISMS

There are three prominent theories about the psychological mechanisms underlying the TABP. Some theorists have asserted that Type A individuals tend to perceive a high proportion of daily occurrences as threats to their personal control. In this perspective, Type A people are motivated to exert extreme control over their environment, and they are often engaged in the struggle to do so. Others have proposed that Type A individuals have exaggerated personal investment in their day-to-day affairs, and that this leads to increased affective and physiological arousal. A third perspective holds that Type A people continually feel the need to prove their self-worth, which leads to intensive striving. As yet, few direct comparisons of these three hypotheses have been conducted, and their relative validity remains uncertain.

Regardless of the motivation, the increased striving and competition of the TABP are thought to influence the pathogenesis of CHD through intensified physiological activation. As Type A behavior is elicited, increased levels of sympathetic arousal are supposedly experienced, and the release of lipids into the bloodstream is promoted. These fats tend to collect in arteries, where they contribute to constricted blood flow. In addition, with increased arousal, heart rate and blood pressure levels fluctuate; this may in turn lead to tears in arterial walls. This tearing results in plaque buildup, which further constricts circulation. Over prolonged periods of excessive and frequent sympathetic activation, arteries supplying the heart may become completely clogged. As a result, heart tissue may be damaged by lack of oxygen, and this damage may ultimately result in infarction.

Consistent with this hypothesis, there are data showing increased autonomic reactivity and arousal in Type A individuals. Type A's tend to have greater arousal than non-Type A's, especially in response to competition- or achievement-oriented stressors. Although Type-A men seem to have higher levels of arousal and reactivity than women, Type A women generally have greater arousal levels than their non-Type A counterparts. Moreover, Type A women seem especially prone to increased sympathetic reactivity and arousal during competitive interpersonal contexts.

Despite reports of greater reactivity and arousal in Type A's than in non-Type A's, a number of studies have failed to demonstrate similar outcomes. It is uncertain what accounts for these inconsistencies, because studies have varied in the method of Type A assessment, type of arousal measured (e.g., blood pressure vs. heart rate), subject characteristics (e.g., age) included, and form of arousal-eliciting challenges employed.

With respect to stress-related illness, the heightened arousal thought to be characteristic of the TABP is believed to be associated with the release of catecholamines and cortisol. These agents have been linked with reduced immune system functioning. Consequently, this may explain why Type A individuals report a higher degree of stress-related illness than non-Type A people. Although there is some evidence of increased catecholamine and cortisol responses to laboratory challenges in Type A individuals, these data are not conclusive.

ASSESSMENT

To assess the TABP, several strategies have been developed. The "gold standard" is the structured interview (SI). During the SI, a trained interviewer interacts with the interviewee in a manner that is intended to elicit Type A responses, such as impatience, frustration, and anger. The content of the individual's statements is not as important as vocal stylistics and nonverbal mannerisms are. The degree to which the interviewee interrupts, speaks quickly or emphatically, has a brief response latency, or responds with heightened emotion is regarded with particular attention.

The SI is considered the most valid method of assessing the TABP. It also has been the most successful method of predicting subsequent CHD. Although it was developed primarily with white middle-class men, with few exceptions, men and women tend to show equivalent Type A characteristics; one difference is that men are prone to talk louder, whereas women are apt to show more verbal competition.

Despite its advantages, the SI does have several potential shortcomings. The SI requires the interviewer to have a relatively high degree of training. Since Type A classifications are based on subjective ratings, they are prone to error and bias. Doubts can also be cast on the SI's reliability, since it is not standardized, and adequate norms do not exist. Moreover, the SI typically takes at least 15 minutes to complete, and only one person can be assessed at a time. Thus, it is costly and time-consuming.

To address these concerns, several self-report measures have been created. In addition to being relatively cheap and quick, TABP questionnaires are objective and not dependent upon subjective interviewer ratings. The questionnaires also provide a wider range of scores to estimate Type A behavior; depending upon its version, the SI provides only four to five classifications of TABP. Consequently, self-report measures may be more likely to capture subtle distinctions in the degree to which individuals show Type A characteristics.

There are three widely used self-report measures of the TABP: the Jenkins Activity Survey (JAS), the Framingham Type A Scale (FTAS), and the Bortner Rating Scale (BRS). Each of these scales is briefer than the SI and can be easily administered with little training. The JAS, BRS, and FTAS were intended to assess the same construct, and they are moderately correlated with one another. However, these questionnaires are not equivalent measures of the TABP. For instance, the JAS seems to assess motivation to exert control over the environment, whereas the BRS and FTAS are associated with neuroticism or anxiety. Hence these scales seem to measure different aspects of the TABP.

Additional problems are particularly evident when considering that the JAS, BRS, and FTAS tend to have relatively weak correlations with Type A classifications made by the SI. Moreover, their relationship with CHD is uncertain. In various studies, scores on the JAS, BRS, and FTAS have been correlated with CHD disease endpoints, but these findings have often not been replicated in subsequent research. Therefore, choosing a self-report TABP measure over the SI should be done with caution.

TREATMENT

Although there is no reliable evidence of a causative role of the TABP in CHD, intervention programs have been developed to diminish Type A behaviors in at-risk individuals. Some initial outcomes have been encouraging. Generally, treatment programs have been patterned after cognitive-behavioral treatment frameworks. Most studies have demonstrated success in significantly reducing Type A behaviors.

Some intervention programs have also decreased recurrent CHD risks. For instance, in one study, patients who had previously sustained a myocardial infarction were assigned to one of two treatments. One condition received cognitive-behavioral therapy, relaxation training, and cardiac counseling over the course of 60 group sessions. Type A behaviors, beliefs, and coping mechanisms were targeted for change. A control condition received cardiac counseling only. At follow-up, 4.5 years after the initiation of treatment, Type A behaviors, cardiac morbidity, and mortality were significantly reduced among individuals in the treatment condition relative to those in the control condition. Hence, there is some support for the use of cognitive-behavioral therapeutic interventions to reduce recurrent CHD.

CONCLUDING CONSIDERATIONS

In tracing the history of the TABP construct, it is interesting to note its initial acclaim. For perhaps the first time, a psychological construct was found to have a reliable relationship with health functioning. Yet, as more recent research has often failed to replicate or support initial findings, the TABP's fame has evolved into a certain notoriety. These recent negative findings may be partially attributed to differences in TABP assessment between the early and later research. Most of the early studies that showed a relationship between TABP and coronary morbidity utilized the SI. Later studies used questionnaires of dubious validity. Consequently, recent negative findings may have been attributable to measurement error.

Nonetheless, even when Type A behavior is assessed with the SI, questions regarding the relationship between the TABP and illness remain. In particular, it appears that disease endpoints have stronger relationships with subcomponents of the TABP than with the global construct. For instance, CHD has been reported to have a stronger association with hostile and angry responses from the SI than with SI-derived global TABP ratings. (For a further discussion of hostility and anger per se, see Smith's chapter.) In other studies, time urgency, impatience, and hard-driving competitive tendencies have accounted for more variance in health complaints than have estimates of global TABP.

These developments may result in a refined understanding of the TABP construct. Distinguishing the "toxic" from the "nontoxic" Type A components may result in improved prediction of disease endpoints. Increasingly valid assessment strategies may be developed by focusing upon more circumscribed constructs, instead of the global TABP, which can be an unwieldy conglomeration of related behaviors. Moreover, intervention outcomes may be enhanced by specifically targeting "toxic" Type A components for change.

Further refinement of the TABP construct may be realized by addressing potential gender differences. Few studies have investigated whether Type A men and women differ in their expression of Type A behaviors, physiological reactivity, cardiac morbidity, or response to therapeutic intervention. Generally, when gender differences have been demonstrated, they have been relatively narrow; however, the empirical base is sufficiently limited and contradictory that conclusive statements cannot be made with great confidence. Paralleling general medical research, psychological research has tended to neglect women's health issues. Hopefully as investigations of the TABP and its component aspects continue, this lack of attention will be addressed.

FURTHER READING

Baker, L. J., Dearborn, M., Hastings, J. E., & Hamberger, K. (1984). Type A behavior in women: A review. *Health Psychology, 3,* 477–497.
This is a relatively early review of findings concerning the TABP in women; it highlights the relative paucity of research in the area.

Harbin, T. J. (1989). The relationship between the Type A behavior pattern and physiological responsivity: A quantitative review. *Psychophysiology, 26,* 110–119.
This is a meta-analysis of psychophysiological research concerning the TABP. Specific findings regarding women are noted.

Houston, B. K., & Snyder, C. R. (Eds.). (1988). *Type A behavior pattern: Research, theory, and intervention.* New York: Wiley.
This is a comprehensive summary of Type A research that documents positive and negative research findings. It also details the beginnings of a "paradigm switch" in Type A investigations.

Strube, M. J. (Ed.). (1990). Type A behavior [Special issue]. *Journal of Social Behavior and Personality, 5*(1).
This is a compendium of research, opinions, and theory regarding the TABP. It includes several interesting experiments, and insightful analysis of epidemiological, assessment, and treatment research.

Thoeresen, C. E., & Low, K. G. (1990). Women and the Type A behavior pattern: Review and commentary. *Journal of Social Behavior and Personality, 5,* 117–133.
This is a more recent review of Type A findings in women; it complements and extends the review by Baker et al. (1984).

22

Hostility

Timothy W. Smith

For centuries, medical writers have speculated that chronic anger and related cognitive and behavioral processes (i.e., hostility and aggression) adversely affect physical health. Although anger and hostility have been discussed primarily in the context of cardiovascular disease, these unhealthy effects have been implicated in a wide variety of serious illnesses. In the last 20 years, scores of empirical studies have addressed this issue, with generally supportive results. In a 1996 meta-analysis of this literature, Miller and his colleagues found that hostility was a reliable predictor of coronary heart disease (CHD), coronary death, and premature death from general causes. However, like much of the research in epidemiology and medicine, the overwhelming majority of studies were conducted on samples that were exclusively or disproportionately male. Thus, this centuries-old question is answered less clearly when it comes to women's health. Nonetheless, the limited evidence available suggests that anger and hostility do pose a potential threat to the health of women. Thus, the prevention and management of illness among women might profitably address these factors.

DEFINITIONS AND ASSESSMENT

The term "hostility" is the most widely used in referring to this area of research. However, it is most accurately reserved for referring to the cognitive component of an interrelated set of phenomena. In this sense, hostility refers to a negative attitude toward others, consisting of enmity, denigration, cynicism, mistrust, and ill-will. Hostility is often—but not always—associated with "anger," an emotional phenomenon varying in intensity from mild irritation to rage. Like all emotions, anger can be considered as a transitory state or a dispositional trait. In this latter meaning, anger refers to a very negative emotion that individuals typically experience with great frequency and intensity. Thus, characteristically or chronically angry persons experience the emotional state of anger often, and when they do it is likely to be more pronounced and prolonged than episodes of anger typically experienced by people lower in this disposition. Closely related emotions include contempt and resentment. "Aggression" refers to attacking, hurtful, or destructive overt behavior, and it is manifested in a wide variety of subtle and obvious, verbal and physical actions. Although these cognitive, emotional, and physical processes often co-occur, their conceptual and empirical distinctiveness is potentially important. It may be that they are differentially related to health, or that they are related through different pathways or mechanisms. Furthermore, there may be sex differences in the relative importance or effects of these processes. In the discussion that follows, I focus primarily on hostility although anger and aggression are also considered to some extent.

Individual differences in hostility (and in anger and aggression) can be assessed through self-report questionnaires, behavioral ratings derived from clinical interviews, and ratings by significant others. Many different assessment devices have been used in this area of research, and the specific instruments vary considerably as to their psychometric quality and the extent to which they have been validated with samples of women. Several of the most widely used questionnaires are among the weakest psychometrically, but their availability in large archival data sets has facilitated the rapid development of a longitudinal literature on the health consequences of hostility. Behavioral ratings are free of many of the self-report biases and artifacts that possibly limit much of the literature on hostility and health, but they require extensive training of raters in order to achieve acceptable levels of reliability and validity. Researchers and clinicians would be wise to consult one of several reviews of these assessment devices, such as the 1994 review by Barefoot and Lipkus or my 1992 article, before making a selection.

ASSOCIATION WITH HEALTH

Until recently, well-controlled, prospective studies of women were sufficiently rare as essentially to preclude all but the most preliminary conclusions regarding the health consequences of hostility in women. One important exception to this trend can be found in a 1995 study of Danish men and women by Barefoot and his colleagues. In a sample of over 400 men and 300 women followed for 25 years, hostility was associated with increased risk of myocardial infarction in both sexes, even when traditional risk factors (e.g., smoking, cholesterol levels, etc.) were controlled for. In addition, hostility was also a significant predictor of all-cause mortality in both men and women, again even when traditional risk factors were controlled for. Cartwright and her colleagues, and Adams, have recently reported similar evidence of prospective effects of hostility on subsequent health in exclusively female samples. However, these studies did not include the unambiguous medical outcomes of myocardial infarction and premature death; instead, they assessed longitudinal changes in self-reported health. As a result, they must be considered less definitive. Thus, although conclusions about the health consequences of hostility must be considered to be less well established in women than in men, the limited data that do exist suggest that chronically angry and hostile women are at increased risk of serious medical illness.

What mechanism accounts for the statistical association between hostility and health? In the general literature on hostility and disease, three primary mechanisms have been suggested. The "psychophysiological reactivity" hypothesis holds that hostile individuals display greater stress-induced increases in blood pressure, heart rate, and circulating levels of stress hormones in response to daily stressors. Recurring activation of these physiological responses over a period of many years, in turn, is expected to initiate and hasten the development of cardiovascular and possibly other diseases. The many studies on the topic generally support this hypothesis, and further demonstrate that hostility is not associated with enhanced reactivity in response to nonsocial stressors, such as cognitive challenges. A few studies have examined this hypothesis in women and had supportive results. For example, Suarez and his colleagues, and Powch and Houston, compared hostile to nonhostile young women; they found that the hostile young women displayed larger increases in blood pressure and other physiological responses when exposed to interpersonal stressors, such as conflict or harassment. As expected, in the absence of relevant interpersonal stress, hostility is not related to women's psychophysiological responsiveness. If this heightened physiological reactivity is characteristic of hostile women's responses to daily stresses and strains, then it is possible that these reactions are an important pathway between hostility and health. However, as in the case of the epidemiological research on the health effects of hostility, research with men predominates in this literature on psychophysiological mechanisms. As a result, conclusions concerning women must be tentative.

A second model of the link between hostility and health ascribes a central role to the psychosocial correlates of hostility. In this view, hostile persons experience less social support and greater interpersonal stress than do nonhostile persons because of the interpersonal consequences of their negative attitudes about others and their disagreeable behavior. The hostile persons' suspiciousness, mistrust, and general animosity are likely to lead them to be cold and unfriendly toward others, and perhaps openly argumentative and antagonistic. Such overt responses are likely to undermine sources of potential social support and to increase the experience of interpersonal conflict. Increased stress and reduced support, in turn, should increase the hostile individual's risk of disease. A number of studies have reported evidence of this type of psychosocial vulnerability in hostile individuals, and several of these studies have included large samples of women. That is, both at home and at their jobs, hostile women experience more interpersonal conflict and less social support than do their nonhostile counterparts.

A third view suggests that unhealthy behaviors, such as smoking, excessive alcohol intake, and poor diet, are the links between hostility and health. Although this literature is somewhat inconsistent, it generally supports the hypothesis that hostility is associated with poor health practices. Women are represented in considerable numbers in several of the important studies of this type, although less well than men are. Thus, one of the ways in which hostility might contribute to disease in women is through its association with unhealthy behaviors, but again conclusions must be tentative.

It is important to note that these mechanisms are by no means mutually exclusive. Rather, hostility may be a robust predictor of adverse health outcomes because it exerts several negative effects on health. In terms of our understanding of psychosocial influences on health and the design of related prevention strategies, hostility may be particularly important because of these multiple adverse factors.

INTERVENTION CONSIDERATIONS

The literature reviewed above suggests that hostility may indeed be a significant risk factor for serious disease in women, and that these effects are likely to be mediated by psychophysiological, psychosocial, and behavioral processes. One implication of these findings is that it may be beneficial to address hostility in disease prevention and health promotion efforts. This suggestion raises two questions. First, can chronic anger and hostility be modified? Second, if it can, does successful reduction in these characteristics lead to improved health among women? Several interventions have been found to be effective in reducing anger and hostility, and they address the emotional, cognitive, and behavioral components of this phenomenon. These include relaxation training, stress management, cognitive restructuring, and assertiveness and communication skills training. Most of the studies documenting the effectiveness of such techniques have relied heavily on male samples, so conclusions regarding their effectiveness in women must be tentative. The selection of specific treatments from the variety typically available depends on the characteristics of the individual case or situation. However, typical elements within most comprehensive approaches include increasing awareness of anger through self-monitoring, relaxation, and disruption of angry emotional responses; cognitive restructuring of hostile thoughts; and training in problem-solving and interpersonal skills that might replace aggressive interpersonal tactics. Thus, the correlated but distinct nature of anger, hostility, and aggressive behavior suggests that several therapeutic strategies can be useful.

As to whether or not such interventions ultimately benefit health, there are very few long-term outcome data for men or women. Certainly many of the interventions listed above have been found useful in the primary and secondary prevention of cardiovascular illness. However, few of the relevant studies have targeted anger and hostility directly, and women are even less well represented in studies of this type than in the literature discussed above. Fortunately, even if ultimate health benefits remain unknown, the reduction of anger and hostility typically results in improved quality of life. That is, successful reduction of anger and hostility is generally its own reward. This is not to say that therapeutic management of these issues is necessarily easy. Angry and hostile individuals are often initially resistant to intervention, partly because they externalize the source of any difficulties they are experiencing. A hostile woman may believe that her only difficulties are the undeserved frustration and mistreatment she suffers as a result of others' selfish and unjust actions. These attitudes and attributions often make the development of a workable therapeutic alliance an essential and difficult challenge in the early phases of any intervention program.

FINAL CONSIDERATIONS

Anger, hostility, and aggressive behavior are closely linked to sex role behaviors and expectations. Although men are generally more angry, hostile, and aggressive than women, the manifestations and functions of these phenomena in men and women may be quite distinct. For example, the expression of anger by women is often intended to serve a constructive function in maintaining relationships, whereas anger expression is more likely to be aggressive or interpersonally controlling among men. Thus, the nature, adaptiveness, and context for the various facets of this interrelated set of psychological characteristics are quite likely to vary for men and women. Therefore, researchers and clinicians alike must exercise caution in conceptualizing, assessing, and changing these potential risk factors. Assumptions based on conceptualizations and research derived from the study of men may be seriously misleading. Future research should include women in sufficient numbers as to permit more definitive conclusions about the nature of hostility, the validity of related assessments, the extent to which it influences health, and the mechanisms underlying such effects. Finally, the effectiveness of primary and secondary prevention strategies must be evaluated in samples of women that are sufficiently large as to permit a more definitive evaluation of the benefits of such efforts for women's health.

FURTHER READING

Adams, S. H. (1994). Role of hostility in women's health during mid-life: A longitudinal study. *Health Psychology, 13,* 488–495.
A prospective study of self-reported health consequences of hostility in women.

Adler, N., & Matthews, K. A. (1994). Health psychology: Why do some people get sick and some people stay well? *Annual Review of Psychology, 45,* 229–259.
An integrative review of psychosocial risk factors, including hostility.

Barefoot, J. C., Larsen, S., Lieth, L. V. D., & Schroll, M. (1995). Hostility, incidence of acute myocardial infarction, and mortality in a sample of older Danish men and women. *American Journal of Epidemiology, 142,* 477–484.
A unique and sound study of the effects of hostility on objective health outcomes in both men and women.

Barefoot, J. C., & Lipkus, I. M. (1994). Assessment of anger and hostility. In A. W. Siegman & T. W. Smith (Eds.), *Anger, hostility, and the heart* (pp. 43–66). Hillsdale, NJ: Erlbaum.
A thorough review of the strengths and weaknesses of current assessment devices.

Cartwright, L. K., Wink, P., & Kmetz, C. (1995). What leads to good health in mid-life women physicians? Some clues from a longitudinal study. *Psychosomatic Medicine, 57,* 284–292.
A well-controlled prospective study of the health effects of hostility and other psychosocial risk factors in upper-socioeconomic-status women.

Deffenbacher, J. L. (1994). Anger reduction: Issues, assessment, and intervention strategies. In A. W. Siegman & T. W. Smith (Eds.), *Anger, hostility, and the heart* (pp. 239–270). Hillsdale, NJ: Erlbaum.
An extensive review of methods for modifying anger, hostility, and aggressive behavior.

Miller, T. Q., Smith, T. W., Turner, C. W., Guijarro, M. L., & Hallet, A. J. (in press). A meta-analytic review of research on hostility and physical health. *Psychological Bulletin.*
A quantitative review of the literature linking hostility and health.

Powch, I. G., & Houston, B. K. (in press). Hostility, anger-in, and cardiovascular reactivity in women. *Health Psychology.*
A recent, well-controlled study of the psychophysiological correlates of hostility in women.

Siegler, I. C. (1994). Hostility and risk: demographic and lifestyle variables. In A. W. Siegman & T. W. Smith (Eds.), *Anger, hostility, and the heart* (pp. 199–214). Hillsdale, NJ: Erlbaum.
A review of the literature on the health behavior correlates of hostility.

Smith, T. W. (1992). Hostility and health: Current status of a psychosomatic hypothesis. *Health Psychology, 11,* 139–150.
A review of conceptual definitions, health consequences, and mechanisms in hostility and health.

Smith, T. W., & Williams, P. G. (1992). Stress reduction in the prevention and management of coronary heart disease. In F. G. Yanowitz (Ed.), *Coronary heart disease prevention* (pp. 427–446). New York: Marcel Dekker.
A review of behavioral treatments for cardiovascular patients, including the integration of hostility-related treatments into general patient management plans.

Suarez, E. C., Harlan, E., Peoples, M. C., & Williams, R. B., Jr. (1993). Cardiovascular and emotional responses in women: The role of hostility and harassment. *Health Psychology, 12,* 459–468.
A recent, well-controlled study of psychophysiological responses in hostile and nonhostile women.

23

Achievement

Sigrid B. Gustafson

*E*ducational, vocational, and developmental psychologists have generally devoted a great deal of attention to fostering academic and career achievement among females. However, because much of this work has compared females to males, as though the male career trajectory were a "standard" against which female accomplishments should be judged, individual differences among girls and women have received less consideration than they perhaps deserve. The purpose of this chapter is to illustrate the very different paths followed by two groups of females—both intellectually gifted—with respect to their scholastic and occupational development from early adolescence to early adulthood.

THE PERSON APPROACH VERSUS THE VARIABLE APPROACH

Research psychologists using nonexperimental designs traditionally investigate associations among variables. In the area of occupational success, for example, psychologists have examined the extent to which intelligence is related to achievement, as well as the degree to which psychosocial variables (e.g., peer and parental support, gender roles, and expectations and values derived from a variety of sources) influence females' selection of and adjustment to academic and career choices. In addition to the significance of psychosocial concepts, we also know that personality variables—such as motivation to achieve, confidence in one's own capability, persistence, tolerance for delayed rewards, and a belief in one's power to effect desirable outcomes—are important aspects of successfully meeting academic and career challenges.

But what psychologists have learned about the relations among variables has not necessarily illuminated the experience of individuals. And because individuals, not variables per se, constitute the focus of this chapter, the material presented here is based on a person approach. The person approach—in this case, applied only to females—describes each individual in terms of her pattern across variables believed to be salient to her functioning in a given domain. Cluster-analytic procedures are used to combine individuals with similar patterns into homogeneous groups. The differential functioning of the individuals who make up these groups can then be assessed with respect to a single outcome measure, or in relation to patterns from another domain.

THE IMPORTANCE OF LONGITUDINAL STUDIES

By its very nature, career achievement is most meaningfully conceptualized as lifetime accomplishment. The stellar performance of a highly intelligent girl in junior high school is lauded primarily because society believes that such behavior predicts continuing success. If the goal of formal education is to prepare students for adult life, findings that reach across significant portions of the lifespan can provide unique insights into the psychological processes underlying long-term achievement. Thus, the further readings listed at the end of this chapter highlight prospective longitudinal studies and, wherever possible, focus on gifted females.

DIFFERENCES AMONG GIFTED GIRLS
IN EARLY ADOLESCENCE

Generally speaking, longitudinal research on gifted children—such as Terman's famous Life-Cycle Study, which began with preadolescents whose IQs were at least 135—has demonstrated that girls (and boys, for that matter) who display high intellectual capability are neither social "misfits" nor emotionally maladjusted. To the contrary, they are frequently better adapted than are their less gifted counterparts. Nevertheless, over the years a few cross-sectional studies have shown a relation, for both sexes, between giftedness and certain personal and social characteristics that bring individuals into conflict with their school and home environments. These characteristics include oversensitivity, resistance to conforming, emotional intensity, isolation, and poor peer relations.

These conflicting results suggest that all gifted individuals do not function in the same manner; however, until the study described here was initiated, research had glossed over individual differences among the gifted—and among gifted females. In contrast, the Swedish longitudinal study of female career development, which Magnusson and I conducted with data gathered regularly from 1968 to 1982, investigated this issue extensively.

The first finding of interest was that two distinct groups of particularly bright 13-year-old girls emerged from a cluster analysis of 403 female subjects whose parents represented the full range of the socioeconomic spectrum. These two groups reflected different patterns across five variables that were selected to capture their intellectual ability and their school adaptation in early adolescence: IQ score, achievement in mathematics, achievement in Swedish, self-perceived ability, and self-reported adaptation to the academic aspects of school life. (All reported means are standardized.)

The girls in the first group ($n = 65$) were labeled the Gifted, High-Adapted Achievers, reflecting the facts that their mean IQ was almost one standard deviation above average (0.85); their achievement means in both math (0.97) and Swedish (1.11) were a standard deviation above average; their mean perception of their own academic ability was as high as the scale allowed; and their school adaptation mean was one standard deviation above average (1.07). In short, these were girls who at age 13 were performing well in and adjusting well to the educational arena, which technically constituted their first full-time "job."

The second group of bright girls, called the Gifted, Low-Adapted Achievers (*n* = 38), displayed a different and somewhat disturbing pattern. Their mean IQ (1.33), as well as their achievement means in both math (1.18) and Swedish (1.31), were all about one and one-third standard deviations above average, and their mean perception of their ability was, like that of the first group, as high as the scale could measure. However, although their intelligence and scholastic achievement exceeded that of the first group, this second group's self-reported adaptation to the academic aspects of the school environment yielded a mean that was one-third of a standard deviation *below* average (–0.34).

Obviously, these two groups were not undergoing the same school experience, despite the high intelligence they manifested in common. The first group had already, in early adolescence, found a stable developmental "niche" that was likely to be strongly reinforced by the reactions of the adult community. No "tension" was evidenced in this pattern. One might logically expect these girls to continue succeeding in school, and ultimately to choose careers commensurate with high academic achievement. By contrast, the pattern characterizing the second group was inherently unstable. The incongruity between intellectual giftedness and lack of adjustment to scholastic demands bespoke an experience that would be likely to change over time. The tension demonstrated by this pattern suggested that if adjustment did not improve, performance (though not intelligence per se) would deteriorate.

STABILITY AND CHANGE IN MIDADOLESCENCE

When ability and school adaptation patterns were clustered for each of 485 subjects at age 16, the expectations of stability and change were confirmed. The variables that defined each girl's pattern were IQ score, achievement in science (the girls were not all enrolled in the same math classes by age 16), achievement in Swedish, self-perceived ability, and self-reported adaptation to the academic aspects of school life. Once again, two groups of gifted girls emerged.

The first group, again called the Gifted, High-Adapted Achievers (*n* = 84), exhibited a mean IQ that was a standard deviation above average (1.07), achievement means in both science (1.31) and Swedish (1.26) that were one and one-third standard deviations above average, a mean level of self-perceived ability (0.85) that was almost a standard deviation above average, and a mean level of school adaptation (0.76) that was three-quarters of a standard deviation above average. As predicted, these girls were also, to a significant extent ($p < .0001$), the *same* girls who had constituted the Gifted, High-Adapted Achievers at age 13. In fact, the *only* group that the age-13 Gifted, High-Adapted Achievers "flowed" significantly into 3 years later was the age-16 Gifted, High-Adapteds.

The second group of gifted girls observed in midadolescence was once more made up of the Gifted, Low-Adapted Achievers (*n* = 40), whose IQ mean was more than a standard deviation above average (1.16), whose achievement means in science (0.81) and in Swedish (1.10) were also about a standard deviation above average, and whose self-perceived ability mean was above average (0.65), but whose mean level of self-reported academic adaptation was three-quarters of a standard deviation *below* average (–0.75). As expected, these girls were, to a significant extent ($p < .0001$), the *same* girls who had formed the group of Gifted, Low-Adapted Achievers at age 13.

It was noteworthy that the age 16 Low-Adapteds' school performance, though certainly respectable, had deteriorated over time and no longer surpassed that of the age-16 High-Adapteds, despite the Low-Adapteds' higher IQ mean. Even the Low-Adapteds' belief in their own ability no longer matched that of the High-Adapteds. Moreover, the Low-Adapteds' school adaptation had decreased markedly by midadolescence.

This overall pattern suggested that the Low-Adapteds' likelihood of continuing formal education beyond the compulsory age of 16, regardless of their intellectual capability, was lower than that of their High-Adapted counterparts. Further investigation provided additional support for this prognosis. At age 13, the Gifted, High-Adapted mean did not differ significantly from the Gifted, Low-Adapted mean on a measure of educational aspiration that asked subjects how many years of postcompulsory education (from "none" to "more than 5") they would accept in order to enter their chosen occupation. At age 16, however, although *all* High-Adapteds and *all* the Low-Adapteds were enrolled in a college preparatory curriculum, the difference was dramatic. On a scale of educational aspiration that included and expanded the measure taken at age 13, the High-Adapteds' mean (1.03) was a standard deviation *above* average, whereas the Low-Adapteds' mean (–0.73) was three-quarters of a standard deviation *below* average.

Finally, in line with the second scenario that was consistent with the inherent instability of the age-13 Low-Adapted pattern, a significant number ($p < .05$) of these 13-year-olds *did* resolve the tension that their ability/adaptation pattern had indicated in early adolescence, and in midadolescence were among the age-16 *High*-Adapteds. No other significant "developmental streams" led into the Gifted, Low-Adapted Achiever group at age 16.

DIFFERENCES IN FAMILY BACKGROUNDS

So far, we know that the Gifted, High-Adapted Achievers had found a compatible "fit" with the school environment in early adolescence, and that their academic commitment had blossomed over time. In contrast, an equally intelligent group of girls had appeared academically unmotivated in early adolescence, and in midadolescence seemed increasingly disinclined to pursue higher education, despite the fact that they were enrolled in all the courses that would prepare them to do so.

To give us a better understanding of the difference between these two groups, the family seemed a promising area to investigate. The first strategy was to cluster the family backgrounds of *all* the girls ($n = 456$) according to the similarity of their patterns across five measures completed by the girls' parents when the girls were age 13. Three of these measures assessed socioeconomic status (SES) (family income, fathers' education, and mothers' education), and two assessed parental values (parents' aspiration for their daughters' education, and parents' evaluation of their daughters' academic capability). The results were as hypothesized: Regardless of their SES, only parents who expressed high aspiration for their 13-year-old daughters *and* a strong belief in their capability were significantly represented among the parents of Gifted, High-Adapted daughters 3 years later. Education-oriented values, *not* SES, defined the early adolescent family patterns of the midadolescent High-Adapteds. And such values occurred in low-, middle-, and high-SES families alike. (Furthermore, with the exception that Sweden has virtually no abject poverty, the SES spectrum is close enough to that of the United States to allow meaningful comparisons.)

Parents' reports of education-oriented values when their daughters were aged 13 were also, to a significant extent, a prerequisite for their parenting 16-year-old *Low-Adapted* daughters. However, SES played a strong role in the family backgrounds of the Low-Adapted Achievers. Only one family background produced a significant number of Gifted, Low-Adapteds: the *highest*-SES parents in the entire sample. It was also noteworthy that the family SES means (income and each parent's educational level) of the age-13 Low-Adapteds who were still Low-Adapteds at age 16 were one-half to one standard deviation *higher* than the comparable means of the age-13 Low-Adapteds who were among the age-16 High-Adapteds.

Actually, the high-SES effect on the Gifted, Low-Adapteds had been hypothesized. The rationale was that the *only* parents who could have successfully maintained the high performance of daughters who seemed to be rejecting education as a long-term commitment at age 13 would be parents who consistently exerted pressure motivated by a desire to see their own achievements reenacted by their offspring. If such were the case, these Low-Adapteds might well be expected to "drop out" of the academic game as soon as they were no longer under their parents' control.

DIFFERENCES IN FAMILY DYNAMICS

That the Gifted, High-Adapteds (at both 13 and 16) seemed to have internalized their parents' values suggested harmonious dynamics between parents and their High-Adapted daughters. In contrast, because the Gifted, Low-Adapteds had rejected their parents' values, but were still under parental control in midadolescence, their family dynamics were expected to be more conflicted. Indeed, further investigation of data collected when the girls were 15 revealed that, compared to the High-Adapteds, the Low-Adapteds identified significantly less with their mothers ($p < .001$), reported significantly poorer relations with their mothers ($p < .05$), and perceived their parents as less approving of them ($p < .01$). However, the Low-Adapteds were significantly more dependent upon their parents to make decisions for them ($p < .01$) than were the High-Adapteds. This last finding supported the earlier conjecture that the parents of the Low-Adapteds exerted considerable control over their gifted but unmotivated daughters over the 3-year period assessed.

ACHIEVEMENT CONSEQUENCES IN ADULTHOOD

As expected, in young adulthood the Gifted, High-Adapted Achievers from supportive families whose values they embraced fared far better in the career domain than did the Gifted, Low-Adapted Achievers, who had not adjusted to scholastic demands since at least age 13, despite parental pressure to excel. By age 26 the High-Adapteds had achieved significantly higher levels ($p < .0001$) of both education and occupation than those exhibited by the Low-Adapteds. Furthermore, the High-Adapteds were overrepresented in occupations that required a university education or the equivalent (e.g., teacher, physical therapist, physician), and underrepresented in occupations that required virtually no academic preparation (e.g., hospital orderly, day care worker). The High-Adapteds were also overrepresented among the women who had no children by age 26.

Finally, and not surprisingly, the High-Adapteds as adults retrospectively evaluated their school experience significantly more favorably ($p < .05$) than did the Low-Adapteds.

These retrospective memories, and their congruence with data gathered prospectively, once again affirm the central theme of this chapter—that over the course of 13 years, two groups of intellectually gifted women experienced powerfully different lives.

FURTHER READING

Eccles, J. S. (1985). Why doesn't Jane run? In F. D. Horowitz & M. O'Brien (Eds.), *The gifted and talented: Developmental perspectives* (pp. 251–300). Washington, DC: American Psychological Association.
Comprehensive review of research on sex differences among the gifted. Covers longitudinal and cross-sectional studies, and proposes and discusses a model of achievement-related choices.

Friedman, H. S., Tucker, J. S., Schwartz, J. E., Tomlinson-Keasey, C., Martin, L. R., Wingard, D. L., & Criqui, M. H. (1995). Psychosocial and behavioral predictors of longevity: The aging and death of the "Termites." *American Psychologist, 50,* 69–78.
Most recent report on the subjects of Terman's Life-Cycle Study. Presents results of a variety of statistical survival analyses and discusses "relative hazards." Addresses sex differences in longevity.

Gustafson, S. B. (1994). Female underachievement and over achievement: Parental contributions and long-term consequences. *International Journal of Behavioral Development, 17,* 469–484.
Concentrates on two groups—underachievers and overachievers—that were part of the overall Swedish longitudinal study of female achievement.

Gustafson, S. B., & Magnusson, D. (1991). *Female life careers: A pattern approach* (Vol. 3). Hillsdale, NJ: Erlbaum.
Comprehensive longitudinal study of the educational, career, and psychosocial development of over 400 Swedish females from 1965 to 1982, using the person approach illustrated here.

Lubinski, D., Benbow, C. P., & Ryan, J. (1995). Stability of vocational interests among the intellectually gifted from adolescence to adulthood: A 15-year longitudinal study. *Journal of Applied Psychology, 80,* 196–200.
A short empirical piece based on the Strong–Campbell Interest Inventory, as adapted to Holland's theory of vocational choice.

Stattin, H., & Magnusson, D. (1990). *Pubertal maturation in female development* (Vol. 2). Hillsdale, NJ: Erlbaum.
A comprehensive longitudinal study of the same female sample investigated in Gustafson and Magnusson (1991). Using more traditional methodology, it emphasizes the interaction of biological and psychosocial influences on development and adjustment, including education and career achievement.

Terman, L. M., & Oden, M. H. (1947). *Genetic studies of genius: Vol. 4. The gifted child grows up.* Stanford, CA: Stanford University Press.
A classic "oldie but goodie." An interesting read in the context of the 1990s.

24

Optimism

Charles S. Carver

*O*ptimists are people who expect good things to happen to them; pessimists are those who expect bad things to happen. Optimists and pessimists experience the events of their lives differently, even if the events are objectively the same. This is because the anticipations these two kinds of people hold can cause them to perceive and interpret events differently. Indeed, by anticipating different outcomes, they may even act in ways that ultimately help create the very outcomes they anticipate.

The idea that optimists and pessimists are very different kinds of people has been part of folk knowledge for centuries. In the past decade or so, however, researchers have begun systematically studying this dimension of individual differences. There is now a substantial accumulation of evidence that optimists do in fact experience life differently than do pessimists; that they cope with adversity in different ways; and that these differences between people have broader implications for mental health, and maybe even for physical health. This chapter briefly summarizes some of that work.

DEFINING AND MEASURING OPTIMISM

Research bearing on this quality of personality has proceeded from several distinct starting points. However, the various theories share some conceptual elements. For example, they all assume that people's behavior is goal-directed. They all assume that efforts at reaching goals stem from the belief that the efforts will be successful, even if the effort is uphill and difficult. The anticipation of eventual success keeps optimists engaged in the struggle.

The theories also assume that if people become convinced that further effort is useless, they will stop trying and give up. Sometimes people can give up without further consequences. But sometimes giving up is not so easy. Sometimes abandoning the attempt to reach a small goal creates a barrier to attaining a larger and more important goal; in this case, giving up leads to distress. When the issues are very important and the giving-up tendency is very strong, so is the distress. Because distress has physiological concomitants, intense distress can have potentially adverse impact on physical aspects of the body.

These adverse consequences all follow from the development of a conviction that further effort toward a goal is useless. This experience of unfavorable expectancies, or doubt, about the future has a number of different labels, including "helplessness," "hopelessness," and yes, "pessimism." Doubt can exist at several levels of abstraction. An unfavorable expectancy can be focused on a particular act (e.g., dunking a basketball, performing a pirouette), on a broad domain of behavior (e.g., performing adequately in exams, making desired impressions on others), or even on the global sense of one's overall life. The generalized sense of positive versus negative expectations for one's future is what most of us mean by optimism versus pessimism.

Good versus bad expectations are embedded in all conceptualizations of optimism versus pessimism, but different theorists emphasize different aspects of the experience; thus they measure this quality in different ways. Our research group's approach has been to measure generalized expectancies directly by self-report, using a brief instrument called the Life Orientation Test. People completing this measure indicate their agreement or disagreement with such items as "I'm always optimistic about my future" and "I hardly ever expect things to go my way." Several other measures exist that use a similar format.

Another approach is to assume that people reveal their expectations for the future in the way they talk about causal forces behind events they have experienced in the past. If you say that an adverse event had causes that are stable (it will still be there tomorrow and next month), you probably expect those causes to operate the next time you engage in a similar kind of behavior. If you think that the cause is also very global (it applies to many situations, not just this one), you probably expect it to operate in many of the behaviors you engage in across the domains of your life's activities. The result is that you expect poorer outcomes in your life than does someone who explains bad outcomes differently.

Using these various definitions and measures of optimism (and related concepts, such as hope and hopelessness), researchers have studied how optimists differ from pessimists. Differences seem to exist in the ways in which people cope with adversity, in the success with which they cope (i.e., in terms of their mental health), and even in some outcomes concerning physical health.

COPING AND MENTAL HEALTH

First, let us consider coping and subjective distress. An assumption behind much of this work is that when confronted with adversity, optimists remain persistent in trying to attain their goals; this is reflected in the coping responses they engage in. Because persistence and goal engagement often pay off, the distress experienced by optimists under conditions of adversity is relatively low. In contrast, pessimists are more likely to respond to adversity by giving up trying to reach their goals. Sometimes the giving-up response cannot be sustained, leaving pessimists in the position of wanting to quit something they cannot really quit. The result is enhanced distress.

There is now a good deal of evidence that optimists and pessimists respond differently when they confront adversity. Optimists are more likely than pessimists to take direct action to solve their problems, are more planful in dealing with the adversity they confront, and are more focused in their coping efforts. Optimists are also more likely to accept the reality of the stressful situations they encounter; moreover, they seem intent on growing personally as a result of negative experiences, and on trying to make the best of even bad situations. (These characteristics of optimists are similar to characteristics of "hardiness," as described in Maddi's chapter of this book.) In contrast to these positive coping reactions, pessimists are more likely than optimists to react to stressful events by trying to deny their reality or by trying to avoid dealing with what is bothering them. Pessimists are also more likely simply to give up and quit trying when difficulties arise.

These differences in coping reactions are reflected in differences in the levels of distress that optimists and pessimists experience when dealing with difficult circumstances. One project bearing on this conclusion examined the process of adjusting to college life. This study collected information about the coping tactics that the students were using, as well as measuring their optimism and eventual adjustment. Optimists relied more on active coping techniques and were less likely to engage in avoidant coping. These two coping orientations were both related to later adjustment, with active coping leading to better adjustment and avoidant coping to poorer adjustment. Further analysis revealed that these two coping tendencies mediated the link between optimism and adjustment. Thus optimists did better than pessimists at least partly *because* they coped in more effective ways with the problems they confronted.

A similar conclusion is suggested by my recent study, with several colleagues, of breast cancer patients. The women in this study reported on their distress and their coping reactions before surgery, 10 days after surgery, and at 3-month, 6-month, and 12-month follow-ups. Throughout this period, optimism was tied to a coping pattern that involved acceptance of the reality of the situation, along with efforts to make the best of it. Optimism was inversely related to attempts to act as though the problem was not real, and to the tendency to give up on the life goals that were being threatened by the diagnosis of cancer. Further analyses suggested that these differences in coping served as paths by which the optimistic women remained less vulnerable to distress than pessimistic women throughout the course of the year.

A number of other studies have also found that optimists and pessimists engage in different coping reactions in response to difficulties as divergent as dealing with infertility problems, coping with a serious disease, and dealing with worries about specific health threats. Yet other studies join with those just outlined to show that pessimists are more vulnerable to distress during trying times than are optimists.

PHYSICAL HEALTH

Optimism appears to act as a buffer against the development of distress under conditions of stress or adversity. But what of its role in physical health? There is less information available on this question, though there is some. In 1995 Scheier and Bridges conducted a broad review of person variables (personality, emotional reactions, and attitudes) to determine whether any such variables had been identified as potential contributors to medical disorders. They found evidence that four clusters of variables appeared to be implicated in multiple diseases.

Of particular interest at the moment is the fourth cluster they identified: a pessimistic or fatalistic attitude toward life and health. Strictly speaking, "fatalism" means something different from "pessimism." It is a belief that outcomes are predetermined. In the context of research on illness, however, fatalism typically implies the belief that one is fated to experience bad outcomes. Thus, in this context the terms "pessimism" and "fatalism" both imply a sense of negativity about the future.

Researchers studying potential health consequences of these orientations have looked at optimism versus pessimism both as a broad disposition and as a domain-specific attitude toward a particular health outcome. There typically are moderate correlations between generalized and specific pessimism, although sometimes the correlation is much lower. Both generalized and specific pessimism appear to have adverse implications for health. There are important limitations to the evidence supporting this conclusion, however, and these should be noted explicitly. First, more of the available data come from research on men than from research on women. Second, most findings bear on cases in which disease already exists; thus, the evidence pertains more to the question of who maintains better health longer than on who comes to have an illness in the first place.

One project by Scheier relevant to the role of optimism versus pessimism examined the experiences of men undergoing coronary artery bypass surgery. Findings from this study hint that pessimism was associated with myocardial infarction during surgery. Pessimists were more likely than optimists to develop new Q-waves on their electrocardiograms as a result of the surgery. Pessimist were also more likely to show a clinically significant release of the enzyme aspartate aminotransferase. Both measures are widely taken as markers for infarction, suggesting that pessimists were more likely to have had an infarction during surgery. This effect of pessimism was independent of the extensiveness of the surgery (i.e., the number of grafts performed), the severity of the coronary heart disease (number of coronary arteries occluded 50% or more), and a composite of coronary risk factors (current smoking status, hypertensive status, and serum cholesterol level).

Optimism was also a predictor of the rate of recovery during the immediate postoperative period. Optimists more quickly achieved behavioral milestones of recovery (e.g., sitting up in bed, walking around the room), and they were rated by medical staff members as showing better physical recovery. The advantages of optimism were also apparent at the 6-month follow-up. Optimists were more likely than pessimists to have resumed vigorous physical exercise and to have returned to work on a full-time basis. Moreover, they tended to return to their activities more quickly. In sum, optimists normalized their lives more fully and more quickly than pessimists did. All of these findings were independent of the subjects' medical status at the outset of the study. Thus, it was not the case that optimists did better simply because they were less sick at the time of their surgery.

Another project examined the experiences of men with AIDS. This study, by Reed and colleagues, examined the effect of what the authors called "realistic acceptance" on AIDS-related mortality. As used here, this phrase denotes a way of coping characterized by a sense of disease-specific pessimism, fatalism, and resignation. In a sample of men with AIDS, having this orientation toward their illness was related to shorter survival over the 50-month period of the study. This effect was independent of self-reported health status, established medical risk factors (e.g., age, number of CD4 lymphocytes ["helper" T cells which are important in immunity], use of the drug AZT [azidothymidine, now called zidovudine]), and health-related behavioral risk factors (e.g., smoking, use of marijuana or cocaine).

A third project, by Schulz and colleagues, examined a group of 238 patients with recurrent cancer who were followed for a period of 8 months. All were receiving radiation treatment for their cancer. By the 8-month follow-up, 70 patients had died. A pessimistic orientation as assessed at baseline proved to be a significant predictor of mortality, even after site of cancer and level of symptomatology at baseline were controlled for.

It is of some interest that this association between pessimism and mortality occurred only among relatively younger patients (ages 30–59). This was one source of information leading Scheier and Bridges to suggest that psychological variables, such as a person's outlook on life, have their greatest influence on physical health during early and middle adulthood. They believe that past that point, biological variables assume a more dominant role, leaving little room for psychological variables to exert much influence.

A final study is important partly because it examined a specific disease, partly because it focused on disease initiation rather than disease progression, and partly because the subjects were all women. This study, by Antoni and Goodkin, examined women who were undergoing further testing after an abnormal Pap smear. This second test revealed the degree of atypical neoplastic growth in the cervix (subjects did not know their diagnosis at the time of psychological assessment). Among the variables assessed were an attitude of helplessness/hopelessness and a sense of future despair (a more focused attitude of hopelessness about the future). Antoni and Goodkin found that these attitudes were significantly related to disease initiation. That is, women whose abnormality was diagnosed as more severe had scores indicating greater pessimism than did women whose abnormality was diagnosed as less severe.

The studies reviewed thus far coalesce around the tentative conclusion that optimism is beneficial for physical well-being. The data are not completely consistent in this respect, however. Some evidence suggests that optimism may relate to poorer immunocompetence. Another study found that "cheerfulness" in childhood, which seems somewhat analogous to optimism, was associated with lower longevity, though no specific cause of death was implicated in the finding. Resolution of the inconsistencies between these findings and those reviewed earlier awaits further research.

RELATED VARIABLES AND HEALTH

Although the focus of this chapter is on optimism per se, I should point out that many other concepts in the psychological lexicon bear a family resemblance to optimism. As a result, it can be hard to know where optimism leaves off and alternative concepts begin. In considering this issue, it is useful to keep in mind the idea from which this discussion of optimism has proceeded—that is, that optimists remain engaged in motivated efforts to attain their goals, whereas pessimists are more likely to give up the attempt. Focusing on this conceptualization brings to mind several additional findings that may be interpreted as also showing the benefits of positive thinking.

For example, Fawzy and colleagues measured active behavioral coping among a sample of malignant melanoma patients, in the context of a study evaluating the effectiveness of a 6-week structured psychiatric group intervention. They found that lower initial levels of active coping were related to higher rates of recurrence and death. "Active behavioral coping" as assessed in that work is a style of coping with illness that is characterized by behavioral engagement. Specifically, patients who show this pattern try to alter aspects of their disease course through such activities as exercising, using relaxation techniques, and consulting frequently with physicians. This pattern is not identical to optimism, but neither is it too far a stretch to suggest that these behaviors reflect a focused sort of optimism and engagement with trying to stay healthy.

These findings are conceptually similar to findings reported by Greer and his colleagues, who examined disease recurrence and death among a group of breast cancer patients. In an initial prospective study of women with nonmetastatic breast cancer, these researchers found that women who reacted to their diagnosis and surgery with what the authors termed "fighting spirit" were significantly more likely to experience recurrence-free survival at a 5-year follow-up than women who reacted with "stoic acceptance" (a kind of fatalism) or feelings of hopelessness and helplessness. A similar pattern of results emerged at a 10-year follow-up and a 15-year follow-up. This kind of focused engagement with the struggle of living and regaining one's strength is just the sort of response that one expects to see from optimists.

I noted earlier that Scheier and Bridges found four clusters of variables that seem to influence disease. Another cluster focuses on depressed mood (ranging from nonclinical dysphoria to clinical depression, depending on the study). Inasmuch as depressed mood is a concomitant and even a consequence of pessimism, one might regard this additional group of findings as being quite relevant to the case of pessimism as well. However, in the interest of brevity (and of not straying too far from the focal subject of this chapter), I refer readers who are interested in this possibility to the Scheier and Bridges article.

IS OPTIMISM ALWAYS GOOD?

The discussion thus far has been fairly explicit in suggesting that optimism is good for people. Are there reasons why it might not always be? There are at least two ways in which an optimistic orientation might lead to adverse outcomes. One derives from the possibility that it is possible to be optimistic in unproductive ways. For example, unbridled optimism might cause people simply to sit and wait for good things to happen, thereby decreasing their chances of success. Although this might occur, I know of no evidence that it actually does occur among people assessed as optimistic by the instruments in this literature. Instead, optimistic people seem to view positive outcomes as partially contingent on their continued effort.

Optimism might also prove detrimental in situations that are not amenable to constructive action. That is, optimists tend to confront problems with efforts to resolve them. Perhaps this head-on approach to problem solving might be maladaptive in situations that are uncontrollable, or that involve major loss or a violation of the person's world view. Data on this question are presently lacking. Yet it is worth noting that the coping arsenal of optimists is not limited to the problem-focused domain. Optimists also use a host of emotion-focused coping responses, including the tendency to accept the reality of the situation, to put the situation in the best possible light, and to grow personally from their hardships. Given these coping options, optimists may prove to have a coping advantage even in the most distressing situations. In short, the evidence thus far is generally consistent with the idea that the optimists of the world tend to have the best outcomes—just as they expected all along.

FURTHER READING

Antoni, M. H., & Goodkin, K. (1988). Host moderator variables in the promotion of cervical neoplasia: I. Personality facets. *Journal of Psychosomatic Research, 32,* 327–338.
Study showing that a pessimistic personality is associated with elevated likelihood that an abnormal Pap smear reflects cancer or a precancerous condition.

Carver, C. S., Pozo, C., Harris, S. D., Noriega, V., Scheier, M. F., Robinson, D. S., Ketcham, A. S., Moffat, F. L., Jr., & Clark, K. C. (1993). How coping mediates the effect of optimism on distress: A study of women with early stage breast cancer. *Journal of Personality and Social Psychology, 65,* 375–390.
Prospective study showing that optimism is related to more adaptive coping and better emotional adjustment among early-stage breast cancer patients.

Carver, C. S., & Scheier, M. F. (1990). Principles of self-regulation: Action and emotion. In E. T. Higgins & R. M. Sorrentino (Eds.), *Handbook of motivation and cognition: Foundations of social behavior* (Vol. 2, pp. 3–52). New York: Guilford Press.
Theoretical summary of how expectancies relate to behavioral persistence.

Fawzy, F., Fawzy, N. W., Hyun, C. S., Guthrie, D., Fahey, J. L., & Morton, D. L. (1993). Malignant melanoma: Effects of an early structured psychiatric intervention, coping, and affective state on recurrence and survival 6 years later. *Archives of General Psychiatry, 50,* 681–689.
Study showing that active coping and engagement in the effort to cope with illness predicted lower recurrence rates and better survival among a group of cancer patients.

Greer, S., Morris, T., & Pettingale, K. W. (1979). Psychological response to breast cancer: Effect on outcome. *Lancet, ii,* 785–787.
Study showing that initial levels of "fighting spirit" in dealing with cancer predicted longer survival 15 years later.

Peterson, C., & Seligman, M. E. P. (1984). Causal explanations as a risk factor for depression: Theory and evidence. *Psychological Review, 91,* 374–374.
Theoretical analysis of how habitual patterns of explanations and events may predispose some people to depression and lower motivation.

Reed, G. M., Kemeny, M. E., Taylor, S. E., Hui-Ying, J. W., & Visscher, B. R. (1994). Realistic acceptance as a predictor of decreased survival time in gay men with AIDS. *Health Psychology, 13,* 299–307.
Prospective study showing that "realistic acceptance" of their deteriorating condition led to sooner death among men with AIDS.

Scheier, M. F., & Bridges, M. W. (1995). Person variables and health: Personality predispositions and acute psychological states as shared determinants for disease. *Psychosomatic Medicine, 57,* 255–268.
Recent thorough review and analysis of the role that personality and such variables as mood states play in predicting who will have health problems or whose health problems will get worse.

Scheier, M. F., & Carver, C. S. (1992). Effects of optimism on psychological and physical well-being: Theoretical overview and empirical update. *Cognitive Therapy and Research, 16,* 201–228.
Review of literature showing that optimism relates to enhanced well-being.

Scheier, M. F., Matthews, K. A., Owens, J. F., Magovern, G. J., Sr., Lefebvre, R. C., Abbott, R. A., & Carver, C. S. (1989). Dispositional optimism and recovery from coronary artery bypass surgery: The beneficial effects on physical and psychological well being. *Journal of Personality and Social Psychology, 57,* 1024–1040.
Study showing that optimistic men did better in several respects than pessimistic men when undergoing bypass surgery and during recovery.

Schulz, R., Bookwala, J., Knapp, J., Scheier, M. F., & Williamson, G. M. (1996). Pessimism, age, and cancer mortality. *Psychology and Aging, 11,* 304–309.
Prospective study showing that pessimism predicts shorter survival among patients being treated for advanced cancers.

25

Hardiness

Salvatore R. Maddi

*I*n these turbulent times, we all need dispositional hardiness. "Dispositional hardiness" is the tendency to address stressful circumstances by (1) accepting them as a natural, even developmentally important, part of life; (2) believing one can transform them into opportunities, rather than letting them become debilitating; and (3) proceeding to cope decisively with them.

CONCEPTUALIZATION OF DISPOSITIONAL HARDINESS

Hardiness derives from the concept of courage in existential psychology. For existentialists, courage is what helps people construct the meaning in their lives when confronted with decisions by choosing the unfamiliar, anxiety-provoking, but developmentally stimulating path rather than the familiar, stultifying one. Hardiness involves beliefs of commitment, control, and challenge. People with a strong commitment component believe that active involvement leads to an interesting and worthwhile life; they experience detachment or alienation as wasteful. Those with a strong control component believe that they can usually influence the outcome of events through struggle; they experience passivity as wasteful. Those with a strong challenge component believe that a sense of fulfillment results when they learn from experiences, whether positive or negative; they view an unchanging environment as stultifying.

Hardiness decreases the likelihood of stress-related physical illnesses, mental illnesses, and performance decrements. Hardiness produces these desirable effects by motivating (1) transformational (active, decisive) rather than regressive (denial-based, avoidant) coping, and (2) beneficial health practices (diet, exercise, relaxation) rather than detrimental ones. Hardiness thus buffers stress via coping and via health practices.

How does hardiness compare to similar concepts, such as "resilience," "coherence," and "optimism"? Resilience refers to constructive reactions to disadvantage, particularly among children (see Wright's chapter in this volume). Hardiness is a personality disposition that increases the likelihood of resilient reactions to disadvantage. Coherence, like hardiness, emphasizes beliefs about the interaction between self and world. Although coherence highlights the person's place in the social fabric as that which lends meaning to existence, hardiness highlights the active construction of one's life through making decisions and implementing them. Optimism emphasizes the generalized expectation of beneficial outcomes to problems, regardless of coping efforts. Optimism may be more likely than hardiness to include elements of naiveté and complacency, such as failure to recognize the seriousness of a stressor or the passive conviction that all will resolve itself automatically. (However, see Carver's chapter.)

DEVELOPMENT OF THE PERSONAL VIEWS SURVEY—II

The Personal Views Survey—II (PVS-II) is an instrument used to measure hardiness. Rating scale items were composed to express specific expressions of commitment, control, or challenge beliefs. Psychometric analysis of 50 items yielded Commitment, Control, and Challenge scores that are internally consistent, moderately intercorrelated with each other, and substantially correlated with the Total Hardiness score. The PVS-II correlates at .91 with the earlier version of this hardiness measure.

The PVS-II has adequate internal consistency (.70 to .75 for Commitment, .61 to .84 for Control, .60 to .71 for Challenge, and .80 to .88 for Total Hardiness) and stability (.68 for Commitment, .73 for Control, .71 for Challenge, and .77 for Total Hardiness). Factor analyses of adults' and adolescents' responses have confirmed that hardiness has three interrelated components. Sample PVS-II items include, for Commitment, "I really look forward to my work," and "Ordinary work is just too boring to be worth doing"; for Control, "What happens to me tomorrow depends on what I do today," and "Most of what happens in life is just meant to happen"; and for Challenge, "It's exciting to learn something about myself," and "The tried and true ways are always the best."

SUMMARY OF RESEARCH

Illinois Bell Telephone Studies

Our research team launched hardiness research in a longitudinal study of Illinois Bell Telephone (IBT) managers that began 6 years before and continued 6 years after the colossal upheavals surrounding the AT&T deregulation and divestiture. The buffering role of hardiness in the stress–illness relationship was first shown in a retrospective design. Next came a prospective demonstration in which stress and hardiness were measured first and illness subsequently, with the added feature of a statistical control for initial illness level. A later study showed that although physical exercise and social support decreased the likelihood of stress-related illnesses, hardiness had virtually twice as large a protective effect. In these studies, hardiness emerged as largely independent of age, gender, education, religion, marital status, ethnicity, and job level. A hardiness training program at IBT taught managers how to cope transformationally, interact supportively, and use the feedback from these efforts to augment one's personal sense of commitment, control, and challenge. This 15-hour, multiple-session training program increased hardiness and job satisfaction, and it decreased such indices of strain as anxiety, depression, blaming others, and blood pressure.

Other Hardiness and Illness Research

Other research has, by and large, supported and extended the pattern of results obtained at IBT. There have been repeated demonstrations that hardiness is (1) a negative predictor of self-reported illness levels, (2) a negative predictor of burnout in the nursing profession, (3) a positive predictor of activity level in the elderly, and (4) a positive predictor of quality of life in sufferers from serious illness. A methodological concern is that the negative relationship between hardiness and self-reported illness might be attributable to the confounding effects of a negative affectivity bias. One rejoinder is that in the IBT studies, the self-report measure of illness was quasi-objective and was validated against physicians' diagnoses. More to the point, at least one study controlled statistically for negative affectivity, with results showing the persistence of the expected pattern of negative relationship between hardiness and the clinical scales of the Minnesota Multiphasic Personality Inventory. Furthermore, there is now evidence that hardiness negatively predicts illness measured objectively.

HARDINESS AND PERFORMANCE STUDIES

The implication that hardiness influences performance as well as illness emerges from several studies. In sports, one study showed that hardiness scores obtained by high school varsity basketball players before the season began positively predicted six of seven indices of performance adequacy throughout the season. In the Israeli military, hardiness levels in men and women predicted successful graduation from grueling officer training and combat training programs. In U.S. military personnel assisting over a period of time with a tragic air disaster, mental and physical health was maintained by those who were high in hardiness. In culture shock studies, initial hardiness level predicted successful recovery from initial stress and subsequent ability to perform effectively in males and females, whether the subjects were U.S. citizens serving in a 2-year overseas training mission in China, or foreigners emigrating to the United States.

FURTHER READING

Florian, V., Mikulincer, M., & Taubman, O. (1995). Does hardiness contribute to mental health during a stressful real life situation?: The roles of appraisal and coping. *Journal of Personality and Social Psychology, 68*, 687–695.
A study of the role of hardiness in maintaining health during combat training.

Funk, S. C. (1992). Hardiness: A review of theory and research. *Health Psychology, 11*, 335–345.
A review of hardiness research.

Maddi, S. R., & Hess, M. (1992). Hardiness and basketball performance. *International Journal of Sports Psychology, 23*, 360–368.
Demonstration that hardiness improves performance in sports.

Maddi, S. R., & Kobasa, S. C. (1984). *The hardy executive: Health under stress.* Chicago: Dorsey Press.
Comprehensive presentation of the hardiness research at IBT.

Orr, E., & Westman, M. (1990). Hardiness as a stress moderator: A review. In M. Rosenbaum (Ed.), *Learned resourcefulness: On coping skills, self-control, and adaptive behavior.* New York: Springer.
A review of hardiness research.

Ouellette, S. C. (1993). Inquiries into hardiness. In L. Goldberger & S. Bresnitz (Eds.), *Handbook of stress: Theoretical and clinical aspects* (2nd ed.). New York: Free Press.
A review of hardiness conceptualization and research.

Westman, M. (1990). The relationship between stress and performance: The moderating effect of hardiness. *Human Performance, 3,* 141–155.
A review of hardiness theory and research, emphasizing its role in military training.

26

Resilience

Margaret O'Dougherty Wright

*H*istorically, clinicians and researchers have sought to identify and understand factors resulting in psychopathology and adaptational difficulties. Consequently, the emphasis in research has been on the study of risk, vulnerability, and illness, rather than on protective factors, adaptive strengths, and health. Yet many people are remarkably resilient when confronting crisis or chronic adversity. Recent research focusing on resilience and protective processes has provided a new conceptual foundation for the investigation of healthy adaptation despite stressful life circumstances. "Resilience" has been described as the capacity for successful adaptation, positive functioning, and competence despite high-risk status, chronic adversity, and exposure to severe stressors. Throughout the research literature, terms such as "risk," "vulnerability," "protective factor," and "resilience" have been used in different and often confusing ways. To enhance understanding of research in this area, a glossary of these terms is provided in Table 26.1.

Theories about resilience, as well as empirical data, emphasize the importance of models that encompass multiple systems in dynamic interaction as they influence and are influenced by the individual. Within this framework, it is important to emphasize that adaptive, maladaptive, or resilient functioning is not viewed as a static condition or a "trait" characteristic of a person; rather, it is the outcome of an evolving transactional process between the individual and the social environment. From this perspective, developmental outcomes are determined by a complex interaction of genetic, biological, psychological, and social factors in the context of particular environments.

However, despite the great need for complex models, rigorous research investigations that have explored the antecedents to and consequences of adaptive performance under severe stress have been rare. Unfortunately, the popularity of resilience as a construct has exceeded the research output associated with it. This chapter summarizes longitudinal research efforts that have involved sufficient time periods to facilitate our understanding of why and how some women are able to function competently despite overwhelming odds or in response to traumatic events. These critical studies provide opportunities to

TABLE 26.1. A Glossary of Individual Risk and Resilience Terminology

Term	Definition
Compensatory factor	A correlate of successful adaptation or development under both favorable and unfavorable conditions that may directly offset or counterbalance the negative effects of risk or adversity.
Cumulative protection	The presence of multiple protective factors in an individual's life, either within or across time.
Cumulative risk	Risk status that is compounded by (a) the presence of multiple risk factors, (b) multiple occurrences of the same risk factor, or (c) the accumulating effects of ongoing risk or adversity.
Protective factor	A correlate of resilience that may reflect preventive or ameliorative influences; a positive moderator of risk or adversity.
Resilience	Successful adaptation or development during or following adverse conditions that challenge or threaten adaptive functioning or healthy development.
Risk	An elevated probability of an undesirable outcome.
Risk factor	A measurable characteristic of individuals that heightens the probability of a worse outcome in the future for groups of individuals who share the risk factor or who have more of the risk variable than a comparison group who do not have the risk factor or have less of the risk variable.
Stress	The state or experience of an imbalance between the demands impinging on an individual and the actual or perceived resources available to meet the challenge, that at some level disrupts the equilibrium of functioning or threatens the organism's adaptive capacity.
Stressors	Events or experiences with the expected potential to trigger stress; stimuli that are believed to cause stress in normative populations.
Vulnerability	Individual susceptibility to undesirable outcomes related to traits or conditions that function to jeopardize adaptation by increasing the probability of exposure to or consequences of risk factors; the diathesis in diathesis–stressor models of psychopathology.
Vulnerability factor	A characteristic that increases the degree of an individual's exposure to or the net negative impact of risk factors or stressors on individual functioning or development; a negative moderator of risk or adversity.

Note. From Masten and Wright (in press). Copyright by Haworth Press, Inc. Reprinted by permission.

understand both progress and setbacks, and they illuminate how the capacity for resilience may develop over time. The longitudinal studies summarized here focused on the risk factors of poverty and economic disadvantage, teenage pregnancy, and sexual victimization.

CHRONIC POVERTY

One of the best-known and illustrative longitudinal projects to explore cumulative risk factors over time is the Kauai study by Werner and her colleagues. In this study, 698 Hawaiian, other Polynesian, and Asian children born on the Hawaiian island of Kauai in 1955 were followed from birth to age 30. The children were studied at birth and at 1, 2, 10, 18, and 30 years of age. Over half of the sample lived in chronic poverty, and many were exposed to multiple risk factors. Approximately one-third of the children experienced four or more risk factors (e.g., moderate to severe perinatal stress, chronic poverty, low maternal education, family instability, parental mental illness, etc.); of this "high-risk" group, one-third (one-tenth of the total sample) were identified as resilient (e.g., adequate academic progress, no delinquency, emotional stability, positive relationships with others) at the 10-, 18-, and 30-year follow-up periods.

These resilient children were compared to a comparable high-risk subgroup of children who had developed problems, in an effort to understand what factors might be important in fostering adaptation despite high risk. As infants, the resilient children displayed positive temperamental characteristics, were able to elicit attention from their caretakers, had a close bond with at least one caregiver, had no major separations in infancy, had no competition from a new baby in the family for at least 2 years, and had fewer physical problems. Both males and females at age 1 were described by their caregivers as very active, although the females were more often described as affectionate and cuddly. Thus, as infants, the resilient children in this study appeared to be both less vulnerable and more protected. As preschoolers, they were cheerful, responsive, self-confident, and independent. They were also advanced in cognitive, motor, social, and language areas. By the elementary school period, they were described as sociable, independent, good at problem solving and communicating, and excellent at getting along with peers. Females in particular had better reasoning and reading skills than those who developed problems. As adolescents, the resilient females were more assertive and more independent than the other females in the cohort, and they tended to have at least one and usually several close friends. Resilient male and female adolescents displayed high self-esteem, an internal locus of control, an achievement orientation, social maturity, and well-internalized values. At age 30, personal competence and determination, support from a spouse or mate, and reliance on faith and prayer were shared qualities of these resilient adults. For females, protective factors within the individuals tended to have a greater impact on the quality of their adult coping; for males, outside sources of support tended to make a greater difference in their lives. High self-esteem, an internal locus of control, and realistic educational and vocational plans were better discriminators for high-risk women who were successful as adults than for high-risk men. Many of the resilient high-risk youths had left the stressful conditions of their childhood homes after high school and sought out environments that were more conducive to their growth.

These findings lend empirical support to theories that address how individuals shape their own environments. A "genotype × environment" theory postulates three types of interaction: a passive stance, in which caregiving is provided directly to a child; an evocative stance, in which responses are elicited by an individual from others; and active interaction, in which an individual actively selects specific people and environmental contexts. This longitudinal study suggests that the resilient individuals shifted from a more passive to a more active response over time. This allowed them the opportunity to find more compatible and supportive contexts for growth. These findings, however, raise important questions about the construct of risk. Although these children had been exposed to comparable risk factors, the child factors that appeared to be protective (easy temperament, good intellectual abilities, positive peer relationships) may also be indicators of lower vulnerability, which may have facilitated both positive parental coping and personal adaptation. Individual contrasts within families where there were differences in adaptational outcome among siblings would be especially useful in furthering our understanding of the child–parent interactional process that promotes positive adaptation.

LONG-TERM OUTCOMES FOR ADOLESCENT MOTHERS

In a 20-year longitudinal study of over 300 teen mothers, Furstenberg and his colleagues have identified characteristics that operated as protective factors resulting in more positive outcomes following teen pregnancy. Successful long-term outcome was associated with a teenager's ability to continue her education, to prevent additional pregnancies within 5 years, to marry after completing high school, and to remain married. Poor outcomes were observed for mothers who had several subsequent pregnancies quickly, were unmarried, lacked family support, did not return to school after the birth of the index child, and became dependent on welfare.

In accounting for differences in adjustment, the researchers found that characteristics of a teenage mother, her career decisions following the child's birth, her participation in intervention programs, and availability of social support were clearly the most striking factors related to good outcome for both the mother and her child. The strongest predictor of eventual economic stability was being at grade level at the time of the pregnancy. A teen who reported higher aspirations was also more likely to remain in school throughout her pregnancy and to finish high school eventually. Level of educational achievement at the 5-year follow-up period was clearly associated with economic success in adulthood, and additional pregnancies were clearly indicative of future economic problems. In addition, academic ability had strong effects even after background and attitudinal variables were controlled for. Finally, the financial support and child care assistance of the primary family often made it possible for a young mother to return to school; thus, family support was a key factor in reducing long-term negative effects of adolescent pregnancy.

The effects of marriage were complex. Although remaining unmarried and living with one's family facilitated a return to high school, women who married after completing schooling were less likely to become welfare recipients. Women who were not married by the time of the 5-year follow-up were over four times more likely to live in poverty and to receive welfare assistance. Early preventive interventions focusing directly on the mother–infant relationship, and providing support to an adolescent mother in her parenting efforts and attempts to complete school, were of critical importance. Provision of adequate health care, and of family planning and counseling that emphasized academic achievement, delaying of marriage, effective use of contraception, and postponement of further childbearing, also increased the likelihood of an adaptive developmental outcome for an adolescent mother.

SEXUAL VICTIMIZATION

One of every four girls in the United States may be sexually abused or assaulted before the age of 18; this can have serious effects on mental health and emotional well-being. Some of these effects include negative self-image, depression, anxiety, feelings of isolation and stigma, substance abuse, problems in interpersonal relationships, and a heightened risk of revictimization. Follow-up studies of women who have survived sexual abuse or assault have identified a number of characteristics and experiences facilitating their recovery. These include the ability to find supportive relationships outside the family, ability to maintain positive self-regard, an external rather than internal attribution of blame for the victimization, and an internal locus of control. Judith Herman, who has written and worked extensively with female trauma survivors, concludes that women can recover from an act of sexual violence through the healing power of relationships. Relationships and connections are vital elements of psychological growth. Positive self-regard is dependent upon the experience of healthy and caring relationships. For some survivors of sexual trauma, a family member, a friend, or another adult has been able to provide such a relationship. Other women benefit from a relationship in psychotherapy. Following sexual victimization, a woman's assumptions about the world's being a safe and just place have often been shattered. However, women who are resilient often have the ability to interpret the experience in a way that leads to personal growth, increased empathy for others, and an ability to move from the experience of victimization to self-empowerment. Although these women often continue to struggle with underlying feelings of sadness or basic questions about their self-worth, they are simultaneously able to maintain positive self-esteem regarding their personal competence, to believe that they do deserve to be loved, and to feel that their trauma has made them more than they might have been otherwise. Again, multiple factors are influential. They include characteristics of the individual (temperament, personality characteristics); characteristics of her environment (social support, response of significant others if the abuse is revealed or detected, availability of treatment); and characteristics of the traumatic event (type of trauma, age at which the trauma occurred, duration, relationship to the perpetrator). All of these characteristics interact and affect outcome.

SUMMARY OF KEY CHARACTERISTICS OF RESILIENT WOMEN

Research in these areas suggests key characteristics that promote resilience. These include (1) an active approach to solving life's problems; (2) an ability to perceive experiences constructively, even if these experiences have caused pain and suffering; (3) an ability from infancy onward to gain other people's positive attention and support; (4) supportive adults within or outside the family who can act as surrogate parents; and (5) a strong reliance on faith or spirituality to maintain a positive view of a meaningful life. A transactional model is particularly helpful in seeing how a woman's disposition can affect her environment in a way that elicits positive responses, reinforces active participation, and enhances competence. However, this research also highlights the importance of viewing the descriptors' "vulnerability" and "resilience" as relative and changing over time, in conjunction with changing life circumstances. Neither is a fixed characteristic or a "trait" of an individual. Rather, at each developmental stage there can be a shifting balance between stressful life events that heighten vulnerability and protective factors that enhance resilience. Under highly stressful circumstances, individuals with the capacity for resilience can also experience a loss of adaptive functioning and deterioration in health.

In order to help those individuals who remain vulnerable, it is important to focus on the protective processes in the lives of resilient women that have resulted in changes in their life path from that of high risk to that of resilience and adaptation. Interventions are particularly needed that (1) reduce risk impact and prevent additional stressors from occurring; (2) foster positive personal coping skills, which can reduce the likelihood of negative chain reactions; (3) promote self-esteem, self-efficacy, and hopefulness; and (4) open up opportunities in education, work, and social relationships. Development of the women's personal resources, competence, and motivation, combined with the support of family or friends, should contribute to positive changes despite poverty, early pregnancy, or victimization. Exploration of factors that promote both recovery and personal growth following extremely stressful events may provide greater insight into the compensatory and protective processes critical to resilience. In future research, it may be useful to examine specific triggering events or turning points that can shift an individual's developmental path toward either greater vulnerability or greater resilience.

FURTHER READING

Furstenberg, F. F., Brooks-Gunn, J., & Morgan, S. P. (1987). *Adolescent mothers in later life.* New York: Cambridge University Press.
A landmark 20-year longitudinal study of over 300 teen mothers, which delineates both risk and protective factors.

Herman, J. L. (1992). *Trauma and recovery.* New York: Basic Books.
A compelling and thought-provoking analysis of the impact of multiple forms of trauma (war, physical abuse, incest) and the process of recovery.

Masten, A. S., Best, K. M., & Garmezy, N. (1990). Resilience and development: Contributions from the study of children who overcame adversity. *Development and Psychopathology, 2,* 425–444.
A comprehensive review article focusing on different aspects of resilience: good outcomes in high-risk children, continued competence under stress, and recovery from trauma.

Masten, A. S., & Wright, M. O. (in press). Cumulative risk and protection models of child maltreatment. In B. B. R. Rossman & M. S. Rosenberg (Eds.), *Multiple victimization of children: Conceptual, developmental, research, and treatment issues.* Binghamton, NY: Haworth Press.
A theoretical and clinical overview of cumulative risk and protection models for understanding the etiology and consequences of child abuse and neglect.

O'Leary, V. E., & Ickovics, J. R. (1995). Resilience and thriving in response to challenge: An opportunity for a paradigm shift in women's health. *Women's Health: Research on Gender, Behavior, and Policy, 1*(2), 121–142.
A conceptual paper that proposes the need for a paradigm shift away from a focus on women's illness and pathology, and toward women's thriving in the face of physical challenges; it reviews the methodological implications of such research.

Rutter, M. (1990). Psychosocial resilience and protective mechanisms. In J. Rolf, A. S. Masten, D. Cicchetti, K. H. Nuechterlein, & S. Weintraub (Eds.), *Risk and protective factors in the development of psychopathology* (pp. 181–214). New York: Cambridge University Press.
Incisive critical analysis of underlying processes or mechanisms that might determine individual variations in response to risk factors.

Schaefer, J. A., & Moos, R. H. (1992). Life crises and personal growth. In B. N. Carpenter (Ed.), *Personal coping: Theory, research and application* (pp. 149–170). Westport, CT: Praeger.
A review article that explores why positive change and personal growth frequently occur among individuals who have experienced life crises.

Werner, E. E., & Smith, R. S. (1992). *Overcoming the odds: High risk children from birth to adulthood.* Ithaca, NY: Cornell University Press.
Landmark 32-year longitudinal study that traced developmental outcomes in a multiracial group of children exposed to multiple risk factors: perinatal stress, chronic poverty, parental mental illness, and family discord.

27

Multiple Roles

Rena L. Repetti

A woman's role as income producer for her family is not new, but the structure of women's employment has changed. Women are now much more likely to work outside of the home for long periods of time each day. This change has been especially dramatic in the case of mothers. In the United States today, a mother's daily work is likely to include an outside job in addition to responsibility for a majority of the housekeeping and child-rearing tasks at home. More and more women simultaneously occupy three major social roles: employee, spouse, and parent. These social changes have raised important questions about their impact on the health and well-being of women, children, and families.

This chapter addresses the question of how functioning in multiple demanding social roles affects women's mental and physical health. Do multiple roles confer a health advantage on women? For example, additional roles bring more social partners who can offer support in times of need, such as physical assistance, a good piece of advice, or just a sympathetic ear. Each role may also add another positive social identity and sense of control, which can act as resources or buffers when things are not going well in a different role. For example, a mother can feel proud of her children when she is passed over for a promotion at work, or a woman can take some comfort in her professional accomplishments or job security when she is facing problems in her marriage. The "role enhancement hypothesis" emphasizes the rights, privileges, and resources that accumulate with involvement in multiple roles.

It is equally easy to see how multiple social roles may be a health liability. The pressures, demands, and physical labor associated with a job, motherhood, and housekeeping may be too much for one person to handle. For example, employed mothers with young children whose husbands do not contribute much to child care and housekeeping, or employed mothers who do not have a partner at home, may suffer from role overload. They simply have too much to do and not enough time to do it all, and their mental and physical health may suffer as a result. Different role demands and responsibilities may also conflict with each other and create daily crises, such as when a child needs to be picked up from day care at the same time that a supervisor asks a mother to complete an important project. The "role strain hypothesis" focuses on role overload and role conflicts; it maintains that, because there are limits on any one person's time and energy, role obligations can easily become exhausting and take a toll on emotional and physical functioning.

ROLE OCCUPANCY AND WOMEN'S HEALTH

What is greater, the strain or the benefits of role accumulation? The initial approach taken to address this question compared women whose lives encompassed different social role combinations. In general, it was found that women who enacted more roles were mentally and physically healthier than women who enacted fewer roles. However, some investigators found that the effects of role accumulation depended not simply on the total number of roles, but also on the particular *types* of social roles that a woman occupied. For example, many studies have reported specific health advantages associated with employment. However, these findings do not necessarily imply that employment has beneficial effects on women's health. The "healthy worker effect" refers to the observation that healthier women are more likely to enter the labor force, and they are more likely to remain employed. The influence of a woman's health on her decision to be employed may account for the better health status enjoyed by employed women. Fortunately, longitudinal studies that control for initial health can separate the impact that employment has on health from the effect that health has on employment status. None of these studies have found negative effects of employment per se on women's mental or physical well-being, and a few have uncovered beneficial effects. As discussed below, the net effect of employment on a woman's health appears to depend on several factors, including the characteristics of her job and other social roles.

Marriage is also associated with better mental and physical health for both men and women. However, these differences may also be attributable to poor health among people who never got married in the first place or who divorced. It is not surprising that most researchers conclude that marital quality is a more important determinant of a woman's well-being than is the simple fact that she has a spouse. Women who say that they are happier in their marriages also tend to report better health.

Interestingly, the impact of parenthood seems to differ from the effects of the other two social roles mentioned here. Some studies find that this role has *negative* mental health consequences for both women and men. At least in its early stages, parenthood is associated with a decrease in marital happiness, which is linked to decrements in mental and physical well-being. Here too, research suggests that the overall impact of one social role may depend on the other roles that a woman occupies. For example, having young children at home may be associated with higher rates of depression for women who are homemakers, but this may not be the case for employed women.

IMPORTANT CHARACTERISTICS OF WOMEN'S SOCIAL ROLES FOR THEIR MENTAL AND PHYSICAL HEALTH

The complex and sometimes contradictory findings of research on mere role occupancy have prompted researchers to focus on specific qualities or characteristics of women's social roles. Working within this paradigm, researchers seek to determine the psychosocial conditions under which a woman's involvement in multiple roles has a positive or negative effect on her health. The search is for role characteristics that may mediate the effects of role occupancy by either straining or enhancing women's health. Recall that according to the role strain hypothesis, multiple roles can easily exhaust a woman's personal resources, with costs to her emotional and physical well being. Two aspects of social roles have been studied for the strain they may produce: the level of responsibilities and demands inherent in a role, and the extent to which interpersonal relationships within that role are distressed. Perceptions of many demands and responsibilities in work or family roles are usually associated with reports of poor mental and physical health outcomes. In particular, many demands at work, combined with perceptions of little job control or autonomy, appear to place some workers at increased risk for coronary heart disease. Descriptions of interpersonal relationships at work that are problematic or conflictual also tend to be associated with greater psychological distress and with reports of more minor physical complaints and illnesses. Similarly, general marital distress and other family problems have been linked to negative health outcomes, including poorer immune functioning.

The role enhancement hypothesis focuses on the benefits which accrue from the psychosocial resources that accumulate with multiple roles. Social support is the best-studied of the potential health-promoting resources associated with social roles. Research has shown that social support can have a direct positive impact on mental and physical health, and that it can act indirectly as a buffer against the debilitating effects of stress. With regard to job-related social support, women and men who describe more supportive relationships with coworkers and supervisors also tend to report better psychological adjustment and fewer health complaints and illnesses. However, studies testing whether support at work can mitigate the effects of job stressors, such as heavy demands, have produced mixed results. Only a limited number of marital studies have addressed health outcomes associated with spouse support. What little research there is suggests that the functional and emotional support provided by a considerate spouse can have direct mental and physical health benefits. Unfortunately, most of what we know about both the strain and support characteristics of work and family roles is based on studies of men's health outcomes.

RESEARCH ALLOWING FOR TESTS OF MORE COMPLEX MODELS

By overcoming significant methodological problems, such as respondent bias and subject selection, some recent studies have allowed for tests of more interesting and complex conceptual models of women's multiple roles. Four new promising trends in this literature are highlighted below.

Studies That Include Objective/Independent Measures

Researchers frequently ask respondents to describe their own physical or mental well-being, as well as the characteristics of the roles they occupy (e.g., daily workload on the job, conflict with a spouse). This approach has a serious shortcoming: Many participants in survey and interview studies demonstrate a bias to respond to questions in a particular way. For example, some people tend to exaggerate the difficulties they are experiencing, whereas others are inclined to downplay their problems. In either case, the result would be an inflated correlation between the role description (e.g., amount of support received from a spouse) and the health report (e.g., symptoms of depression or pain during the last week). Some recent studies have incorporated objective indicators of role characteristics and health, or they rely on others as sources of information. Examples of objective measures that have been used include daily records of the number and types of calls by police dispatchers to assess their workload; Federal Aviation Administration records of air traffic volume at the airport to assess air traffic controllers' workload; and the use of blood tests to assess health outcomes. Other individuals can also act as independent sources of information. For example, coworkers' ratings have been used to assess the social climate of a workplace; spouses have been used to characterize key aspects of a marriage and household; and physicians or nurses have been asked to describe an individual's health.

Studies that avoid respondent biases generally support the same basic conclusions about the effects of certain role characteristics on women's health; however, the effects are often weaker than those found in studies that rely solely on an individual's own reports. Although results based on self-reports may in some cases be inflated by respondent biases, in other cases the stronger correlations may reflect the importance of an individual's appraisals in determining health outcomes.

Longitudinal Studies

Prospective longitudinal studies follow a sample of people over time, usually 1 year or more, to assess patterns of change in certain biopsychosocial variables. As mentioned above, this type of study has significantly improved research on multiple roles by allowing investigators to control for initial health status when estimating the impact that occupying a particular role (e.g., the role of employed worker) has on the course of women's health. Studies of the health effects of specific role characteristics also benefit from longitudinal designs. With this approach, researchers can ask whether particular characteristics of social roles predict changes in mental or physical health over time. Unfortunately, there are not many published longitudinal studies of role characteristics and women's health. The Framingham Heart Study suggested that having a nonsupportive supervisor may be a risk factor for future coronary heart disease, at least among married clerical workers. More investigations of this type are needed before researchers can accurately estimate the effects of role characteristics on women's health outcomes.

Tests of Interactive Models of Multiple Role Involvement

Studies of multiple role involvement have led to a new set of questions about how combinations of social roles with different characteristics might influence women's health. Two basic types of models have been investigated. "Additive models" are fairly simple; they predict that work and family roles have direct, independent effects on health. For example, an unpleasant or conflictual social climate at work is expected to have the same impact on health, regardless of the quality of a woman's marriage. According to an additive or direct-effects model, a happy marriage enhances a woman's health and an unhappy marriage detracts from her total well-being, but the health effects of the social environment at work remain constant. In contrast to an additive model, an "interactive model" predicts that the impact of a social role on health can actually be shaped or modified by experiences in another role. Interactive models can describe opposite kinds of interactive effects among roles. A buffering effect occurs when experiences in one role serve to attenuate or reduce the impact of another role. An exacerbating effect occurs when experiences in one role serve to strengthen or amplify the effects of another role. Investigations of interactive models of multiple roles have focused almost exclusively on women's mental health outcomes. Little is known about how the interaction of experiences in different social roles may influence women's physical health.

According to some interactive models, the mere occupancy of one social role can shape the impact of characteristics of another role on mental health. For example, some research suggests that marital problems are less likely to be associated with depression among employed women as compared to women who are homemakers. In this case, it appears that simply being in the role of paid worker may help to buffer women from the depressive effects of an unhappy marriage. More complex interactive models consider the interaction of specific characteristics of different social roles. Among these models, buffering effects demonstrate that a positive or health-promoting characteristic in one role can reduce or attenuate the impact of strain in another role. In other words, experiences in one role that are psychologically enhancing (e.g., the provision of social support) are assumed to make one more resilient when confronted with negative experiences in another role. For example, there is evidence that having supportive wives can buffer the negative effects of work stress on men's mental health. Interestingly, although researchers have tested for buffering effects of supportive husbands in samples of employed women, they have not been found.

Exacerbating effects are usually tested to examine the interaction of negative, or role strain, characteristics of different roles (e.g., high workload or interpersonal problems at work and at home). The assumption here is that straining experiences in one role can leave one more vulnerable to the debilitating effects of negative experiences in another role. Some research suggests that inequity and conflict in the marital relationship, or heavy home labor or child care responsibilities, can amplify the psychological impact of stressors at work. These studies indicate that an unhappy marriage or too much work at home intensifies the effects of job stress on rates of depression and psychological distress among women. However, not all studies that have tested for these types of exacerbating effects have found them. So far in the research literature, interactive effects in general have been fairly elusive. They are sometimes found, and sometimes not. One reason for this may be the statistical power that is needed to detect interactive effects, as compared to the power that is needed to detect a simple addictive effect. In fact, interactive effects are typically tested only after controlling for any addictive effects in the data.

Conceptually, investigations of interactive effects are much more appealing than studies that examine characteristics of a single role at a time or those that test only for simple additive effects. Interactive models more accurately reflect the real-life experiences of most women in multiple roles today, and they consider the possibility of "spillover" effects from one role to another. On methodological grounds, these models avoid two of the key problems in the research literature that have been highlighted above. First, because they begin with women who occupy the same set of multiple roles and focus on variations in the characteristics of those roles, interactive models are not subject to the "healthy worker effect" or other problems associated with respondents who have selected themselves into different role combinations. Second, the multiple-regression analyses that are used in this field first control for the independent impact of role characteristics on health, and only then test for interactive or multiplicative effects. This means that even if the data are based entirely on self-reports, all respondent biases are eliminated before the interactions are tested. Future research on the mental health consequences of multiple roles is likely to focus much more on interactive models. However, there has been little use of these types of models to study women's physical health outcomes. To the extent that the specific characteristics of women's multiple roles are important contributors to their health profiles, interactive models should also be incorporated into research focusing on physical health outcomes in women.

Daily-Diary Studies

Daily-diary or daily-report studies represent another promising new direction for research on multiple roles. These are sometimes regarded as short-term longitudinal studies because subjects are followed over a limited period of time, anywhere from a few days to a few months. The "health outcomes" that are measured are usually short-term changes in mood or minor health complaints that are associated with increases in role-related stressors and supports. Among women, friendliness of coworkers is associated with more positive emotional states, and stress resulting from simultaneously juggling the demands of work and family roles is associated with short-term increases in negative mood. Interestingly, both women and men appear to adapt quite well to the impact of daily role stressors on mood and to recover fairly quickly. That is, there does not appear to be a carryover of negative mood from a stressful day to the following day. However, there are significant individual differences in reactivity to role stressors. People who are low in self-esteem, and those who experience chronically high levels of negative affect, show more extreme responses to daily increases in role stressors.

ACKNOWLEDGMENT

I would like to acknowledge the support of my first award (R29-48593) from the National Institute of Mental Health.

FURTHER READING

Baruch, G. K., & Barnett, R. (1986). Role quality, multiple role involvement, and psychological well-being in mid-life women. *Journal of Personality and Social Psychology, 51*, 578–585.
This empirical paper suggests that a focus on role quality, rather than role occupancy, may be more useful for understanding the relationship between role involvement and well-being.

Burman, B., & Margolin, G. (1992). Analysis of the association between marital relationships and health problems: An interactional perspective. *Psychological Bulletin, 112*, 39–63.
This review of the empirical literature concludes that marital variables probably have indirect, nonspecific effects on health, and provides a hypothetical model of the association between marriage and health.

Crosby, F. J. (1987). *Spouse, parent, worker: On gender and multiple roles.* New Haven, CT: Yale University Press.
This book contains an interdisciplinary collection of chapters focusing on the benefits and costs of multiple roles for women, and emphasizing the importance of studying role quality.

McLanahan, S., & Adams, J. (1987). Parenthood and psychological well-being. *Annual Review of Sociology, 5,* 237–257.
This review of the empirical literature suggests that parenthood is associated with lower levels of psychological well-being, and discusses possible explanations for this finding.

Repetti, R. L. (1993). The effects of workload and the social environment at work on health. In L. Goldberger & S. Breznitz (Eds.), *Handbook of stress* (2nd ed., pp. 368–385). New York: Free Press.
This chapter reviews existing studies of the short-term and long-term effects of two psychosocial job characteristics on mental and physical health.

Repetti, R. L., Matthews, K., & Waldron, I. (1989). Employment and women's health. *American Psychologist, 44,* 1394–1401.
This review of the empirical literature highlights methodological issues and concludes that employment does not have a negative effect on women's health, on average.

Waldron, I., & Jacobs, J. A. (1989). Effects of multiple roles on women's health: Evidence from a national longitudinal study. *Women and Health, 15,* 3–19.
This empirical study finds that involvement in multiple roles generally contributes to better health, due to the beneficial effects of paid employment and marriage for some women.

Williams, K. J., Suls, J., Alliger, G. M., Learner, S. M., & Wan, C. K. (1991). Multiple role juggling and daily mood states in working mothers: An experience sampling study. *Journal of Applied Psychology, 76,* 664–674.
This empirical study presents evidence that role juggling has negative effects on working mothers' moods within a day, but not across days.

28

Life Events

Helen Sweeting

*T*he basic supposition of life events research is that experiences that disrupt or threaten to disrupt an individual's everyday life can result in disturbing psychological or physical reactions. The area has attracted a great deal of research attention over the past 20–30 years; a computer search among medical journals using the key words "life changes" or "life events" would identify several thousand articles published within the past decade. With respect to women's health, two strands of interest can be distinguished. First, some studies focus on disorders that solely or predominantly occur among women, some present results separately by sex, and others choose to restrict their samples to women. The second broad approach is the attempt to explain observed differences between the health (almost exclusively limited to psychological distress) of men and women in terms of differential exposure or differential reactions to life events or life stress.

This chapter aims to cover four issues. First, for readers unfamiliar with the subject, a brief overview of the methodologies and pitfalls of life events research is presented. Second, recent studies (the majority published within the past several years) of life events and both mental and physical disorders are presented as examples of work in this area. This is followed by a description of older work highlighting the associations between socioeconomic status, life events, and depression in women. Finally, a review of research on sex differences in exposure or vulnerability to life events is given.

LIFE EVENTS RESEARCH: AN OVERVIEW

The most popular approach in life events research involves the use of questionnaires or checklists. This method originates from the work by Holmes and Rahe in the 1960s that resulted in the publication of the Social Readjustment Rating Scale, a list of events regarded as requiring adaptive or coping behavior on the part of subjects. The "size" of each event and a rating of whether it is positive or negative may be obtained as a consensus from an objective panel or from the respondents themselves. The former method can be criticized on the grounds that it assumes that respondents from a variety of backgrounds and cultures will each assign the same meaning to a certain event; the latter can be criticized on the grounds that it may cause an artifactual association between life events and illness, since the ratings given to events may be influenced by current mood.

With respect to event desirability, the initial assumption that it is simply *change* that leads to stress in a subject has generally been abandoned in favor of the notion that it is only *undesirable* life events that are potentially damaging. Perhaps somewhat surprisingly, the literature on life event scoring suggests that assigning objective weightings to events does not markedly improve associations with illness, compared with the results obtained from simply counting numbers of events.

An alternative approach to obtaining information on life events via questionnaire is the more complex Life Events and Difficulties Schedule (LEDS), developed by Brown, Harris, and their colleagues in the United Kingdom. This involves detailed interviews by members of a research team who, taking into account the context in which each event occurred, rate the degree of threat each event represented. This rating is based on the likely response of an average person to such an event in such circumstances. The advantages of objectivity and of the impressive reliability and validity that may be obtained via this procedure must be balanced against the fact that it is quite time-consuming and labor-intensive. Rather different traditions of research have developed around the interview-based LEDS and the questionnaire- and checklist-based life event methodologies.

Further issues that have to be addressed within life events research are those of event "contamination" and "dependence." Life event scales may contain (be contaminated by) items that reflect health status directly (e.g., items asking about personal injury or illness, change in sleeping habits, etc.). In addition, events reported via either checklist or interview may be dependent upon the actions or well-being of the subject (e.g., marital separation). Each type of problem may artificially create or inflate an association between life events and illness.

Many papers are available that further detail potential pitfalls in the methodology of life events research. Despite the hazards, a great deal of useful work has been conducted, and significant advances have been made in our understanding of the relationship between events and illness.

LIFE EVENTS AND HEALTH

Psychological Well-Being

The majority of empirical studies have focused on the relationship of stressful life events to the onset, course, and outcome of a variety of psychiatric disorders. Most of these studies have found associations between events and disorders, but the correlations, though significant, are usually fairly low. To focus on studies of women, a recent example conducted among 100 women in Turkey obtained a correlation of .24 between number of life events and depression inventory score. An alternative to correlating events with distress is found in a study that compared mother-only families referred to a child guidance clinic with non-clinic-referred mother-only families. The clinic-referred families experienced more objectively rated negative events and more severe events, whereas non-clinic-referred families reported more positively rated events. The symptomatic families were clearly experiencing greater stress.

Such results must always be interpreted with caution, however. An investigation that collected data from a sample of materially disadvantaged mothers at two time points 1 year apart serves to highlight the complex and bidirectional associations between life events and depressive symptomatology. Increased depressive symptoms were associated with current health stress, family fights, and financial stress after earlier symptomatology was controlled for. In addition, depressive symptoms themselves predicted a wide range of stressful life events over the following year.

The results of a number of other studies suggest that certain events may predictably happen more frequently to certain people. One study found that self-critical women (defined as organized, controlled, and valuing reason over emotion) reported a greater number of academic events *and* were significantly more depressed. The authors hypothesize that this arises because self-critical individuals set themselves very high standards, which they fail to meet (life events), and therefore become depressed. Similarly, they found that more dependent women (defined as emotional and sensitive to interpersonal issues) experienced a greater number of relationship stressors *and* were significantly more depressed than less dependent women. Not only do individuals actively enter some situations and avoid others; they may also create events by evoking responses or influencing their environment in other ways.

In addition to evidence linking particular types of people to particular types of events, there are indications that outcome subsequent to stressful events is mediated by individual characteristics. A recent study investigated recovery from the single life event of rape among a sample of women. Behavioral and characterological self-blame and thinking more often about why the rape occurred were related to poorer long-term recovery, whereas the belief that future rapes are unlikely (i.e., a sense of control) was associated with better outcome.

Physical Well-Being

The notion that stress may play a role in the onset of physical illness, as well as in psychological well-being, is an old one. Some theorists suggest that physical illness occurs when emotional responses are denied or blocked; others suggest that intense emotional distress may have a direct physical outcome. A series of studies has shown that psychological stress, bereavement, and psychiatric illness can impair immunological function. (Diseases closely associated with immunological mechanisms include infection, malignancy, and AIDS.) It is obviously possible that in individuals with already weakened immune systems, stress may particularly increase the risk of illness. Another mechanism may be autonomic nervous system reactivity, as suggested by those studies showing an association between life events, or prolonged (particularly work-related) stress, and myocardial infarction. Certain responses, such as altered dietary or exercise patterns, may also play an intervening role with regard to life events and physical illness.

A number of recent studies show a relationship between adverse life events, or particular adverse events (e.g., death of a spouse), and the onset or relapse of breast cancer among women. It has been suggested that a family history of breast cancer may act as a vulnerability factor and a severe event as the provoking agent. Life stress has also been implicated in disorders of menstruation. Here there is some evidence of specificity: Menorrhagia is preceded by increased rates of severe events or major difficulties and is associated with depression, whereas secondary amenorrhea is preceded by minor events or challenge experiences and associated with tension and fatigue.

Some studies report results for men and women separately. One study found that the experience of many life events in the preceding year was associated with a gain in body mass (called "reactive obesity") for both sexes. However, the weight gain for women was not apparent after a second year of follow-up, suggesting that it was effectively counterbalanced by regulatory mechanisms. Another study—unusual in that positive rather than negative events were implicated—found that among women with insulin-dependent diabetes mellitus, positive events were associated with an improvement in measures of glucose metabolism. No statistically significant correlations were found for males.

Also relevant here are investigations of the associations between life events and physical illnesses that disproportionately affect women, such as unexplained abdominal pain, which can lead to the removal of a normal appendix. Severe events have been found to be more common in patients with pain but without acute inflammation than in those with inflammation or comparison subjects. It is possible that such events cause abdominal pain via contraction of the colon, or, alternatively, that associated psychiatric symptoms alert others to a need for medical treatment.

LIFE EVENTS AND DEPRESSION IN WOMEN

The careful work of Brown and Harris on the social origins of depression, conducted 20 years ago, was carried out solely among samples of women. Women were chosen for the strategic reason that they suffer more depression than men. The study identified three broad groups of factors: "provoking agents," "vulnerability factors," and "symptom formation factors."

Provoking agents—severe events involving long-term threat or long-term difficulties—were found to influence when the depression occurred. However, not all women who experienced such life events became depressed; vulnerability factors acted as moderating variables, increasing the chance of developing depression in the presence of a provoking agent, but otherwise having no effect. Four factors were identified as vulnerability factors (or, if reversed, protective factors): death of a woman's mother before the woman reached age 11, three or more children under age 14, absence of a confiding relationship with a husband or partner, and lack of a job. It is suggested that these factors acted by lowering a woman's self-esteem and increasing her sense of hopelessness. Finally, symptom formation factors influenced the type and severity of symptoms once a woman was depressed. A severe event after the first onset, a previous episode of depression, and any past loss increased the severity of symptoms. In addition, psychotic conditions were related to loss by death (more common in older women), and neurotic conditions to loss by separation.

Among the women studied, each of these groups of factors was unequally distributed according to socioeconomic status. Lower-status women experienced more severe events and difficulties, and were also more likely to have lost a mother, to have young children at home, and to be without a confiding relationship. These inequalities explained the social class difference in risk of depression among women with children.

CAN LIFE EVENTS EXPLAIN SEX DIFFERENCES IN HEALTH?

Differential Exposure?

Research on sex differences in psychological distress suggests that women are at greater risk than men for such problems as anxiety and depression. Some studies suggest that this arises because women are exposed to a greater number of stressful life events than men. One study using social readjustment ratings, for example, found that women had higher scores for all events and for events probably beyond the respondents' control. However, other studies have produced inconsistent results with regard to differential male–female event exposure. One reason may be differences or biases in the types or domains of life events sampled. Stressors may be unique to certain roles; thus, for example, scales containing larger numbers of events relating to work or finance issues may well result in higher scores for males.

Another strategy has been to examine whether women experience more of certain types of events than men. There is some evidence that women report greater numbers of "network" or "interpersonal" events. This may be because of differential practices in sex role socialization; perhaps women define a wider range of people as significant others than men do, or perhaps they are more aware than men are of network or interpersonal events (or perceive them more) as crises. Once again, findings in this area are inconsistent.

Differential Vulnerability?

The next stage of this research process has involved models hypothesizing that women may be more vulnerable to the psychological consequences of stressful life situations. The bulk of studies suggest that women are indeed more vulnerable to the effects of life events, or at least to particular types of events, and that accounting for this reduces the sex differences in psychological distress. An early study found that although men's psychological symptom levels were most strongly related to scores for all life events, those of women were most closely related to scores for events they did not control. A number of investigations have demonstrated that women more frequently become depressed over disruption and conflict in close relationships, whereas men become depressed over the loss of an ideal or an achievement-related goal. Identity-relevant events are thus more disturbing than identity-irrelevant events. For example, one recent study found women to be more distressed by exposure to negative events within the family, and men by work and financial events. Another found that high interpersonal distress was related to self-reported depression and suicidality more strongly among women than among men.

Differences in Social Support?

One reason for differing vulnerabilities may be that the personal and social mediating resources an individual can mobilize in the face of life events vary by gender. Principal among these mediators is social support (emotional, material, or informational). A distinction needs to be made between perceived and received support, because the two are only weakly related. Much of the literature suggests that social support enhances resilience to stressful events, and most studies find that women are more likely than men to perceive support as available and to recall receiving support. How can these findings be reconciled with women's apparently greater vulnerability to life events, particularly people-focused events? The answer may lie in the fact that not all relationships are supportive; moreover, women may face greater demands from their social network than men do. A recent investigation found that women in untroubled marriages experienced more emotional problems in response to their husbands' job problems than did women in marriages marked by tension and discord. The authors suggest that a woman in an untroubled marriage has a stronger emotional involvement with her husband and so is more adversely affected by his problems.

FURTHER READING

Brown, G. W., & Harris, T. O. (1978). *Social origins of depression: A study of psychiatric disorder in women.* London: Tavistock Publications.
A study of depression among women in which detailed accounts of their daily lives, experiences, and symptoms were collected and from which the authors conclude that clinical depression is largely the result of psychosocial influences.

Brown, G. W., & Harris, T. O. (Eds.). (1989). *Life events and illness.* New York: Guilford Press.
An overview of the research tradition based on the LEDS; results are presented for both psychological and physical disorders.

Conger, R. D., Lorenz, F. O., Elder, G. H., Simons, R. L., & Ge, X. (1993). Husband and wife differences in response to undesirable life events. *Journal of Health and Social Behavior, 34,* 71–78.
A study of married couples showing gender differences in the types of life events reported, and in distress in response to different types of events.

Frazier P., & Schauben, L. (1994). Causal attributions and recovery from rape and other stressful life events. *Journal of Social and Clinical Psychology, 13,* 1–14.
A survey of female students (21% of whom reported an experience that met the legal definition of rape) to determine how self-blame and perceptions of future control were related to recovery.

Geyer, S. (1993). Life events, chronic difficulties and vulnerability factors preceding breast cancer. *Social Science and Medicine, 37,* 1545–1555.
A survey of women admitted to a hospital for removal of a suspicious breast lump; the author suggests an inherited "vulnerability" factor, causing elevated susceptibility to the triggering of breast cancer after the experience of severe life events.

Holmes, T. H., & Rahe, R. H. (1967). The social readjustment rating scale. *Journal of Psychosomatic Research, 11,* 213–218.
A study in which subjects were given a list of 43 life events to rate in terms of the "social readjustment" which each would require. Events judged most "stressful" in this sense were death of a spouse (scoring 100) and divorce (73); least were Christmas (12) and minor violations of the law (11).

Kessler, R. C., & McLeod, J. D. (1984). Sex differences in vulnerability to undesirable life events. *American Sociological Review, 49,* 620–631.
Analyses based on five epidemiological surveys of the general population, which show that women are not more vulnerable to the effects of all undesirable events but are to "network" events, that is, those that happen to a significant other.

Paykel, E. S. (1987). Methodology of life events research. *Advances in Psychosomatic Medicine,* *17,* 13–29.
A review of some of the difficult issues encountered in conducting studies of recent life events.

Pianta, R. C., & Egeland, B. (1994). Relation between depressive symptoms and stressful life events in a sample of disadvantaged mothers. *Journal of Consulting and Clinical Psychology, 62,* 1229–1234.
An investigation suggesting that the relationship between stressful life events and depressive symptomatology is complex and bidirectional.

Rook, K., Dooley, D., & Catalano, R. (1991). Stress transmission: The effects of husbands' job stressors on the emotional health of their wives. *Journal of Marriage and the Family, 53,* 165–177.
A study showing husbands' job stressors to be associated with significantly elevated symptom levels in their wives, their impact being moderated by marital tension.

29

Social Comparison

Lisa G. Aspinwall

The need to know oneself—one's capabilities, opinions, and emotions—is powerful, especially during times of stress or illness. In many situations, few objective indicators are available. For example, a woman who wishes to know whether she is coping well while awaiting breast cancer biopsy results ("How upset should I be? Are my fears normal or irrational? What should I do while I wait?") has little more to go on than the opinions and experiences of other people.

The process by which people seek such information from other people has been extensively studied. According to social comparison theory, if people are uncertain about themselves and objective information is unavailable, they will evaluate their opinions and other attributes in reference to those of similar others. That is, they will use other people as benchmarks for evaluating themselves. As it turns out, social comparisons are powerful predictors of how individuals feel about themselves. In many surveys, people's beliefs regarding how they compare to others are the single best predictors of satisfaction in many different life domains. For example, comparisons to others are better predictors of how satisfied people are with their standard of living than are objective indicators, such as income.

SOCIAL COMPARISONS AND COPING WITH STRESS

A great deal of research has been devoted to understanding why social comparisons are so important to us and what functions comparisons to others may serve among people facing new and threatening situations. In studies conducted in the 1950s, research participants were told that they would receive some painful electric shocks and were given the opportunity to wait alone or with other participants. Most participants chose to wait with others, leading the researcher to speculate that participants wanted to use the emotional reactions of other people to determine whether their own feelings about the upcoming shock were appropriate. Because the situation was stressful and participants had little information about it, they turned to others facing the same situation to evaluate their own reactions.

Since then, researchers have examined social comparisons in a variety of stressful situations, especially those involving threats to physical and mental health. When one's well-being is challenged by stress or illness, the need to understand one's situation and to know how to handle it increases. Ample evidence suggests that individuals obtain such information from other people at virtually all stages of confronting a threat to health—from the interpretation of symptoms and the decision to seek health care, to awaiting and recovering from surgery, and/or to making lifelong adjustments to chronic illness and pain. Some of the most influential studies have been conducted with women participants.

EXAMPLES OF SOCIAL INFLUENCES ON HEALTH

Three examples illustrate the impact of social comparisons on people in new and threatening situations. First, women college students whose views on abortion were strongly challenged by other women had lower blood pressure and had heart rates 8 beats per minute lower in the presence of a single stranger who supported their views than did women who argued their views without another person to support them. Second, research participants who had just received the news that they tested positive for an enzyme disorder rated their illness as more serious if they were told that they were the only person to test positive in a group of five than if they were told that four out of the five people in their group tested positive. Finally, men awaiting major heart surgery who were assigned roommates who had already had their surgery were less anxious and were released from the hospital sooner than other patients.

WHAT DO PEOPLE LEARN FROM SOCIAL COMPARISONS?

In the preceding examples, people's emotions (anxiety), beliefs (about the seriousness of their illness), and even their health (cardiac reactivity, discharge from the hospital) were influenced by other people. Why are the opinions, experiences, and even simply the agreement of other people so influential? The answer may lie in the ability of social comparison information to answer four critical questions: (1) "What is happening?" (2) "Is it normal?" (3) "How am I doing?" and (4) "What should I be doing?" Let us examine each of these in turn.

"What Is Happening? (And Is It Serious?)"

Social comparison theory suggests that conditions of uncertainty increase people's need to know what is happening. The emergence of somatic symptoms is one such circumstance. Many symptoms are ambiguous and require interpretation. Is that twinge of pain in one's side indigestion, appendicitis, a muscle strain, or something else? If people have little direct experience with that symptom, they may compare themselves to others. Both role-playing studies and experiments find that the opinions of other laypeople about whether symptoms are serious are just as important as more seemingly objective information (e.g., diagnostic tests) in determining whether people believe that their symptoms require medical attention. In some cases, social information actually seems to override more objective information. For example, even when a diagnostic test suggested that participants in one study were fine, they said that they would be likely to see a doctor if friends and family suggested they should. Social influence works the other way, too. In studies in which participants received test results suggesting the presence of illness, the presence of another person—even a stranger—who minimized the seriousness of their condition was enough to make participants report that they were less likely to seek follow-up care.

"Is It Normal?"

Social comparison theory also states that people want to know whether their feelings are appropriate. Information that one's feelings, symptoms, opinions, or experiences are shared by others is called "normative information." In the previous examples, people who believed that many others had tested positive for the same disorder were less worried about it, and the women college students who had someone present who supported their views faced disagreement from others more calmly. Normative information conveys reassurance that one is not alone in one's difficulties and that one's opinions are not out of line.

Although normative information may confer many benefits, a great deal of research suggests that people under stress find it difficult to obtain such information. This may be especially true when people are facing severe physical illness, mental illness, or other negative life events (e.g., bereavement and rape). It may be difficult to find other people with the same experience, and one's friends and family may know little about it. Often people facing serious illness do not discuss their fears and concerns, for fear of upsetting others. In some studies, more than 80% of cancer patients reported keeping their distress and uncertainty to themselves. In addition, friends and family members may discourage distressed persons from expressing negative thoughts and feelings in order to cheer them up, to calm them, to avoid an awkward interpersonal exchange, or to put on a brave front for the distressed persons. The net effect of such behaviors is that people often do not receive information that their fears and concerns are valid and shared by others. Failure to obtain normative information may intensify feelings of difference, isolation, and inadequacy. The potential of support groups composed of other people managing the same illness or stressor to provide normative information is therefore very important.

"How Am I Doing?" and "What Should I Be Doing?": Using Social Comparisons to Meet Coping Needs

In addition to getting information about what they are facing and whether they are responding normally, people use information about other people to meet two different kinds of coping goals—problem solving and the regulation of emotion. People want to learn how to manage a stressor, and they also want to feel better about a stressful situation. In the study of hospital patients mentioned earlier, seeing someone who had gone through the experience of major heart surgery may have provided both kinds of benefits. Specifically, someone who had just gone through such surgery may have provided information about how to handle the sensations and procedures a patient might experience (information useful in problem solving), and may also have provided living evidence that people survive the surgery (information useful in regulating emotions, such as anxiety). The following sections examine how two different kinds of social comparisons, downward comparisons and upward comparisons, may be used to meet these coping needs.

DOWNWARD COMPARISONS AND SELECTIVE EVALUATION

Although the original social comparison theory suggested that people would compare themselves to similar others, researchers rapidly found that people under stress compared themselves to people worse off than themselves—a "downward comparison." What stressed people seem to do is to identify areas in which they are relatively advantaged, and, in doing so, to make the best of a difficult situation.

Downward comparisons have been extensively studied among people coping with chronic illness. Some of the best evidence comes from interviews of breast cancer patients. In a study by Taylor, Wood, and Lichtman, 78% of the women interviewed said that they were better off than other women with breast cancer. How did they reach this conclusion? As the following examples illustrate, these women were quite skilled in using downward comparisons to highlight ways in which the experience of breast cancer could have been worse. One older woman observed, "The people I really feel sorry for are those young gals. To lose a breast when you're so young must be awful. I'm 73, what do I need a breast for?" A young woman said, "If I hadn't been married, I think this thing would have really gotten to me. I can't imagine dating or whatever knowing you have this thing and not knowing how to tell the man about it."

In examining how women were able to arrive at the conclusion that they were better off than others, the researchers identified several strategies for selective self-evaluation: comparing oneself with less fortunate others, focusing on attributes that give one an advantage, creating hypothetical worse worlds, and manufacturing normative standards of adjustment. This last strategy involves inventing a dimension on which one is faring well. An example would be the coach of a kids' softball team who gives an award for every conceivable aspect of the game, such as "best slider" or "best spirit." Interestingly, these different ways of making oneself feel better were not restricted to the women managing breast cancer, but also appeared among their husbands. Husbands compared their adjustment to that of "all those animals who left their wives," when in reality only a tiny proportion of marriages had dissolved after the wives' surgery.

Since this classic study, dozens of other studies—including studies among people with rheumatoid arthritis, women experiencing failure with *in vitro* fertilization, and women facing age-related declines in health—have supported the idea that people manage stress by making downward comparisons. Similarly, experiments that provide downward comparisons (either by telling a story about someone with extreme difficulties or by manipulating the performance of a fellow participant who performs poorly) find that people under stress report improvements in mood, better evaluations of their own performance, and greater hope for the future, compared to people for whom no downward comparison information is available.

It is important to note, however, that there may be some exceptions to the general finding that downward comparisons are beneficial to people under stress. In particular, under some conditions, downward comparisons may be depressing or may raise fears that one's own situation will decline. Studies of adjustment to cancer and chronic pain find that this may be especially true if patients do not believe they have control over the course of their illness.

UPWARD COMPARISONS AND PROBLEM SOLVING

Whereas downward comparisons most often serve one's needs for emotional regulation, comparisons to people adjusting better than oneself on some dimension, termed "upward comparisons," may provide important information about how to do better. Information about people adjusting successfully to chronic illness may also serve as a source of hope or inspiration. Unfortunately, information about people doing better than oneself may lead to jealousy and frustration as well. For example, a mother who wishes to learn how to handle the stress of working and raising young children may look to a "supermom" for both inspiration and information. However, such a comparison may make her feel inferior. In addition, the "supermom" may enjoy some advantages the "regular mom" does not, such as the ability to hire assistance or a partner who will help around the house. For these reasons, researchers find that people often avoid upward comparisons. For example, in studies of pay equity, women tend to compare their pay to that of other women, rather than to the pay of men in similar positions, because comparisons to men may make women's compensation seem inferior. As a result, women may feel subjectively satisfied with outcomes that are objectively unfair.

As the "supermom" and pay equity examples illustrate, upward comparisons may provide useful information, but this information may make people feel bad. What makes social comparison research exciting is that a single comparison rarely meets both of the two coping goals of problem solving and emotional regulation. Instead, it is more likely that a comparison helps in one way, but hurts in another. How people direct their attention to certain aspects of comparisons—that is, how they juggle different comparisons on different dimensions, in order to feel good about themselves and also to learn from successful others—is a lively research area. What seems to be important in upward comparisons is to learn from successful people, but to avoid explicit comparisons to them. In addition, individuals must consider any special advantages the successful others have that may account for their superior standing, so as to avoid setting unrealistic standards for themselves.

SOCIAL COMPARISONS AND SUPPORT GROUPS

Serious illness and other negative life events generate needs for both information and emotional support. The idea behind support groups is that information about similar others can best meet both of these needs. Surprisingly, little research on social comparison processes in support groups exists, largely because of researchers' concerns about sensitizing support group members to explicit comparisons among themselves. Instead, researchers have created experimental groups and situations, manipulated the information presented about other group members, and assessed participants' feelings and beliefs. Although these studies clearly do not recreate the settings of real support groups, they do offer some interesting findings about the impact of other people's experiences on how individuals feel about themselves. In particular, these studies support the idea that the presence of persons with difficulties is encouraging to other people under stress, especially to people with low self-esteem.

In one of the few studies to examine social comparisons in actual support groups, researchers studied middle-aged men and women in smoking cessation groups. Group members were surveyed at different times about their preference for different types of people in their group. At the start of treatment, people who were heavy smokers preferred to have someone with worse smoking problems than themselves as a fellow group member. Such a person might provide a downward comparison that would make the heavy smokers' own difficulties with smoking and quitting seem less severe. As people quit smoking, their preference for such a person as a group member decreased. Interestingly, there was no evidence that people made downward comparisons to actual group members (which might be awkward); they seemed instead to compare themselves to a mental image of the "typical smoker." Just like the husbands of breast cancer patients who believed that other men were handling the situation poorly, the smokers who were quitting maintained a mental image of someone who was worse off. In sum, these studies suggest that the presence of another person experiencing difficulties—whether the person is actually present or is imagined—helps people feel better about their own situation. A clear task for future research is to examine how such dynamics work in actual support groups and how people may learn from those who are coping well without loss of self-esteem.

FURTHER READING

Buunk, B. P., & Gibbons, F. X. (Eds.). (1997). *Health, coping, and well-being: Perspectives from social comparison theory.* Mahwah, NJ: Erlbaum.
A new volume of current research and theory on social comparisons and health, with chapters on the following topics: depression, burnout, adolescent risk behavior, risk judgments, lay referrals, AIDS prevention, stress, chronic pain, coping, and cancer.

Coates, D., & Wortman, C. B. (1980). Depression maintenance and interpersonal control. In A. Baum & J. E. Singer (Eds.), *Advances in environmental psychology: Vol. 2. Applications of personal control* (pp. 149–182). Hillsdale, NJ: Erlbaum.
A fascinating discussion of what happens when people who are distressed express negative feelings to others and do not receive the support and validation they desire. This chapter focuses specifically on the problems depressed people may encounter when they express negative feelings to others.

Croyle, R. T. (1992). Appraisal of health threats: Cognition, motivation, and social comparison. *Cognitive Therapy and Research, 16,* 165–182.
A review of laboratory experiments and other studies of how other people influence individuals' appraisals of and emotional reactions to information suggesting that the individuals are at risk for illness. Discusses how these social sources of information may be incorporated in broader theories of illness representation and stress and coping.

Gibbons, F. X., Gerrard, M., Lando, H. A., & McGovern, P. G. (1991). Social comparison and smoking cessation: The role of the "typical smoker." *Journal of Experimental Social Psychology, 27,* 239–258.
A rare longitudinal study of adults in smoking cessation groups. Changes in preferences for downward comparisons, and views of the "typical smoker," were found to be related to people's ability to quit smoking.

Swallow, S. R., & Kuiper, N. A. (1988). Social comparison and negative self-evaluations: An application to depression. *Clinical Psychology Review, 8,* 55–76.
An examination of the importance of social standards of self-evaluation and some of the difficulties depressed people have in applying such standards fairly to themselves. Excellent treatment of social comparison theory, with a focus on upward comparisons.

Taylor, S. E., Aspinwall, L. G., Giuliano, T. A., Dakof, G. A., & Reardon, K. (1993). Storytelling and coping with stressful events. *Journal of Applied Social Psychology, 23,* 703–733.
People facing difficult situations are often inundated with unasked-for advice and stories about other people. Unfortunately, most of these stories are negative—describing, for example, people who battled unsuccessfully with cancer or who flunked out of college. Using interviews and experiments, this study examined how cancer patients and college students responded to upward and downward comparisons provided by other people, with emphasis on the conditions under which such information provides hope and conditions under which comparisons are seen to provide unwanted advice.

Taylor, S. E., Buunk, B. P., & Aspinwall, L. G. (1990). Social comparison, stress and coping. *Personality and Social Psychology Bulletin, 16,* 74–89.
An integration of social comparison theory with research on stress and coping; reviews the effects of upward and downward comparisons on people facing threats to well-being.

Taylor, S. E., Wood, J. V., & Lichtman, R. R. (1983). It could be worse: Selective evaluation as a response to victimization. *Journal of Social Issues, 39*(2), 19–40.
A classic and influential interview study of women with breast cancer, in which respondents showed remarkable flexibility and creativity in reevaluating their situation following surgery.

Tesser, A. (1988). Toward a self-evaluation maintenance model of social behavior. In L. Berkowitz (Ed.), *Advances in experimental social psychology* (Vol. 21, pp. 181–227). Orlando, FL: Academic Press.
Unwanted upward comparisons may come from close others (an overachieving sibling, a neighbor's new house and charming children, etc.); unfortunately, the closer the person, the more painful the comparison. Examines how people choose their activities and their close relationships to avoid painful upward comparisons and to preserve self-esteem. Also examines cases in which people associate with successful others to "bask in reflected glory."

Wills, T. A. (1981). Downward comparison principles in social psychology. *Psychological Bulletin, 90,* 245–271.
A thorough and important examination of when and why people compare themselves to others who are worse off. Examines the darker side of downward comparisons, such as prejudice, hostile humor, and scapegoating.

30

Positive Mental Health

Carol D. Ryff

Mental health has been routinely conceptualized as the absence of illness (i.e., not suffering from depression, anxiety, etc.), rather than as the presence of wellness. The program of research summarized in this chapter rests on a positive formulation of psychological functioning. Key dimensions of well-being are defined, and their theoretical origins are noted. Descriptive studies dealing with age, gender, class, and cultural variations in well-being are then summarized. A final section targets women's life experiences and their interpretations of them as factors influencing well-being. The research shows that when the positive side of mental health is considered, women show unique psychological strengths. Thus, the prevailing research emphasis on dysfunction tells an incomplete story about women's health. Furthermore, the findings document women's adaptive capacities as they deal with life's challenges.

THE MEANING OF PSYCHOLOGICAL WELL-BEING

Six key dimensions of positive psychological functioning constitute the model of well-being described herein: autonomy, environmental mastery, personal growth, positive relations with others, purpose in life, and self-acceptance. Definitions for each dimension are provided in Table 30.1. The constructs emerged from the integrations of three literatures. Developmental psychology, particularly lifespan developmental psychology, offers numerous depictions of wellness, conceived as progressions of continued growth across the life course. Included are Erikson's model of the stages of psychosocial development, Buhler's formulation of basic life tendencies that work toward the fulfillment of life, and Neugarten's descriptions of personality change in adulthood and old age. Clinical psychology offers further formulations of well-being, such as Maslow's conception of self-actualization, Rogers's view of the fully functioning person, Jung's formulation of individuation, and Allport's conception of maturity. The literature on mental health,

TABLE 30.1. Definitions of Theory-Guided Dimensions of Well-Being

Self-acceptance
  High scorer: Possesses a positive attitude toward the self; acknowledges and accepts multiple aspects of self, including good and bad qualities; feels positive about past life.
  Low scorer: Feels dissatisfied with self; is disappointed with what has occurred in past life; is troubled about certain personal qualities; wishes to be different from what he or she is.

Positive relations with others
  High scorer: Has warm, satisfying, trusting relationships with others; is concerned about the welfare of others; capable of strong empathy, affection, and intimacy; understands the give and take of human relationships.
  Low scorer: Has few close, trusting relationships with others; finds it difficult to be warm, open, and concerned about others; is isolated and frustrated in interpersonal relationships; is not willing to make compromises to sustain important ties with others.

Autonomy
  High scorer: Is self-determining and independent; is able to resist social pressures to think and act in certain ways; regulates behavior from within; evaluates self by personal standards.
  Low scorer: Is concerned about the expectations and evaluations of others; relies on judgments of others to make important decisions; conforms to social pressures to think and act in certain ways.

Environmental mastery
  High scorer: Has a sense of mastery and competence in managing the environment; controls complex array of external activities; makes effective use of surrounding opportunities; is able to choose or create contexts suitable to personal needs and values.
  Low scorer: Has difficulty managing everyday affairs; feels unable to change or improve surrounding context; is unaware of surrounding opportunities; lacks sense of direction; does not see purpose in past life; has no outlooks or beliefs that give life meaning.

Purpose in life
  High scorer: Has goals in life and a sense of directedness; feels there is meaning to present and past life; holds beliefs that give life purpose; has aims and objectives for living.
  Low scorer: Lacks a sense of meaning in life; has few goals or aims; lacks sense of direction; does not see purpose in past life; has no outlooks or beliefs that give life meaning.

Personal growth
  High scorer: Has a feeling of continued development; sees self as growing and expanding; is open to new experiences; has sense of realizing his or her potential; sees improvement in self and behavior over time; is changing in ways that reflect more self-knowledge and effectiveness.
  Low scorer: Has a sense of personal stagnation; lacks sense of improvement or expansion over time; feels bored and uninterested with life; feels unable to develop new attitudes or behaviors.

though guided largely by absence-of-illness definitions of well-being, includes significant exceptions, such as Jahoda's formulation of positive criteria of mental health and Birren and Renner's conception of positive functioning in later life.

The six qualities that make up the model of psychological well-being represent the points of convergence in these diverse attempts to articulate the meaning of positive functioning. Empirical studies have been conducted to operationalize these components of well-being with structured self-report procedures. Multiple investigations document the reliability and validity of scales constructed to measure these six constructs.

VARIATIONS ON THE DIMENSIONS OF WELL-BEING

Our research group's findings also describe differences between men and women, age differences, class differences, and (more recently) cultural differences on the dimensions of well-being.

Sex Differences

Multiple data sets have shown that women of all ages consistently rate themselves higher on positive relations with others than do men; in a number of studies, women scored higher than men on personal growth. The remaining four aspects of psychological well-being consistently show no significant differences between men and women. Such findings are particularly relevant in the context of prior mental health research, which repeatedly documents a higher incidence of psychological problems (particularly depression) among women. When the positive end of the mental health spectrum is examined, however, women are shown to have greater psychological strengths compared to men in certain aspects of well-being, and comparable profiles with regard to others. To miss these differences is to convey an incomplete picture of the psychological functioning of women.

Age Differences

Our cross-sectional studies with young, middle-aged, and elderly adults have shown diverse and replicable patterns of age differences on the six dimensions of well-being. Some features of wellness, such as environmental mastery and autonomy, show incremental age patterns (only from young adulthood to midlife for the latter). Others, such as personal growth and purpose in life, show decremental patterns (especially from midlife to old age). Self-acceptance, by contrast, shows no age differences across the three life periods. The interpersonal dimension, positive relations with others, varies between showing age increments and showing no age differences. These overall patterns have been evident in community samples as well as in nationally representative samples. Together, they point to a differentiated profile of well-being in which some qualities appear to improve with time, others seem to decline, and still others are stable.

Longitudinal research is necessary to clarify whether the patterns reflect true maturational processes or cohort differences. In either case, the recurrent reports of lower self-ratings among older adults on purpose in life and personal growth warrant attention. Such findings point to the important psychological challenges of later life, and relate to growing arguments that contemporary social structures lag behind the added years of life many people now enjoy. Opportunities for continued development and meaningful existence may be restricted for present cohorts of older persons—a situation compounded by our findings that older adults, like their younger counterparts, aspire to these aspects of well-being.

Class Differences

The link between social class and profiles of well-being has been examined in the Wisconsin Longitudinal Study of educational and occupational aspirations and achievements. Based on a sample of midlife adults who have been studied since their senior year in high school, the research shows higher well-being for those with higher occupational standing. Higher well-being is also evident among those with greater educational attainment. These differences are most strongly evident for reported levels of purpose in life and personal growth, particularly for women. Viewed in terms of the growing literature on class and health, these findings indicate that lower social class standing not only increases the likelihood of negative outcomes, but also decreases chances for positive well-being. Such psychological strengths may provide valuable protective factors in the face of life's difficulties, although their role in maintaining positive mental health is largely unexplored.

Cultural Variation

Much current social-scientific discussion revolves around distinctions between individualistic/independent cultures and those that are more collectivistic/interdependent. These suggest that more self-oriented aspects of well-being (e.g., self-acceptance and autonomy) may be salient in Western cultural contexts, whereas other-oriented dimensions (e.g., positive relations with others) may be prominent in Eastern, interdependent cultures. These ideas were examined with a midlife sample of adults from the United States and a sociodemographically comparable sample from South Korea. U.S. respondents had higher well-being—a finding consistent with prior findings that Westerners attribute greater positive qualities to themselves. Analyses within cultures revealed that Koreans showed highest self-ratings on the measure of positive relations with others, and lowest ratings for self-acceptance and personal growth. Among U.S. respondents, personal growth was rated highest, especially for women; autonomy, contrary to the purported emphasis on self-determination in the West, was rated lowest. In both cultures, women rated themselves significantly higher than men on positive relations with others and personal growth. Qualitative data showed that Koreans placed greater emphasis on the well-being of others (e.g., children) in defining their own well-being than did U.S. respondents.

UNDERSTANDING THE VARIATION: LIFE EXPERIENCES AND INTERPRETIVE MECHANISMS

In addition to the examination of variation in psychological well-being via broad sociodemographic variables (gender, age, class, culture), we have studied more proximal life experiences and individuals' interpretations of them as influences on their mental health. Three such experiences are briefly noted here: parenthood, community relocation in later life, and the emergence of physical health problems with aging. With regard to the first of these, we interviewed midlife parents about how their grown children had "turned out." The guiding idea was that children's accomplishments and adjustment would influence parents' assessments of themselves (i.e., their levels of self-acceptance, purpose in life, environmental mastery, etc.). We further hypothesized that parental well-being would be influenced by social comparison and attributional processes (i.e., how their children's lives compared with their own, the extent to which they saw themselves as responsible for their children's lives). The latter constitute theory-guided psychological "interpretations" of the parental experience.

The findings indicated that multiple aspects of parental well-being (particularly those dimensions noted above) were strongly predicted by children's adjustment (personal and social), and less so by their attainment (educational and occupational). These effects were evident for mothers as well as fathers of both sons and daughters, although mothers' well-being was more strongly tied to the lives of sons, particularly their personal and social adjustment. The findings further indicated that social comparisons with children had negative links to parents' self-evaluations. That is, parents had lower levels of well-being when they perceived children had done better than themselves—an effect that occurred primarily with regard to comparisons about adjustment. In the attainment domain, mothers, but only those with higher levels of education, felt more positive about themselves when their children exceeded their own achievements. The attributional results revealed that parents with the lowest profiles of well-being were those whose children who had not done well and for whom they had exercised little parental responsibility (i.e., support, involvement). Collectively, these findings point to the diverse avenues through which parenthood (a status occupied by approximately 90% of midlife U.S. adults) is linked with positive mental health.

Raising children represents an enduring (if not chronic) life experience, although we have also studied discrete life transitions, such as community relocation. We are currently tracking a sample of aging women through the increasingly normative transition of moves from a private residence to a retirement community or apartment. We are investigating how specific relocation factors (e.g., reasons that "push" the women to move, factors that "pull" them to particular new settings, and the fit between these two), as well as an array of interpretive processes (e.g., quality of ties to friends and family), affect the mental and physical health of the respondents. Results to date have documented that both relocation factors and interpretive mechanisms are linked to multiple aspects of psychological well-being. Longitudinal findings have underscored women's adaptive capacities—for example, how in the course of this transition they change core aspects of their identities to maintain positive profiles of well-being, and how they partake of and benefit from "unexpected gains" in the relocation process.

A final example pertains to ongoing studies on the dynamic nature of the relationship between the physical and mental health of aging women. In this work, the targeted life experience pertains to the emergence or persistence of physical symptoms and chronic conditions that accompany growing old, and the ways in which these (as mediated by an array of interpretive processes) affect mental health. Findings in this work show that the effects of physical conditions on psychological functioning are mediated by social comparisons and perceived integration with the social structure. This research under-scores the adaptive features of their interpretations: Women with poorer physical health conditions, for example, maintain positive mental health profiles by engaging in favorable social comparisons.

The story emerging from this work about women is that they have unique psycho-logical strengths, particularly with regard to the quality of their relations with others and their sense of self-realization through time. The findings underscore women's varied experiences, as mothers and as aging widows confronting health problems. From an adaptational perspective, the work shows the benefits that follow from the interpretive lenses women bring with them to their life experiences.

FURTHER READING

Allport, G. W. (1961). *Pattern and growth in personality*. New York: Holt, Rinehart & Winston.

Birren, J. E., & Renner, V. J. (1980). Concepts and issues of mental health and aging. In J. E. Birren & R. B. Sloane (Eds.), *Handbook of mental health and aging* (pp. 3–33). Englewood Cliffs, NJ: Prentice-Hall.

Buhler, C., & Massarik, F. (Eds.). *The course of human life*. New York: Springer.

Erikson, E. (1959). Identity of the life cycle. *Psychological Issues, 1,* 18–164.

Heidrich, S. M., & Ryff, C.D. (1993). Physical and mental health in later life: The self-system as mediator. *Psychology and Aging, 8,* 327–338.
Study showing how late-life relationships between physical and mental health in women are mediated by social comparison processes, self-discrepancies, and social integration.

Heidrich, S. M., & Ryff, C. D. (1993). The role of social comparison processes in the psychological adaptation of elderly adults. *Journal of Gerontology, 48,* 127–136.
Study showing that older women in poor physical health who engage in positive social comparisons have mental health profiles similar to those of older women in good physical health.

Jahoda, M. (1958). *Current concepts of positive mental health*. New York: Basic Books.

Jung, C. G. (1933). *Modern man in search of a soul* (W. S. Dell & C. F. Baynes, Trans.). New York: Harcourt, Brace, and World.

Kling, K. D., Ryff, C. D., & Essex, M. J. (1997). Adaptive changes in the self-concept during a life transition. *Personality and Social Psychology Bulletin, 23,* 989–998.
Longitudinal study showing that changing what is central to one's self-definition can protect psychological well-being during the experience of community relocation.

Maslow, A. H. (1968). *Toward a psychology of being* (2nd ed.). New York: Van Nostrand.

Neugarten, B. (1973). Personality change in late life: A developmental perspective. In C. Eisdorfer & M. P. Lawton (Eds.), *The psychology of adult development and aging* (pp. 311–335). Washington, DC: American Psychological Association.

Rogers, C. R. (1961). *On becoming a person*. Boston: Houghton Mifflin.

Ryff, C. D. (1989). Happiness is everything, or is it? Explorations on the meaning of psychological well-being. *Journal of Personality and Social Psychology, 57,* 1069–1081.
Original validation study for development of the multidimensional approach to the assessment of psychological well-being.

Ryff, C. D. (1995). Psychological well-being in adult life. *Current Directions in Psychological Science, 4,* 99–104.
Provides an overview of our program's research on well-being, including descriptive studies of sociodemographic variations (age, gender, class, culture) as well as explanatory life experience studies.

Ryff, C. D., & Keyes, C. L. M. (1995). The structure of psychological well-being revisited. *Journal of Personality and Social Psychology, 69,* 719–727.
Study documenting the six-factor structure of the well-being model in a national probability sample, and replicates prior findings of gender and age differences.

Ryff, C. D., Lee, Y. H., Essex, M. J., & Schmutte, P. S. (1994). My children and me: Mid-life evaluations of grown children and of self. *Psychology and Aging, 9,* 195–205.
Study reporting middle-aged parents' views of how think their grown children have "turned out," and relates these assessments to their own psychological well-being.

Ryff, C. D., Schmutte, P. S., & Lee, Y. H. (1996). How children turn out: Implications for parental self-evaluation. In C. D. Ryff & M. M. Seltzer (Eds.), *The parental experience in mid-life* (pp. 383–422). Chicago: University of Chicago Press.
Chapter summarizing the larger program of research on the midlife parental experience and its effects on parents' well-being via social comparison and attribution processes.

Section III

PREVENTION

31

Section Editor's Overview

Abby C. King

*T*he significant public health and medical gains made in combating and controlling infectious disease during the first half of the 20th century served to usher in a new era of optimism about the control men and women could potentially wield over disease processes that had plagued humankind for centuries. Such optimism has since given way to alarm and frustration in the face of the major challenges that currently occupy health professionals in the United States and other Western nations—the various chronic diseases that remain largely unharnessed, and the devastating illness that is AIDS. Although significant advances have been made in the diagnosis and treatment of a number of the major chronic diseases plaguing the United States, including cardiovascular disease, cancer, pulmonary disease, and a range of metabolic diseases, the rising health care costs accompanying these advances have been staggering, resulting in the current U.S. health care crisis. What is even more sobering is the fact that roughly two thirds of all U.S. deaths from these and other diseases are preventable. Moreover, clear behavioral pathways for preventing HIV infection have been elucidated, although a cure for AIDS itself remains elusive.

These dramatic statistics are at odds with the budgeting of U.S. health care dollars, fewer than 1% of which are typically earmarked for health promotion and disease prevention activities. Yet there is an increasing consensus that most of the premature morbidity and mortality caused by the leading killers of U.S. women as well as men—cardiovascular disease and cancer—are preventable through changes in cigarette smoking, alcohol use, diet, physical activity, and environmental exposures, as well as behaviors leading to early detection (e.g., breast self-examinations, Pap smears). One of the reasons for this disparity may stem from the fact that prevention is among the basic (and often unglamorous) public health activities that have provided the principal means for keeping U.S. residents well (e.g., public sanitation, control of environmental exposures and communicable infections, education in personal hygiene and risk factor reduction). Technological advances in science and medicine have meanwhile led to a primarily treatment-oriented medical approach to health care, which has fired the public's imagination and increasingly fueled the health care industry; in turn, less attention has been paid to more "upstream" public health approaches to chronic disease prevention and control.

191

COMPARING THE MEDICAL AND THE PUBLIC HEALTH APPROACHES TO INTERVENTION

The medical model and the public health model of intervention involve different philosophies, perspectives, and goals. In the medical approach, the target for intervention is typically the individual, and the professional stance of the health care provider is often a "waiting" stance, in which the provider chooses a location, schedule, and intervention philosophy suited primarily to his or her needs and preferences. The intervention is typically biologically based, and is aimed at treating disease that has already become evident (i.e., a "downstream" approach).

By contrast, in the public health approach, the target for investigation and intervention is the community or population at large. The health care professional takes a "seeking" stance to identify and better understand the factors influencing the disease process, with the goal of developing effective strategies in order to keep the disease from manifesting itself (i.e., primary prevention), in addition to preventing or minimizing recurrences of disease states (i.e., secondary prevention). A multiple-level approach to intervention is often developed, with intervention goals typically expanded beyond individual behavior change to include changes in social networks and structures, organizational norms, regulatory policies, and the physical and social environment as a means for enhancing long-term maintenance of the target behaviors. Theories and perspectives relevant to such aims (e.g., social marketing, communication theories, diffusion, community organization, and systems approaches), in addition to those theories and strategies relevant to individual behavior change, are brought to bear. Instruments of program delivery are expanded beyond the health care professional to include other community professionals, agencies, and organizations, such as the mass media. The "location" of program delivery expands accordingly beyond the confines of the health care provider's setting to encompass other community settings as well as the more general environment. The expansion of program delivery channels and locations improves the program's access to those sectors of the community that may be able to benefit particularly from preventive programs, but that typically are not reached through traditional clinical settings (e.g., the homeless, ethnic minority populations).

In public health or community-based approaches to intervention, other groups of people in the community, in addition to those segments at risk for a specific disease or condition, become useful targets for intervention. These other groups consist of those persons who probably have the greatest influence on the community at large or on the population segments of particular interest. They include a variety of health professionals, persons working in the mass media, and politicians, as well as other community opinion leaders (e.g., chief executive officers of major businesses, owners of small businesses, school board members, leaders of religious institutions or service organizations).

PREVENTION AND WOMEN'S HEALTH: BASIC CONCEPTS

This section begins with chapters on the prevention of specific conditions affecting women (HIV, breast cancer, osteoporosis), and then moves on to chapters concerning the modification of various lifestyle factors (smoking and alcohol use, nutrition, oral health, exercise, and relaxation). As reflected by this description, the scope of preventive efforts in the area of women's health is potentially huge, although the promise that prevention offers women—in terms not only of reduced morbidity and mortality, but of enhanced quality of life—has to date been little realized in most areas of women's health. The promise of prevention for women is based on a number of basic concepts. These include the notions that preventive strategies for most diseases, particularly those of a chronic nature, should begin early in a woman's life, ideally in childhood or conceivably earlier (i.e., during the prenatal period); that with few exceptions, preventive activities and behaviors typically require ongoing vigilance throughout a woman's life; and that such activities need to take into account a woman's demographic, biological, developmental, behavioral, psychosocial, and environmental milieus (i.e., population segmentation is critical for the development of effective preventive interventions). The chapters in this section serve to highlight these varying milieus.

THE DEMOGRAPHIC MILIEU

It has become increasingly clear that in addition to sex, demographic factors such as age, educational level, socioeconomic status (SES), marital status, ethnic or racial group, and religious affiliation are strongly associated with a range of diseases, conditions, and health behaviors in both women and men. Such factors can be utilized to identify those subgroups of women at particular risk for certain diseases, or those who have to date been underserved in important health areas. This issue is highlighted in the chapter by Mantell and Susser on homeless women as important targets for HIV prevention activities. As pointed out by these authors, families headed by women are among the fastest-growing homeless groups in the United States, and the challenges of homelessness create an environment that may make women vulnerable to HIV risk behavior. Mantell and Susser make it clear that homeless women are a diverse group and need to be understood as such, although it appears unlikely that HIV prevention programs aimed at women in general, described in the chapter by Sikkema, will reach this underserved segment of women.

As pointed out by Mayer and Kaplan in their respective chapters on breast cancer screening, age is another demographic factor that can be used to organize and target subgroups of women for prevention activities. Both these authors note that breast cancer mortality could be diminished considerably if all women aged 50 years and older obtained regular mammograms (i.e., every 1–2 years). In addition to providing a means for differentiating those groups of women who are at generally increased risk of certain diseases, age can also provide a means for identifying groups of women with increased risk because of certain deleterious health behaviors. One such negative health behavior, discussed in Dubbert's chapter on exercise, is physical inactivity. Older women have been generally found to be less active than either younger women or older men. At the other end of the age spectrum, Killen points out in his chapter on cigarette smoking prevention that adolescent girls may be at particular risk for smoking adoption.

Race and ethnicity have also been used to identify subgroups of women who may have an increased likelihood of contracting a disease, and thus may become important targets for preventive efforts. A striking example of this is found in Sikkema's chapter, in which she notes that although African-American and Hispanic women constituted 21% of all U.S. women in 1995, they accounted for 76% of AIDS cases among women diagnosed in the United States. It is important to note, however, as a growing number of researchers have done, that ethnicity is often confounded by SES. The conditions found in a low-SES environment, as opposed to cultural variables reflected by racial and ethnic differences, may be the important predisposing factors responsible for increased vulnerability in contracting disease; these factors, therefore, should become the targets in public health efforts.

THE BIOLOGICAL MILIEU

The presence of biological vulnerabilities provides an important means of classifying women for purposes of delivering preventive interventions. The utility of this approach is demonstrated in the chapters by Brunner and St. Jeor on nutrition and women's health. As these authors point out, U.S. national nutrition recommendations have been organized around different health conditions and diseases, including heart disease, cancer, hypertension, and non-insulin-dependent diabetes mellitus. Although the nutrition messages developed for the prevention and control of this range of diseases are generally consistent with one another, they do tend to emphasize different parts of the nutrition message. For example, the message described for the prevention of heart disease tends to focus on decreasing certain nutrients (e.g., saturated fat), whereas the message described for the prevention of cancer tends to emphasize an increase in fruits, vegetables, and fiber. This may help to explain, at least in part, the U.S. public's confusion concerning the best diet to maintain good general health and decrease the chances of disease. Brunner and St. Jeor note that several of the recommendations that have received the widest scientific support (e.g., keeping total dietary fat below 30% of total energy intake, including at least five servings of fruits and vegetables per day) continue to be unmet by the majority of U.S. women.

Some of the methods that have been evaluated to help women change their diets to decrease their risk of chronic diseases such as breast cancer are described in the chapter on nutrition education by Glanz. The Women's Health Trial Vanguard Study described in Glanz's chapter represents an example of how biological vulnerabilities (e.g., family history of breast cancer) have been used to target subgroups of women who may be able to benefit most from preventive efforts.

THE DEVELOPMENTAL MILIEU

Glanz's chapter also provides an example of how developmental transition periods or milestones can be used to shape and tailor preventive strategies in order to optimize their effects. Her discussion of the importance of adequate nutrition during pregnancy underscores the critical nature of appropriate health practices for the health and well-being of the developing infant, in addition to the health of the mother. Other health practices that can have potentially devastating effects during this important developmental milestone are maternal cigarette smoking and alcohol use, as noted in the chapters by Killen and Tucker, respectively.

In addition to pregnancy, other important transition periods or developmental milestones in the lives of women include puberty, entry into college or the work force, marriage, retirement, menopause, and family caregiving episodes (i.e., caring on a regular basis for a sick or frail relative). Adolescence, for example, is a time when girls' concerns about body weight and body image typically increase; yet physical activity, a healthful weight control strategy, is often low, as noted in Dubbert's chapter. Meanwhile, it appears that adolescent girls may seek out unhealthy strategies for controlling their weight, such as cigarette smoking. As discussed in Killen's chapter, thoughts about weight, eating disorder symptoms, and weight control attempts have been found to be prospectively related to smoking initiation in adolescent girls but not boys; these findings underscore the need to address weight control strategies in smoking prevention efforts aimed specifically at girls.

Epidemiological evidence also indicates that adults in their early 20s show a disproportionate amount of weight gain during the subsequent decade, making them an important population segment for obesity prevention efforts as well. Although it makes sense that such periods of change may influence as well as provide opportunities related to preventive health practices among women, relatively few systematic investigations of many of these life stages and their potential impact in the prevention area currently exist.

THE BEHAVIORAL MILIEU

Because all of the health practices discussed in this section consist of behaviors that are to a large degree volitional (i.e., individuals must take active steps to improve their health), behavioral capabilities and skills, as well as knowledge, become important areas to assess in promoting changes in these health areas. In contrast to past public health efforts such as the purification and fluoridation of water supplies, which have utilized a passive prevention approach (i.e., individuals are not required to enact any specific behaviors to reap the health benefits), today's major killers require largely active prevention strategies. Even areas such as nutrition, in which some passive prevention approaches have been enacted (e.g., reduction or elimination of sodium from baby foods), continue to present individuals with a plethora of choices. As noted in many of the chapters in this section, the successful ongoing enactment of HIV prevention behaviors (e.g., safe sex), breast self-examination, a healthful diet, and an appropriate physical activity program all require a level of knowledge and behavioral skill that many women currently lack. The challenges continue to be the development of methods to teach such knowledge and skills in a manner that is relevant to specific subgroups of women, and the use of delivery channels that can reach at-risk women.

THE PSYCHOSOCIAL MILIEU

Just as the presence or absence of preventive behaviors can be influenced by a woman's behavioral capabilities and skills, a woman's perceptions of her body, health, and related concepts can have an impact on her psychological readiness for making health behavior changes. An example of how such psychosocial variables may affect participation in preventive activities is provided by Douthitt's chapter on exercise for adolescents, in which she points out that adolescent girls have been found to use exercise as a means of improving their perceived self-worth as well as perceptions of their physical appearance. As Douthitt notes, exercise adherence in this population improves with increases in the "fit" between a girl's psychological profile (i.e., personality style) and the demands of the physical activity or sport in which she is engaged.

THE ENVIRONMENTAL MILIEU

Although much of the prevention work undertaken by behavioral scientists and public health professionals to date has focused on individual-oriented approaches to health behavior change, it remains the case that major strides in all of these prevention areas are likely to require an increased focus on population-oriented strategies aimed at reaching a broader segment of the U.S. public. The need for such a multilevel approach is critical in light of the population prevalence of many of the health-related behaviors of interest, as well as the important role the environment plays in shaping these health behaviors.

An excellent example of what such a multilevel approach to a preventive activity might look like is described in Mayer's chapter on promoting adherence to breast cancer screening. In such an approach, individual-oriented strategies (e.g., public education campaigns, counseling, prompts for appointments, and the use of incentives) are supplemented with population-oriented strategies (e.g., federal, state, and local laws and policies that facilitate mammographic screening through such avenues as changes in insurance coverage). An additional environmental strategy involves the use of the mass media to set the stage for and reinforce such health behaviors.

CONCLUSION

As noted in all of the chapters in this section, factors influencing the probability that a woman will engage in a preventive health behavior are varied and complex. No one strategy, approach, or perspective is likely to be effective by itself in achieving the level of risk factor change required to produce enduring public health effects in disease prevention across all subgroups of U.S. women. Rather, combinations of approaches based on the differing milieus described above, and requiring the collaboration of a diversity of professional disciplines and interests (both public and private), are strongly indicated.

FURTHER READING

American Heart Association. (1987). *Heart facts.* Dallas, TX: Author.
Summarizes the risk factors associated with heart disease.

Califano, J. A., Jr. (1986). *America's health care revolution: Who lives? Who dies? Who pays?* New York: Random House.
Discusses the emerging issues facing the United States as health care is reformed.

Choi, K. H., & Coates, T. J. (1994). Prevention of HIV infection. *AIDS, 8,* 1371–1389
This article discusses recent approaches to the prevention of HIV.

Cushner, I. M. (1981). Maternal behavior and perinatal risks: Alcohol, smoking, and drugs. *Annual Review of Public Health, 2,* 201–225.
This article reviews the myriad effects of iatrogenic maternal health behaviors on the developing child.

Farquhar, J. W., Fortmann, S. P., Flora, J. H., & Maccoby, N. (1991). Methods of communication to influence behavior. In W. W. Holland, R. Detels, & G. Knox (Eds.), *Oxford textbook of public health* (2nd ed., Vol. 2, pp. 331–344). Oxford: Oxford University Press.
A comprehensive review of the potential influence of mass media and other communication strategies on health-related behaviors.

Forge, W. H. (1987). Public health: Moving from debt to legacy—1986 presidential address. *American Journal of Public Health, 77,* 1276–1278.
Discusses the importance of a preventive, "upstream" orientation in combating the major public health problems currently facing the United States.

Forge, W., Amler, R., & White, C. (1985). Closing the gap. *Journal of the American Medical Association, 254,* 1355–1358.
Provides a discussion of the chronic disease epidemic and the potential utility of preventive approaches.

French, S. A., Perry, C. L., Leon, G. R., & Fulkerson, J. A. (1994). Weight concerns, dieting behavior, and smoking initiation among adolescents: A prospective study. *American Journal of Public Health, 84*, 1818–1820.
Provides prospective evidence of the link between weight concerns and smoking initiation among adolescent girls.

Hanlon, J. J., & Picket, G. E. (1984). *Public health: Administration and practice* (8th ed.). St. Louis, MO: C. V. Mosby.
Provides an overview of the major public health issues facing the nation and the importance of applying a preventive perspective in combating these issues.

Kahn, H. S., & Williamson, D. F. (1990). The contributions of income, education and changing marital status to weight change among U.S. men. *International Journal of Obesity, 14*, 1057–1068.
This epidemiological study provides evidence of the relationship between changes in marital status, as well as other demographic variables, and weight change among a population-based sample of U.S. men.

Kelly, J. A., Murphy, D. A., Sikkema, K. J., & Kalichman, S. C. (1993). Psychological interventions in the prevention of HIV infection are urgently needed. *American Psychologist, 48*, 1023–1034.
Presents an overview of the behavioral pathways that are currently available for preventing HIV infection.

King, A. C. (1991). Community intervention for promotion of physical activity and fitness. *Exercise and Sport Sciences Reviews, 19*, 211–259.
Provides an overview and critique of the forms of community intervention that have occurred to promote physical activity.

King, A. C. (1994). Community and public health approaches to the promotion of physical activity. *Medicine and Science in Sports and Exercise, 26*, 1405–1412.
Compares the approaches used in individual versus community-focused intervention for physical activity promotion, and highlights promising intervention strategies for increasing physical activity.

King, A. C., Blair, S. N., Bild, D. E., Dishman, R. K., Dubbert, P. M., Marcus, B. H., Oldridge, N. B., Paffenbarger, R. S., Jr., Powell, K. E., & Yeager, K. K. (1992). Determinants of physical activity and interventions in adults. *Medicine and Science in Sports and Exercise, 24*(Suppl. 6), S221–S236.
This review, developed via an expert panel, summarizes the physical activity determinants and intervention literature as it applies to adults.

Umberson, D. (1992). Gender, marital status and the social control of health behavior. *Social Science and Medicine, 34*, 907–917.
Presents evidence of the relationship between changes in marital status and its effects on health behaviors.

Williamson, D. F., Kahn, H. S., Remington, P. L., & Anda, R. F. (1990). The 10-year incidence of overweight and major weight gain in US adults. *Archives of Internal Medicine, 150*, 665–672.
Presents epidemiological data indicating the critical age groups (young adulthood) when weight gain is prevalent.

Winett, R. A., King, A. C., & Altman, D. G. (1989). *Health psychology and public health: An integrative approach.* Elmsford, NY: Pergamon Press.
Provides a conceptual framework that combines the perspectives of two major disciplines—health psychology and public health—along with applications of this framework to the understanding of current health issues facing industrialized societies.

Winkleby, M. A., Fortmann, S. P., & Barett, D. C. (1990). Social class disparities in risk factors for disease: Eight-year prevalence patterns by level of education. *Preventive Medicine, 19*, 1–12.
This article demonstrates the inverse relationship between educational levels and chronic disease risk factors in a community sample.

32

HIV Prevention

Kathleen J. Sikkema

AIDS is now the fourth leading cause of death among adult U.S. women under the age of 45, and the incidence of AIDS is increasing more rapidly among women than among men. Similar to the historical pattern of HIV infection among men, risk for the disease is not equally distributed across the entire population of women, but is disproportionately high among impoverished minority women in U.S. inner cities. Approximately three-fourths (76%) of AIDS cases among women diagnosed in the United States in 1995 occurred among African-American and Hispanic women, although African-American and Hispanic women made up 21% of all U.S. women in that year. The epidemiology of HIV infections among women is also changing, with heterosexual transmission rather than a woman's own injection drug use (IDU) now accounting for the majority of new infections. Women at highest risk for heterosexually transmitted HIV infection include those whose heterosexual partners engage in high-risk behaviors (e.g., IDU), adolescents and young adults with multiple sexual partners, commercial sex workers, and those with sexually transmitted diseases (STDs).

A significant number of studies have contributed to a descriptive understanding of psychosocial factors related to risk-taking behaviors. Across studies with various samples, such factors as perceived norms supporting behavior change, perceived self-efficacy for behavior change, accurate estimation of personal risk, intentions to practice safer sex, sexual negotiation or assertiveness skills, condom use attributions, and alcohol or recreational drug use patterns have been identified as significant predictors of sexual risk reduction among gay men, adolescents, and heterosexual adults. In contrast to the extensive literature on psychosocial correlates of HIV risk behaviors, relatively few published studies have reported on risk behavior change outcomes in controlled intervention trials. Moreover, the majority of the descriptive research has been conducted with gay men; less is known about women's HIV risk behaviors, and only a handful of intervention trials targeted specifically at women have been evaluated.

PSYCHOSOCIAL FACTORS RELATED TO
HIV RISK BEHAVIORS AMONG WOMEN

Several populations have been studied to identify factors associated with HIV risk behaviors among women. The populations include women with IDU sexual partners, women in drug treatment, women in primary care and obstetrical clinics, women living in low-income housing developments, and women in homeless shelters. (The characteristics of the homeless population are discussed in greater detail by Mantell and Susser in their chapter.) The majority of women in these studies have been African-American or Hispanic/Latina, and even though slightly distinct psychosocial factors have emerged as predictive of HIV risk behaviors, the critical significance of culturally sensitive prevention programs is commonly concluded.

Various social and cultural factors—such as patterns of traditional sex role socialization, lack of power in dyadic sexual relationships, social and economic dependence on a male relationship partner, male resistance to condom use, and life problems associated with impoverishment—all constitute barriers to women's ability to take protective steps against sexually transmitted HIV infection. In a national sample of women with IDU sexual partners, women with multiple partners who exchanged sex for drugs or money were at higher risk for HIV than were women with single or multiple partners. These higher-risk women led lives that were the most chaotic, the least healthy, and the most risky, as evidenced by a much greater likelihood of being homeless, having been incarcerated, and having to engage in illegal activities as a way to survive. However, in contrast to patterns observed in men, in which sexual HIV risk is often conferred through having large numbers of different partners, a woman may be more frequently at risk because of her main or single partner's IDU or sexual activity outside of their relationship.

Normative beliefs concerning condom use have been found to be salient influences on minority women's intentions to use condoms, whereas substance use, greater severity of concerns, more depression, and less self-esteem were reported as determinants of high levels of HIV risk behaviors among homeless and drug-addicted minority women. Sexual communication skills and enjoyment of condom use have also been shown to influence condom use among sexually active urban women. HIV/AIDS knowledge has not been shown to differentiate levels of behavioral risk among women living in inner-city housing developments, but indices of social norm perception, strength of risk reduction behavioral intention, and beliefs about self-efficacy of behavior change and condom use have been shown to be linked to risk levels.

The results of these descriptive studies indicate that interventions to promote risk behavior change among women should focus on strengthening behavioral intentions and self-efficacy through skill development of proper condom use and sexual communication. Such interventions must be appropriately tailored for women, particularly impoverished minority women. Culturally and personally relevant prevention messages may emphasize cultural pride, community concern, and family responsibility. Sexual negotiation skills also need to be tailored to relationship type: Women with multiple partners, women who trade sex for money or drugs, and women with single high-risk partners have qualitatively different relationships that require different approaches. Group interventions focused on managing factors (especially substance use) related to high-risk behaviors, developing problem-solving and sexual communication skills, and receiving social and peer support for behavior change efforts have been proven effective with other populations and show promise with inner-city women. A challenge to this type of intervention is to incorporate prevention approaches that take into account the social, psychological, economic, and relationship barriers to change among many women.

INTERVENTIONS TO REDUCE HIV RISK BEHAVIORS

HIV risk behavior change outcomes in controlled intervention studies have primarily described the effect of cognitive-behavioral group interventions that intensively develop risk reduction skills in gay men and adolescents, and more recently in high-risk inner-city women. Evaluations of community-level interventions for behavior change are limited, and are focused on gay men and IDUs. Interventions for IDUs, commercial sex workers, and adult heterosexuals include women, but are not necessarily gender-specific.

Interventions for IDUs have included HIV educational information, drug treatment, HIV counseling and testing, needle exchange programs, street outreach, and media campaigns. The intervention trials have shown mixed results, although drug treatment and community-based interventions are believed to have had a beneficial impact on injecting behavior. The modification of sexual behavior in IDU populations has been more difficult.

Many programs targeted at commercial sex workers exist, but these have received little or no evaluation. The majority of such interventions have been implemented in African countries and have involved HIV counseling and testing or community-based peer education and outreach. Condom use appears to have increased with clients, but interventions with commercial sex workers' steady partners are recommended, because condom use seems to be less frequent in personal than in professional relationships.

Interventions designed for adult heterosexuals have included programs for HIV-serostatus-discordant couples, who received educational information and group counseling, HIV testing, condoms and spermicide supplies. The effectiveness of these studies implemented in African countries was evidenced by increased condom use and decreased rates of gonorrhea and HIV infection at follow-up. One intervention trial with STD clinic patients that included condom use information, sexual negotiation skill development, and free condoms resulted in decreased rates of STD reinfection for male but not female participants. Skills training interventions emphasizing cognitive-behavioral techniques, negotiation skills, peer support, and empowerment approaches, targeted specifically at inner-city and minority women, have been evaluated in the United States. These programs have been shown to be effective in reducing HIV risk behaviors, as assessed by increased condom use, increased condom-seeking behavior, decreased number of partners, and decreased drug use.

SPECIFIC ELEMENTS OF EFFECTIVE HIV PREVENTION PROGRAMS FOR WOMEN

Two examples of controlled intervention trials evaluating HIV-related skills training interventions for inner-city women will be briefly described. One study compared the effects of a five-session HIV/AIDS intervention group to those of a three-session group intervention on health topics unrelated to AIDS but relevant to low-income women. Women attending an urban primary care clinic were eligible for the study on the basis of any of these risk factors: multiple male partners, diagnosis of an STD, or unprotected sex with a high-risk partner (e.g., an IDU partner) during the preceding 12 months. HIV/AIDS intervention components included detailed information on HIV risk; skills training (including role-play practice and feedback) in condom use and sexual assertiveness; self-management of risk triggers; group problem solving; and peer support for behavior change. Women in the HIV/AIDS intervention group exhibited significantly increased sexual communication and negotiation skills, reduced frequency of unprotected sexual intercourse, and increased condom use (from 26% of intercourse occasions at baseline to 56% at follow-up) at the 3-month follow-up assessment. Comparison group women showed little corresponding change in condom use or other skills related to HIV/AIDS.

Another study compared the effectiveness of a four-session AIDS prevention group, a health promotion group, and a no-intervention group. Participants were single, pregnant women who sought obstetrical care at clinics for low-income women. The group interventions provided information, behavioral competency training, social support, and empowerment; however, only the AIDS prevention group focused on AIDS-specific knowledge and skills. The AIDS prevention group produced increases in knowledge, risk reduction intentions and conversations, condom and spermicide usage, and condom and spermicide acquisition. These effects were maintained at the 6-month follow-up assessment.

Important elements of HIV risk reduction interventions for women thus include skills training, peer and social support, empowerment approaches, and the incorporation of HIV prevention into important issues in the women's lives. Skills training should include sexual assertiveness and negotiation, problem solving, risk behavior self-management, condom use, coping skills, and relapse prevention. Skills training techniques are considered to have an impact on HIV risk behaviors because the approach involves practice (e.g., proper condom placement on an anatomical model), role playing of sexual assertiveness, problem solving with reinforcement and feedback, cognitive rehearsal, and the encouragement of a sense of mastery. Skills training and empowerment approaches are also likely to enhance a woman's self-esteem and sense of control.

Cultural specificity and sensitivity are considered further key elements of HIV risk reduction interventions for women, particularly minority and impoverished women. The promotion of cohesion and the development of support with intervention groups cannot be underestimated. The use of culturally diverse and genuinely committed staff members also provides the opportunity for role models, mutual respect, and connectedness. In addition, it is imperative that a program be integrated into the problems of daily living faced by most of these women and individualized to their needs. Consideration should be given to transportation, child care, and scheduling concerns in relation to the economic, gender, and ethnic realities of these women's lives. A benefit of the skills training approach is that although the process is similar across groups of women, the specific content for role playing and problem solving is presented by the women from their individual situations, and plans for behavior change are generated through a supportive group process. This type of approach provides the opportunity for behavior change in the context of the women's lives, and is made relevant to the women themselves, their families, and their community.

It should be noted that HIV counseling and testing (following state guidelines) have been found to have limited effects on sexual risk behavior for seronegative women. HIV counseling and testing are considered critical for early intervention and referral to medical care, but couple, group, or more intensive individual interventions are seen as potentially more effective for HIV prevention than is HIV testing alone.

FURTHER READING

Amaro, H. (1995). Love, sex, and power: Considering women's realities in HIV prevention. *American Psychologist, 50,* 437–447.
Discussion of how gender, women's social status, and women's roles affect sexual risk behavior and examination of factors that should be considered on HIV prevention programs.

Choi, K. H., & Coates, T. J. (1994). Prevention of HIV infection. *AIDS, 8,* 1371–1389.
Critical review of the scientific literature on AIDS prevention programs to determine efficacy of behavioral interventions for reducing risk behaviors.

DiClemente, R. J., & Wingood, G. M. (1995). A randomized controlled trial of an HIV sexual risk-reduction intervention for young African-American women. *Journal of the American Medical Association, 274,* 1271–1276.
Evaluation of a community-based social skills HIV prevention intervention to enhance consistent condom use.

Exner, T. M., Seal, D. W., & Ehrhardt, A. A. (in press). A review of HIV interventions for at-risk women. *AIDS and Behavior.*
Review of published reports on primary prevention of sexual transmission of HIV with women, including methodological critique and recommendations for future research.

Hobfoll, S. E., Jackson, A. P., Lavin, J., Britton, P. J., & Shepherd, J. B. (1994). Reducing inner-city women's AIDS risk activities: A study of single, pregnant women. *Health Psychology, 13,* 397–403.
Controlled study showing effectiveness of an AIDS prevention group intervention with inner-city, pregnant women.

Ickovics, J. R., Morrill, A. C., Beren, S. E., Walsh, U., & Rodin, J. (1994). Limited effects of HIV counseling and testing for women. *Journal of the American Medical Association, 272,* 443–448.
Study suggesting that the behavioral and psychological impact of HIV counseling and testing for women at risk is small.

Kelly, J. A., Murphy, D. A., Washington, C. D., Wilson, T. S., Koob, J. J., Davis, D. R., Ledezma, G., & Davantes, B. (1994). The effects of HIV/AIDS intervention groups for high-risk women in urban clinics. *American Journal of Public Health, 84,* 1918–1922.
Randomized study demonstrating the effectiveness of a skills training group intervention for high-risk women in reducing HIV risk behaviors.

Nyamathi, A., Bennett, C., Leake, B., Lewis, C., & Flaskerud, J. (1993). AIDS-related knowledge, perceptions, and behaviors among impoverished minority women. *American Journal of Public Health, 83,* 65–71.
Description of AIDS-related knowledge, perceptions, and risk behaviors among minority women residing in homeless shelters and drug recovery programs; the need for culturally sensitive prevention programs is emphasized.

Sikkema, K. J., Heckman, T. H., Kelly, J. A., Anderson, E. S., Winett, R. A., Solomon, L. J., Wagstaff, D. A., Roffman, R. A., Perry, M. J., Cargill, V., Crumble, D. A., Fuqua, R. W., Norman, A. D., & Mercer, M. B. (1996). HIV risk behaviors among women living in low-income, inner-city housing developments. *American Journal of Public Health, 86,* 1123–1128.
Description of the prevalence and psychosocial predictors of HIV risk behaviors among inner-city women.

33

HIV Prevention among Homeless Women

Joanne E. Mantell
Ezra S. Susser

*T*his chapter focuses on the risk of HIV infection among homeless women, and on the need for preventive interventions among them. Women currently represent 15–30% of the adult homeless population in the United States. This proportion is likely to increase, however, because families with children, headed by women, are among the fastest-growing homeless groups.

HIV seroprevalence has been reported to be 3.6% in a representative sample of homeless women in San Francisco. A study by Allen and colleagues of 11 cities found prevalences ranging from 1.2% (Dallas) to 15.4% (Miami). Unfortunately, homeless women's exposure to HIV infection has been studied inadequately, and this impedes efforts at prevention. We propose that the risk of HIV among homeless women can be understood best within the context of these women's interactions with the adverse conditions in their environment. Thus, the confluence of person-level variables (e.g., cognitive impairments, attention deficits, poor impulse control, interpersonal skill deficits, and low income) and setting-level factors (e.g., residential instability, inaccessibility to private places to have sex, inaccessibility to condoms, ideology of service providers) contributes to homeless women's vulnerability to HIV infection.

CHARACTERISTICS OF HOMELESS WOMEN

For HIV prevention to be effective among homeless women, their characteristics need to be understood. The portrait of homeless women is diverse, varying by age, ethnicity, patterns of drug and alcohol use, degree and chronicity of psychological impairment, locality, patterns of mobility, length of homelessness, and type of shelter setting. Some characteristics do appear, however, to be associated with a high risk of homelessness. In regard to demographic characteristics, two associations are relatively consistent. First, women under the age of 40 years appear to be at greater risk for homelessness than older women. Second, African-Americans are disproportionately represented among both homeless women and those with HIV/AIDS, compared with other ethnic groups. Of course, both of these factors are associated with poverty, and this may well account for their association with homelessness, which may be considered an extreme form of poverty.

Among health states, mental illness and substance abuse are strongly associated with homelessness among women. Epidemiological studies indicate that about one-third of women in adult women's shelters are mentally ill. Conversely, about one-third of chronically mentally ill women have been homeless. Similarly, about one-third of homeless women are estimated to be substance users.

Homeless women living in family shelters are distinctly different from homeless women who are housed in single-adult shelters. Women housed in single-adult shelters are more likely than women housed in family shelters with their children (1) to have mental health problems, (2) to have been hospitalized for a psychiatric problem, and (3) to have had a substance abuse problem. They also tend to be older than homeless women in family shelters.

THE SOCIAL CONTEXT OF HOMELESSNESS AND ITS RELATION TO HIV RISK BEHAVIORS

The causal relationship between HIV and homelessness is unclear. Because most studies of homeless persons are cross-sectional, it is difficult to disentangle whether HIV is an antecedent or a consequence of homelessness. Some health problems coincide with homelessness, whereas other health problems are associated with the psychosocial burdens of homelessness. It does seem clear, however, that the social context of homelessness promotes vulnerability to HIV.

First, homeless women may sell or trade sex for drugs, money, food, or shelter, because they may perceive sex as the only saleable asset they possess. Although this may be adaptive economically, it is maladaptive in that it is deleterious to mental and physical health. Second, homeless women are vulnerable to physical assault and to sexual abuse by men. They may be deterred from raising the issue of HIV risk reduction out of fear of rejection or further abuse from their sexual partners. Moreover, homeless women are more likely than housed women to have been abused during childhood, and such childhood experience may affect their current response to abuse. Third, the sexual partners of homeless women are often homeless men; these men are at high risk for HIV infection. Finally, unemployment, job inequality, substance abuse, disaffiliation, and fragmented social networks exacerbate homeless women's efficacy in health promotion. These factors make it extremely difficult for them to adopt behaviors that could reduce their exposure to a complex array of health risks, including HIV infection.

BARRIERS TO HEALTH CARE

HIV-infected homeless women may have limited involvement with health services. Seeking medical care for gynecological problems, in particular, has been noted to be a primary stressor for such women. When services are accessible, the quality of care may be substandard or inconsistent. Moreover, negative attitudes of health care providers may be a major deterrent for some women.

Because of competing priorities, such as obtaining adequate food and clothing, finding permanent housing, and (often) procuring drugs, homeless women are among the least likely to comply with recommended treatment and to keep appointments for medical care. Although one study by Schlosstein and colleagues found homeless women to be no different from low-income women with regard to referral keeping for medical conditions, the proportion of homeless women keeping referrals for preventive care was much lower (22% vs. 44–51%). Those who use drugs may avoid prenatal care, out of fear that child welfare authorities will take away their children after birth. Distrust of authority may further undermine their ability to seek not only prenatal care, but health care in general. Even when health services are accessible, they may be underutilized or inappropriately utilized. For example, homeless women have been noted to be heavy users of hospital emergency rooms because they lack a regular source of care. This in turn contributes to their lack of continuous health care.

As a result of these barriers to health care and the distinct patterns of service use by homeless women, standard approaches to HIV prevention will not be sufficient for this population. Effective prevention will first require some means of entering the social settings in which homeless women are found. Then the task will be to integrate prevention methods into the natural life of these settings.

IMPLEMENTING HIV PREVENTION

As yet, HIV prevention for homeless women has not been a high priority. Research in this area has been minimal, so that little is known about what attempts these women make to protect themselves from becoming infected, and about what could motivate them to change their risk behaviors. The characteristics of homeless women and the barriers to health care that they experience suggest, however, that they are unlikely to be reached through programs targeted at the general population of women. At the same time, few institutions that specifically serve the homeless have made HIV prevention activities a primary focus.

First, to reach homeless women in residential settings, system-wide interventions must be implemented. Shelters, community residences, and psychiatric hospitals with special services for the homeless are venues with "captive audiences" of homeless women. These settings also offer the opportunity for promoting social norms for safer sex and shaping residents' behavior. Changing the behavior of the residents undoubtedly requires changing the behavior of the staff. Organizational commitment to making HIV preventive interventions a top priority is essential to promote and reinforce residents' adoption and maintenance of HIV risk reduction methods. Various individual-level interventions for residents are also needed, including cognitive-behavioral skills training and support groups.

Second, to reach homeless women who do not use shelters and other congregate facilities, aggressive outreach is needed. Mobile health vans may be effective in bringing health care to the people who are least likely to seek help—that is, homeless HIV-infected women. HIV risk reduction education could also be provided as part of outreach efforts, as has been done with injection drug users. Anchoring services, especially case management linkage, in a user-friendly, community-based climate may enhance continuity of primary care and prevention services for homeless women.

HIV prevention programs should be framed within the gender-specific context of homeless women's lives, especially the cultural constructions of relationships and sexuality. This is critical, since these constructions shape women's perceptions of HIV risk. Women-centered preventive interventions should be directed toward preventing violence and abuse by partners, addressing the power imbalance in sexual relationships, and reproductive behavior. Regarding the reproductive needs of homeless women, interventions should focus on increasing their awareness of HIV-related gynecological manifestations, offering HIV testing to those who are pregnant or who intend to become pregnant, and informing HIV-infected women of the benefits of taking zidovudine (formerly called azidothymidine or AZT) during pregnancy. Because many homeless women may have difficulty in convincing their sex partners to use condoms, HIV preventive interventions need to offer a hierarchy of female-initiated prevention methods, including the female condom, microbicides, and the diaphragm with microbicides. These methods may be especially critical for women who use drugs and those who are unwilling or unable to ask their partners to use condoms. The high rates of pregnancy and certain sexually transmitted diseases, of delayed (or no) prenatal care, of lower-birth weight babies, and of infant mortality among homeless adult women and teens underscore the need for comprehensive reproductive services that integrate family planning with HIV prevention and primary care. Programs designed to increase knowledge of contraception, as well as access to and use of contraceptive services, are needed.

A diffusion approach using small print media can be used as an HIV prevention strategy. Printed stories with HIV behavioral change messages and accounts of homeless women's HIV risk-reduction experiences are created. These stories are designed to be credible to homeless women so that they can identify with story characters who have successfully lowered their risk behaviors. Homeless women can be recruited and trained as peer educators to deliver role model stories that can be used as the catalyst for discussion. Story lines should be anchored in the lives of the women and should address such topics as refusing unprotected sex, introducing female-initiated methods, reducing partner violence, and developing supportive networks for safer sex and drug use. Evaluation must be an essential component of these initiatives, in order to determine such programs' effectiveness and to facilitate the replication with other populations of homeless women of those proven to be effective.

A few researchers have begun to develop preventive interventions for women. The Homeless Prenatal Program in San Francisco draws upon an empowerment model, providing professional and peer support, case management, and advocacy through the use of community health outreach workers to enhance women's bonds with their children, improve birth outcomes, and ultimately transform their lives. We have initiated an HIV environmental risk reduction intervention for homeless women in New York City residential settings. This is a multilevel intervention, adapted from models that emphasize diffusion of innovation and community-based rehabilitation. It seeks to promote community-wide norms for safer sex and sexual risk reduction by (1) working with program staff members to develop HIV prevention plans; (2) enhancing direct service and ancillary support staff members' ability to integrate HIV prevention into their professional and spontaneous contacts with residents; (3) providing group-based cognitive-behavioral skills training workshops to residents; (4) training homeless women to deliver HIV prevention messages to other residents; and (5) maximizing use of the physical environment to introduce HIV prevention messages and barrier devices. These programs and others around the United States provide some hope for improved services to homeless women.

FURTHER READING

Allen, D. M., Lehman, J. S., Green, T. A., Lindegren, M. L., Onorato, I. M., Forrester, W., & the Field Services Branch. (1994). HIV infection among homeless adults and runaway youth, United States, 1989–1992. *AIDS, 8,* 1593–1598.
A national survey of homeless populations in 14 cities.

Bassuk, E. L., & Rosenberg, L. (1988). Why does family homelessness occur?: A case control study. *American Journal of Public Health, 7,* 783–788.
One of the first case–control studies to examine the factors placing women at risk for homelessness.

Breakey, W. R., Fischer, P. J., Kramer, M., Nestadt, G., Romanoski, A. J., Ross, A., Royall, R. M., & Stine, O. C. (1989). Health and mental health problems of homeless men and women in Baltimore. *Journal of the American Medical Association, 262,* 1352–1357.
A comprehensive survey of the physical and mental health problems of homeless men and women in Baltimore.

Institute of Medicine. (1988). *Homelessness, health, and human needs.* Washington, DC: National Academy Press.
A comprehensive review of the health problems of homeless men and women.

Link, B. G., Susser, E., Stueve, A., Phelan, J., Moore, R. E., & Struening, E. (1994). Lifetime and five-year prevalence of homelessness in the United States. *American Journal of Public Health, 84,* 1907–1912.
Paper examining the national prevalence of homelessness in the United States.

Schlosstein, E., St. Clair, P., & Connell, F. (1991). Referral keeping in homeless women. *Journal of Community Health, 16,* 279–285.
A survey of referral keeping for health care needs among homeless women in Seattle emergency shelters.

Susser, E., Moore, R., & Link, B. (1993). Risk factors for homelessness. *Epidemiologic Reviews, 15,* 546–556.
This paper reviews the studies of risk factors for homelessness in women as well as in men.

Weitzman, B. C., Knickman, J. R., & Shinn, M. (1992). Predictors of shelter use among low-income families: Psychiatric history, substance abuse, and victimization. *American Journal of Public Health, 82,* 1547–1550.
One of the most comprehensive studies of risk factors of homelessness among women with children.

Zolopa, A. R., Hahn, J. A., Gorter, R., Miranda, J., Wlodarczyk, D., Peterson, J., Pilote, L., & Moss, A. R. (1994). HIV and tuberculosis infection in San Francisco's homeless adults. *Journal of the American Medical Association, 272,* 455–461.
A study of HIV and tuberculosis in a representative sample of homeless men and women in San Francisco.

34

Breast Cancer Screening: Improving Adherence

Joni A. Mayer

*B*reast cancer is a woman's disease; fewer than 1% of the estimated 181,600 cases that will be diagnosed in the United States in 1997 will be men. As the most common cancer and the second leading cause of cancer-related mortality in U.S. women, breast cancer will be responsible for the deaths of 43,900 women in 1997. The lifetime incidence of the disease is currently one in eight.

Commonly accepted risk factors fall into the "nonmodifiable" category and include female gender, increasing age, family history of the disease, earlier menarche, later menopause, and no or delayed childbearing. A recently discovered gene, BRCA1, is highly predictive of breast cancer when a mutation is present. To date, the combined results of prospective observational studies suggest that the relationship between dietary fat intake during adulthood and breast cancer is negligible, although this is a controversial point (for differing views, see the chapters in this volume by Brunner and St. Jeor on nutrition and disease, and by Glanz on nutrition education). Alcohol intake and breast cancer may have a positive association, but this research is in its early stages. Thus, as this book goes to press, few if any scientifically verified primary prevention strategies are available.

MAMMOGRAPHIC SCREENING: RECOMMENDATIONS AND TRENDS

Because treatment of breast cancer at its earliest stages offers women the best chances for survival, promoting early detection through screening has been a top priority of cancer control specialists. Screening includes mammography, clinical breast exam, and breast self-examination at age-specific intervals; this chapter's focus is on mammography. Encouraging women under age 50 (without additional risk factors) to have regular screening mammograms has been criticized, because clinical trials generally have shown no mortality reductions for ages 40–49 years. (For a fuller discussion of this controversy, see Kaplan's chapter on screening.) In contrast, based on strong scientific evidence, the majority of health organizations recommend that women 50 and older have regular mammograms; the definition of "regular" ranges from every 12 to every 24 months, depending on the organization. Breast cancer mortality could be reduced by an estimated 30% if all women in this age group obtained regular mammograms. Population-wide screening for women aged 50 and over is justified, because the large majority of breast

TABLE 34.1. Possible Approaches to Achieving Annual Mammographic Screening

Approaches	Examples
Population-oriented	
Federal and state laws/ordinances, etc.	Congress passes the Breast and Cervical Cancer Mortality Prevention Act of 1990 (Public Law 101-354): States are awarded grants and matching funds for screening services for underinsured/uninsured women. Some states mandate that insurance policies cover screening at specific intervals.
Policies (e.g., reimbursement, etc.) of health organizations, regulatory agencies, and health care providers	Health maintenance organizations provide screening at specific intervals. Medicare covers (capped) amount for screening at specific intervals. Mammography facilities implement "inreach" strategies that increase their profitability.
Scientific/technological innovations	Tests are developed that identify "high-risk" women, rendering population-wide screening unnecessary.[a] New screening methods are developed that replace existing ones, with higher predictive value, less discomfort, lower costs, etc.[a]
Individual-oriented	
Public education campaigns[b]	American Cancer Society annually sponsors Breast Cancer Awareness Month (e.g., public service announcements, discounts on screenings).
Prompting	Each patient receives reminder for appointment.
Counseling	Woman who has missed several appointments receives phone call from provider; barriers are identified and addressed.
Social influence	Physician discusses screening with patient and refers her. Woman is contacted by a specially trained peer in her social network who encourages participation in screening.
Positive reinforcement/incentive systems	Woman receives gift from the mammography facility after receiving her annual mammogram.

[a]Hypothetical.
[b]Also may be conceptualized as population-oriented.

cancer cases would be missed if only "high-risk" women were targeted. For example, only a small proportion of women with breast cancer report any family history of the disease, and the BRCA1 gene may account for fewer than 5% of all breast cancer cases.

U.S. women aged 50 and older have shown substantial increases in the past 10 years in the rates of having had one mammogram, and in the rates of recent screening. Three trends that emerge with consistency are as follows: (1) Rates of annual screening continue to be fairly low; (2) beyond age 50, screening adherence and age are inversely related (whereas breast cancer and age are positively related); and (3) referral for mammography by a physician is a strong predictor of adherence to regular mammography. These trends are addressed below.

APPROACHING THE ADHERENCE PROBLEM

In 1989 Robert Jeffery lucidly contrasted population-oriented and individual-oriented strategies for defining and solving public health problems, and recommended a combined approach. The need to integrate these "levels" of interventions is particularly relevant to the issue of promoting adherence to regular mammographic screening. Table 34.1 illustrates selected discrete approaches, categorized according to population versus individual orientation. The population-oriented approaches generally involve something other than the individual woman in the intervention per se, even though changes in mammography-obtaining behavior may be the desired outcome. This type of approach may be more likely to change the societal norm or climate, or the context in which individuals behave. The individual approaches generally intervene directly with individuals or groups, attempting to modify knowledge, attitudes, and behaviors.

Mammographic screening at regular intervals involves an interplay among the primary (or referring) physician, the patient, and the mammography provider. Both physicians and mammography providers have various motives (e.g., ethical, quality-of-care, financial) for promoting annual screening of patients. This interplay occurs in an ever-changing context of policies and laws, which influence screening guidelines for women, quality assurance guidelines for providers, and reimbursement opportunities and restrictions. The topics and examples in Table 34.1 and the discussion below are in no way exhaustive, but I hope that they will promote brainstorming of additional intervention and research ideas.

Combining population- and individual-oriented strategies may serve to strengthen an intervention. In fact, one type of strategy alone may be futile in certain situations. For example, following the passage of a law in California mandating that insurance policies cover screening mammograms in accordance with American Cancer Society age guidelines (e.g., annually for women 50 and over), a survey indicated that many women who had the coverage were not aware that they had it. This deficit indicated the need for educational campaigns specific to the new benefit. Likewise, educating women about and motivating them for regular screening (individual-oriented strategies) in the absence of available, affordable screening services (population-oriented strategies) would also be impractical, as well as unethical.

A second example that combines approaches is an "inreach" program with mammography facilities to promote annual mammograms among women 50 and older. The program, which is part of my own research, is based on the following premises. First, in an urban area, facilities are highly competitive; maintaining high levels of annual return rates among current patients is economically desirable. Second, many facilities routinely use mailed reminder systems; this method of intervention is acceptable to them. Third, physician involvement in achieving mammography adherence is important, probably because of the physician's roles as gatekeeper to the services and as a credible, influential advisor. However, many physicians do not make referrals at the recommended intervals, even though they may endorse the guidelines.

Our current study is comparing the effects of a physician reminder, a facility reminder, and no reminder on annual return rates. The burden on physicians is minimized by the mammography facilities; physicians give the facilities a supply of their letterhead stationery and signature stamps. To date, approximately half of the referring physicians associated with the initial four participating facilities have joined the program. In a pilot study, physicians were pleased with the system, and the physician reminder produced significantly higher return rates than no reminder. Outcome data from the current study will be available in 1998. The system, if successful, has the potential (1) to allow a mammography facility to provide a service to a referring physician; (2) to strengthen the link between the facility and the physician; and (3) to remind each patient to schedule her appointment. From a health perspective, the patient's appointment adherence is of course the most important outcome. Nevertheless, the first and second outcomes may help ensure that the program will be institutionalized and maintained. In fact, an increase in the probability of institutionalization is a major advantage of combining population- and individual-oriented approaches, both within and outside of the breast cancer screening arena.

AN IMPORTANT ROLE FOR BEHAVIORAL SCIENCE

Behavioral medicine practitioners and researchers, particularly those trained as clinical psychologists, are likely to be more comfortable in working with clinical (or high-risk) populations, using individual-oriented intervention approaches. However, in the area of mammography adherence, there is still a great need to work with the general population and to incorporate population-oriented approaches. Behavioral medicine specialists have contributed much to the understanding and promotion of breast cancer screening adherence. Areas still needing further investigation with this expertise, to name a few, are (1) factors associated with low referral rates by physicians of healthy elderly women; (2) patient-based factors associated with low adherence rates of elderly women; and (3) interventions that reduce or offset the punishing consequences of mammograms. But, to reiterate, individual-oriented interventions resulting from these lines of inquiry should be consolidated with population-oriented strategies.

ACKNOWLEDGMENT

Preparation of this chapter was supported, in part, by the U.S. Army Medical Research and Materiel Command under DAMD-17-94-J-4360. The contents of the chapter do not necessarily reflect the position or the policy of the government, and no official endorsement should be inferred.

FURTHER READING

American Cancer Society. (1997). *Cancer facts and figures—1997.* Atlanta: Author.
Annual update of U.S. cancer statistics, including morbidity and mortality rates, nationwide and by state.

Anderson, L. M., & May, D. S. (1995). Has the use of cervical, breast, and colorectal cancer screening increased in the United States? *American Journal of Public Health, 85,* 840–842.
Comparisons between 1987 and 1992 of data from the National Health Interview Survey Cancer Control Supplements.

Elder, J. P., Geller, E. S., Hovell, M. F., & Mayer, J. A. (1994). *Motivating health behavior.* Albany, NY: Delmar.
A basic how-to guide for health professionals, describing behavior change technologies as applied to health promotion programs.

Jeffery, R. W. (1989). Risk behaviors and health: Contrasting individual and population perspectives. *American Psychologist, 44,* 1194–1202.
An excellent examination of health risk behaviors from two contrasting perspectives.

Mayer, J. A., Clapp, E. J., Bartholomew, S., & Elder, J. (1994). Facility-based inreach strategies to promote annual mammograms. *American Journal of Preventive Medicine, 10,* 353–356.
Paper describing a series of three randomized, controlled intervention studies.

Mayer, J. A., Jones, J. A., Eckhardt, L. E., Haliday, J., Bartholomew, S., Slymen, D. J., & Hovell, M. F. (1993). Evaluation of a worksite mammography program. *American Journal of Preventive Medicine, 9,* 244–249.
Paper describing a multicomponent intervention and its impact on mammography adherence among university employees.

The NCI Breast Cancer Screening Consortium. (1990). Screening mammography: A missed clinical opportunity? *Journal of the American Medical Association, 264,* 54–58.
Data from seven studies on (then) current rates of breast cancer screening and its correlates.

Rimer, B. K. (1994). Mammography use in the U.S.: Trends and the impact of interventions. *Annals of Behavioral Medicine, 16,* 317–326.
An excellent review of interventions for promoting mammography adherence.

35

Breast Cancer Screening: When to Begin?

Robert M. Kaplan

*C*ancer is perhaps the disease that women fear most. Breast cancer, for example, is believed to have reached epidemic proportions. The incidence of detected cancer has increased significantly for both white and black women (see Figure 35.1). There was a sharp increase in the number of cases detected in 1974, following the diagnosis of breast cancer in Betty Ford and Happy Rockefeller, the wives of the president and vice-president of the United States at that time. These cases received significant publicity and heightened awareness of the epidemic.

Some evidence suggests that the perceived risk of breast cancer exceeds the actual risk. For example, the American Cancer Society reports that one woman in eight will develop breast cancer. However, the incidence data are complicated and difficult to interpret. Among a birth cohort in which everyone lives to age 95, the odds may be one in eight of developing breast cancer. For a woman aged 20 to develop breast cancer in the next decade, the odds are between 1 in 2,500 and 1 in 1,000. A woman who has not developed breast cancer by age 95 will have less than a 1-in-100 chance of ever suffering from the disease. Women in their 40s overestimate their risk of developing breast cancer by over 20-fold, and may overestimate the absolute risk reduction in death attributable to mammography by over 100-fold.

Early detection has been promoted as the best weapon in the war against cancer, and there has been a substantial campaign to include mammography for all women in basic benefits packages. In its 1994 testimony on health care reform, the American Cancer Society argued that all women aged 40–49 should have a mammogram every 1–2 years. The organization took issue with statements in the initial Clinton administration health care reform proposal, which indicated that screening should begin at age 50. According to the American Cancer Society, the Clinton administration proposals were based on "economic considerations rather than good science." The American Cancer Society does acknowledge that there should be practice guidelines, but it emphasizes that the practice guidelines should be created by itself, not by any other group.

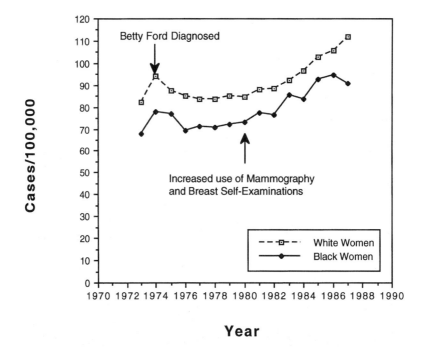

FIGURE 35.1. Breast cancer cases for white and African-American women, 1973–1987. Data from National Cancer Institute Surveillance Epidemiology End Results (SEER) Program (Miller et al., 1992).

WHY IS THERE CONTROVERSY?

There is strong reason to believe that mammographic screening is valuable. If cancer is present even in a small number of women, it seems reasonable that detection efforts should be supported, because early detection leads to early treatment. However, the U.S. push for early detection has not been matched by other industrialized countries. Various countries around the world have examined the evidence. Virtually all developed nations, except Sweden, have recommended that mammographic screening begin at age 50. The United States is unique because at least some authorities have recommended that such screening begin at age 35. In 1994, the American Cancer Society and the National Cancer Institute were split in their opinions. The suggestion that screening begin at age 50 is consistent with the recommendations of the American College of Physicians and the U.S. Preventive Services Task Force. The National Cancer Institute, after reviewing the evidence, has suggested that screening begin at age 50, but the American Cancer Society still insists that screening begin at age 35–40. The controversy accelerated in early 1997. In January of 1997, the National Institutes of Health convened a consensus panel to consider mammographic screening for women 40 to 49 years of age. New evidence had emerged from an unpublished Swedish study that suggested early screenings may be valuable. However, a careful review of the evidence continued to raise questions. For example, some of the studies supporting early use of mammography did not begin screening until age 45, and the average age of the women screened was about 47 or 48 years. Further, on average, there appeared to be no health benefit associated with early screening. The committee recognized that the issue remained controversial. On the one hand, women who undergo regular screening take a significant risk of having a false–positive test. The consensus committee argued that the evidence was, indeed, quite conflicted. They suggested that the ambiguity be communicated to women so that consumers could make an informed choice. The media immediately reacted and suggested that these recommendations were inappropriate. Shortly after the media reaction, the United States Senate approved a "Sense of the Senate" resolution. In contrast to the expert panel, the senate concluded that evidence supported the use of mammographic screening for all women and urged the National Cancer Advisory Board (NCAB) to recommend screening for all women.

The American Cancer Society reacted by forming its own review panel. The NIH panel was made up of respected scientists who themselves had not contributed to the literature on mammographic screening. These selections were made to minimize the chances that the panel would be biased by preconceived notions. In contrast, the American Cancer Society created a panel made up of individuals who had already published arguments in favor of mammographic screening. The American Cancer Society Panel, which met in February 1997, concluded that mammographic screening for women 40 to 49 years of age was appropriate. Further, the American Cancer Society panel recommended that screening be done every year rather than every other year. In response, the NIH and the NCAB decided to disregard the advice of their own panel and to endorse the recommendations of the American Cancer Society. President Clinton immediately backed the American Cancer Society recommendations. He suggested that the Medicare Program and programs for federal employees pay for mammographic screening for all women older than 40 years of age. The recommendation for Medicare will have only a small effect since Medicare covers relatively few women who are less than 65 years of age.

In order to understand this controversy, it is necessary to consider two types of biases: lead time bias and length bias.

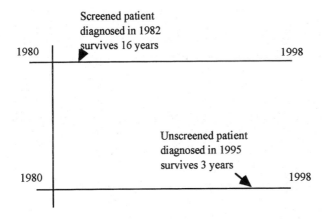

FIGURE 35.2. Example of lead time bias. Two patients develop cancer in 1980 and die in 1998. The patient screened in 1982 appears to survive cancer longer even though the true interval between cancer initiation and death is identical for both patients (see text).

Lead Time Bias

Cancer screening may result in early detection of disease. Survival is typically calculated from the date that disease is documented until death. Since screening is associated with earlier disease detection, the interval between detection and death is longer for screened cases than for unscreened cases; epidemiologists refer to this as "lead time bias." Figure 35.2 illustrates this bias.

Imagine that two women each developed breast cancer in 1980 and died in 1998. Hypothetically, the progression of the cancer was identical in these two women. The woman whose case is illustrated on the upper line of Figure 35.2 was screened in 1982, and the cancer was detected. After this diagnosis, she lived 16 additional years before her death in 1998. The woman whose case is shown on the lower line did not receive screening and detected a lump herself in 1995. After this, she lived 3 additional years. Survival for the woman on the top appears in the figure to be much longer than that for the woman on the bottom, even though the interval between developing cancer and dying was exactly the same. In several major studies of breast cancer, it has been suggested that increased survival associated with screening can be attributed to lead time and not to early detection and treatment. The only way to eliminate lead time bias is to perform clinical trials in which women are randomly assigned to either treatment or control groups and followed for many years. These trials have many methodological problems, but they remain our best way of determining the value of screening.

Length Bias

Tumors progress at different rates. Some cancers are very slow-moving, whereas other tumors progress very rapidly. Some cases may regress, remain stable, or progress so slowly that they never produce a clinical problem during an ordinary lifetime. These cases might be described as "pseudodisease," because they are not clinically important. The probability that disease will be detected through screening is inversely proportional to the rate of progression; epidemiologists refer to this as "length bias." For example, early detection may not produce a clinical benefit with rapidly progressing disease, because cases are detected too late. On the other hand, diseases with very long preclinical phases are more likely to be detected by screening. However, diseases that are progressing extremely slowly may never cause clinical problems. Ironically, advances in screening technology have a greater likelihood of detecting cases for which a clinical manifestation will never materialize.

THE HEART OF THE CONTROVERSY

It is possible that some of the apparent benefits of screening and treatment for cancer are actually attributable to lead time and length bias. If this were true, then the greater incidence of detected disease (see Figure 35.1) would not be reflected in reduced mortality rates. Figure 35.3 shows changes in breast cancer mortality between 1973 and 1992. Current data suggest that despite increases in screening, rates for breast cancer death have remained constant over the last two decades. The same holds for ovarian cancer, colon cancer, and most other malignancies (except lung cancer). The center of the controversy is a set of experimental trials evaluating the benefits of screening. These trials are important because they eliminate lead time and length bias.

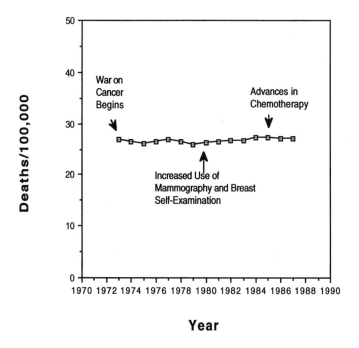

FIGURE 35.3. Change in breast cancer mortality, 1973–1987. Data from National Cancer Institute Surveillance Epidemiology End Results (SEER) Program (Miller et al., 1992).

The effects of screening have been evaluated in at least eight studies. Figure 35.4 summarizes the relative risk of breast cancer death by age at entry for these eight key studies. Mortality data included in the analyses constitute the latest follow-up data that were reported in the respective studies. Risk ratios less than 1.0 imply a benefit of screening, while those greater than 1.0 imply a negative consequence. All the studies included women under the age of 50; however, only six of the studies presented the results broken down by age. To the extent that the information was available in the primary studies, the results are shown separately for women under age 50 and women over age 50. As the figure shows, there is a substantial benefit for screening women 50 years of older. This is essentially noncontroversial. However, there appears to be little benefit of breast cancer screening for women less than 50 years old in any study. One study (the Health Insurance Plan Trial, or HIP) did suggest some benefit among younger women if they were followed for a longer period of time (18 years). Also, the Florence study reported lower breast cancer mortality rates for women younger than 50 who had received mammography screening than for those who had not. However, these differences were not statistically significant.

Several aspects of the data for women 40–49 years of age must be considered. Although these studies on average show no benefit of screening for this age group, the studies differ by length of follow-up. Studies with follow-ups of 7–9 years tend to show a very small increase in the risk of breast cancer among women who were screened. However, two studies (the Swedish two-county study and the HIP) have suggested a benefit of screening for women who were followed 9 years or longer. These findings are not statistically significant. It has been argued that the failure to find a significant effect

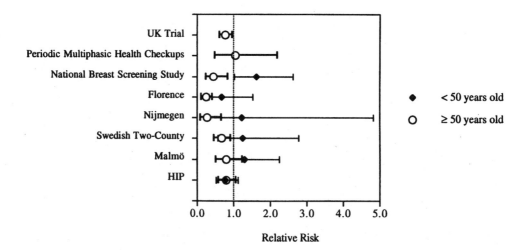

FIGURE 35.4. Summary of breast cancer screening trials. From Navarro and Kaplan (1996). Copyright 1996 by Lawrence Erlbaum. Reprinted by permission of the authors and publishers.

of screening results from low statistical power. It is possible that larger studies would show statistically significant benefit for screening.

On the other hand, there are at least two arguments to the contrary. First, averaged across all studies, the effect size is very small. Thus, the sample size required to detect this small statistical effect would be enormous. A second argument is that the effect for women with 7–9 years of follow-up should be similar to that reported for women with longer follow-up. The difference in statistical power would be reflected in different widths of the confidence interval. Examination of the data does not support this hypothesis. In fact, women with longer follow-ups may have had a greater reduction in deaths associated with breast cancer because they were older at the time of follow-up assessments. These women may have been screened closer to age 50 or after age 50, and the observed benefit may be that commonly reported for women of postmenopausal age. Certainly, this issue deserves further evaluation. In particular, we need more data on women screened during their 30s and evaluated 10–20 years after their initial screening.

To date, the most positive results have been reported by Tabar and colleagues from the Swedish two-country program. Focusing exclusively on the Tabar et al. results, Kattlove and colleagues performed a cost-effectiveness analysis for screening and treatment of early breast cancer. They considered the effect of screening upon disease-free survival and health-related quality of life. In addition, they evaluated the costs of screening in relation to other alternatives. Even using the most optimistic assumption about the benefits of screening for breast cancer, Kattlove et al. have also concluded that basic benefit packages should not include screening of premenopausal women.

Cost-utility analyses consider the cost to produce the equivalent of a year of life. Almost all of the analyses considered here suggest that mammography should not be part of a basic benefit package for women aged 40–49, because there is essentially no benefit. With the denominator of the ratio as zero, the cost-effectiveness ratio will be large to infinite. Using the more optimistic estimates of the effectiveness of screening makes it possible to get a cost-effectiveness ratio. The Kattlove et al. analysis shows that the cost to save one potential life within 10 years by screening premenopausal women is $1,480,000. The equivalent cost to save a life for women greater than 50 years of age is $183,000. To place this in perspective, the cost to save the equivalent of a life year with hypertension screening is about $20,000.

CONCLUSIONS

Problems in health care are complex. Consumers have assumed that the more health care they receive, the more benefit they achieve. Cost-effectiveness studies of mammography have caused particular concern, because they often suggest that women may be denied a benefit that they feel is valuable. However, the increases in U.S. health care costs threaten consumers' willingness to pay, and huge costs may have significant negative impacts on the economic viability of the United States. As a result, policy analysts suggest that it is important to enact policies that produce the most health for the most people.

Advocates for mammographic screening suggest that screening all women is a good use of health care funds, and that even one missed cancer is too many. A society can choose to enact any policy. The option to have mammographic screening for all women is one alternative. However, there are consequences. Enacting this policy will either increase the health care costs that will be paid by consumers or taxpayers, or require that we disregard the opportunities to offer other services. Virtually all analysts agree that women over age 50 should be screened. Opponents of screening believe that screening women without other breast cancer risk factors will offer no health benefit. Screening programs targeted by age have the potential to produce more health at a lower cost. The savings may be used to support other effective services for women or for other citizens. It is unlikely that this issue will be resolved in the near future. Moreover, as time passes, it becomes more difficult to perform systematic experimental trials that will further clarify the issues.

FURTHER READING

American Cancer Society. (1994). *American Cancer Society position—Clinton health reform plan.* Atlanta: Author.
This offers the American Cancer Society's position on cancer screening. The statement emphasizes the need to screen women beginning at age 40, and is in conflict with statements by other groups, including the National Cancer Institute.

Black, W. C., Nease, R. F., & Tosteson, A. (1995). Perceptions of breast cancer risk and screening effectiveness in women younger than 50 years of age. *Journal of the National Cancer Institute, 87,* 720–731.
A study of 145 women who were asked to estimate their risks of dying of breast cancer within the next 10 years. The women overestimated their risk by more than 20-fold. The study suggests that women may not have a clear understanding of the true risks of breast cancer.

Black, W. C., & Welch, H. G. (1993). Advances in diagnostic imaging and overestimations of disease prevalence and the benefits of therapy. *New England Journal of Medicine, 328*(17), 723–743.
Review of the issues related to the use of diagnostic tests. The authors argue that advances in diagnostic testing may result in an increase in procedures that provide no health benefit to patients.

Carter, R., Glasziou, P., van Oortmarssen, G., de Koning, H., Stevenson, C., Salkeld, G., & Boer, R. (1993). Cost-effectiveness of mammographic screening in Australia. *Australian Journal of Public Health, 17,* 42–50.
A study from Australia that used a computer model to estimate the benefits of mammographic screening. The model suggested clear benefits for screening women over age 50, but unclear benefits for screening younger women.

Fletcher, S. W., Black, W., Harris, R., Rimer, B. K., & Shapiro, S. (1993). Report of the International Workshop on Screening for Breast Cancer. *Journal of the National Cancer Institute, 85,* 1644–1656.
Summary of the National Cancer Institute's International Workshop on Screening for Breast Cancer. A review of the data suggested little benefit of mammographic screening for women 40–49 years of age, but a significant benefit of screening women older than age 50.

Kattlove, H., Liberati, A., Keeler, E., & Brook, R. H. (1995). Benefits and costs of screening and treatment for early breast cancer: Development of a basic benefit package. *Journal of the American Medical Association, 273,* 142–148.
A review of the evidence on the cost-effectiveness of mammographic screening. The authors conclude that screening of women 40–49 years of age should not be a necessary component of a basic benefits package.

Kerlikowske, K., Grady, D., Rubin, S. M., Sandrock, C., & Ernster, V. L. (1995). Efficacy of screening mammography: A meta-analysis. *Journal of the American Medical Association, 273,* 149-154.
A meta-analysis of experimental studies on the effects of mammographic screening. The analysis suggests that women can increase their chances of surviving if they are screened after age 50, but that screening women 40–49 years of age produces no health benefit.

Kopans, D. B., Halpern, E., & Hulka, C. A. (1994). Statistical power in breast cancer screening trials and mortality reduction among women 40–49 years of age, with particular emphasis on the National Breast Screening Study of Canada. *Cancer, 74,* 119–123.
Considers the statistical concerns in evaluations of mammography. The authors suggest that the failure to detect a benefit for women 40–49 years of age may be attributable to low statistical power.

Miller, B. A., Ries, L. A. G., Hankey, B. F., & Edwards, B. K. (1992). *Cancer statistics review 1973–1989* (NIH Publication No. 92-2789). Washington, DC: National Cancer Insitute.
The publication summarizes cancer morbidity and mortality in the United States.

Navarro, A. M., & Kaplan, R. M. (1996). Mammography screening: Prospects and opportunity costs. *Women's Health: Research on Gender, Behavior, and Policy, 2*(4), 209–233.
Reviews the controversy surrounding mammography and presents a meta-analysis of the major studies. The authors consider alternative uses of health care funds if screening mammography would be delayed.

Tabar, L., Fagerberg, G., Duffy, S. W., Day, N. E., Gad, A., & Grontoft, O. (1992). Update of the Swedish two-county program of mammographic screening for breast cancer. *Radiology Clinics of North America, 30,* 187–210.
Reports results from the Swedish two-county study, which showed a significant benefit of mammographic screening. In addition, the study demonstrated that women with small tumors detected early had a better chance of survival than those whose tumors were detected at a more advanced stage.

36

Osteoporosis Prevention

Heidi D. Nelson

Osteoporosis afflicts 25 million people in the United States, resulting in 1.3 million fractures per year. Osteoporosis and resultant fractures are common among older women, and some estimate that one of every six white women will experience a hip fracture during her lifetime. Hip fractures increase mortality and lead to disability, loss of function, and independence. Risk factors for osteoporosis have been evaluated through multiple epidemiological studies and are useful for evaluating patients' risks. Although some risk factors are not modifiable, many can be modified by altering lifestyle and behavior. Preventive measures enlist different strategies at different stages of the life cycle for optimal effectiveness.

RISK FACTORS FOR OSTEOPOROSIS

Bone undergoes a continual process of remodeling, in which bone resorption is coupled with bone formation. Eighty percent of skeletal bone is composed of cortical bone, most commonly found in the shafts of long bones; the other 20% is composed of trabecular bone, found in the flat bones, vertebrae, and ends of long bones. Trabecular bone is more responsive to changes in mineral homeostasis and undergoes more active remodeling. Osteoporosis and osteoporotic fractures affect primarily trabecular bone.

Age and estrogen deficiency are two major risk factors for osteoporosis. Bone mass changes throughout the life cycle, accumulating most substantially during the first 18 years, and continuing to be built and restructured until the late 30s. During this period, bone mass reaches its lifetime maximum, which is influenced heavily by estrogen status (including both endogenous sources and exogenous sources, such as oral contraceptives) and heredity. From this point, loss of bone mass begins and persists throughout the remaining life cycle, with the most rapid losses for women occurring during menopause. In response to reduced levels of estrogen at menopause, bone turnover increases, with the balance shifting to increased bone resorption and decreased bone formation. When bone mass reaches a critical low threshold, fractures are more likely. Unfortunately, other factors predisposing postmenopausal women to falls—such as increased general debility, loss of neuromuscular function, and impaired vision—contribute to fracture risk at a time when bone mass may be critically reduced.

Calcium and vitamin D are essential for bone formation. However, many women consume inadequate amounts of calcium, particularly during the important bone growth years. After menopause, absorption of calcium is diminished, and dietary requirements rise. In addition, many older women have an increased likelihood of vitamin D deficiency. Inadequate consumption of calcium and vitamin D is associated with osteoporosis, particularly when this coexists with other risk factors.

Bone is formed in response to physical stress. The effects of gravity and muscular activity promote bone formation by stimulating osteoblast function. Women who engage in weight-bearing activities and lead an active lifestyle are able to maximize formation of bone and reach a higher bone mass than those who lead a sedentary lifestyle. These effects are observed with even moderate weight-bearing exercise, such as brisk walking 45–60 minutes per day for 3 days per week.

Consumption of certain substances on a regular basis has deleterious effects on bone. Most associations demonstrate dose–response effects, whereby the longer periods of use and higher amounts consumed result in worse bone mass outcomes. Cigarette smoking decreases the bioavailability of estrogen to bone, and has systemic antiestrogenic effects that may also compromise bone mass. Excessive alcohol use produces multiple effects related to acute and chronic ingestion. These include decreasing bone formation by hindering calcium absorption, decreasing the activity of osteoblast cells, and decreasing bone remodeling secondary to a direct toxic effect. Caffeine increases osteoclast bone resorption, increases urinary calcium losses, and may produce a negative calcium balance. Corticosteroid use inhibits bone formation and increases excretion of calcium. All of these influences promote osteoporosis.

Certain medical conditions, such as hyperthyroidism, are associated with osteoporosis. Hyperthyroidism, including that induced by overly high doses of exogenous thyroid, increases bone turnover and remodeling and stimulates bone resorption.

Thin body mass is also associated with osteoporosis. Part of this influence may be related to the reduced gravitational forces on bone because of less body mass. In addition, thin women have less peripheral conversion of estrogen, resulting in exposure to a lower total level of estrogen than that seen in women with higher body mass.

Hereditary risk factors are associated with osteoporosis as well. Although women cannot modify these factors, a positive family history can be helpful to identify who is at higher risk for developing osteoporosis and fractures. Women whose relatives have osteoporosis are more likely to develop it as well, and they may want to take a more aggressive preventive approach earlier in the process. Women of European or Asian ancestry are more likely to develop osteoporosis than women of other races; however, this does not mean that other groups are spared.

RISK FACTORS FOR FRACTURE

Osteoporotic fractures occur when a combination of conditions exceeds a critical threshold. These conditions include not only compromised bone strength, but also mechanical force from a fall or other physical stress, as well as lack of protective responses. Research to identify risk factors for osteoporotic fractures has focused on these components in order to prevent fractures, particularly of the hip.

The Study of Osteoporotic Fractures is a prospective multicenter study of nearly 10,000 white women 65 years and older, designed to identify risk factors associated with fractures. After 4 years of follow-up, Cummings and colleagues identified several factors associated with hip fracture. The nonmodifiable factors included advancing age, history of maternal hip fracture (especially if it occurred when a mother was under 80 years of age), history of previous fractures after the age of 50 (including those at wrist, spine, hip, or other sites), and tall stature at age 25. Potentially modifiable factors included weight loss since age 25, overall health self-described as poor to fair, previous hyperthyroidism, current use of long-acting benzodiazepines, current use of caffeine, low calcaneal bone density, reduced physical activity (e.g., spending 4 or fewer hours per day on one's feet and not walking for exercise), inability to rise from a chair without using one's arms, visual impairment (measured as poor depth perception and contrast sensitivity), and resting pulse rate of 80 beats per minute. Several factors associated with osteoporosis and fractures in previous studies were not identified in these models for various reasons, including adjustment of these effects with other variables in the multivariate model, and low frequency of certain conditions (e.g., history of previous stroke).

The list of risk factors for hip fracture resulting from this study included ones associated specifically with low bone mass, as well as ones associated with debility and unsteadiness. Data from another study support the observation that women with impaired physical function are vulnerable not only to falls, but also to fractures associated with these falls. When elderly women with hip fractures were compared to a control group of women without fractures, lower-limb dysfunction, use of ambulatory aids, visual impairment, previous stroke, and Parkinson's disease were associated with increased risk of falls and fractures. Also, increased body mass was associated with decreased risk, as reported by Grisso and colleagues. Since over 90% of hip fractures are the result of a fall, it is essential to determine the degree of a woman's physical debility when one is assessing her risks for fracture.

Although age-specific incident rates for hip fractures in black women are half those of white women, fractures are still a significant concern among black women. Studies of risk factors for black women indicate many similarities with results based on white women. Black women at increased risk for hip fractures were those with low body mass, those with a history of stroke, those who used aids in walking, and those who consumed seven or more alcoholic drinks per week. Postmenopausal estrogen therapy has been found to protect against hip fractures in black women under age 75.

Several additional prospective and case–control studies focusing on specific risk factors and their relationships to osteoporosis confirm the findings in these studies. Of particular interest to fracture prevention are the studies evaluating risk factors modifiable by lifestyle and other behavioral changes. Regular physical activity (e.g., walking or gardening) protected against hip fractures in a case–control study of British women, independent of other known risk factors, according to Cooper and colleagues. Strength of hand grip was also protective and was correlated with physical activity. These findings have been corroborated in several other prospective studies. Activity and muscle strength may protect against hip fracture either by preserving bone mass or by reducing the risk and severity of falls.

Use of certain substances on a regular basis has also been found to be associated with fractures, although these associations vary among studies. Data from the Framingham Study associated consumption of 2½ or more cups of coffee per day, or an equivalent amount of caffeine, with a significantly increased risk of hip fracture. This relationship was also seen in the Nurses' Health Study cohort, where women consuming more than 4 cups of coffee per day had a threefold increase in risk of hip fractures. Use of alcohol at levels of 7 or more ounces per week was associated with modestly increased risk of hip fracture in some of the studies. Current use of long-acting benzodiazepines, defined as those with an elimination half-life of 24 hours or more, was associated with an increased risk of hip fracture in a case–control study of Canadians older than 65 years.

PREVENTION STRATEGIES

Research results indicate that osteoporosis and resultant fractures are multifactorial in etiology. Prevention therefore also requires a multifactorial approach, with emphasis on different strategies at different points in the life cycle (see Figure 36.1).

During the premenopausal years, bone mass is being built up. The strategy at this time of life is to maximize peak bone mass. Weight-bearing exercise and adequate calcium and vitamin D intake are essential for healthy bone development. Adolescents and postmenopausal women need 1,500 mg/day of elemental calcium, and adult pre-menopausal women need 1,000 mg/day as a minimum requirement. Dietary surveys indicate that the majority of adolescent and adult women are deficient in calcium during these crucial bone-building years of their lives. Other lifestyle choices during these years

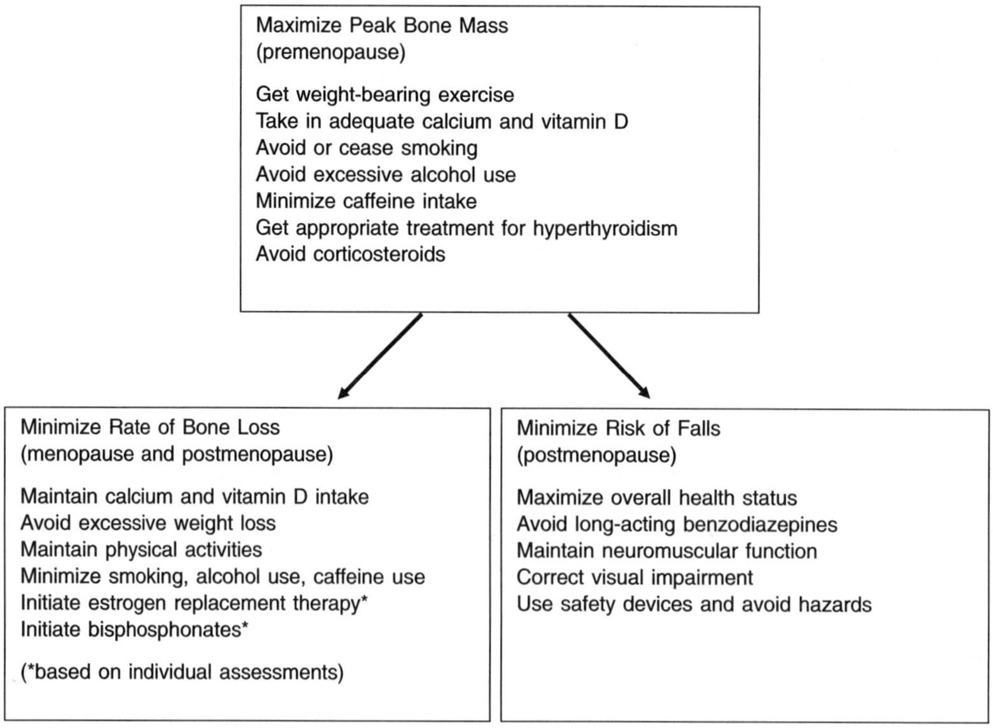

Maximize Peak Bone Mass
(premenopause)

Get weight-bearing exercise
Take in adequate calcium and vitamin D
Avoid or cease smoking
Avoid excessive alcohol use
Minimize caffeine intake
Get appropriate treatment for hyperthyroidism
Avoid corticosteroids

Minimize Rate of Bone Loss
(menopause and postmenopause)

Maintain calcium and vitamin D intake
Avoid excessive weight loss
Maintain physical activities
Minimize smoking, alcohol use, caffeine use
Initiate estrogen replacement therapy*
Initiate bisphosphonates*

(*based on individual assessments)

Minimize Risk of Falls
(postmenopause)

Maximize overall health status
Avoid long-acting benzodiazepines
Maintain neuromuscular function
Correct visual impairment
Use safety devices and avoid hazards

FIGURE 36.1. Osteoporosis prevention strategies.

can also compromise attainment of maximal bone mass. Smoking, alcohol use, and caffeine use should be minimized to prevent their contributing to osteoporosis.

During the menopausal and postmenopausal years, the strategy shifts to minimizing the rate of bone loss. Maintaining calcium and vitamin D intake and keeping up a moderate level of physical activities remain important to maintaining bone density. However, these goals become more difficult at this time of life. Calcium absorption is less efficient for postmenopausal women, and vitamin D deficiencies become more common as women have less sun exposure. Therefore, calcium recommendations are increased, and vitamin D supplements should be added if indicated. Weight loss below a healthy baseline should be avoided.

Menopausal women may want to consider initiation of estrogen replacement therapy in the perimenopausal period. Its many health benefits include proven effectiveness in the prevention of bone loss and osteoporotic fractures. Estrogen stabilizes bone structure by reducing the resorption of trabecular plates. Its use was associated with a 50% decrease in risk for wrist fractures and for all nonspinal fractures, compared to no estrogen use, among the 9,701 postmenopausal women in the Study of Osteoporotic Fractures. These outcomes were similar regardless of use of progestin, age above or below 75 years, and current smoking status. Maximal benefits were demonstrated among estrogen users who started estrogen within 5 years of menopause and who continued it for longer than 10 years; these women had a significantly decreased risk for hip fractures, in addition to wrist and nonspinal fractures.

As with all medical therapies, the risks and benefits of estrogen need to be assessed for each woman on an individual basis. A clinician can effectively do so by assessing a woman's risk factors and, when indicated, evaluating bone mineral density with bone densitometry. In one survey of older women, women who underwent densitometry and were found to have bone density measurements below normal were more likely to begin some type of fracture prevention measure, to start hormone therapy, and to take precautions to avoid falling than were women with normal results. Bone densitometry can be particularly helpful in situations where the results may identify a high-risk individual, influence a decision for estrogen therapy, or monitor rates of bone loss in selected individuals.

Bisphosphonates are analogues of pyrophosphate that act as potent inhibitors of bone resorption. These agents show great promise for treatment and prevention of osteoporosis, and are being assessed in several ongoing clinical trials. Although currently they are most often used by women who cannot take estrogen, bisphosphonates are predicted to become the main form of therapy during the next few years. Regimens of bisphosphonates alone or in combination with estrogen are expected to provide the most effective outcomes, with proven significant increases in hip and vertebral bone mineral content and decreases in vertebral and other type of fractures after 2–3 years of treatment.

Calcitonin has been available as an alternate therapy for women who cannot tolerate estrogen or for whom estrogen is contraindicated. It is a peptide synthesized in parafollicular cells of the thyroid and works by inhibiting osteoclast activity. Its effects on fractures are currently under investigation. Use of parathyroid hormone, sodium fluoride, vitamin D metabolites, or growth factors for routine therapy of osteoporosis is not supported by clinical trials, although investigations are continuing.

Optimizing bone mass is not the only goal in prevention of osteoporotic fractures. During the postmenopausal years, women must also minimize their risks for falls. Maintaining good overall health is important for prevention of fractures and of resulting disability and mortality. Avoiding sedative medications, especially long-acting benzodiazepines and anticonvulsants, will decrease risks for falls and fractures. Maintaining neuromuscular function, particularly strength, agility, and coordination of the lower extremities, will also protect against falls. Vision should be evaluated regularly, and any impairments should be corrected. Use of safety devices during ambulation and in the home, and avoidance of hazards, can diminish risks of falls and should be encouraged in appropriate individuals.

This preventive approach, enlisting specific strategies at different times of the life cycle, may provide the best chance to reduce risks of osteoporosis. Many of these preventive measures require active involvement of women themselves in order to alter behavior and lifestyle. Assessing individuals and informing them of their risks are valuable first steps in the lifetime prevention of this chronic, potentially debilitating condition.

FURTHER READING

Cauley, J. A., Seeley, D. G., Ensrud, K., Ettinger, B., Black, D., & Cummings, S. R., for the Study of Osteoporotic Fractures Research Group. (1995). Estrogen replacement therapy and fractures in older women. *Annals of Internal Medicine, 122,* 9–16.
Results from the Study of Osteoporotic Fractures, a large prospective study, indicated that postmenopausal women who were currently using estrogen replacement therapy had decreased risks for fractures.

Cooper, C., Barker, D. J. P., & Wickham, C. (1988). Physical activity, muscle strength, and calcium intake in fracture of the proximal femur in Britain. *British Medical Journal, 297,* 1443–1446.
This case–control study indicated that increased daily activity and muscle strength protected against fractures.

Cummings, S. R., Nevitt, M. C., Browner, W. S., Stone, K., Fox, K. M., Ensrud, K. E., Cauley, J., Black, D., & Vogt, T. M., for the Study of Osteoporotic Fractures Research Group. (1995). Risk factors for hip fracture in white women. *New England Journal of Medicine, 332,* 767–73.
The Study of Osteoporotic Fractures found that older women with multiple risk factors and low bone density had an especially high risk for hip fracture, which could potentially be reduced by modification of risk factors.

Grisso, J. A., Kelsey, J. L., Strom, B. L., Chiu, G. Y., Maislin, G., O'Brien, L. A., Hoffman, S., & Kaplan, F., for the Northeast Hip Fracture Study Group. (1991). Risk factors for falls as a cause of hip fracture in women. *New England Journal of Medicine, 324,* 1326–1331.
This case–control study of women with hip fractures concluded that a number of previously identified risk factors for falls are also associated with fractures.

Karpf, D. B., Shapiro, D. R., Seeman, E., Ensrud, K. E., Johnston, C. C., Adami, S., Harris, S. T., Santora, A. C., Hirsch, L. J., Oppenheimer, L., Thompson, D., for the Alendronate Osteoporosis Treatment Study Groups. (1997). Prevention of nonvertebral fractures by Alendronate—A meta-analysis. *Journal of the American Medical Association, 277,* 1159–1164.
This study evaluated the results of five completed prospective, randomized, placebo-controlled trials of am aminobisphosphonate, alendronate sodium, in older women with osteoporosis and found that it significantly reduced the risk of nonverbal fractures over at least 3 years.

Kiel, D. P., Felson, D. T., Hannan, M. T., Anderson, J. J., & Wilson, P. W. F. (1990). Caffeine and the risk of hip fracture: The Framingham Study. *American Journal of Epidemiology, 132,* 675–684.

Consumption of 2.5 or more units of caffeine per day significantly increased the risk of hip fractures in subjects from the Framingham Study.

Riggs, B. L., & Melton, L. J. (1992). The prevention and treatment of osteoporosis. *New England Journal of Medicine, 327,* 620–627.

This paper, a comprehensive review of osteoporosis treatment regimens and prevention recommendations, also describes physiological mechanisms.

Rubin, S. M., & Cummings, S. R. (1992). Results of bone densitometry affect women's decisions about taking measures to prevent fractures. *Annals of Internal Medicine, 116,* 990–995.

Older women who underwent bone densitometry and then were surveyed were found to be influenced toward preventive measures by their test results.

37

Smoking Prevention

Joel D. Killen

Smoking kills about 400,000 people in the United States each year. Although the prevalence of smoking among adults has declined sharply, significant numbers of adolescents continue to adopt the smoking habit despite three decades of health warnings. Presently, about 60% of high school seniors report lifetime exposure to cigarettes, and 28% report smoking cigarettes in the previous 30 days. In one recent study, daily smoking prevalences were 7%, 12%, and 17% in grades 8, 10, and 12, respectively. These rates would be even higher if high school dropouts were included in study samples.

Large-scale survey data indicate that the prevalence of "current smoking" (smoking in the past month) among adolescents has remained comparatively steady over the last decade. Although smoking was somewhat more common among adolescent females than among males by the early 1980s, today the prevalence of current smoking for both sexes is roughly equivalent. Pooled data from the 1985–1989 Monitoring the Future survey of high school seniors provide estimates of current smoking by gender and ethnicity. Current smoking prevalence was highest among Native American adolescents (males, 37%; females, 44%) and lowest among Asian-Americans (males, 17%; females, 16%) and African-Americans (males, 16%; females, 13%).

WHY ADOLESCENTS START SMOKING: DO FEMALES START FOR DIFFERENT REASONS?

There is some evidence that smoking onset among males and females may be controlled by different sets of variables. For example, in reviewing the case for gender differences, Clayton found that although smoking among both sexes was strongly influenced by social-environmental variables (e.g., peer and parent smoking behavior), some evidence suggests that adolescent males may use smoking to cope with social insecurity. In contrast, adolescent female smokers tend to be more self-confident and socially adept than their peers. As Clayton has pointed out, to the extent that many prevention efforts emphasize self-esteem building and social skills development, they may not be optimal for females.

228

One factor that may be more important for the onset of smoking among adolescent females is concern for weight and body shape. Weight and shape concerns have become normative in Western culture. In response, many adolescent females may employ smoking as a weight control strategy. Cross-sectional, community-based studies have shown that adolescent females who report high levels of weight concern and disordered eating symptomatology also report higher levels of cigarette smoking. Intriguing evidence that weight concerns and dieting behavior are prospectively related to smoking in adolescent females was presented in a recent prospective trial. French and colleagues found that over a 12-month period, thoughts about weight, eating disorder symptoms, and weight control attempts were prospectively related to smoking initiation in females. Since these factors were not predictive of smoking onset among males in this study, the authors suggest that smoking may indeed serve as a weight control strategy for females, and that this issue may need to be addressed specifically in smoking prevention efforts.

The social environment may play the most important role in promoting the adoption of cigarette smoking by both sexes and in most ethnic groups. The social environment may include peers, family members, teachers, and mass media figures who model various attitudes and behaviors and are in a position, through their own actions, judgments, or social position, to influence the behaviors of others. Among both males and females, perceptions of peer attitudes and behaviors probably represent the strongest influences on substance use, including cigarette smoking. For example, in a study of 1,447 students in grade 10, increased level of substance use by both males and females was most strongly predicted by friends' marijuana use. For males, this was followed by perceived safety of cigarette smoking, poor school performance, and parents' education. Together, these factors accounted for 44% of the overall variation in males' substance use. For females, friends' marijuana use was followed by poor school performance; self-induced vomiting for weight control; perceived safety of cigarette smoking; use of diet pills, laxatives, or diuretics for weight control; parents' education; and perceived adult attitudes about cigarettes. These factors together accounted for 53% of the overall variance for females. Separate multiple-regression analyses by Robinson and colleagues for cigarette smoking, alcohol, and marijuana use produced similar results.

THE NEED FOR SMOKING PREVENTION PROGRAMS

Effective smoking prevention programs are needed for several reasons. First, most smokers begin using tobacco in adolescence; comparatively few start smoking as adults. Second, heavier smoking is associated with age of onset. Those who begin to smoke at younger ages are more likely to become heavier users in adulthood, and research indicates that heavy smokers are at increased risk for cancer, heart disease, and other illnesses. Overall mortality ratios increase with amount smoked. Third, once the habit is established, nicotine dependence may develop among adolescent smokers. Research suggests that addiction processes in adults and adolescents are fundamentally the same. For example, Henningfield and colleagues reported that 84% of 12- through 17-year-olds who smoked a pack a day or more felt that they were dependent upon cigarettes. Other research shows that young smokers develop tolerance and dependence to nicotine. Fourth, despite recent advances in treatment, relapse continues to be the scourge of smoking cessation research. In published cessation studies, most smokers relapse within 1 year of treatment termination. Thus, as the recent U.S. Surgeon General's report on preventing tobacco use concluded, "Preventing smoking and smokeless tobacco use among young people is critical to ending the epidemic of tobacco use in the United States."

The effects of maternal smoking during pregnancy underscore the importance of developing effective smoking prevention programs for females. Numerous studies have shown that smoking increases fetal mortality, decreases fetal growth, and increases death in newborns. Furthermore, exposure to smoke may diminish intellectual function and increase behavioral problems in children who survive the first 4 weeks of life.

SMOKING PREVENTION: DOES ANYTHING WORK?

The bulk of the scientific literature on the effects of smoking prevention programs has focused on information-only and psychoeducational interventions, delivered primarily through the schools. Although some research suggests that adolescent females may respond more favorably to prevention efforts in general, the development of gender-specific program components will require better understanding of factors (e.g., the afore-mentioned weight concerns) that may have a differential influence on the susceptibility of the sexes to smoking initiation.

Early smoking prevention education emphasized the harmful long-term health effects of cigarette smoking. Although some studies reported positive changes in knowledge and attitudes, most found little or no effect on students' reported smoking behavior. Smoking prevention programs that emphasize long-term health effects may miss the mark because the perceived positive benefits associated with smoking may outweigh the long-term negative health effects. For example, most adolescents believe the traditional health education message that smoking is dangerous to their physical health. Despite this knowledge, sources of social influence may exert considerable pressure on adolescents to adopt the smoking habit.

Better results have been achieved with interventions designed to equip adolescents with cognitive and behavioral skills to resist the diverse social influences that promote tobacco use. The social influence resistance approach is derived from McGuire's social inoculation theory, which was developed in the context of work on processes influencing persuasive communications. Social inoculation is viewed as analogous to physiological inoculation (immunization). Physiological immunizations provide resistance to infections by introducing weakened, noninfectious forms of organisms to the body; this primes the production of antibodies to those organisms that will be present in increased numbers if true infection eventually occurs. Social inoculation theory suggests that beliefs can be protected from persuasive appeals by pretreating persons with weak forms of those appeals. Evidence from a variety of studies suggests that inoculation will be effective to the degree that persons are motivated to acquire a defense for beliefs and to practice defending beliefs against attack.

In smoking prevention programs based on social inoculation theory, adolescents are presented with a variety of inducements to smoke, followed by opportunities to invent and practice overt and covert counters to these inducements. The primary training objectives are (1) to acquaint students with the powerful social influences that may trigger smoking (e.g., advertising, peer smoking), as well as with the proximal negative consequences of smoking; and (2) to provide adolescents with coping skills and a strong sense of self-efficacy to resist these influences when they encounter them in the future. The results of numerous studies (backed up by the conclusions of several meta-analyses) indicate that school-based prevention programs based on the social influence resistance model can reduce the incidence of smoking, relative to control conditions. For example, in my study with Telch and colleagues, the rate of regular smoking among control students (16%) at a 33-month follow-up was about three times higher than the rate reported by students receiving a social influence resistance curriculum (5.5%). The general consistency of effects achieved by social influence resistance approaches across studies led the National Cancer Institute (NCI) to convene a panel of experts to establish a consensus regarding the essential elements of effective smoking prevention programs. The panel identified eight features that could be considered both necessary and sufficient for effective smoking prevention programs:

1. Classroom sessions should be delivered at least five times per year in each of 2 years in grades 6 through 8.
2. Programs should emphasize the social factors that influence smoking onset, short-term consequences of smoking, and social influence resistance skills.
3. Programs should be integrated into the existing school curricula.
4. Programs should be introduced during the transition from elementary school to junior high or middle school.
5. Students should be involved in the presentation and delivery of programs.
6. Parental involvement should be encouraged.
7. Teachers should be adequately trained.
8. Programs should be socially and culturally acceptable to communities.

Despite the promise associated with school-based social influence resistance skills training, it has become clear in the years following the NCI panel's recommendations that the effects of these programs may dissipate over time. For example, researchers at the University of Waterloo reported that intervention effects stemming from a program delivered in grades 6 through 8 had all but disappeared by a 5-year follow-up assessment. Such limitations associated with the resistance skills training approach have forced investigators to acknowledge the need to develop interventions that can account for a broader range of determinants. For example, the efficacy of school-based prevention programs may be enhanced by extending intervention beyond the classroom curricula. Behavior changes may be more durable and of greater magnitude when most students have bonded with the school and when peer group support exists for the goals of prevention programs. One potentially useful approach to facilitate school bonding and to enlist peer group support is to engage students in prosocial activities that can compete successfully with substance use and other problem behaviors.

It may be unrealistic to expect school-based programs to address all of the influences that affect young people's health behaviors. First, since school dropouts have higher rates of unhealthy behaviors than youths who stay in school, school-based programs are not able to reach some of the highest-risk youths. Second, because of limited classroom time, curricula may not always be implemented comprehensively or intensively. Third, health-related behaviors occur in numerous community settings, outside of school, that often support unhealthy action and thus counteract the effects of a school-based program. Larger and more durable smoking prevention effects might be achieved if classroom-based interventions were to combine social influence resistance skills training with opportunities for students to mobilize the larger community in support of cigarette smoking prevention and cessation activities.

Finally, much of our knowledge base on the efficacy of smoking prevention approaches is derived from studies with predominantly white, middle-class adolescents.

Despite the NCI recommendations to develop socially and culturally acceptable prevention interventions, significant research efforts in this area have been slow to develop. It is essential that workers in the field of cigarette smoking prevention turn their attention to the design of interventions that are culturally appropriate for high-risk and minority groups.

FURTHER READING

Clayton, S. (1991). Gender differences in psychosocial determinants of adolescent smoking. *Journal of School Health, 6,* 115–120.
Review of the literature examining gender differences in determinants of adolescent smoking.

Flay, B. R., Ryan, K. B., Best, J. A., Brown, K. S., Kersell, M. W., d'Avernas, J. R., & Zanna, M. P. (1985). Are social psychological smoking prevention programs effective?: The Waterloo study. *Journal of Behavioral Medicine, 8,* 37–59.
Report of the long-term effects of a smoking prevention program based upon the social influence resistance model.

French, S. A., Perry, C. L., Leon, G. R., & Fulkerson, J. A. (1994). Weight concerns, dieting behavior, and smoking initiation among adolescents: A prospective study. *American Journal of Public Health, 84,* 1818–1820.
Prospective study of risk factors for smoking initiation in a sample of 1,705 girls in grades 7 through 10.

Glynn, T. J. (1989). Essential elements of school-based smoking prevention programs. *Journal of School Health, 59,* 181–188.
Survey recommendations of an expert panel on the prevention of youth smoking.

Henningfield, J. E., Clayton, R., & Pollin, W. (1990). Involvement of tobacco in alcoholism and illicit drug use. *British Journal of Addiction, 85,* 279–292.
Conference report summarizing evidence indicating that tobacco use is associated with the initiation of other addicting substances.

Johnston, L. D., O'Malley, P. M., & Bachman, J. G. (1993). *Drug use, drinking, and smoking: National survey results from high school, college, and young adult populations.* Rockville, MD: National Institute on Drug Abuse.
Reports of the results of a large-scale survey of drug use prevalence among adolescents.

Robinson, T. N., Killen, J. D., Taylor, C. B., & Telch, M. J. (1987). Perspectives on adolescent substance use: A defined population study. *Journal of the American Medical Association, 258,* 2072–2076.
Report of a cross-sectional study of factors influencing adolescent substance use.

Telch, M. J., Killen, J. D., McAlister, A., Perry, C. L., & Maccoby, N. (1982). Long term follow-up of a pilot project on smoking prevention with adolescents. *Journal of Behavioral Medicine, 5,* 1–8.
Report of the long-term effects of a smoking prevention program based upon the social influence resistance model.

U.S. Department of Health and Human Services. (1994). *Preventing tobacco use among young people: A report of the Surgeon General.* Atlanta: U.S. Department of Health and Human Services, U.S. Public Health Service, Centers for Disease Control, and the Office on Smoking and Health.
Surgeon General's report, which provides a detailed look at smoking in young people.

38

Preventing Alcohol Problems

Jalie A. Tucker

As summarized in Table 38.1, interventions to prevent excessive drinking and its negative consequences have spanned the continuum from individual approaches to community and population-based approaches, and have variously employed educational, legal, economic, and environmental strategies. Selecting an approach will depend on one's purpose, target audience, behavior change goals, resources, and expertise. The approaches are not equally well developed, nor do they have comparable empirical foundations. Indeed, research-based prevention efforts are in their infancy, the proliferation of school-based educational programs notwithstanding.

ORIENTING ASSUMPTIONS AND DECISIONAL ISSUES

Basic assumptions guiding alcohol prevention (as well as treatment) efforts are (1) that discontinuities often exist between quantity/frequency measures of drinking practices and negative health, legal, and other psychosocial problems related to drinking; and (2) that both dimensions lie along a continuum with respect to severity. Thus, when a prevention approach is being chosen, basic decisions must be made concerning which dimension is relatively more important for program goals, where along the severity continuum the intervention should be targeted, and over which population or subgroup a program's cost–benefit analysis should be calculated.

For example, even though very heavy drinkers are at relatively greater risk for many alcohol-related problems, they constitute only a small subset of persons who drink. Thus, at a population level, those who drink less heavily can contribute more occurrences of serious alcohol-related consequences, such as drunk driving. In such cases, they are more

TABLE 38.1. Selective Summary of Interventions to Prevent Alcohol-Related Problems

Intervention type	Goals	Methods	Outcomes
School-based programs	Reduced substance use and substance-related problems in youths	Alcohol and drug education, peer resistance training, changing social norms	Positive changes in attitudes and knowledge more common than reduced substance use
Warning labels on alcoholic beverages	Reduced alcohol use, especially during pregnancy and while driving	Labels mandated by law	Many drinkers have not noticed the labels
Environmental restrictions on alcohol availability	Reduced per capita consumption and associated problems	Higher liquor prices and taxes, restricted outlet hours, lower outlet density	Restrictions, especially higher prices, reduced consumption
Legal restrictions on availability	Reduced alcohol use and associated problems in youths	Raising the legal drinking age (to 21 years)	Reduced alcohol use and alcohol-related driving fatalities in target age group
Dram shop liability laws	Responsible beverage service, reduced customer involvement in alcohol-related accidents	Legal liability for injuries involving intoxicated customers, server training, server interventions	Some reductions in alcohol-impaired driving noted, but consistency of implementation is an issue
Drunk driving deterrence	Reduced drunk driving, change in social norms about drinking and driving	Random roadside breath testing, automatic license suspension, MADD[a]	Modest reductions in drunk driving, but random tests raise constitutional concerns
Worksite programs	Reduced job-related substance use, accidents, and lost productivity	Drug and alcohol testing programs	Deterrence value insufficiently evaluated
Relapse prevention	Reduced drinking episodes after alcohol treatment	Cognitive-behavioral interventions to promote effective coping in high-risk situations for relapse	Outcome data mixed, but some evidence for reduced relapse episodes

[a] Mothers Against Drunk Driving.

appropriate intervention targets than are problem drinkers. This is an effect known as the "preventive paradox."

Decisions about optimal levels and targets of interventions are further complicated by the complex economic considerations involved in cost–benefit analyses. Such analyses may reveal recommendations that run counter to common-sense notions about the benefits of early prevention. They may indicate, for instance, that it is cheaper to wait to intervene until a subset of individuals develops risk factors or problems than it is to mount a universal prevention program for the population at large.

RISK FACTORS FOR THE DEVELOPMENT
OF ALCOHOL PROBLEMS

Another core issue concerns the degree of connection between risk factors and prevention activities. Universally applied programs do not discriminate on the basis of risk factors except at a very general level (e.g., programs aimed at youths), are fairly cursory in scope, and are of modest effectiveness at the individual level, although the aggregated effects over the population may be considerable. In contrast, selectively applied programs target subgroups or individuals with known risk factors and often are more intensive in nature. When risk factors are known, the latter approach allows intervention resources to be concentrated on fewer individuals, which is appropriate when intensified interventions produce increments in positive outcomes to a degree that justifies their usually greater cost.

Research on risk factors for alcohol problems has accrued sufficiently to support focused prevention programs. These factors include the following:

1. *Age.* Alcohol use and abuse peak in early adulthood and decline over the lifespan. Earlier onset of drinking is associated with a higher probability of later problems.

2. *Gender.* Male problem drinkers outnumber female problem drinkers by a ratio of about 3:1.

3. *Family history of alcoholism.* Research has not fully determined the extent to which familial transmission is genetically or environmentally determined, and both routes appear to be contributory, especially in males. However, many persons with a positive family history do not develop drinking and other adjustment problems, and variables that may mediate the relationship are being investigated.

4. *Exposure to social norms that promote substance use and abuse.* This probably operates to some extent across the lifespan, but appears especially important for youths.

5. *Ready availability of alcoholic beverages* (e.g., low prices, high liquor outlet density, liberal hours of outlet operation). The effects of this risk factor are heightened when coupled with constraints on the availability of valued nondrinking alternative activities.

Additional risk-related considerations that are unique to women include the following:

1. Women drinkers may develop alcohol-related problems at lower levels of drinking than men, in part because of sex differences in ethanol metabolism.

2. The development of alcohol-related problems, including dependence, from the onset of heavy drinking appears to occur more rapidly in women than in men (i.e., development is "telescoped"), and reproductive and sexual dysfunctions are often prominent features.

3. Women who drink to intoxication and women problem drinkers are socially stigmatized to a greater degree than their male counterparts, and they have a higher probability of being sexually or criminally victimized.

4. Many forms of substance use, including alcohol consumption, are known to have adverse effects on fetal development and to impair parenting skills after birth. Although heavy drinking during pregnancy does not inevitably result in fetal alcohol syndrome or less pervasive fetal alcohol effects, intake risk thresholds for such defects have not been

well established; hence most authorities make the conservative recommendation that pregnant women abstain.

PREVENTION PRIORITIES FOR WOMEN

Both males and females should be targeted in prevention programs aimed at groups with known risk factors that apply to both sexes; these groups include young people, drunk drivers, and persons with a positive family history of alcoholism. Additional prevention priorities for women as a selected group are to (1) reduce or eliminate drinking and other substance use (including smoking) during pregnancy; (2) improve parenting skills and family environments after birth; and (3) reduce sexual and criminal victimization associated with drinking.

Intervening during pregnancy entails many complex issues, including (1) ethical and legal issues related to the rights of the mother as opposed to the needs of the fetus; (2) difficulties in accurately assessing substance use before and during pregnancy, because accurate reporting may result in punitive rather than therapeutic consequences; (3) issues related to HIV testing if drug use is revealed; (4) medical management of substance withdrawal (e.g., abrupt withdrawal from some drug classes can cause seizures in the fetus); and (5) the fact that pregnant women who are substance abusers may not receive prenatal care until late in pregnancy, if at all, which reduces intervention opportunities.

Given these complexities, perhaps it is not surprising that programs to prevent (and treat) substance abuse in pregnant women are only now being developed and evaluated. A related, but often overlooked, prevention issue concerns the consequences for children of being raised by a substance abusing parent(s). In many cases, the postpartum home environment may have a more malignant effect on child development than any direct *in utero* effects of maternal drug use. Prevention programs thus should broaden their scope beyond the gestation period. Finally, women's increased vulnerability to sexual and criminal victimization when drinking has been virtually unaddressed. Recent increased awareness about preventing date rape has probably had some impact on this issue, but substance-related victimization deserves more attention in prevention programs.

LOOKING AHEAD

Traditional boundaries between prevention and treatment are becoming increasingly blurred in the addictions area. Intensive treatments have proven to add little to positive outcomes beyond what can be achieved with briefer interventions. As a result, intervention resources are being redistributed away from intensive treatments for the small subset of severe, chronic substance abusers, and toward providing briefer interventions for the larger, underserved majority of individuals with less severe problems. This change has been accompanied by a growing appreciation of a public health (as contrasted with a clinical) perspective on addictive behavior change. Prevention activities are central to a public health model. They are likely to increase as the field strives to develop a more complete continuum of intervention options that are better matched to meet the heterogeneous needs of persons with substance use problems.

FURTHER READING

Ennett, S. T., Tobler, N. S., Ringwalt, C. L., & Flewelling, R. L. (1994). How effective is Drug Abuse Resistance Education? A meta-analysis of Project DARE outcome evaluations. *American Journal of Public Health, 84,* 1394–1401.
Documents the very limited effectiveness in preventing or reducing drug use of police-delivered DARE programs, which are widely used in U.S. schools, and suggests that interactive programs that emphasize social competencies produce better outcomes.

Hilton, M. E., & Bloss, G. (Eds.). (1993). *Economics and the prevention of alcohol-related problems* (NIAAA Research Monograph No. 25). Rockville, MD: U.S. Department of Health and Human Services.
Presents contemporary research aimed at preventing alcohol-related problems from a health economic perspective, which is a dominant approach, but one that may be unfamiliar to many health and mental health professionals.

Mrazek, P. R., & Haggerty, R. J. (Eds.). (1994). *Reducing risks for mental disorders: Frontiers for preventive intervention research.* Washington, DC: National Academy Press.
Articulates a comprehensive approach to prevention research for mental disorders, including but not limited to alcohol problems.

U.S. Secretary of Health and Human Services. (1993). *Eighth special report to the U.S. Congress on alcohol and health.* Rockville, MD: U.S. Department of Health and Human Services.
One in a series of regularly issued reports to Congress; these provide an excellent overview of contemporary basic and applied research findings related to alcohol and health.

39

Nutrition: Diet and Disease

Robert L. Brunner
Sachiko T. St. Jeor

*I*n this chapter, we consider the evidence that particular dietary patterns of intake can be related to major diseases affecting adult women in developed countries. This technical review considers the relationship of dietary goals or guidelines to cardiovascular disease (especially coronary heart disease, or CHD), cancer, osteoporosis, and non-insulin-dependent diabetes mellitus (NIDDM).

The present understanding of how nutrition quality is related to health maintenance and disease has been formed from the scientific study of nutrient shortage and excess balance. Table 39.1 lists health outcomes that have well-established correlates with nutrition quality for black and white women in the United States and other developed countries. Cardiovascular disease and cancer account for about two-thirds of all deaths in women. Although most diseases have multiple determinants, age of onset, morbidity, mortality, and prevention of the disorders discussed here are feasibly modified by lifestyle factors. Because of differences in nutrition quality and many other factors, chronic health problems are more prevalent and damaging among the poor, especially among minorities.

ENERGY (CALORIE) INTAKE

Studies of calorie intake, as a factor separate from weight, in cancer and heart disease rates are infrequent. A multiple-regression analysis of Food and Agriculture Organization (FAO) intake data and World Health Organization (WHO) mortality statistics produced significant contributions of dairy and lard fat to breast, colon, rectal, and lung cancer and to ischemic heart disease in women. The addition of total caloric intake, or the total minus the dairy/lard calories, did not show any contribution independent of caloric intake. In other studies, increased energy intake is a risk factor for colon cancer, after adjustment for body mass. Total calories and amounts of specific nutrient levels contributing calories do not exist in isolation and have perhaps a more intricate

TABLE 39.1. Prevalent Health Outcomes with Significant Nutrition Components in Their Etiology

Outcome	Black women	White women
CHD (age-adjusted death rate per 100,000)	88.8	68.8
Hypertension (% prevalence)	43[a]	25
NIDDM (age-adjusted death rate per 100,000)	25.4	9.5
Breast and colorectal cancer (age-adjusted death rate per 100,000)	43.0	33.8
Osteoporotic hip fractures (% lifetime risk)	5.4+	14.7+

[a]Mortality 6 to 13 times greater in blacks.

relationship than might first appear to be the case. In both rural and urban Japanese adult men and women, the percentages of calories from fat and cholesterol rose by 7–15% (more for rural residents) during the period 1960–1990, but total energy intake declined about 10% in both groups. Changes in fish, milk, and meat intake were responsible for the increase in fat, yet the shift toward a "Westernized" diet was not accompanied by an increase in calories. Similarly, immigration from Japan to the United States (as studied in the Honolulu Heart Program) produces a doubling or more of dietary fat intake and an increase in risk factors without a commensurate change in calories. Three large-cohort studies (the Framingham, Honolulu, and Puerto Rico studies) are consistent with benefits from diets that emphasize lowering fat intake, but higher rates of myocardial infarction and CHD were associated with lower caloric intake. Nevertheless, metabolic studies show inherited differences in the predisposition to store energy as fat or as lean tissue. The Iowa Women's Health Study found a reduced risk of colon cancer with increased vegetables (and dietary fiber), which remained statistically significant after adjustment for total energy intake. Energy intake was not positively associated with risk in this study.

INTAKE OF BREADS, GRAINS, AND OTHER STARCHES

The attribution of health effects to specific constituents of breads, grains and legumes is complicated by the multiple dietary differences inherent in their consumption. Grain products contribute more carbohydrates than other food groups (41%). However, both starch and sugar are also contributed, the latter particularly in many baked products. Dietary fiber is highest in grains and their products, in other starches, and in vegetables/fruits, seeds, and nuts. Recent food consumption data from households in Europe indicate that cereals and their derivatives contributed half of total dietary fiber. In addition to the fact that these foods make contributions to both carbohydrates and fiber, they may displace foods with various health effects, such as meat or eggs. Thus, the relative contributions to health and disease of the foods added or taken away is ambiguous. It is widely believed that the "diseases of civilization," including CHD, colorectal and breast cancers, and perhaps NIDDM, are affected by inadequate fiber intake. A large case–control study found a "weak" protective effect from fiber against colon cancer, but none from vitamins A or C. The correlations between dietary fiber and disease endpoints have been somewhat weak and controversial, and/or have been explained by body weight. Studies have variously supported or refuted ideas that only vegetable-derived fiber is protective and that low fat must accompany high fiber.

Starch from peas and beans has been shown to have a particularly strong relationship to reduced CHD risk. In addition to being sources of fiber, legumes are high in vitamin B_6, vitamin B_{12}, and folate, important in the clearing of plasma homocysteine. In a new research development, several studies have recently found that high homocysteine levels were more predictive of atherosclerosis than was the plasma lipid profile; this has increased researchers' interest in the role of these vitamins in cardiovascular disease.

FAT INTAKE

Cross-cultural and migration studies provide evidence linking consumption of high-fat diets to the etiology of CHD and of colorectal, breast, and lung cancers. In the Seven Countries Study, as one example, saturated fat intake in particular correlated strongly with CHD mortality rates. A study of WHO and FAO data concerning dietary fat and breast cancer in 30 countries found relationships between age-specific breast cancer rates and animal fat minus fish fat intake, which increased with age. The hypothesis that implicates total fat intake in cancer is more controversial, partly because clear risk markers such as blood lipids do not exist for cancer. The literature on diet and breast cancer suggests that studies have not consistently shown effects of saturated fat or total fat intake on primary prevention, although lowered fat seems to improve prognosis once breast cancer is diagnosed. (For a fuller discussion of this issue, see Glanz's chapter on nutrition education in this volume.)

Randomized trials of cholesterol lowering for the primary prevention of heart disease have included too few women for a convincing effect to be obtained in healthy women. However, observational data suggest that dietary interventions to improve lipid profile should benefit both women and men. Many years of feeding studies have generally led to the conclusion that diets in which the fat component is mainly saturated lead to plasma cholesterol levels significantly higher than those resulting from diets high in polyunsaturated fatty acids. A simple relationship suggests that saturated fatty acids are twice as effective in raising plasma cholesterol as polyunsaturated fatty acids are in lowering it. However, certain saturated fats (beef tallow, cocoa butter, coconut and palm kernel oils, and milk fat) are not effective in raising cholesterol. Also, the individual sensitivity of blood cholesterol to saturated fat intake varies greatly.

The non-Asian developed countries have average diet in which about 34% of calories come from fat. Experts have recommended that fewer than 30% of calories should come from fat. Fat is either saturated and harmful or unsaturated and less harmful; although recommended healthy diets have conventionally replaced saturated fat with polyunsaturated fat, the picture has recently become less simple. Monounsaturated fat (e.g., olive oil) is the cornerstone of the Mediterranean diet. The use of olive oil may underlie the lower-than-expected rates of CHD and cancer, given the relatively high total fat intake, in that region of the world. To deepen the confusion, other oils have been promoted as beneficial, or at least less harmful than the saturated fats. Those that have drawn interest are the omega-3 fatty acids (found in fish) and alpha-linoleic fatty acids (found in canola and soybean oils, and in some vegetables and nuts). Consensus has not been achieved on either of these issues. A third issue arose when studies involving women, one prospective and one case–control, found the risk of CHD to be predicted by intake of trans-fatty acids, which raise the level of harmful lipoproteins and lower the level of those that protect, and thus may increase disease risk. In addition to margarine, these hydrogenated oils often are found in commercial fried and baked snacks. Finally, on this point, a debate is underway as to whether it is preferable to replace saturated fats with natural oils (nonhydrogenated) or with carbohydrates.

Serum low-density lipoprotein (LDL) concentrations are less in vegetarians than in meat eaters, providing one mechanism by which fruit and/or vegetable intake may have a beneficial impact on CHD and cancer. Most of the research on cholesterol and CHD has been restricted to men. Nevertheless, associations between elevated cholesterol (particularly LDL) and the risk of morbidity and mortality from CHD have been demonstrated in women, both white and nonwhite. Substantial data from epidemiological studies and clinical trials have established an association between consumption of "prudent" low-fat diets and reduced CHD and cancer rates, but again men have largely made up these cohorts. Large-cohort studies have related dietary cholesterol intake to both all-cause mortality and CHD. A meta-analysis of large cholesterol reduction trials has provided a rule of thumb in which each 1% reduction in serum cholesterol achieves a 1.7% reduction in heart attack and a 2% reduction in mortality; however, too few women have been included for these figures to be definitive for females, especially since the mortality effect assumes a reduction in breast cancer. In addition to cholesterol lowering and general fat reduction, fruit and vegetable sources may provide their own advantages.

Diets high in saturated fat intake, which leads to increases in LDL concentrations in the blood, may be particularly problematic in NIDDM because harmful lipoprotein synthesis is enhanced by elevated plasma insulin.

FRUIT AND VEGETABLE INTAKE

Fruits and vegetables are rich in antioxidant vitamins and in fiber, both of which are thought to protect against cancer and heart disease. An examination of the influence of fruit and vegetable intake on relative risk of cancer found significant protection in 128 of 156 studies. Mortality from cardiovascular disease has statistically significant negative relation to consumption of fruit and green vegetables.

Although studies have reported a moderate beneficial effect of a vegetarian diet on cancer and all-cause mortality, most have concluded that the benefits are not attributable the strict avoidance of meat, but to sound nutritional principles. It has also been suggested that benefits of higher fruit and vegetable intake may derive from other unmeasured or unknown components, correlated lifestyle factors, or the resulting lower consumption of certain other foods or nutrients. The components of individual foods can be extensive, and these may interact to produce an effect different from those of single components in isolation. Also, it is no simple matter to determine whether the replacement of other foods—for example, those that contain fat and cholesterol or are calorie-rich—is responsible for some of the health benefits observed in high-vegetable/fruit (and/or other high-carbohydrate) diets.

Vegetarians were found to have significantly reduced standardized mortality ratios for all cancers after adjustment for the effects of smoking, body mass index, and economic level, but no firm conclusion could be made about deaths from heart disease. A cohort study of Seventh-Day Adventists (n = 34,198), half of whom were lacto-ovo-vegetarians, found that fruit consumption was the one dietary constituent that showed a strong, statistically significant protective association with lung cancer that was independent of smoking. There was a 70% lower risk with consumption of three or more fruit portions per week, compared with fewer than three. Other studies have assessed the effects of supplemental vitamins A,

E, and/or beta-carotene on cancer and heart disease in men and women. In the beta-carotene and retinol efficacy trial, lung cancer and overall mortality were significantly increased in those taking the supplement. In the Alpha-Tocopherol Beta-Carotene Cancer Prevention Study (men only), lung and other cancers were increased in the beta-carotene treatment group. The results were less clear for vitamin E as some cancer rates increased (stomach) and others decreased (colorectal, prostate).

Fruits and vegetables are high in dietary fiber, and in epidemiological studies higher intake has had modest correlations with lower colorectal and breast cancer rates. Diets high in these foods have been associated with reductions in breast cancer rates in some studies but not in others. However, some studies have suggested that fiber (whether from fruits and vegetables or from grains) is only protective in diets that are high in fat, and that specific fibers and certain vegetables, particularly soybean products and garlic, may be more protective than others. This suggests that studies of the positive effects of fiber need to consider the type and sources of fiber, as well as the composition of the total diet.

SODIUM, CALCIUM, SUGAR, AND ALCOHOL INTAKE

Average sodium consumption in the United States is between 4 and 6 grams per day (2–3 teaspoons of salt)—an amount much higher than that needed for normal functioning. The relationship of sodium or salt to high blood pressure is a major health concern of nutritionists, who suggest moderate or reduced salt intake. The issue is controversial: Only a specific group (i.e., salt-sensitive individuals) may be at risk, but sensitive individuals are not easily identified; thus, the recommendation has population implications, especially since low-sodium diets have not proven harmful. The debate also concerns sodium's rank on the list of factors affecting blood pressure and whether it is only significant within the context of other constituents, particularly potassium, calcium, magnesium, chlorine, and protein. The largest of the population studies of sodium's relationship to health was the INTERSALT Study, which compared the blood pressure of both women and men (n = 10,079) in 32 countries. International comparisons are important, because nutritional variability within countries is often too small to provide sufficient statistical power without extremely large sample sizes. Sodium excretion (which mirrors intake) was significantly related to blood pressure across populations and to increasing blood pressure with age, independent of body mass, alcohol consumption, and gender. Extrapolation showed that a modest decrease in sodium and a small increase in potassium intake would reduce the population increase in systolic blood pressure with age by 9 mm Hg, and that the reduction in CHD mortality would be more than 5%.

The Trial of Antihypertensive Interventions and Management (n = 878) to reduce mild hypertension found that a low-sodium/high-potassium diet lowered blood pressure, but not as well as diuretic drugs did. Adding a low-sodium/high-potassium diet to drug therapy did not enhance change, but reducing body weight did. The Trial of Hypertension Prevention is a study of women and men (n = 2,164; 30% women) with high normal blood pressures. Dietary reduction of sodium (–1.5%) caused drops in both systolic (–1.7 mm Hg) and diastolic (–0.9 mm Hg) pressure, which were maintained at a 18-month follow-up. The results were the same when analyses were adjusted for gender, age, race, and baseline blood pressure. Body weight was not significantly reduced. Some critics feel that changes of these magnitudes are of no practical significance in public health. Supplements of calcium, magnesium, or potassium were of minor or no effect in reducing blood pressure—a finding repeated in other studies.

NIDDM is often accompanied by hypertension, and this association is independent of age and obesity. With the insulin resistance found in NIDDM, sodium retention increases, which is in part responsible for the hypertension. This apparently makes the recommendations for limited sodium intake particularly relevant to those with or at risk for NIDDM.

Osteoporosis is a disorder associated with bone fractures in women, particularly postmenopausal women. Many factors, a number of which are poorly understood, affect bone mass. It appears that adult bone mass in women is related to calcium intake and utilization in childhood and adolescence, and that this intake is inadequate in the majority of young women. Some data suggest that the relationship between calcium intake and peak bone mass is not linear, instead requiring only that a critical threshold be exceeded. In older women, bone loss depends on the integrity of ovarian hormone function. Bone loss may be reduced by higher calcium intake after menopause, but the effect is delayed by a matter of years. Moreover, most studies have not been able to relate calcium intake (primarily from dairy products) directly to the risk of fracture. The Women's Health Initiative, a large-scale study of women over 50, has a treatment arm that supplements calcium (not through food intake); this should help in resolving some issues in the area of calcium's relationship to hormone function, bone loss, and fractures. (For a further discussion of osteoporosis, see Nelson's chapter in this volume.)

In the United States, the combination of naturally occurring and added sugar contributes about 21% of total calorie intake. Added sugar consumption accounted for 4.8–11.6% of the energy intake for women in a community cohort in Scotland ($n = 11,626$), similar to the 9% generally quoted in the United States—findings suggesting that it is not an insignificant component of the diet. Sucrose is traditionally restricted in the diets of diabetics, although recent recommendations of the American Diabetic Association have liberalized its inclusion in the diabetic diet. Increased sucrose in the context of a high-carbohydrate diet has been demonstrated to increase serum triglycerides in some individuals, independent of diabetic status. A link to heart disease resulting from sucrose consumption has not been shown, although triglycerides have been associated with risk of heart disease. Of perhaps more direct importance, sucrose contributes "empty calories" (i.e., it lacks other nutrients) and may thus be deleterious for weight control, which is a major concern in women's health.

A full discussion of alcohol use and health is beyond the scope of this chapter. However, some studies—the Nurses' Health Study in particular ($n = 85,526$)—find better cardiovascular disease endpoints with moderate alcohol intake than with abstention. The same U-shaped curve for alcohol consumption is not as clearly established for the other health outcomes. At the high end of consumption, alcohol potentiates heart disease, high blood pressure, cancer risk, and NIDDM, in addition to its widely acknowledged effects on psychosocial, gastrointestinal, and hepatic disease.

CONCLUSIONS

The subject of what and how much to eat so as to promote good health is made complex by the interactions of the various constituents of the total diet, as well as by the subtle, long-term cumulative nature of the relevant outcomes. In addition, the effect sizes may be relatively small; that is, they may involve only modest increases in the average number of years of healthy life. Furthermore, the clustering of diet with nondiet factors that also affect health again means that large numbers of observations and complex statistical analyses are necessary to identify independent dietary influences. All these difficulties mean that large and rigorous research efforts are necessary if scientifically exact answers to primary prevention questions are demanded before behavior will change with regard to nutrition. Up to this point, correlational studies are the major sources of information about eating behaviors and health, and seem to have been sufficiently convincing to inspire large-scale changes in the commercial food supply of the United States and other developed Western nations. The wide use of unsaturated fats and oils, and now the introduction of a fat substitute, are the prime examples of this sequence. Interestingly, however, the substitution of synthetic sweeteners for sugar, now so widely accepted and pervasive, has a rationale with very minimal ties to health or disease. The information from correlational studies seems to have resulted in an attempt to preserve the current diet through manipulation of identified constituents, rather than the adoption of an apparently healthier diet. Unfortunately, evidence is scarce that such a "micromanagement" approach to the diet improves health or reduces disease in a meaningful way. The problem may be in part attributable to a premature emphasis by health experts on a plausible intervening risk factor (i.e., serum cholesterol, in the case of saturated fat intake) rather than on the actual behavioral–nutritional difference (i.e., the diet as eaten). The objective of psychologists and other behavioral researchers may be to learn how the diet can be more pervasively and permanently changed within individuals and groups. Research of this type is beginning to be undertaken; if successful, it should stimulate the demand for similar enterprises.

FURTHER READING

American Diabetic Association. (1997). Nutrition recommendations and principles for people with diabetes mellitus and diabetic care. *Journal of Clinical and Applied Research and Education, 20*(514).
Position statement of the American Diabetic Association with respect to nutritional factors leading to heart disease and hypertension.

Anderson, K. M., Wilson, P. W. F., Odell, P. M., & Kannel, W. B. (1991). An updated coronary risk profile: A statement for health professionals. *Circulation, 83,* 356–362.
Updated risk equations for CHD based on the Framingham sample were similar for women and men except for aging differences.

Block, G., Patterson, B., & Subar, A. (1992). Fruit, vegetables, and cancer prevention: A review of the epidemiologic evidence. *Nutrition and Cancer, 18,* 1–29.
A scholarly and comprehensive consideration of the evidence concerning specific foods and cancer prevention.

Boonen, S., & Dequeky, J. (1996). Strategies for the prevention of senile (type II) osteoporosis: An update. *Journal of Internal Medicine, 239,* 383–389.
The beneficial effects of most prevention strategies have not been adequately documented, although risk factors are potentially preventable.

Chu, K. C., Tarone, R. E., Chow, W. H., & Alexander, G. A. (1995). Colorectal cancer trends by race and anatomic subsites, 1975 to 1991. *Archives of Family Medicine, 10,* 849–856.
Decline of age-adjusted breast cancer mortality rates in the past 10 years in women aged 40 to 70 cannot be explained by screening or medical treatment alone.

Chu, K. C., Tarone, R. E., Kessler, L. G., Ries, L. A., Hankey, B. F., Miller, B. A., & Edwards, B. K. (1996). Recent trends in U.S. breast cancer incidence, survival, and mortality rates. *Journal of the National Cancer Institute, 88,* 1571–1579.

For white women and men, colorectal cancer incidence rates declined after 1985, although for black women and men rates were unchanged.

Das, B. N., & Banka, V. S. (1992). Coronary artery disease in women. *Postgraduate Medicine, 91,* 197–206.

Prevention strategies for women center around smoking cessation, aspirin therapy, diet modification, and estrogen replacement.

Francis, C. K. (1990). Hypertension and cardiac disease in minorities. *American Journal of Medicine, 88*(Suppl. 3B), 3B–3S.

Recent decreases in mortality from hypertension through efforts like the National High Blood Pressure Education Program have been less in blacks and Hispanics than in whites.

Harris, M. I. (1985). Prevalence of non-insulin dependent diabetes and impaired glucose tolerance. In National Diabetes Data Group (Eds.), *Diabetes in America: Diabetes data compiled 1984.* (U.S. Department of Health and Human Services Publication No. PHS 85-1468, pp. 1–31). Bethesda, MD: National Institutes of Health.

Prevalence of undiagnosed diabetes (3.2%) was nearly equal to that of diagnosed diabetes (3.4%), with rates equal in women and men and higher in blacks than whites.

Manson, J. E., Colditz, G. A., Stampfer, M. J., Willett, W. C., Krolewski, A. S., Rosner, B., Arky, R. A., Speizer, F. E., & Hennekens, C. H. (1991). A prospective study of maturity-onset diabetes mellitus and risk of coronary heart disease and stroke in women. *Archives of Internal Medicine, 151,* 1141–1147.

Diabetes onset afater 30 is a determinant of cardiovascular disease in women and is further increased by obesity, hypertension, or smoking.

National Research Council. (1989). *Recommended dietary allowances* (10th ed.). Washington, DC: National Academy Press.

Nutrient intake goals (recommended dietary allowances) are discussed.

Riggs, B. L. (1995). The worldwide problem of osteoporosis: Insights afforded by epidemiology. *Bone, 17,* 505S–511S.

In the United States, 1.5 million fractures annually are attributable to osteoporosis, with up to 20% mortality in the next 6 months. Lifetime risk is 40% in white women after the age of 50, compared with 13% in men.

Rodriguez, J. G., Sattin, R. W., & Waxweiler, R. J. (1989). Incidence of hip fractures, United States, 1970–1983. *American Journal of Preventive Medicine, 5,* 175–181.

For each age group, women had hospitalization rates twice those of men; rates for women rose exponentially by age decade.

Roussouw, J. E. (1994). The effects of lowering serum cholesterol on coronary heart disease risk. *Medical Clinics of North America, 78,* 181–195.

A review of findings with regard to dietary fat reduction, cholesterol reduction, and heart disease.

Stamler, J., Rose, R., Stamler, R., Elliott, P., Dyer, A., & Marmot, M. (1989). INTERSALT Study findings: Public health and medical care implications. *Hypertension, 14,* 570–577.

Necessary reading to understand the complex results of this major study of salt intake and blood pressure.

Steinmetz, K. A., Kushi, L. H., Bostick, R. M., Folsom, A. R., & Potter, J. D. (1994). Vegetables, fruit, and colon cancer in the Iowa Women's Health Study. *American Journal of Epidemiology, 139,* 1–15.

This study examined specific foods and their relationship to cancer in women.

Willett, W. C. (1994). Diet and health: What should we eat? *Science, 264,* 532–537.

A provocative general discussion of the role of foods in disease by a widely quoted researcher.

40

Nutrition: Guidelines, Attitudes, and Behaviors

Robert L. Brunner
Sachiko T. St. Jeor

*O*f the lifestyle factors affecting health and disease, probably none surpass nutrition in sparking discussion and research ideas. In this chapter, dietary goals proposed by major health education and policy groups are first described. Where relevant data are available, there is discussion of how closely women's intake generally conforms with these recommendations. Research on relevant attitudes in women is then described; such research should help answer some of the many remaining questions in all areas of women's health and nutrition. Finally, some group behavior change efforts are outlined.

NUTRITION QUALITY GUIDELINES

The prevention and treatment of chronic disease are affected by food intake, which is often poor in quality, despite availability and adequacy of the food supply. Conceptions of nutrition quality are fairly consistent in the dietary recommendations made by government, advisory, and special interest groups. The Recommended Dietary Allowances (RDAs) are widely used in the evaluation of nutrition adequacy or quality. They are specific levels recommended by the Committee on Dietary Allowances of the Food and Nutrition Board of the National Research Council "to meet the known nutritional needs of nearly all healthy people" and are not levels specific to disease prevention or therapeutic intervention. Table 40.1 shows the 1989 RDAs for selected dietary constituents for women. Only those constituents with established epidemiological links to prevalent and significant health outcomes are listed in Table 40.1. Midpoints of ranges and approximate amounts are used where applicable. For comparison of recommended

TABLE 40.1. The National Research Council's 1989 RDAs of Selected Dietary Constituents for Women Aged 19–50 Years

Constituents	RDA
Energy[a]	2,000 calories
Fat	30% of calories
Saturated fat	< 10% of calories
Dietary fiber	Not specified; eat fiber-containing foods
Calcium	800–1,200 mg
Salt	< 6.0 grams
Vitamin A plus carotenoids[a]	4,000 IU or 800 μ RE[b]
Vitamin C[a]	60 mg
Folate[a]	180 μg
Vitamin B$_6$	1.6 mg
Vitamin B$_{12}$	2 μg

Note. The data are from National Research Council (1989).
[a]This RDA was met by women, according to NHANES III data.
[b]Vitamin A is now expressed in retinol equivalents as the standard unit.

and actual intake, data from the third National Health and Nutrition Examination Survey (NHANES III) are used. Selected constituents for which the RDAs and NHANES III data are in apparent conformity are footnoted in Table 40.1. A comparison of data from NHANES I and II with those from NHANES III suggests that between 1970 and 1980 energy intake only increased, and not markedly so, in black women. However, between 1980 and 1990 black women continued this increase, and smaller increases were also seen in white women. It has not yet been determined whether parallel increases in body weight and in obesity of 6–7% may be partially explained by these small increases in energy intake or by a combination of factors, including subtle changes in sampling procedures, physical activity, nutrient apportioning, and eating patterns. Women's diets in general continue to have excess fat, saturated fat, and salt, and are below RDAs for fiber-containing fruits and vegetables and for calcium.

It has been emphasized that the RDAs are recommendations rather than requirements, and that they, like most general standards of nutrition quality, assume that individuals are within the normal range of metabolic and physiological variability. In view of the complex interactions among constituents of the diet, individual variability, and need, all health-related recommendations regarding specific nutrients need to be made carefully. It is essential to recognize that dietary intake studies examine nutrients not alone but as foods, without eliminating the possibility that another element in the foods besides the one being focused upon may also take an active part. Thus, the total diet over time may be a vital consideration in understanding the link of nutrition quality to health.

The Dietary Guidelines for Americans, developed jointly by the U.S. Department of Agriculture (USDA) and the U.S. Department of Health and Human Services (DHHS), were most recently published in 1995. The Dietary Guidelines represent a consensus of experts based upon scientific evidence, and are written so as way to be of practical use. They are applicable within a range of eating patterns affected by cultural, economic, and individual factors. They state that one should eat a variety of foods; maintain a healthy weight; choose a diet low in fat, saturated fat, and cholesterol; choose a diet high in grain products, vegetables, and fruits; and choose a diet with sugars, salt, sodium, and alcohol in moderation.

The Dietary Guidelines offer authoritative advice and a framework for improving nutrition quality. The Food Guide Pyramid was developed by the Human Nutrition Information Service of the USDA to help U.S. residents put the Dietary Guidelines into action and make the best food choices. The base of the pyramid, which represents the largest proportion of the diet in terms of number of daily servings, consists of breads and grains. Fruits and vegetables occupy the next largest subdivision and are second highest in number of servings. The dairy and meat groups are next on the pyramid, as their recommended number of servings is fewer. The smallest part of the pyramid (at the tip) is made up of fats, oils, and sweets, which should be "used sparingly." Accompanying literature specifies that sodium intake (salt is 40% sodium, and 1 teaspoon contains about 2,000 mg of sodium) should not be in excess of 3,000 mg/day. Food Guide Pyramid serving units are cups, ounces, or "pieces" (fruit or bread slices), and what counts as one serving in each food group is described. Also, an approximate number of daily servings is recommended for small, medium, and large calorie levels. The Food Guide Pyramid emphasizes reducing fat intake, because the average U.S. dietary intake of fat is too high.

The NHANES III data discussed thus far refer to nutrients and do not provide a means of assessing observance of Food Guide Pyramid recommendations, which are given in terms of foods. The Nationwide Food Consumption Surveys (NFCS), conducted every 10 years by the USDA, permit relevant comparisons to be made because several food groups are presented as percentages of total energy intake. The NFCS conducted in 1985 indicated that women averaged 4.5 servings of fruits and vegetables per day, compared to the recommended 5–9 servings (depending on the total calorie level). Women of low income averaged 2 servings of fruits and vegetables. Women of all income groups were similar in obtaining 29% of food energy from grains, slightly below recommendations. Dairy intake for women overall was consistent with the Food Guide Pyramid, but was slightly lower for low-income women. The contribution of the meat group to total calories was marginally higher for low-income women than for all women, but was in line with the Food Guide Pyramid. Another analysis of these same data indicated that increases in dietary variety (number of foods or varieties within or between food groups) improved nutrition quality to a greater degree in women than in men.

Healthy People 2000 is a document in which the U.S. Public Health Service (a branch of the DHHS) outlines a national strategy to improve health through disease prevention. A significant portion of this initiative focuses on nutrition. Decreased fat (both total and saturated) and salt, and increased complex carbohydrate, fiber, and calcium, are overall goals. Goals specific to infants, children, pregnant/lactating women, and the aged, and to education, food availability, and medical delivery, are also included in *Healthy People 2000*. Among these goals are reducing iron deficiency in vulnerable populations, promoting breastfeeding, widening healthy food opportunities, increasing product label awareness, promoting school/worksite nutrition education, and providing nutrition services in primary care settings.

Organizations like the American Heart Association have guidelines for dietary quality consistent with those of the USDA/DHHS. They add maintenance of a desirable body weight, 2 or fewer ounces of alcohol per day, and no more than 7.5 grams of salt per day. The American Heart Association's Nutrition Committee states that only 10–12% of the U.S. population meets these recommendations. The National Cancer Institute and the American Cancer Society both advise against foods processed by means of salt, smoking, or other curing methods. The National Cancer Institute has a fiber intake goal of 20–30 grams/day, and both these groups recommend avoiding obesity. The National Heart, Lung, and Blood Institute's National Cholesterol Education Program (NCEP) began in 1984 to highlight the links of dietary saturated fat and blood lipids to coronary heart disease. Clinical judgments of high levels of blood lipoproteins trigger stepwise interventions, which begin with diet modification. The aim of the diet is to lower intake of saturated fat and cholesterol, and thereby to lower blood cholesterol and low-density lipoprotein to the cut-points or below which initiated treatment. It has been suggested that in women, more emphasis should be placed on high-density lipoprotein. The NCEP Step 1 diet is very similar to the USDA/DHHS Dietary Guidelines, but more specific (fewer than 30% of calories from fat, fewer than 10% of calories from saturated fat, and under 300 mg of cholesterol per day). The Step 2 diet is more stringent (saturated fat < 7% and cholesterol < 200 mg/day). Like the Food Guide Pyramid, the NCEP suggests 6 ounces or less of meat per day, 6–8 teaspoons of added oil or fat per day, no more than 3 egg yolks per week, and 2+ servings of very-low-fat dairy foods per day for calcium. According to the NHANES III and NFCS data, fat recommendations have been exceeded in the U.S. diet. The dairy and egg recommendations are complex to track, but in the NFCS the mean amount of low-fat or skim milk consumed did not reach the NCEP criterion of 2 cups and was especially low in low-income women. Analysis of the NFCS data base shows that pregnant and lactating women consume larger amounts of dairy products than nonpregnant women, yet still less than the recommended 3 cups (or the equivalent) per day. Vegetables and fruits were also consumed more during pregnancy and lactation but at levels below recommendations, especially vegetables high in folate and vitamin A.

Two further issues arise with regard to nutrition quality. First, what is known about women's concepts of nutrition quality, and how do these compare with recommendations? Second, are behavior change efforts, whether on a large scale or a modest scale, successful in bringing women's attitudes and behaviors into greater conformity with better nutrition quality?

PUBLIC PERCEPTION OF DIET IN HEALTH SURVEYS

Health beliefs or attitudes and health behaviors are closely tied in all prominent explanatory theories. Messages to the public about improving food choices do not ensure that habits will be changed, or will be maintained once changed. Many factors beyond knowledge are involved in the process of change. These include the belief that diet is important to health; a sense of one's own levels of risk and benefits, as well as a sense that these are at least partly controllable; the influences of important others (i.e., social norms); and a complex web of individual factors encompassing personality, sociodemographics, and self-efficacy. These components have begun to be scrutinized, so that improved nutrition interventions can be designed and delivered. However, pertinent data regarding influences on women's nutrition- and health-related knowledge, attitudes, and behavior are rare.

Knowing the status and trends of diet and health beliefs in target groups should help in the design of programs and interventions that will modify behavior in the desired direction. Several recent studies offer consistent views. In its survey of

American dietary habits, the American Dietetic Association interviewed men and women 25 years of age and older (n = 1,000). A minority (26%) were "nutrition-conscious"—that is, sought information, purchased low-fat foods, and felt they did everything they could to eat a healthy diet. At the other end of the spectrum, 36% did not consider nutrition to be of importance and did not attempt to manage their eating habits. A middle group believed nutrition to be important, although they sensed they were not doing enough to eat a healthy diet. Women were more likely than men to consider diet and nutrition to be very important. Without prodding, subjects cited eating more vegetables, fruit, poultry, grains, and fish, in that order, as healthy eating behaviors. When women were asked about health concerns, about two-thirds mentioned concern about "general health maintenance." One-third cited weight maintenance or loss, and 10% or fewer specified another health problem. Dietary constituents cited by women for surveillance were fat, cholesterol, vitamins, calories, salt or sodium, and fiber, in that order. Women cited fat and calories more often and fiber and cholesterol less often than men.

In a study of preventive health attitudes, one-third of medical, dental, and nursing students (n = 835) were only slightly concerned or not concerned about dietary fat consumption—the most often targeted aspect of dietary quality in all nutrition guidelines. Nurses (almost entirely women in this study) were 10% more likely than medical or dental students (primarily men) to report being very concerned about fat consumption. In the Pawtucket Heart Health Program (n = 1,250), belief that reducing fat intake would help prevent coronary heart disease increased from 28% to 64% over a 5-year interval. Belief in the positive effects of less salt rose from 13% to 19%, while belief in the positive effect of fewer calories was stable at about 6–8%. Belief in weight control to help prevent heart disease dropped from 32% to 28%. The Stanford Five-City Project also showed that reducing high-fat foods had the largest increment as an identified heart disease risk factor. Weight declined as an identified risk factor. Salt, fiber, meat, and cholesterol all significantly increased as risk factors identified by subjects, whereas general diet did not. In the RENO Diet–Heart Study, women's scores were higher than men on a "Nutrition Concern" factor representing health consciousness in nutrition. Women had lower scores on a factor termed "Meat Preference," which represented the central importance of meat in most meals. Similarly, in the Stanford Five-City Project, more women than men were vegetarians (the ratio was approximately 3:2). Higher income, more education, and younger age were also associated with vegetarianism. Body mass and cholesterol were significantly lower in vegetarians, suggesting two benefits that have several health ramifications.

In more than 3,000 Australians, women and men who ate low-fat diets (26% calories from fat) were more nutrition-conscious, with more women than men eating such diets. Women in the low-fat quintile ate fewer meats, eggs, snack foods, sweets, and dairy products, but two times greater amounts of rice, fruit, and fruit juice, and 50% more alcohol and soft drinks. Various specific nutrients reflecting dietary quality were more favorable in the low-fat consumers, including fiber, sodium, beta-carotene, vitamin C, and folate, but not vitamins A, B_6, B_{12}, or calcium.

These findings suggest that components of various nutrition quality guidelines are recognized and endorsed by the public to varying degrees. Women are generally more aware of nutrition quality than men, although the data presented in the next section indicate that the difference does not encompass all facts and advice.

GROUP BEHAVIOR CHANGE

Behavior change programs include efforts targeting a population—that is, essentially everyone in a country, state, or town (e.g., randomized trials in a diverse sample); worksite interventions; and clinical interventions in a high-risk group (e.g., reducing salt consumption among black women). Information campaigns in the mass media, or changes in nutrition labeling, are not strictly behavioral programs. Clinical programs by practitioners do not reach much of the public and are not considered here, although programs that promote the use of behavioral techniques to change dietary habits within a health care entity of significant size (e.g., a health management organization) are increasing.

Women are more likely than men to report having made voluntary changes in their diets suggested by the USDA/DHHS Dietary Guidelines. "Changers" differ from those not making changes on the basis of their sense of personal susceptibility to diet-related disease, overall health orientation, perceived benefits from change, and attention to mass media messages or valued peers. More involvement in purchasing and preparing food—functions more often performed by women—also predicts positive dietary change.

Knowledge of guidelines may be slight, yet many in Washington State believed in a diet–disease connection ($n = 1,971$). Although only very general responses were required, 22% of women (and 33% of men) had no knowledge of the National Cancer Institute's guidelines with reference to fat and fiber. About 26% of women mentioned both lower fat and more fiber as being recommended. The number of healthful changes was predicted by beliefs, knowledge, and the influence of valued others. About two-thirds of the Pawtucket Heart Health Program cohort (gender not specified) limited fat and salt intake, while about half tried to lose weight. Neither of these behaviors increased in the 1980s. In addition to the limited success many people experience in changing such habits, a recent study adds that having fat consumption measured, being told that it is high, and being told how it may be lowered produce emotional distress. Those told that they had the highest fat intake were actually *least* likely to report intentions to lower dietary fat. Providing risk factor information also has emotional and belief-related consequences that may not promote desired change.

Worksite nutrition education efforts are included in the *Healthy People 2000* recommendations. A randomized trial at 13 worksites (5 intervention, 8 control; $n = 2,365$) targeted reduction in fat and increase in fiber. Interventions included classes, point-of-purchase education, and taste tests during this 15-month program. Significant differences in the intervention group were observed in consumption of vegetables (increased) and of margarine and butter used as spreads (decreased). Twelve other food items specific to the messages did not differ significantly. Women's results were not separately presented.

The Women's Health Initiative is underway at 40 centers in the United States to study the health of women between the ages of 50 and 79 for a period of 12 years. The research design includes a low-fat (20% of calories as fat) diet arm, which was tested for its feasibility at the three sites. Women ($n = 333$) with a mean baseline intake of 39% of calories from fat were randomly assigned to treatment (20 sessions) and control conditions. Four follow-up assessments from 3 to 24 months showed that 77% of the treatment group met the 20% criterion after 6 months, and that 66% were still at that level after 24 months. Controls did not significantly change their nutrient intake over the

2-year period. The low-fat group reduced calories by more than 20% and body weight by 3%. Micronutrients (vitamins A, B_6, B_{12}, and C, as well as iron, calcium, and protein) were not adversely affected in adherents to the low-fat diet. Greater success in reduction of fat was predicted by significantly greater reductions in fat from all four food groups (fats and oils, red meats, dairy products, and grains/baked goods) at the 6-month assessment. Those who had less success showed more slippage in the use of fats and oils.

The National Cancer Institute has begun a "five-a-day" campaign to recommend more daily servings of fruits and vegetables, with the developing knowledge that these foods offer protection against colorectal, lung, and breast cancers. Several studies are now underway to test and improve the effectiveness of the campaign, and to tailor it to specific target groups or settings.

CONCLUSIONS

It has been made clear in cross-cultural studies that a diet can be relatively flexible while still achieving health benefits. Also, in developed countries a great many dietary options are available, some of which may be different from the cultural norm. Despite the fact that they come from various interest groups and government agencies, healthy eating guidelines are surprisingly consistent with one another. However, several of the recommendations with the widest scientific support remain unmet by the majority of women. These include keeping total fat below 30% of total energy intake, keeping saturated fat below 10% of energy intake, and eating five servings of fruits and vegetables each day. Research questions abound concerning which nutrients are protective and harmful, and how these interact with age, gender, and lifestyle factors. Although studies to answer these intriguing questions are underway, a major effort should be made in the behavioral realm to achieve meaningful progress toward motivating women to meet the goals and recommendations that have already been established and validated.

FURTHER READING

American Cancer Society. (1984). *Nutrition and cancer: Cause and prevention. American Cancer Society Special Report.* New York: American Cancer Society.
Nutritional guidelines provided that may modulate the development of several cancers of the gastrointestinal tract.

American Dietetic Association. (1991). *Survey of American dietary habits: Executive summary.* Chicago: Author.
Conducted by The Wirthlin Group.

American Heart Association. (1993). American Heart Association Nutrition Committee: Rationale of the diet–heart statement of the American Heart Association. *Circulation, 88,* 3009–3029.
Position statement of the American Heart Association.

Carleton, R. A., Dwyer, J., & Finberg, L. (1991). Report of the expert panel on population strategies for blood cholesterol reduction: A statement from the National Cholesterol Education Program, NHLBI, NIH. *Circulation, 83,* 2154–2232.
A description of and rationale for the institution of cholesterol-lowering treatments, both dietary and nondietary.

Carleton, R. A., Lasater, T. M., Assaf, A. R., Feldman, H. A., & McKinlay, A. (1995). The Pawtucket Heart Health Program: Community changes in cardiovascular risk factors and projected disease risk. *American Journal of Public Health, 85,* 777–785.
Disease risk factors were assessed in 15,261 people in an education program to reduce cardiovascular disease. Risk factors dropped but the program's impact diminished after it ended.

Fortmann, S. P., Taylor, C. B., Flora, J. A., & Winkleby, M. A. (1993). Effect of community health education on plasma cholesterol levels and diet: The Stanford Five-City Project. *American Journal of Epidemiology, 137,* 1039–1055.

A long-term health education intervention trial in men and women, aged 25–74 years brought modest but sustained reductions in risk in treatment compared to control cities.

Kristal, A. R., White, E., Shattuck, A. L., Curry, S., Anderson, G. I., Fowler, A., & Urban, N. (1993). Long-term maintenance of a low-fat diet: Durability of fat-related dietary habits in the Women's Health Trial. *Journal of the American Dietetic Association, 92,* 553–559.
The results of the feasibility study for reducing dietary fat on which the Women's Health Initiative design was based.

National Cancer Institute. (1987). *Diet, nutrition, and cancer prevention: A guide to food choices* (NIH Publication No. 87-2878). Washington, DC: U.S. Public Health Service, U.S. Department of Health and Human Services.

NCI guidelines to lower cancer risk suggest maintenance of appropriate body weight, from fat, less than 30% of calories intake of fruits and vegetables containing vitamin A, and 20–30 grams of fiber per day.

National Research Council (1989). *Recommended dietary allowances* (10th ed.). Washington, DC: National Academy Press.

Nutrient intake goals (recommended dietary allowances) discussed.

Shrapnel, W. S., Calvert, C. D., Nestel, P. J., & Truswell, A. S. (1992). Diet and coronary heart disease: The National Heart Foundation of Australia. *Medical Journal of Australia, 156,* S9–S16.
Position statement of the National Heart Foundation of Australia with respect to nutritional factors leading to heart disease and hypertension.

St. Jeor, S. T. (Ed.). (1997). *Obesity assessment: Tools, methods, interpretations. A reference case: The RENO Diet–Heart Study.* New York: Chapman & Hall.

The RENO Diet–Heart Study, which observed diet, physiology, psychology, and behavior in about 500 women and men over the course of 8 years, is described.

U.S. Department of Agriculture (USDA). (1987). *Nationwide Food Consumption Survey: Continuing survey of food intakes of individuals. Women 19–50 years and their children 1–5 years, 4 days, 1985* (Report No. 85-4). Hyattsville, MD: Human Nutrition Information Service.
This is an important source of information about the food intake of U.S. women.

U.S. Department of Agriculture (USDA). (1988). *Nationwide Food Consumption Survey: Continuing survey of food intakes of individuals. Low-income women 19–50 years and their children 1–5 years, 4 days, 1985* (Report No. 85-4). Hyattsville, MD: Human Nutrition Information Service.
This is an important source of information about the food intake of U.S. low-income women.

U.S. Department of Agriculture (USDA). (1992). *The Food Guide Pyramid.* (Home and Garden Bulletin, No. 252). Hyattsville, MD: USDA Human Nutrition Information Service.
This educational tool is helpful in visualizing the recommended number of portions from various food groups to maintain a healthy diet.

U.S. Department of Agriculture (USDA). (1995). *Nutrition and your health: Dietary guidelines for Americans* (4th ed.) (Home and Garden Bulletin No. 232). Hyattsville, MD: Human Nutrition Information Service.

Nutrient intake goals (recommended dietary allowances discussed.

U.S. Public Health Service. (1991). *Healthy people 2000: National health promotion and disease prevention objectives.* (DHHS Publication No. PHS 91-50212). Washington, DC: U.S. Government Printing Office.

This document sets forth health goals for achievement by the year 2000.

41

Nutrition Education

Karen Glanz

*T*hroughout the past century, women have had the major responsibility for food preparation and shopping in industrialized countries. This continues to be the case, despite the increase in women in the work force and shifting gender roles. More recently, over the past three decades, attention has been focused on women's unique nutritional needs and the impact of nutrition on their health and the health of their children. This chapter discusses preventive nutrition and nutrition education for women at different points during the life cycle: during pregnancy, and during middle age and older adulthood. Much recent scientific research has focused on these time periods, when pregnancy outcomes can be influenced favorably and there is the potential to prevent breast cancer.

Nutritional recommendations for pregnant women focus on dietary adequacy (maternal weight gain; adequate intake of vitamins and minerals) and preparation for breastfeeding. Most of the nutrition education research focusing on these issues concerns high-risk women: adolescents, minorities, and the economically disadvantaged. Dietary guidelines for cancer prevention emphasize moderation (eating patterns that are low in fat, and high in fruits, vegetables, and starches; avoidance of obesity). Up to now, however, published nutrition education research on breast cancer prevention through diet has been largely within clinical trials, with predominantly middle-class, white participants. Much has been learned about nutrition education both for pregnant women and for breast cancer prevention, but the bodies of research contrast sharply with each other. This review highlights current findings and gaps that warrant attention.

NUTRITION DURING PREGNANCY

Association of Women's Nutrition with Pregnancy Outcomes

Adequate nutrition during pregnancy is associated with delivery of a healthy, full-term infant of appropriate size, and hence with a reduction in infant mortality. Sufficient weight gain and intake of vitamins and minerals contribute to optimal pregnancy outcomes, and alcohol should be avoided. However, various medical, social, behavioral, and dietary factors both before and during pregnancy contribute to the risk of a low-birthweight (LBW) infant. In addition, breast milk is the food of choice for infants, and a pregnant woman should begin to prepare for breastfeeding by consuming sufficient and appropriate foods even before her child is born. It is important to note that although less is known about the effect of prepregnancy nutritional status, it is generally recognized that nutrition both before and beyond the months of pregnancy is also important.

Historical Perspective

Over the past 30 years, scientific knowledge and recommendations about nutrition during pregnancy have changed markedly. The most dramatic change is that health care providers have begun to recommend greater gestational weight gain; recommendations have increased from 8–9 kg (18–20 pounds) to an average of 11 kg (24 pounds). During this period, health policy, guidelines for the public, increased emphasis on prenatal care, and medical and food assistance programs for mothers, infants, and children have become widespread. In addition, there have been recommendations and initiatives to reduce smoking among pregnant women (another contributor to LBW), and more recently to avoid alcohol consumption during pregnancy.

Also during this period, there has been a renewed interest in dietary adequacy with respect to vitamins and minerals, and hence an increase in the use of nutrient supplements. A balanced diet can provide sufficient amounts of all nutrients except iron, but not all women consume an adequate and varied diet. Also, the role of folate in preventing birth defects has come to the forefront. Finally, a trend toward promoting breastfeeding has pointed to the importance of preparing women for breastfeeding while they are pregnant.

At-Risk Populations

Women who are underweight or of short stature before becoming pregnant are at higher risk of insufficient gestational weight gain. Also, adolescents, smokers, and substance abusers are at high risk of nutritional deficiency. Demographic risk factors include low educational levels and low income, which are often associated with minority ethnic status. Because of these risk factors, food assistance programs such as the Supplemental Food Program for Women, Infants, and Children (WIC) have been established. WIC programs are often conducted in conjunction with prenatal care at public health clinics. Interestingly, in WIC programs have been the most frequent sites for evaluation of research aimed at assessing the impact of nutrition education in pregnancy.

Impact of Nutrition Education

Several dozen studies of the impact of nutrition education for pregnant women have been conducted; as noted above, the majority have targeted disadvantaged or high-risk women and adolescents in public health clinic settings. In these studies, individualized nutrition counseling that includes dietary assessment and personalized information about how to improve diet has been shown to increase maternal weight gain and decrease the prevalence of LBW. Group classes, especially when combined with counseling, have also been effective, though in some cases participants have improved knowledge without adopting behavior changes. Prenatal nutrition education for breastfeeding has also been shown to be effective. One study of 159 low-income African-American women found that classes and counseling significantly increased the proportion of mothers who initiated breastfeeding. Programs for adolescents have typically been less effective.

The strength of the research literature on nutrition education in pregnancy is its emphasis on high-risk mothers and its conduct in real-world community settings. But this strength also accounts for many weaknesses in the studies. Many lack controlled designs, have high attrition rates, and do not distinguish between nutrition education and other services (e.g., prenatal care, smoking cessation, and income assistance programs).

BREAST CANCER PREVENTION

Association of Women's Nutrition with Breast Cancer Risk and Prognosis

Breast cancer is the most common women's cancer and the second most common cancer killer in women. Emerging research over the past two decades suggests that dietary factors may hold promise for preventing breast cancer and its progression. Although the data remain inconclusive (see below), there is mounting evidence that (1) a diet low in fat and saturated fat, and high in fruits, vegetables, and starches, and (2) avoidance of over-weight, can reduce breast cancer risk and improve prognosis. This focus on controlling overnutrition has been met with enthusiasm, because it offers a low-risk means of preventing a major women's disease, is also likely to help prevent other chronic diseases, and may even improve quality of life. Recent and current research efforts include clinical trials of healthful diets for cancer prevention, promulgation of guidelines to the general public (see Brunner and St. Jeor's chapter on nutrition guidelines), and community intervention studies.

Guidelines and the State of the Science

The National Cancer Institute has established specific dietary objectives that include (1) reduction in average consumption of dietary fat from about 37% to 30% or fewer of total calories; (2) increase in average consumption of fiber to 20–30 grams/day; (3) consumption of five or more servings of fruits and vegetables daily; (4) alcohol consumption in moderation or not at all; and (5) avoidance of overweight. Much recent nutritional/epidemiological research on diet and breast cancer has focused on the roles of dietary fat and obesity. Although the evidence remains controversial, many scientists say that the data are inconclusive because the goal of 30% of energy from fat is too high; they feel that diets with between 15% and 25% calories from fat are much more likely to influence prevention. Hypotheses about the mechanisms by which diet causes breast cancer are now focusing on the interaction of dietary constituents with female sex hormones—suggesting, for example, that dietary fat can increase the level of circulating estrogens, which in turn affect the development of breast cancer. Exciting new research in both animals and humans, and the well-known differences in diet–cancer associations between premenopausal and postmenopausal women, support these hypotheses.

Some research has examined the association of nutritional status at different periods in the life cycle with breast cancer incidence. This research suggests that adult weight gain and obesity at the time of diagnosis contribute to increased incidence of, and poorer prognosis in, postmenopausal breast cancer. However, there is a dearth of research addressing the question of which periods in life are most suitable for intervention. Clinical trials are focusing on middle-aged and older women, even though there is suggestive evidence for an influence of diet and physical activity earlier in life. Former athletes (in high school and college) have been found to have a significantly lower lifetime occurrence of breast cancer.

Women's Health Trial: Impact of Nutrition Education

Clinical trials of dietary change to explore the feasibility of dietary means of preventing breast cancer in middle-aged women (aged 45–69) at high risk for breast cancer began in the late 1980s with the Women's Health Trial (WHT) vanguard study and its extension. The aim of the WHT was to reduce total dietary fat intake in the intervention group from about 39% to 20% of energy. This group was encouraged to follow a low-fat eating plan through a multicomponent intervention, which included nutrition instruction, behavioral counseling, self-monitoring, feedback, and educational materials. The intervention was designed to be flexible and adaptable to individuals' different eating patterns. Women in the intervention group were successful in achieving initial fat reduction goals, in achieving concurrent reductions in weight and cholesterol, and in maintaining most of the changes at 24 months. The nutrition intervention methods of the WHT have been adopted for the Women's Health Initiative, a 10-year multicenter trial (1994–2004) of women's health that is studying a broad range of factors associated with prevention of cancer, heart disease, and osteoporosis.

The WHT vanguard study showed clearly that significant dietary change is possible in selected, highly motivated participants. The study used an intensive, multicomponent educational and behavioral intervention, which was much more intensive than typical outpatient nutrition education interventions. The greatest limitation in generalizing from this study involves the restrictive procedures for recruiting subjects into the trial: Because high levels of adherence were needed to accomplish the study's ultimate goal of testing the efficacy of diet for prevention, the methodology limits the generalizability of findings about educational and behavioral strategies. In fact, when women in the WHT were asked to identify their most important motivations for participating, the reason most often stated was helping in a scientific research project. This clearly raises the question of how feasible the successful nutrition intervention strategies might be outside the context of a controlled trial.

From Clinic to Community

Although there have not yet been intervention studies of breast cancer prevention through diet in health care settings and other community organization settings, nutrition education for cardiovascular risk reduction suggests common elements in successful programs. These nutrition education strategies provide assistance to motivated and high-risk persons. Screening, personalized advice, and the use of behavioral strategies based on social-cognitive theory have been found to produce effective short-term behavior change and risk reduction (e.g., lower blood cholesterol). A key predictor of success has been the level of a person's initial risk, which may be more influential than the strategies used.

Community-based interventions for primary prevention that use a public health or population-based approach are also beginning to emerge. These strategies incorporate promising clinical strategies, but go beyond them to interventions that include environmental change, community organization, and diffusion efforts. Examples include multi-level worksite health promotion programs, policy interventions, and point-of-choice nutrition information. Results of studies to date suggest that these methods can achieve small but significant population-wide dietary changes.

Gender Differences

Although the focus of this chapter is on nutrition education for specific women's health problems, findings from mixed-gender research are useful in identifying how women may differ from men in their predisposition to make nutritional changes. Studies of preventive nutrition behavior have shown that women, more educated persons, and older adults are more likely to be interested in, aware of, and knowledgeable about healthful eating habits. Our recent research within a large worksite cancer prevention trial examined gender differences in readiness to make dietary changes, which was operationalized in terms of the construct of stages of change. Women were consistently found to be less likely to be in the precontemplation or contemplation stages (unaware of, uninterested in, or only thinking about change) with respect to fat, fiber, and fruits/vegetables; they were more likely to be in the action or maintenance stages (actively changing or working to maintain changes). This suggests that women constitute a motivated audience for nutrition education; however, further research should help pinpoint differences among subgroups of women.

RESEARCH GAPS

Our understanding of nutrition education for women's health concerns is relatively recent, and many important questions remain unanswered. For both nutrition during pregnancy and breast cancer prevention through diet, there are clear gaps. In fact, nutrition education research on these two concerns is a study in contrasts. Nutrition education in pregnancy has mainly been studied among disadvantaged and minority women, in natural clinical settings. Breast cancer prevention through diet has primarily been the focus of clinical trials whose subjects are mostly white, middle-class, middle-aged women, who are highly motivated to contribute to scientific research.

Prenatal nutrition education has relied mainly on an informational or a knowledge dissemination model. Some attention has also been given to cultural tailoring for unique ethnic minorities and poorer women. What is needed is research that examines nutrition education both as part of, and as separate from, other components of prenatal care and health education. Small-scale controlled trials of both informational and behavioral strategies would be informative, as would in-depth, qualitative, ethnographic studies. Finally, both descriptive and intervention studies of nutrition education for pregnant middle-class and majority women can help refine clinical practice beyond public health settings.

Despite the lack of conclusive proof that healthy diets can prevent breast cancer, nutrition holds the greatest promise for prevention at this time; thus, research should extend beyond the ongoing clinical trials. In particular, preventive nutrition education for high-risk women of all ages should be developed and tested. Likewise, strategies to influence minority and disadvantaged women are needed. Nutrition education as a part of general health promotion deserves study, as does nutrition education combined with efforts to reduce excess alcohol consumption and tobacco use.

Nutrition is an important contributor to women's health throughout the life cycle, and a better understanding of ways to encourage healthful eating can be valuable to both clinicians and public health practitioners. There is mounting evidence that behavioral and educational concepts and strategies can improve the success of nutrition education; there is also a need for further investigation.

FURTHER READING

Bowen, D. J., Henderson, M. D., Iverson, D., Burrows, E., Henry, H., & Foreyt, J. (1994). Reducing dietary fat: Understanding the success of the Women's Health Trial. *Cancer Prevention International, 1,* 21–30.
This article reviews the methods and findings of nutrition intervention in the WHT, and discusses factors associated with successful reduction of dietary fat in a feasibility trial for a large randomized clinical trial.

Glanz, K. (1994). Reducing breast cancer risk through changes in diet and alcohol intake: From clinic to community. *Annals of Behavioral Medicine, 16,* 334–346.
This article reviews evidence for breast cancer prevention through diet, and illustrates the variable success rates of a range of nutrition interventions as studied in settings ranging from clinical trials to community-wide trials.

Glanz, K., & Eriksen, M. P. (1993). Individual and community models for dietary behavior change. *Journal of Nutrition Education, 25,* 80–86.
This article articulates and illustrates the application of various behavior change theories (social cognition, stages of change, consumer information processing, and diffusion of innovations) to dietary change.

Glanz, K., Patterson, R. E., Kristal, A. R., DiClemente, C. C., Heimendinger, J., Linnan, L., & McLerran, D. F. (1994). Stages of change in adopting healthy diets: Fat, fiber, and correlates of nutrient intake. *Health Education Quarterly, 21,* 499–519.
This paper reports on data from the Working Well Trial, examining the association of stages of dietary change for fat, fiber, and fruits/vegetables to actual dietary intake and psychosocial factors, such as motivation, self-efficacy, and weight loss experience.

Hankin, J. H. (1993). Role of nutrition in women's health: Diet and breast cancer. *Journal of the American Dietetic Association, 93,* 994–999.
This is a comprehensive review of nutritional/epidemiological studies of diet and breast cancer.

Institute of Medicine. (1990). *Nutrition during pregnancy.* Washington, DC: National Academy Press.
This book presents the state-of-the-art rationale and guidelines for nutrition during pregnancy, addressing such issues as weight gain, nutrient requirements, and recommendations concerning vitamin and mineral supplements.

Institute of Medicine. (1992). *Nutrition during pregnancy and lactation: An implementation guide.* Washington, DC: National Academy Press.

This guide is a follow-up to the 1990 publication just described; it includes practical guidance for clinicians working with women to implement the guidelines for healthful nutrition during pregnancy and lactation.

Kistin, N., Benton, D., Rao, S., & Sullivan, M. (1990). Breastfeeding rates among black urban low-income women: Effect of prenatal education. *Pediatrics, 86,* 741–746.

This article reports on a study of prenatal nutrition education for low-income African-American women, which showed that classes and counseling significantly increased the proportion of women who initiated breastfeeding.

42

Oral Health

John W. Osborne

*D*entistry is faced with a unique anatomical situation, in that hard bony tissue (teeth) protrudes through soft tissue (gingiva or gums). This boundary between hard and soft tissue, by its very nature, is highly susceptible to bacterial infection. Because this oral environment is dark, damp, and warm, bacteria of many varieties thrive. Oral health involves many facets, but the two main disease processes are dental caries (tooth decay) and periodontal disease. Caries affects the teeth and generally occurs between the ages of 6 and 20 and in older individuals (those age 60 and over). Periodontal disease affects the supporting tissues of the teeth and is prominent after age 35.

Diseases of the oral structures, if left untreated, can cause many problems: an unsightly appearance; halitosis (bad breath); soreness, sensitivity, and discomfort, which can affect diet; extreme pain that can keep one awake at night; and even the loss of teeth. Although caries and periodontal disease are the main topics covered in this chapter, they are by no means the only issues related to oral health that women must confront. A few of the others are discussed later.

DENTAL CARIES

Dental caries, the process by which the tooth is demineralized, is the most common disease in the population. Interestingly, few people had this problem prior to the 16th century; with the advent of refined sugar and flour, however, the tooth decay rate skyrocketed. There are several theories of why teeth decay, but fundamental to all are that four components need to be present for the caries process: (1) bacteria, (2) susceptible teeth, (3) food sources, and (4) time.

Bacteria and Plaque

Bacteria and some of the constituents of saliva (but not all; see below) form a network of what the dentist calls "plaque." Plaque consists of bacteria, food debris, amino acids, organic acids, carbohydrates, and cells from the oral lining. The plaque is initially loosely organized, but if left undisturbed it will become firmly attached to the teeth as it matures. When the bacteria in the plaque are given sugar, they produce organic acids, which will demineralize the teeth. This demineralization takes place at about a pH of 5.5 or lower, and the process of demineralization begins about 20 minutes after eating. The persistent exposure to organic acids leads to the dissolution of the enamel and dentin.

Prevention and Reduction of Caries

Three factors will greatly lower the rate of tooth decay: (1) decreasing the solubility of the teeth, (2) reducing the sugar sources, and (3) disturbing the plaque/bacteria mass.

Decreasing Teeth's Susceptibility

It is well understood that fluoride in tooth enamel will decrease its susceptibility to decay by making the enamel less soluble. Fluoride is most effective when incorporated into the tooth as it is developing. Since teeth are developing *in utero,* expectant mothers should consult with their physician as to the need for a fluoride supplement during pregnancy. The use of a fluoride supplement can depend upon where a mother lives. Some areas have no fluorides; other areas have natural fluorides in the water, or fluoride is added to the water supply. In cases of adequate fluoride in the water, no prenatal fluoride may be needed. When the baby is born, the need for fluoride should be discussed with the pediatrician, and supplementation should be given as necessary (again, depending upon the area). Tooth enamel are forming up to the age of 6, so the systemic addition of fluoride until this time is necessary to obtain maximum benefits. Later, fluoride can be given topically by the dentist or hygienist, as well as through toothpastes and mouth rinses that contain fluorides to decrease acid solubility of teeth. Systemic uptake and topical applications of fluorides have been shown to reduce the tooth decay rate by as much as 40%.

Reducing Sugar Sources

Frequency of eating plays a significant role in tooth decay. People who snack regularly will have a greater potential for decay. More frequent sources of sugar produce more acid, and thus there is a greater potential for demineralization. Even items with few calories (e.g., breath mints and diet soft drinks) can contribute to the decay process. It is best to eat three meals a day and not to snack in between. Although sugars are well known to increase decay, the amount of sugar is not as important as when it is ingested. Limited amounts of sweets after a meal are less harmful to the teeth than a sugar source in between meals.

    Diet content is important as well, for there are many foods that have anticaries activity. Cheeses such as aged cheddar, Swiss, mozzarella and Brie consumed after a meal have been shown to reduce tooth decay. On the other hand, peanuts may not cause acid formation and demineralization, but peanut butter may cause an increase in decay because of its sugar content and it sticks to the teeth.

Disturbing Plaque and Bacteria

Removal of the plaque through good home care (brushing and flossing) is highly effective in reducing caries. Plaque removal is particularly critical, for what is important is not how often teeth are brushed, but how thoroughly it is done. It should be strongly emphasized that most people spend too little time brushing. Brushing once a day for 3–5 minutes is better than brushing two to three times per day for 30 seconds each. Brushing for 3–5 minutes with a soft toothbrush, making sure that the plaque is disrupted so that it cannot mature and adhere to the teeth, is one of the most effective oral remedies. Flossing disrupts plaque in between the teeth that cannot be reached by a toothbrush. Research on antiplaque mouth rinses has noted a certain amount of success; new toothbrush systems using ultrasonic applications also show promise in aiding plaque removal. Good home care and dietary measures will reduce caries another 30%.

The Role of Saliva

Saliva is a complex mixture of water, salts, proteins, and other inorganic and organic substances that play an important role in maintaining normal oral health. Saliva lubricates the mouth and aides in chewing, swallowing, and digestion. It dilutes and buffers the acids produced by the bacteria. Saliva has antibacterial, antifungal, and antiviral capacities. Two compounds within saliva, calcium and phosphates, have the capacity to remineralize teeth. The longer teeth are bathed in saliva, the more remineralization occurs, thus reducing the chance of decay. An increase in salivary flow immediately after eating, through chewing gum that is sugar-free or contains aspartame, sorbitol, or xylitol, will help reduce dental caries. On the other hand, if the flow of saliva is diminished, not only can this produce the sensation of a dry mouth (xerostomia), the loss of taste, and severe discomfort; it also increases the risk of dental caries. Any condition that reduces saliva—such as therapeutic radiation of the head and neck, the taking of certain medications (e.g., some antihistamines and certain tranquilizers), removal of the salivary glands because of a tumor, or specific salivary gland diseases—can have a dramatic effect on an individual's oral health. As a consequence of the loss of quality and quantity of saliva, decay rates go up and this dental decay tends to occur in areas that are difficult for the dentist to treat, and recurrence of the decay is very rapid.

PERIODONTAL DISEASE

"Periodontal disease" is the overall term for a complex group of diseases that affect the supporting tissues of the teeth. Periodontal disease, unlike caries, has plagued humans since the beginning of time. Even ancient Egyptian and Chinese writings discussed this disorder. Periodontal disease is usually divided into two groups: "gingivitis," which affects the gingival tissue, and "periodontitis," which affects the underlying structures of the bone, the tooth root, and the ligament that holds the tooth to the bone. It has long been recognized that both gingivitis and periodontitis are caused by plaque on the teeth and under the gingiva. We now know that specific bacteria, not the same ones involved with caries, are causative agents in these disease processes.

Gingivitis

Gingivitis can either be an acute or a chronic infection that is characterized by redness, swelling of the gingival tissue, and gums that bleed easily when brushed. Gingivitis affects a high percentage of people; however, it is not considered as serious a problem as periodontitis, in which the underlying structures are affected.

The most effective way to reduce gingivitis is to remove the bacterial plaque through brushing and flossing. Since bacteria in the plaque will release enzymes and toxins, the removal of the bacteria will get rid of the offending agents. Dentists and hygienists can clean and polish teeth, which will greatly facilitate the home care procedures, but this periodic professional cleaning cannot replace daily brushing and flossing.

A particularly severe form of gingivitis is acute necrotizing ulcerative gingivitis. This is also called "trench mouth" and is characterized by sudden onset and pain, spontaneous bleeding, tissue necrosis, and bad breath. Brushing even with a soft toothbrush can be very uncomfortable in these cases. The patient should see a dentist immediately, for tissue necrosis can be severe. The dentist can cleanse the area and may possibly prescribe a special mouthwash. If the patient has severe pain, a nonsteroidal analgesic may be given to alleviate the discomfort, and antibiotics may be prescribed if the patient has a fever and swollen lymph glands.

Periodontitis

More teeth are lost in adult life because of periodontitis than for all other reasons combined. This infection causes the destruction of the underlying bone, modifies the roots of the teeth, and aggravates the loss of the ligaments holding the teeth in the bone. It is a general rule that the more destructive the periodontal disease, the more challenging it is for the dentist to diagnose and treat. Although this condition is most common in adults, it can be found in adolescents. In periodontitis, not only do the bacteria release enzymes, toxins, and substances that interfere with cell function; they may also be cytotoxic, and the bacteria may inhibit the normal defense mechanisms of the body.

The treatment for periodontitis is directed at slowing the progress of the disease and preventing recurrence. Again, the most important single factor is the removal of the plaque. One complicating factor about plaque is that it will mature and later mineralize. This mineralized plaque forms "calculus" (tartar). The calculus not only makes brushing difficult and reduces its effectiveness, but must be removed by a dental professional. The effective removal of the plaque may be extremely difficult in situations where so much bone has been lost that there are deep pockets next to the teeth. In deep pockets, the site of infection may no longer be effectively cleaned by either the patient or dental personnel, and this accelerates the destructive progress. At this point, surgical intervention may be necessary to facilitate the plaque removal process. Surgery may also be used in bone-grafting and regeneration procedures.

A high level of meticulous home care to remove the plaque may not be realistic for all patients. Adjunct therapy with antibacterial rinses to reduce the plaque, and use of small doses of tetracycline, may change collagen functions in the tissue to alter the course and progress of the disease. It should be reemphasized that clinical studies have shown that when mechanical removal of plaque and bacteria was achieved, periodontal disease did not recur after treatment by the dentist. It is a good rule that if the gingival tissue bleeds, the plaque has not been effectively removed for 3 days.

OTHER DENTAL CARE ISSUES FOR WOMEN

In the majority of cases, women are the ones who take the major responsibility for children's dental health. Several issues occur with regard to dental care for children. Prenatal and early postnatal fluoride uptake has already been discussed. One of the more serious problems in infancy and early childhood is called "baby bottle tooth decay." When a child holds a bottle of milk, juice, or sugar-based drink in the mouth while sleeping, this causes an explosion of tooth decay that can affect all surfaces of the teeth. Not only are infants and young children difficult to treat because of their age, but teeth can be severely damaged and require extensive work. This early, destructive tooth decay is very uncomfortable, and any premature tooth loss can lead to misaligned teeth later in life. The simple solution is not to allow a child to go to sleep with a bottle of milk or juice in the mouth. In rare but documented cases, this type of decay has been known to occur in nursing infants, and the solution for them is the same as above.

One of the questions that arises is when to take a child to the dentist for the first time. Interestingly, the *parents* should see the pediatric dentist (children's dentist) when the child's first tooth erupts. The dental staff can demonstrate how to clean the child's teeth and help head off later problems. Care should be taken when a toothpaste containing fluoride is used, for most small children swallow the toothpaste. Excessive fluoride uptake can cause tooth discoloration.

Unfortunately, but frequently a tooth is knocked out of a child's mouth, and the parents are confused about what to do. The answer to this is to put the tooth back in the socket after a gentle rinse, and to get the child to the dentist as soon as possible. The dentist can examine for other oral–facial injuries and splint the teeth. If the tooth cannot be placed back in the tooth socket, the parents should place the tooth in a glass of milk and take the child and tooth to the dentist. Even if no tooth is found, the child should see the dentist as soon as possible because the tooth could be driven into the gums. The key in any case is to see the dentist as soon as possible.

Hormonal differences in women can create certain oral manifestations. During menstruation and pregnancy the gingival tissues are more sensitive, and the so-called "pregnancy tumor" can occur. This is a bump on the gum that may bleed and be slightly uncomfortable. Other problems, such as herpes labialis and apthous ulcers (cold sores), are more common in women during menstruation. Burning tongue is more common in postmenopausal women. For whatever reason, severe discomfort in the joints of the jaw (temporomandibular joint pain) is more common in young women than in any other group. Women with any of these conditions should see the dentist for an examination and recommended treatment.

Orthodontic treatment is another consideration, both for older children/adolescents and (increasingly) for adult women. Straight teeth and a nice smile can play a critical role in anyone's self-concept. Like all long-term care, orthodontia can be a financial burden to a family. There are many conditions during orthodontic treatment that the patient needs to take responsibility for. Home care, through good brushing and other aids to reduce plaque and to care for the appliances, is essential. Most patients will need to wear an appliance for some time after treatment at the office has been completed, in order to prevent collapse of the teeth. Noncompliance may hasten relapse or even lead to retreatment of the mouth.

Aesthetic appearance is becoming more important to the public. A dentist has in his or her armamentarium many procedures and techniques that can improve a patient's smile and tooth color. Teeth can be bleached, discolored spots can be abraded away, and veneers can be used to correct spaces or give a natural look to deeply stained teeth. Women who are unhappy with the appearance of their teeth should consider cosmetic dental care.

FURTHER READING

American Academy of Pediatric Dentistry. (n.d.). *Oral health: You and your baby* and *Check list for infants and toddlers.* (Availability from the Academy at 211 E. Chicago Ave., Suite 1036, Chicago, IL 60611)
Two informative pamphlets that should be sent for by every woman who has or is expecting a child.

Mandel, I. D. (1989). The role of saliva in maintaining oral homeostasis. *Journal of the American Dental Association, 119,* 298–304.
Excellent review by the leading authority in oral biology on saliva's critical part in oral health.

Neville, B. W., Damm, D. D., Allen, C. M., & Bouquot, J. E. (1995). *Oral and maxillofacial pathology.* Philadelphia: W. B. Sanders.
Text used in many dental schools for teaching oral diseases and pathology.

Williams, R. C. (1990). Periodontal disease. *New England Journal of Medicine, 332,* 373–379.
A classic paper reviewing the broad aspects of periodontal disease.

43

Exercise

Patricia M. Dubbert

HEALTH BENEFITS OF PHYSICAL ACTIVITY AND EXERCISE

Regular physical activity (body movements that expend energy) and exercise (planned, repetitive, structured, and purposeful physical activity) build and maintain physical fitness. Fitness contributes importantly to women's health by enhancing the safety and efficiency of self-care, household, occupational, and recreational activities.

Understanding of the role of physical activity in women's health remains incomplete. Until recently, many trials and existing data sets on the benefits of activity and exercise did not include any women or had insufficient numbers of women for separate analyses. Nevertheless, a growing body of evidence from epidemiological and experimental studies has led experts to believe that sedentary lifestyles contribute to many chronic conditions that have a negative impact on women's lifespans and quality of life. Heart disease, high blood pressure, some forms of cancer, diabetes, obesity, and osteoporosis are all associated with low levels of endurance-type activity and fitness. Notably, low levels of physical fitness in women are associated with a greater risk of death from cardiovascular disease, cancer, and all causes combined. Depression and anxiety also appear to be related to inactivity. Other aspects of fitness, including muscle strength and flexibility, may have protective effects against disabling low back pain and falls in the elderly.

HOW MUCH EXERCISE DO WOMEN NEED?

The most recent recommendation from the Centers for Disease Control and Prevention and the American College of Sports Medicine (ACSM) on physical activity for health is for every adult in the United States to accumulate 30 minutes or more of moderate-intensity physical activity on most, preferably all, days of the week. This recommendation represents an emerging consensus that vigorous-intensity, sustained sessions of 20–30 minutes or more may not be required for many health benefits. It also reflects an understanding that many adults are unwilling or unable to adopt or maintain more vigorous exercise regimens.

The most familiar example of the moderate-level activity targeted in the new recommendation is brisk walking (3–4 miles per hour). Walking is an ideal exercise for most adults, but the variety of other activities within the moderate intensity range (e.g., racquet sports, active fishing, many home cleaning and repair activities, gardening and lawn mowing, moderate swimming) allows women and men to identify recreational and occupational activities compatible with their interests and lifestyles. It is important to note that the recommendation allows for an accumulation of activity over the course of a day; for example, a woman can meet her daily goal by playing actively with her children for 10 minutes, sweeping a floor or sidewalk for 10 minutes, and walking briskly for 10 minutes on an errand at the grocery store. Some women will prefer and be able to set aside 30 minutes or more for continuous moderate or vigorous exercise, such as aerobics classes. Regular and more vigorous exercise is still strongly encouraged. To build cardiorespiratory endurance, the ACSM recommends a program of exercise involving large muscle groups for 20–60 continuous minutes at 60–90% of maximum heart rate, from 3 to 5 days per week. To build muscle strength, the ACSM recommends 8–12 repetitions of 8–10 resistance exercises 2 days per week. Exercise above this amount yields rapidly diminishing returns and is more likely to result in injury.

CAN EXERCISE BE HARMFUL FOR WOMEN?

Women with conditions that complicate or limit physical activity, such as heart disease, high blood pressure, asthma, obesity, diabetes, peripheral vascular disease, and arthritis, need to work closely with their physicians to develop a physical activity plan tailored to their needs. Women who are pregnant can usually continue types of activities to which they are adapted, but may need to reduce the intensity of these activities. Exercise does not interfere with successful breastfeeding. Women of any age who begin exercising at very low levels of fitness, or who try to progress too rapidly in the frequency and intensity of their workouts, increase their risk of musculoskeletal injury.

Two unique and important potential adverse effects of exercise for women are exercise-related menstrual dysfunction and estrogen deficiency. Girls and women engaged in intense athletic training, in combination with attempts to maintain an unnaturally low body weight, seem most vulnerable. Regular exercise also may delay puberty, but unusually late menarche probably occurs mainly in girls who are successful in athletics because they are genetically predisposed to be late maturers. Exercise-induced amenorrhea is a serious condition. It increases the risk of premature osteoporosis, stress fractures, and perhaps heart disease. Most women are too inactive to be concerned about these effects, and can be reassured that exercise-related menstrual dysfunction and infertility can usually be rapidly reversed with decreased training and/or an increase in weight and body fat.

EPIDEMIOLOGY AND DETERMINANTS
OF WOMEN'S ACTIVITY

Data from surveys in the early 1990s indicated that fewer than one-third of U.S. women and men engaged in leisure-time activity at the targeted levels of at least 30 minutes of moderate-intensity activity 5 days per week, or at least 20 minutes of vigorous activity

3 days per week. The prevalence of sedentary lifestyles increased for both genders with advancing age, lower levels of education and income, and minority racial and cultural status. Women were somewhat less likely to report vigorous activity and sports participation than men, but gender differences in prevalence of sedentary lifestyles were not significant when moderate-level activities were included.

Experts agree that activity estimates, such as public health surveys, are subject to considerable measurement error. Current measures that focus on leisure-time and higher-intensity activities may be even less accurate for women than for men. Even so, it is clear that the prevalence of sedentary lifestyles is a major public health problem. Although there is no evidence that adolescent physical activity continues into adulthood, it is also a matter of concern that U.S. adolescents, especially young women, are very inactive. Patterns generally mimic those of adult populations, with marked decreases from early to middle adolescence, and a higher prevalence of inactivity in young women of color and those of lower socioeconomic status. (For a fuller discussion of exercise for adolescents, see Douthitt's chapter.)

Understanding of the biological and psychosocial factors associated with varying levels of physical activity has lagged far behind the rapidly increasing body of knowledge linking activity to health outcomes. Nevertheless, there has been some progress in identifying variables that appear to be consistently correlated with physical activity status in women as well as men. Identification of these "determinants" of physical activity and exercise does not imply discovery of cause-and-effect relationships, but is an important preliminary step in the design of well-controlled studies of activity promotion interventions.

Early studies of determinants of exercise and activity were typically limited to theoretical observations of variables associated with dropout from supervised exercise programs for men with cardiovascular disease. Recent studies, however, have extended the literature to include data on women, healthy individuals, men and women exercising on their own in the community; different stages of physical activity participation; and more systematic attempts to test cognitive and behavioral theories of health-related behavior.

Studies of community exercisers suggest that a single, cross-sectional survey paints an incomplete picture of exercise and activity. A significant percentage of men and women engaged in vigorous activity, for example, will no longer be active at that level 6 months or a year later, but some of those who were inactive will have adopted a regular activity program. Moderate activity (which, as noted earlier, tends to be favored by women) seems to be more stable across time. Understanding the factors that encourage or inhibit change from one level of physical activity participation to another is an important priority in this area of research.

For both women and men, adoption and maintenance of vigorous activity appear to be consistently associated with high levels of exercise self-efficacy, or confidence in the ability to continue activity despite various barriers and distractions. Social support for exercise from family members and friends is also a consistent predictor of exercise adoption for women. In one large-scale community study, the most frequently reported cause of vigorous exercise relapse was injury; however, lack of time and loss of interest are also consistently reported as factors in the interruption of sustained programs of activity. Although they are consistent negative predictors of vigorous exercise participation, perceived and objective barriers have not yet been adequately examined by gender and socioeconomic status. Lack of time, interest, self-discipline, companionship, and enjoyment were reported as important perceived barriers to vigorous exercise in one community survey, along with lack of exercise knowledge, equipment, and facilities. In general, childhood or adolescent exercise and sports participation have not been reliably associated with greater activity in adulthood. Depressed mood is associated with lower levels of activity, as would be expected.

As noted earlier, demographic variables, including female gender, are reliable predictors of physical activity. Thus far, it has not been possible to separate out the effects of differences in education, health knowledge and access to health care providers, financial situation, occupational physical activity and time demands, child care responsibilities, access to attractive and safe places for physical activity, and other variables that are confounded with socioeconomic and ethnic status in the United States today.

PROMOTION OF HEALTH ACTIVITY FOR WOMEN: RECOMMENDATIONS FOR CLINICIANS

Various interventions, primarily derived from behavioral and cognitive theories, have been evaluated in quasi-experimental and experimental studies of exercise promotion. In general, the results suggest that these theories are applicable to exercise and physical activity, and that the same kinds of interventions that have been effective in modifying other lifestyle factors (e.g., diet, smoking, and alcohol use) may also be effective in modifying physical activity. Most of the studies of exercise and physical activity interventions published to date, however, have important limitations, including small sample sizes, brief intervention phases, and small to moderate effects in comparison to control conditions. Investigators have often relied only on self-report to assess behavior change, and have rarely measured change in fitness or other physiological outcomes. The need for larger-scale, better-controlled studies of methods to promote healthy physical activity has been recognized, and at the time this chapter was written, major clinical trials designed to evaluate activity interventions were in progress.

Despite these limitations, the available data provide support for a number of specific recommendations to guide activity promotion efforts. Suggestions that can be adapted to a variety of different intervention settings are summarized in this final section.

1. An intervention should begin with an assessment of a woman's activity experience, interests, and readiness to change her current level of physical activity. Women who indicate no plans to alter a sedentary lifestyle can be encouraged to think about why they are inactive, and they can be assisted in identifying physical and psychological benefits of even small increases in activity. Those who express interest in changing in the near future can be assisted in developing more specific plans and reinforced for taking steps toward increasing activity. Those who are already active may benefit from continued shaping to reach beyond minimal levels of recommended activity, and from reinforcement and assistance in avoiding relapse.

2. In keeping with recent public health recommendations, clinicians should provide specific guidance about the value of moderate as well as vigorous activities of different types for fitness and health, and focus particularly on assisting women who are very inactive to become at least a little more active.

3. Interventions should include such behavioral management strategies as goal setting, selecting activity types and schedules that are most likely to be successful and

rewarding, keeping a diary or log of progress, and providing for reinforcement of success. These strategies can be used in face-to-face counseling and in a variety of minimal-contact interventions mediated by telephone, mail, computer, the mass media, and other resources.

4. Clinicians should take advantage of "teachable moments" when women may be particularly receptive to activity interventions. Unique opportunities are available in health care settings, schools, worksites, and communities.

5. It is important to be sensitive to the substantial barriers many women face in trying to increase their physical activity. Some of these barriers may be difficult to overcome, particularly for women from educationally and economically disadvantaged backgrounds, without community-level and policy interventions (e.g., provision of worksite facilities for exercise and cleanup, improved safety in public parks). However, motivational enhancement and creative problem solving can help every woman to achieve physical activity goals consistent with current public health recommendations.

FURTHER READING

American College of Sports Medicine (ACSM). (1990). The recommended quantity and quality of exercise for developing and maintaining cardiorespiratory and muscular fitness in healthy adults. *Medicine and Science in Sports and Exercise, 22,* 265–274.
The ACSM's official recommendations, based on available scientific evidence.

Bouchard, C., Shephard, R. J., & Stephens, T. (Eds.). (1994). *Physical activity, fitness, and health.* Champaign, IL: Human Kinetics Press.
A comprehensive edited compilation of chapters summarizing current knowledge in almost every area of exercise and physical activity.

Dishman, R. K. (Ed.). (1994). *Advances in exercise adherence.* Champaign, IL: Human Kinetics Press.
An edited book with sections on exercise adherence, theories and models for activity research, interventions, and physical activity in special populations.

Dubbert, P. M. (1992). Exercise in behavioral medicine. *Journal of Consulting and Clinical Psychology, 60,* 613–618.
A brief summary of progress in physical activity research relevant to behavioral medicine in the preceding decade, with recommendations for future research.

King, A. C. (1994). Biobehavioral variables, exercise, and cardiovascular disease in women. In S. M. Czajkowski, D. R. Hill, & T. B. Clarkson (Eds.), *Women, behavior, and cardiovascular disease* (NIH Publication No. 94-3309, pp. 69–88). Washington, DC: U.S. Government Printing Office.
Summarizes research on exercise and cardiovascular disease in women, including an excellent commentary on important areas for further study.

King, A. C., Blair, S. N., Bild, D. E., Dishman, R. K., Dubbert, P. M., Marcus, B. H., Oldridge, N. B., Paffenbarger, R. S., Jr., Powell, K. E., & Yeager, K. K. (1992). Determinants of physical activity and interventions in adults. *Medicine and Science in Sports and Exercise, 24,* S221–S236.
Review of biological, psychological, and social variables that have been correlated with physical activity, with specific recommendations for future study.

Marcus, B. H., Dubbert, P. M., King, A. C., & Pinto, B. M. (1995). Physical activity in women: Current status and future directions. In A. Stanton & S. Gallant (Eds.), *The psychology of women's health* (pp. 349–379). Washington, DC: American Psychological Association.

A chapter describing benefits of physical activity for women, barriers to increasing activity, interventions that have been demonstrated to increase activity, and commentary on future directions in this area of study and practice.

Pate, R. R., Pratt, M., Blair, S. N., Haskell, W. L., Macera, C. A., Bouchard, C., Buchner, D., Ettinger, W., Heath, G. W., King, A. C., Kriska, A., Leon, A. S., Marcus, B. H., Morris, J., Paffenbarger, R. S., Jr., Patrick, K., Pollock, M. L., Rippe, J. M., Sallis, J., & Wilmore, J. H. (1995). Physical activity and public health. *Journal of the American Medical Association, 273,* 402–407.

The most recent public health recommendations for physical activity for U.S. adults, with an excellent summary of supporting research.

44

Exercise for Adolescents

Vicki L. Douthitt

Many behavioral patterns manifested in adulthood are established in childhood, and exercise behavior may be no exception. According to a study by the Centers for Disease Control, the typical U.S. school-age child in 1992 displayed fitness and activity profiles well below the levels believed to be necessary to lower health risks significantly. In fact, only 19% of all school-age children in the United States meet minimum activity standards, and researchers have found that one out of every five U.S. children will develop clinical symptoms of coronary heart disease before age 16.

A wide array of factors can affect behavior in youth and in adults. Intrapersonal and environmental factors can combine in a myriad of ways to produce a given behavioral action. Thus, an individual's decision to exercise or not has best been explained by interactional models in which influences from several areas are considered. Environmental influences such as peer or coach support, as well as intrapersonal factors such as self-motivation and perceived athletic competence, have been found to have a significant impact on exercise behavior. Motivational factors have varied across the gender, age, and level of competitiveness of research participants.

In any discussion of factors affecting exercise motivation or adherence, it is necessary to consider a multidimensional paradigm. In the early to mid-1970s, sport psychologists debated whether the basis for sport or exercise motivation was centered more in a "trait" or in a "situationist" paradigm. Trait psychology is the study of personal individual characteristics that are consistent across time and different environmental situations. The situationist approach to psychology seeks to explain an individual's behavior in terms of his or her reactions to a particular situation or circumstance. Although the trait paradigm garnered more initial support from sport psychology researchers, it became clear that such a narrow focus could not explain the multifaceted nature of human sport behavior. What evolved from this debate was the interactionist approach to the study of exercise adherence and motivation; that is, the view of exercise behavior as a synthesis of the two paradigms. Contemporary models of exercise adherence and motivation have as their components stable personological or trait variables, environmental variables, and the interaction that occurs between these two sets of constructs.

Considered from an interactional perspective, the questions addressed in this chapter include the following: What are the primary motivating factors for adolescents who choose to participate in exercise or sport behavior? What are the differences in these factors for males and females? Are competitive and noncompetitive populations active for different reasons, and if so, what are the reasons for each group? Recommendations are also included for encouraging lifelong active lifestyles in adolescents, particularly females.

FACTORS RELATED TO ADOLESCENTS' EXERCISE MOTIVATION/ADHERENCE

Although research on exercise adherence and exercise motivation suffers from inconsistencies in the behavioral definition of these constructs, some consistent patterns have nonetheless emerged. For most adolescent populations, intrinsic factors seem to be more important than extrinsic ones. "Having fun" has consistently been stated by the youths themselves as the top reason why they participate in physical activity. Additional intrinsic factors include improving one's skills, being with and making new friends, enjoying the thrill and excitement, and becoming physically fit. Although less important, extrinsic factors given by adolescents for their physical activity include pleasing a coach, parents, or a physical education teacher; winning games; and winning prizes.

A number of studies have taken a descriptive, correlational approach to assessing how such personality factors as perceived self-competence relate to sport or exercise motivation. Most research probing participants for this factor has found that youths with higher levels of perceived self-competence are more likely to be active. Of course, correlational research does not establish cause and effect; therefore, it is not known whether higher levels of competence motivate individuals to participate in sports, or whether the perceived higher levels of competence are results of sport participation.

The competence motivation theory posits that individuals seek opportunities to demonstrate mastery in many different domains, such as the physical, academic, and social domains. Youth with high levels of perceived physical competence tend to view sport or exercise as an opportunity to perfect athletic skills, while those with high perceived social competence identify social affiliation reasons as important motivators.

GENDER DIFFERENCES IN ADOLESCENT EXERCISE MOTIVATION

In the 19th century, the United States was a young country where women's roles were primarily dependent and domestic. Life in a rural environment was hard and physically demanding, and there was very little time for recreational pursuits of any kind. What few moments were afforded to recreational sport activities were dominated by things that allowed women some feeling of physical empowerment, but encouraged them to retain their societally defined grace and femininity. Sports like horseback riding, dance, ice skating, and light calisthenics were popular. In the early 20th century, reports on motivational factors for female sport participation noted such things as the simple joy of physical movement, the feeling of exerting productive effort, the delight of experiencing nature, the health benefits of exercise, contact with people interested in sports, and body weight or body fat reduction.

Traditional societal stereotypes still exert an influence on female sport motivation today, although the definition of femininity is changing. It is more commonly accepted in contemporary society for women of all ages to exhibit aggressive or assertive behavior, both in athletic circles and in other life roles. Recent investigations into sport or exercise motivation for young women have found that appearance factors such as body weight or body fat reduction are still important reasons for pursuing an active lifestyle. However, having fun, being with and making new friends, and improving athletic skills also motivate physically active young women today. Older women who are juggling careers, marriages, and motherhood report an enhancement in their general sense of empowerment and well-being, as well as stress reduction and other health benefits, as motivational determinants of exercise behavior.

An interesting psychological determinant of both male and female exercise behavior has received some attention in the last few years: a match between an individual's personality type and the type of sport in which he or she is participating. According to the theory of personality–sport congruence, if people are participating in a sport that allows them to "be themselves" in terms of their psychological characteristics (e.g., level of aggression, sociability, spontaneity, and self-discipline), they will enjoy the exercise experience much more and want to continue. Studies with college students and adolescents have found the personality–sport congruence construct to improve the physical activity level of participants.

Both male and female adolescents tend to focus more on intrinsic factors (e.g., having fun, improving skills) than on extrinsic factors (e.g., pleasing a coach or parents, winning a game). However, more male adolescents report an interest in the competitive and achievement aspects of sport participation, whereas females tend to place more of an emphasis on the health benefits and social aspects of exercise.

MOTIVATION IN COMPETITIVE AND NONCOMPETITIVE POPULATIONS

Considerably more attention has been given to competitive than to noncompetitive sports and exercise participants of both genders and all ages. Competitive groups or teams are a more "captive audience" and allow researchers easier access to them for data collection. As one might expect, competitive athletes place more emphasis on winning, measuring their skills against those of others, improving their skills, and pleasing significant others (coaches, teammates, and parents) than do their noncompetitive counterparts. Noncompetitive populations seem to be more concerned with having fun, the health and appearance benefits of exercise, and spending time with friends.

The personality–sport congruence construct seems to be a stronger motivator for noncompetitive than for competitive populations. In one recent study where the participants were divided into competitive and noncompetitive groups, the competitive athletes did not consider the degree of match between their chosen sports and their personalities to be important. By contrast, those adolescents in a less structured, noncompetitive environment did increase their level of activity as the degree of personality–sport match increased.

RECOMMENDATIONS FOR INCREASING ADOLESCENTS' ACTIVITY LEVELS

Just as adolescents are not considered to be physiologically mature adults, so should their motivations for behavior not be assumed to be emotionally or cognitively similar to those of adults. For example, the research that has consistently identified self-motivation as an important determinant of exercise behavior in adults has not proven to be true for adolescents. Hence, external motivators (e.g., behavioral contracting) that have been helpful with adults whose self-motivation is low will not necessarily work with adolescents.

When planning interventions for increasing adolescents' activity levels, fitness professionals need to consider behavior motivation from the perspective of the people they are trying to serve. Basing physical education curricula and other youth sport programs on the psychological needs and perspectives of the adults guiding the experiences will not necessarily have the intended effect on the adolescent participants—that is, increased long-term activity levels. Whereas adults usually consider the health benefits of exercise as strong reasons for physical activity, the primary motivator for competitive and noncompetitive male and female adolescents is the desire to have fun.

Most other important factors in youth sport motivation are intrinsically rather than extrinsically based, and those supervising and designing programs should take this information into account as well. Fitness professionals should ensure that adolescents have ample opportunities to experience success in their sport or exercise pursuits, so as to enhance their perceived self-competence and feelings of skill mastery.

Females seem to be particularly motivated by the social and physical appearance benefits of sport participation. Therefore, consideration should be given to team-building and friendship-enhancing activities; moreover, acknowledgment of and education about the body weight and body fat reduction advantages of exercise should have a positive influence on female adolescents. Finally, both genders seem to respond positively to experiences where there is a greater match between the type of sport and the personality profile of the person engaging in the sport. Therefore, fitness practitioners may have more success with adolescents if consideration is given to assessing personality profiles and doing some exercise counseling as to the types of sports that will constitute the best match for each profile.

FURTHER READING

Centers for Disease Control and Prevention. (1992). *The Surgeon General's Report on Physical Activity and Health: Adolescents and young adults. National Health Interview Survey/Youth Risk Behavior Survey*: Washington, DC: U.S. Government Printing Office.
U.S. Government report on the population's progress toward 1990's fitness goals.

Costa, D. M., & Guthrie, S. R. (1994). *Women and sport: Interdisciplinary perspectives.* Champaign, IL: Human Kinetics Press.
Provides an overview of women's sport participation from a variety of disciplines including social, psychological, and physiological perspectives.

Dishman, R. K., & Dunn, A. L. (1988). Exercise adherence in children and youth: Implications for adulthood. In R. K. Dishman (Ed.), *Exercise adherence: Its impact on public health* (pp. 155–200). Champaign, IL: Human Kinetics Press.

Exercise motivations for youth and the resulting adherence implications for adult populations.

Douthitt, V. L. (1994). Psychological determinants of adolescent exercise adherence. *Adolescence, 29*, 711–722.
Detailed analysis of original research regarding the psychological exercise motivations of male and female adolescents.

Douthitt, V. L., & Harvey, M. A. (1995, May/June). Exercise counseling: How physical educators can help. *Journal of Physical Education, Recreation, and Dance*, 31–35.
Provides suggestions for physical educators in schools to enhance the long-term exercise adherence of their students.

Gavin, J. (1988). *Body moves: The psychology of exercise*. Harrisburg, PA: Stackpole Books.
Comprehensive discussion of the personality/sport congruence theory of exercise motivation.

Gerber, E. W., Felshin, J., & Berlin, P. (1974). *The American woman in sport*. Reading, MA: Addison-Wesley.
Historical account of the evolution of women's participation in sports.

Gould, D., & Horn, T. (1984). Participation motivation in young athletes. In J. Silva & R. Weinberg (Eds.), *Psychological foundations of sport* (pp. 359–370). Champaign, IL: Human Kinetics Press.
Analysis of the sport motivations of both male and female athletes participating in a variety of sports.

Martens, R. (1975). The paradigmatic crisis in American sport personology. *Sportwissenschaft, 1*, 9–24.
Comprehensive review regarding the conceptual framework for characterizing sport participation personological factors in American athletes.

Weiss, M. R., & Frazer, K. M. (1995). Initial, continued, and sustained motivation in adolescent female athletes: A season-long analysis. *Pediatric Exercise Science, 7*, 314–329.
In-depth examination of female adolescent basketball players' motivations for continued participation over an entire sport season.

45

Relaxation

Mary Banks Jasnoski Gregerson

Relaxation, like prevention itself, comes in many forms. Women use myriad methods of relaxation in everyday life; relaxation also has an abundant therapeutic and research history in primary, secondary, and tertiary prevention. In much of preventive therapy, relaxation is rarely produced by a single activity, but rather a sundry collection of activities. Even in preventive research, relaxation can be an independent or dependent variable, but always signaling an end state of reduced arousal. These multiple means to relaxation cloud precise meaning and, thus, use.

DIMENSIONS OF RELAXATION

In all types of prevention, relaxation is recreation. Leisure in its different activity levels produces a respite from the usual work and routine. There is general agreement that this "break" helps people to manage stress and prevent illness. Successful relaxation techniques can be categorized by their primary dimensions—that is, "cognitive," "emotional," "behavioral," or "physiological." Within each dimension, a number of techniques have been developed. The emotional dimension includes guided affective imagery and music. The behavioral dimension includes thermal biofeedback, electromyographic biofeedback, voluntary respiratory pattern, progressive muscle relaxation, and diaphragmatic breathing. Finally, the physiological dimension includes such techniques as the restricted environmental stimulation flotation tanks (REST), baths, physical exercise, and pharmacology. In some research a comparison of two or more different relaxation techniques shows no difference, but in other research significant differences among techniques do exist. In these latter cases, parsimony and efficacy indicate which technique to use with which problem in primary, secondary, and tertiary prevention.

RELAXATION AND THE THREE TYPES OF PREVENTION

In "primary prevention," the aim is to include relaxation in healthy persons' lives and to avert problems through lifestyle management. For instance, relaxation aids proper digestion. By providing important nutrients in the most efficient fashion for high energy, healthy living becomes an easier reality. In "secondary prevention," relaxation techniques are taught to specific at-risk populations, with the aim of neutralizing prodromal symptoms. In "tertiary prevention," the goals are to restore health to ill populations, to reverse illness indices, and to ward off other complications. In this type of prevention, for example, essential hypertension may be counteracted, with high blood pressure lowered to normal ranges. No further injury occurs, and the disease state disappears.

WHO RELAXES BEST WITH WHICH TECHNIQUES?

One person's relaxation may be another's stimulation. A particular form of relaxation also must match the characteristics of the person doing the relaxation; otherwise, the target of end-state reduced arousal may not occur. For example, one person finds exercise immediately arousing, but relaxing in the final analysis. After exercise, this person's stimulation signs dip below preexercise "resting" baseline levels. For another person, no ultimate reduction may occur; arousal may stay high without subbaseline descent after exercise.

Within the category of women, few special groups have been studied. Minorities have included African-Americans, working-class Latinas, and French-speaking Canadians. Some work has examined older women (e.g., women in senior center recreation programs), children, and early adolescents. The generalizability of findings among these different categories of women needs to be studied; include age, socioeconomic status, ethnicity, geographical region, educational level, family constellation, and professional/occupational status.

Thus, individual differences and preferences need to be considered. For instance, the degree to which a person possesses the characteristic of "absorption" determines whether biofeedback or an internally focused technique such as imagery is preferable. Absorption is an intense concentration ability that evokes more than normal physiological responsiveness to mental and actual events. Biofeedback is contraindicated for high absorbers, who prefer and physiologically respond better to internal, imaginal techniques for relaxation.

Another example of the match between characteristic and technique comes from the anxiety literature. Anxiety is hyperarousal to a nonspecific or otherwise innocuous "threat." Some years ago, the distinction between "cognitive" and "somatic" anxiety indicated that these two types responded differentially to relaxation techniques. Cognitive (or mental) anxiety responded better to meditation, whereas somatic (or physical) anxiety responded better to exercise. Thus, a cognitive relaxation technique more effectively reduced cognitive anxiety, and somatic relaxation was indicated to work better for somatic anxiety. In relaxation therapy, person specificity needs to be recognized and utilized.

Individual differences such as the ones just described (i.e., absorption and anxiety) should be used to pinpoint the most efficacious technique for a specific client. Comprehensive prescreening assessment can determine the most appropriate technique. Then treatment outcome evaluations can monitor and verify the effectiveness of an intervention uniquely designed for a particular client.

Monitoring can also be used to check for a curious and disturbing anomaly: Sometimes clients may actually increase rather than diminish their anxiety while performing relaxation techniques. This single general contraindication has occurred in the research efficacy literature. The documented list of ailments eased by relaxation, though, includes both physical and mental problems.

PROBLEMS THAT RESPOND TO RELAXATION

After relaxation-inducing techniques, physical health improvements have been documented for cardiovascular, neurological, urinary, obstetrical/gynecological, and sexual problems. Cardiovascular ailments responding to various relaxation techniques include angina pectoris, myocardial infarction recurrence, hypertension, and other heart and vascular irregularities as well as recovery from cardiac surgery. Neurological problems palliated by relaxation approaches include the symptoms and seizure rate of epilepsy, as well as pain problems (e.g., migraine and menstrual headaches; upper limb, lower back, neck, and shoulder pain). Urinary difficulties ameliorated with relaxation interventions include functional urinary coordination and incontinence. Obstetrical/gynecological difficulties that respond to relaxation therapies include infertility, premature labor, postterm delivery, premenstrual syndrome, spasmodic dysmenorrhea, pain resulting from punch biopsy of the cervix, and pain secondary to vaginal hysterectomy. Relaxation has also been used in prenatal education. Sexual dysfunctions treated successfully with relaxation include vaginismus, foot fetishism, situational orgasmic difficulty, preorgasmic problems, problems related to childhood incest, and sexual arousal difficulty.

The number of physical health problems responding positively to relaxation techniques mounts daily. Central mechanisms of health seem triggered by these techniques. Recent research has demonstrated that the immune system itself responds to the relaxation techniques. However, the recentness of this field of inquiry, has precluding tying symptomatology to these immune alterations. Most of this physical health research has also documented mental health improvements as well. Another body of work, though, has examined mental health specifically.

Mental problems, both psychosomatic and more purely psychological, have also responded well to relaxation approaches. Psychosomatic problems treated with relaxation include alcohol dependency, arthritis, bronchial asthma, eating disorders (bulimia and food aversion), hyperactivity associated with mental retardation, hyperemesis gravidarum (hysterical vomiting), insomnia, rheumatoid arthritis, and Type A coronary-prone behavior. Psychological difficulties ameliorated with relaxation include abuse, academic underachievement, anxiety, depression, hyperfunctional dysphonia, occupational stress, performance impairment (for athletes and musicians), and phobias (animal and social). Various relaxation techniques have documented effectiveness with this range of mental problems, as well as with the range of physical problems.

RESEARCH ISSUES

Research findings are complex. In the literature, "relaxation" may mean a single therapeutic session or a multiple-session treatment program. Relaxation may be the target intervention or only one component of a multifaceted stress management program. In either instance, relaxation is the independent variable by which relaxation and non-re-laxation conditions are compared.

On the other hand, relaxation as an outcome variable, has been a manipulation check, a covariate, a desired outcome, or a spurious confound. As a manipulation check, relaxation demonstrates empirically that the technique, whether alone or in combination with other stress management procedures, has lowered arousal. As a covariate, relaxation level is correlated with the pretreatment distress, in order to uncover causal indicators. Relaxation itself, though, may be the nondistress state enhanced as an outcome variable. Finally, in combined techniques, the relaxation could be an epiphenomenal confound or "red herring," obscuring accurate and precise attribution of causation to, say, guided imagery or REST. Researchers and clinicians using particular evidence need to carefully determine relaxation's roles in theoretical investigations and its applications to therapeutic situations.

FURTHER READING

Harmon, T. M., Hynan, M. T., & Tyre, T. E. (1990). Improved obstetric outcomes using hypnotic analgesia and skill mastery combined with childbirth education. *Journal of Consulting and Clinical Psychology, 58,* 525–530.
Sixty nulliparous women demonstrated that those receiving hypnosis and those highly suggestible compared to the controls reported less pain; those receiving hypnosis had shorter Stage 1 labors and more spontaneous deliveries, used less medication, and had higher Apgar scores; those highly suggestible who received hypnosis reported the lowest depression.

Humphrey, J. H. (1987). *Stress in coaching.* Springfield, IL: Charles C Thomas.
This book includes progressive relaxation, meditation, and biofeedback as suggested stress management techniques not only for use in athletes' performance training, but also for coaches' own personal enhancement and improved effectiveness.

Larsen, H., & Pagaduan-Lopez, J. (1987). Stress-tension reduction in the treatment of sexually tortured women: An exploratory study. *Journal of Sex and Marital Therapy, 13,* 210–218.
In this study, three sexually tortured Filipina women with histories of social, sexual, and psychomatic difficulties responded to a nonverbal stress reduction program with less psychomotor tension, more relaxed body language, and improvements in ability to express emotions.

Lehrer, P. M., Carr, R., Sargunaraj, D., & Woolfolk, R. J. (1994). Stress management techniques: Are they all equivalent, or do they have specific effects? *Biofeedback and Self-Regulation, 19,* 353–401.
This review strongly supports the contention that specifically cognitive, or autonomic, muscular stress management techniques produce cognitive, autonomic, or muscular effects, respectively, and thus are differentially indicated for disorders more predominantly cognitive, autonomic, or muscular.

Long, B. C., & Haney, C. J. (1988). Coping strategies for working women: Aerobic exercise and relaxation interventions. *Behavior Therapy, 19,* 75–83.
A comparison of jogging and progressive relaxation programs for 8 weeks showed that both programs significantly and nondifferentially reduced trait anxiety and improved self-efficacy (effects that were both maintained at an 8-week follow-up), but did not affect coping strategies.

O'Leary, A., Shoor, S., Lorig, K., & Holman, R. (1988). A cognitive-behavioral treatment for rheumatoid arthritis. *Health Psychology, 7,* 527–544.

Compared to a self-help control group, women with rheumatoid arthritis who received a combined treatment program in self-relaxation, cognitive pain management, and goal setting showed greater perceived self-efficacy, less pain and joint inflammation, and enhanced psychosocial functioning.

White, S., & Winzelberg, A. (1992). Laughter and stress: Humor. *International Journal of Humor Research, 5,* 343–355.

This study among college students showed that relaxation training, more than humor, significantly reduced physiological but not psychological measures of stress.

Section IV

HEALTH CARE PARADIGMS, POLICIES, AND SETTINGS

46

Section Editor's Overview

Lewayne Gilchrist

Women receive their health care in contexts shaped by political and social processes that in themselves affect the type, quality, and effectiveness of the care. The chapters in this section provide a glimpse of the many issues related to these contexts of care. Some of the chapters outline concerns about current practices, such as the lack of training for physicians in women's health. Other chapters illustrate trends that, although currently small, offer directions for the future that may improve the accessibility, sensitivity, and effectiveness of health services for women. The chapters cluster into two overlapping domains: (1) health care policies and paradigms that affect women; and (2) nontraditional settings and methods for delivering more effective and responsive health care to and for women.

HEALTH CARE POLICIES AND PARADIGMS

The sheer diversity and apparent lack of connections among the chapters in this section are not accidental. Even strong advocates for women's health as a much-needed specialization in health care voice concern about lack of coordination, coherence, and cooperation as this fledgling field evolves. As Edmunds noted in a 1995 article, and as she notes here in her chapter on U.S. health care policy, the diverse landscapes of public health, biomedical research, and behavioral and psychosocial research have evolved in the United States as separate and distinct cultures with unique communication and work styles, sources of funding, research interests, professional incentives, and public images. All of these cultures are developing their own particular specialties and subspecialties related to women's health, resulting in fragmentation and competition for available resources. In her chapter, Edmunds stresses the need for all researchers and clinicians involved in behavioral medicine and women's health—whatever their particular disciplines and loyalties—to acquaint themselves with federal, state, and local policies affecting women's health care; to get involved in the policy-making process by communicating with their legislators and by serving on government panels and committees that determine funding priorities; and to become involved likewise in their professional organizations and relevant groups in the private sector.

Other recent commentary on health care for women highlights the fragmentation not only within the developing field of women's health, but within existing systems and services. Clancy and Massion have labeled the field "a patchwork quilt with gaps." Gender-specific barriers exist in both access to and quality of care for U.S. women. Although women use health services more frequently than men do, they are more likely than men to encounter financial barriers to obtaining care; to fail to receive preventive services; to have their health concerns dismissed by a male physician as "merely" emotional; to have serious medical conditions misdiagnosed and mistreated by physicians who have received no training in women's health; to have serious health-affecting conditions (e.g., eating disorders, chemical dependency, depression, and sexual dysfunction) missed or ignored by their care providers; and to face an especially confusing service system, with unclear boundaries defining which type of provider (gynecologist, family/primary care physician, internist) they should turn to as their appropriate source of care.

The social and the biological in human lives are inextricably linked. Women differ from men not just in the biological sense. Increasingly, psychosocial influences are recognized as important contributors to health and disease. Economics and larger social structures affect women differently from men. For example, regardless of income, women have greater family responsibilities than men do. Moreover, although both men and women perform in multiple roles, women—particularly working women—often experience greater interrole conflict and overload. Krieger and colleagues have argued that the field of women's health must move beyond seeing women as different from men only biologically and only with regard to reproductive functions. Risk and protective factors affecting health are embedded in a web of social-structural relations—relations that have not only psychological but actual physiological (i.e., health) consequences. For example, stress is a known correlate of disease, but the stresses associated with gender, race, and social class inequities are all too rarely incorporated into the explanatory models and methods used to treat women.

As Levy notes in her chapter, the emerging paradigm of "accountability" in health care should—if it is not undercut by diminishing health care resources—help to reduce gender bias in research and treatment. Accountability (also referred to as "evidence-based health care," "empirically validated treatment," and "data-based practice" in various disciplines) is the use of information searches to locate interventions. According to Levy, the increased demand for accountability should encourage greater precision in the diagnosis and treatment of women, as well as the conducting of research that takes women's biological and psychosocial characteristics more precisely into account and covers more questions of relevance to women.

A traditional health care paradigm that is increasingly seen as inadequate in regard to women's health is the model of training and preparation for physicians. Wallis, in her chapter, discusses the gaps and deficiencies in the traditional medical school curriculum and model of training. She then describes various curricular initiatives and other improvements at all levels of medical education that have taken place in the 1990s. Wallis emphasizes that women's health is a comprehensive discipline and must be viewed as such; it is not merely a currently fashionable label for gynecology with a few "extras."

Substance abuse and chemical dependency constitute a specific women's health issue that traditional health care policies and paradigms do not effectively recognize. As Wallen's chapter notes, women with substance abuse problems use health services far more than women without such problems, yet the vast majority of substance abusers rarely report their abuse or identify it as underlying their reasons for seeking treatment. They speak instead of digestive or sleep problems, depression, anxiety, obstetrical or gynecological problems, or other symptoms. Stigma and social condemnation for substance abuse are greater for women than for men, and women are understandably reluctant to be identified as substance abusers or as chemically dependent. Even when the issue of substance abuse arises in the course of care, physicians and other health care practitioners may regard such abuse as a psychological problem outside their realm of expertise and leave the issue unexplored and unaddressed, with lingering health consequences for the women involved.

INNOVATIVE HEALTH CARE SETTINGS AND PRACTICES

The next group of chapters in this section examines unusual or neglected environments for delivering more responsive health care to women. The constant and increasing theme in all discussions of health care is cost control. Beyond that important theme, health policy analysts note that current specialized health care environments and settings can overlap in confusing ways for women, are not readily accessible for many women, are not tailored to address the needs of special groups of women (e.g., the very young and the elderly), and are often so narrowly focused that preventive services in particular are difficult to obtain or are unavailable to many women. One theme in these chapters is the desire to address the needs of special populations of women more efficiently and effectively by taking services to sites and contexts where such women actually spend their time. Mary Lou Balassone's chapter outlines the success of school-based clinics in improving adolescent women's access to and use of health care services, especially preventive services. In addition to financial barriers, very young women may stay away from traditional health care settings because they are afraid of or feel demeaned by staff members unaccustomed to adolescents; because they lack knowledge about what services exist; because they lack the skill or the resources to access such services on their own; because they simply lack transportation; or because they are afraid to reveal their sexual activity (and their resulting need for contraceptives, pregnancy exams, exams and treatment for sexually transmitted diseases, or treatment for the aftermath of sexual assault) to their parents. School-based clinics bring specialists in adolescent health concerns into the major community institutions—public schools—where adolescents are. The notion of lodging age-tailored health services in settings that contain a single age group is also seen in retirement homes, where the needs of older women are the special focus. Access, acceptability, and effectiveness of services are all shown to increase in these cases. Less information is available on the long-term efficiency and cost containment of these setting-specific services.

Another special setting for health services for women is the workplace. U.S. women now work outside their homes in record numbers. Although employment may increase health insurance and financial resources for health care for some women, employment also creates barriers to obtaining care. Such barriers include inability to take time off from a job and difficulties in arranging child care to seek health services outside the job. These factors in particular reduce women's use of prevention and health promotion services, which may be judged dispensable in the face of important logistical difficulties. Maheu's chapter outlines recent trends in health promotion programs for women in worksites, with nicotine treatment programs as the primary examples. The chapter by

Pierce examines one particular worksite for women: the military. Pierce's chapter suggests that environments that once served only men are slowly beginning to recognize and respond to the needs of increasing numbers of women. There is much to be learned about meeting the special health needs of women in the armed forces and in other professional settings, as women assume roles and responsibilities that are increasingly indistinguishable from those of their male counterparts. Another social system that is newly and uneasily recognizing the health care needs of unprecedented numbers of women is the law enforcement/correctional system. Jails, prisons, and reformatories rarely have policies, facilities, or resources in place to deal smoothly with pregnancy, eating disorders, gynecological problems, or other women's health issues.

Although Brown's chapter on prenatal care does not describe a shift in the settings in which such care is provided in the United States, it describes a number of attempts to improve access to this care in other ways. Brown describes four types of barriers that may prevent pregnant women from seeking prenatal health care: financial barriers, limits on the health care system's capacity, inhospitable practices, and women's own personal and attitudinal issues. She then describes efforts in both the public and private sectors to address these barriers, and notes that the rise in pregnant women's levels of participation in prenatal health care between the late 1960s and the 1990s may be attributable in part to these initiatives.

The final two chapters in this section address changes in the content of health care services themselves, rather than changes in the settings in which such services are provided for women. (Indeed, the changes described in these chapters are sufficiently sweeping that they could be described as paradigm shifts in health care.) Black and Scott build upon recent changes in communication technology to suggest a structure and means for broader and more extensive use of self-administered health-promotive interventions as an effective enhancement of traditional services. The potential exists to create a web of accessible resources for improving women's health. Certainly easy access to accurate and helpful information about steps to improve one's own health is attractive from the perspectives of efficiency and cost containment. Public health research has shown that information alone can effect health-promotive behavior change. Such research also shows that information accompanied by socially supportive interpersonal contacts is even more effective, especially for women. Electronic media (including computerized links to electronic mail and information services), and even old-fashioned telephone links to health care providers, can efficiently provide both information and supportive contacts. This could be a considerable boon to women in rural areas, women who are house- or bed-bound, and women whose concerns about privacy and confidentiality may make them reluctant to seek out and be identified within more traditional health care settings and environments.

Finally, Cornman's chapter on alternative medicine addresses a rapidly growing movement in the United States away from traditional medicine and toward holistic health care practices associated with Eastern traditions and philosophies. Although this movement has arisen in part out of concern for the rising costs of traditional Western-style health care, the appeal of alternative medicine involves more than economic concerns. A clear disillusion with traditional settings, policies, and practices is reflected in the popularity of nontraditional approaches to healing. Nontraditional and alternative medical practices involve blended and intuitively appealing considerations of both physiological and psychosocial issues in people's lives. Thus the real complexities of women's lives are considered in planning treatment procedures that focus on achieving wellness through holistic balance, rather than on "curing" an isolated symptom. Finally, these practices emphasize self-responsibility and include women as active participants in their own care—an appealing approach for women whose needs may never have been adequately recognized or addressed by traditional medical settings and methods.

CONCLUSION

In conclusion, health care policies, paradigms, settings, and practices, as well as health care availability, costs, and effectiveness, will continue to be issues of high-level debate and concern. Commentators on women's health note the necessarily multidisciplinary nature of the women's health field. The policies, paradigms, settings, and practices involved in the delivery of responsive health care to women reflect this diversity. Findings from research illustrated or at least suggested by chapters in this section must be responsibly integrated into treatment approaches and public policy to reduce the gender biases in health status, health research, health care, and health policies that currently remain for U.S. women.

FURTHER READING

Clancy, C. M., & Massion, C. T. (1992). American women's health care: A patchwork quilt with gaps. *Journal of the American Medical Association, 268*(14), 1914–1920.
The commentary paper emphasizes women's special health care needs and the fragmentation of health care services for women in the U.S.

Council on Ethical and Judicial Affairs, American Medical Association. (1991). Gender disparities in clinical decision making. *Journal of the American Medical Association, 266*(4), 559–562.
The article is an abridged version of a report adopted by the American Medical Association. It covers gender differences across a variety of symptoms, diagnoses, and therapeutic interventions. The report also summarizes stereotypes, prejudices, and other social attitudes that may affect the delivery of health services to women. Finally, the report addresses the role of the medical profession in examining gender disparities and in eliminating biases in services.

Edmunds, M. (1995). Policy research: Balancing rigor with relevance. *Women's Health: Research on Gender, Behavior, and Policy, 1*(1), 97–119.
The author reviews 20 years of national policy and national policy research relating to women's health care.

Krieger, N., Rowley, D. L., Herman, A. A., Avery, B., & Phillips, M. T. (1993). Racism, sexism, and social class: Implications for studies of health, disease, and wellbeing. *American Journal of Preventive Medicine, 9*(Suppl. 6), 82–122.
The authors provide an encyclopedic review of medical and health services research that, by conflating race and sex with ethnicity and gender and by ignoring social class issues, disserve or misrepresent women in literature that forms the basis for clinical and political decision making related to health care.

Rodin, J., & Ickovics, J. R. (1990). Women's health: Review and research agenda as we approach the 21st century. *American Psychologist, 45*(9), 1018–1034.
The authors review past research and project future needs regarding women's health. The article addresses declining differences in mortality rates between men and women and examines variables that appear to contribute to this decline.

47

Health Care Policy

Margaret Edmunds

As a field, behavioral medicine has traditionally been underinvolved in health care policy. There are several reasons why this might be the case. On the one hand, behavioral and psychosocial clinicians and researchers tend to be more familiar with biomedical institutions than with government and other institutions associated with public policy. Conversely, health policy-makers have not been aware of the extent of research showing the effectiveness of interventions involving behavioral changes and personal health practices. Behavioral change strategies often focus on individuals, whereas health policy as a field within public health tends to address population-based strategies (e.g., laws about the legal age to purchase alcohol and cigarettes, or regulations to post warnings about smoking cigarettes or drinking alcohol when pregnant).

Women's health is a cross-cutting field with roots in public health, biomedical research, clinical practice, and the consumer movement; nevertheless, it still has had relatively little involvement in public policy development. This chapter first describes the policy process, with an emphasis on U.S. federal agencies concerned primarily with women's health and behavioral medicine. Next, some of the current national trends influencing health policy are described. Finally, strategies are suggested for clinicians and researchers in behavioral medicine and women's health to increase their involvement in the policy process.

KEY FEDERAL AGENCIES

In 1990, the Office for Research on Women's Health (ORWH) was established at the National Institutes of Health (NIH) to address the gaps and inequities in funding for research on women's health, to ensure that women are included in clinical studies, and to promote biomedical career opportunities for women. It was the view of the national leadership in women's health at that time that the field would never receive full recognition by the medical profession, policy makers, and the public without the stature of an NIH agency. In 1992, the ORWH set a research agenda addressing four developmental stages (birth to young adulthood, young adulthood to perimenopausal years, perimenopausal to mature years, and mature years) and identifying six areas for research: reproductive biology, early developmental biology, cardiovascular diseases, malignancies, immune and infectious diseases, and the aging process. Recently funded studies have addressed the prevalence of risk factors among women of racial and ethnic subgroups, violence against women, the relationship of depression to other health problems, and many other areas. The ORWH actively participates in national conferences on a variety of issues, and serves as a focal point for women's health issues at the federal level.

In 1995, the NIH Office of Behavioral and Social Sciences Research (OBSSR) became operational. In response to advocacy from a variety of scientific and other professional organizations, the OBSSR was formed to provide national leadership through integrating behavioral and social sciences into the biomedical research studies at the NIH. The agency was mandated by Congress to develop a definition of what is included in the term "health and behavior," which will be used to assess and monitor NIH support of the behavioral and social sciences. Experts from the behavioral and psychosocial fields, including behavioral medicine and research staff members of the various NIH institutes, assisted in developing the consensus definition as well as in developing a strategic plan to help establish OBSSR's priorities. Researchers on women's health were among those included in these processes. As of the spring of 1997, the definition was being tested in order to see that is accurate before using it to assess the NIH research portfolio in a report to Congress.

Because every federal agency's budget must be approved by Congress, the direction of public funds for women's health and for behavioral and psychosocial research is influenced by the political climate. Most legislators are not well informed about research methodologies, but they are interested in findings that can help them make policy-relevant decisions. For example, given two equally effective interventions, the lower-cost intervention is usually preferred. Behavioral researchers can do far more to increase public awareness of the clinical value and cost-effectiveness of behavioral interventions to reduce such high-risk behaviors as substance abuse, unsafe sex, poor nutrition, and sedentary lifestyles.

THE CURRENT HEALTH POLICY CONTEXT

The National Health Care Reform Debate

Unlike nearly all other industrialized countries, the United States does not have a national health policy. For several months during the national health care reform debate initiated by the Clinton administration, there seemed to be widespread agreement that all citizens should have access to health care. In the area of women's health, there were questions about what kinds of care should be covered, such as whether obstetricians/gynecologists should be considered as primary care providers. There were also questions about what services should be included in a basic benefits package, such as whether mammograms should start at age 40 or 50, and how frequently they should be given. It was acknowledged that most people could lose their health insurance if they lost their jobs or sustained a major illness, and that "the uninsured" are not a permanent economic underclass, but people whose life experiences are not out of the mainstream.

After many elements of the business community began to protest the proposed national health insurance plan because they did not want to be overburdened by paying for it, the national agreement on access to health care began to unravel. Not enough taxpayers and consumers realized that the costs of uncompensated care would be passed along to the insured in the form of higher premiums. The debate then began to shift to the restructuring of the two national public insurance programs, Medicare and Medicaid, which cover individuals who are elderly, disabled, and poor. These programs became targets in an overall strategy to balance the budget—not only because their costs were growing faster than the overall budget, and they needed streamlining and better accountability, but also because they are entitlements. This means that they raise fundamental philosophical issues about the role of government: Should anyone who meets eligibility criteria be entitled to health care when he or she needs it, or is a "safety net" a costly, unnecessary, and undesirable form of welfare?

In the fall of 1996, the Health Insurance Portability and Accountability Act was passed by Congress, with an implementation date of July 1997. Viewed as a modest and incremental effort to improve access to health care, the Act was introduced by Senators Nancy Kassebaum and Ted Kennedy in order to prohibit health plans from limiting or denying coverage for individuals with certain medical conditions and also to reduce disparities in coverage for medical and mental health coverage. In the spring of 1997, Congress began to consider ways to expand insurance coverage for the estimated ten million uninsured children who lack private insurance coverage from parents' employers and who are also not eligible for Medicaid. Achieving consensus on how to finance insurance expansion will be a major challenge for Congress, state government, and other policy-makers.

Managed Care

In the absence of a national health care policy, many decision makers are moving Medicaid and Medicare populations into managed care, in the belief that taxpayers will spend less on health care. At its best, managed care provides coordinated, integrated health care services that emphasize primary care, prevention, and health education; there is evidence that managed care can provide efficient, high-quality care at a lower cost than traditional fee-for-service systems serving comparable patient populations. In the more common forms of managed care, a health maintenance organization (HMO) contracts with or employs a group or groups of physicians, hospitals, and other providers to deliver services to its members for a fixed monthly premium or capitated payment. Often several different types of services (e.g., primary and specialty care, well-baby clinics, optometry, laboratory tests, etc.) are located at a single HMO site. In a preferred provider organization (PPO), the health plan negotiates lower rates for its members among a network of providers. These networks may include hundreds of providers who work out of their own offices, may participate in more than one PPO, may or may not also accept Medicaid and Medicare patients, and have varying degrees and types of practice patterns and referral networks.

Because the managed care organizations (MCOs) receive fixed monthly premiums, they must work within the financial constraints of these preset amounts. Some have found that managed care lowers costs primarily by decreasing the use of unnecessary proce-dures, contrary to the inherent incentives in a fee-for-service system to order more procedures to increase the providers' revenue. However, there is ample evidence that some MCOs deny needed services or make it difficult for members to receive services, such as by enrolling new members before there are enough providers in a network to meet the demand. In some cases, pregnant women have been unable to make an appointment for prenatal care for several weeks or months into their pregnancies. Thus, there is growing pressure from consumers, employers, and other purchasers of health care to develop report cards and other indicators of quality assurance activities. There is also a trend to provide a separate or "carved-out" benefits package for managed mental health and substance abuse (known as behavioral health care), and to carve out other "big-ticket" items (e.g., cancer care).

OPPORTUNITIES FOR INVOLVEMENT IN THE POLICY PROCESS

As informed citizens, researchers and clinicians should know who represents them in the Senate and in the House of Representatives, whether these individuals sit on any committees that handle health issues, and what their voting records have been. Researchers and clinicians should correspond with legislators or meet with them to discuss research findings and clinical experiences that can inform decision makers about funding priorities for research, clinical services, and prevention. Legislators on health-related committees have staff members who are usually receptive to researchers who provide clear and concise information on health issues—for example, the effectiveness of school-based behavioral interventions to prevent substance abuse, or evidence of disparities in health status for women of color in a particular congressional district. In election years, researchers and clinicians can volunteer for political campaigns for national, state, and local offices.

National professional organizations—the American Psychological Association, the American Nurses Association, and the American Public Health Association, to name a few—have task forces that develop policy statements on areas such as health care access, substance abuse, HIV/AIDS, and other issues related to women's health. Behavioral medicine should undertake a similar process by developing statements on the clinical effectiveness, cost-effectiveness, and cost offsets of behavioral interventions to manage chronic illness; reduce consumption of alcohol, tobacco, and illicit drugs; and improve nutrition and fitness. If such statements were endorsed by national professional organizations such as the Society of Behavioral Medicine, they could provide a basis for developing standardized behavioral interventions in MCOs, which have thus far underutilized behavioral medicine strategies.

Federal agencies such as the ORWH, the OBSSR, the National Institute on Drug Abuse, the National Institute on Alcohol Abuse and Alcoholism, the Agency for Health Care Policy Research, and the Centers for Disease Control and Prevention have research programs that include women's health and are concerned with behavioral risks. Interested clinicians and researchers can be nominated by their professional organizations to serve on grant review panels and on advisory committees that help public agencies determine their research priorities.

Many of these agencies have newsletters and public affairs departments, which help to inform the field of their current and proposed activities. At the state and local levels, there are also opportunities to be involved in public policy development. For example, the state of California now requires citizen input in its planning process for programs for HIV/AIDS, and many coalitions and consortia have been organized to coordinate strategies among several professional, community-based delivery, and consumer organizations. Health departments, mental health departments, and substance abuse agencies frequently have advisory committees or task forces on issues of local concern, such as teen pregnancy, domestic violence, gangs, or gun control. In the private sector, hospitals and clinics have advisory boards for public awareness campaigns and other programs, and also sponsor health education activities and support groups. Researchers and clinicians can contribute their expertise to all of these efforts in a variety of ways.

With Medicaid waivers and block grants increasing states' decision-making authority, it is important for researchers and clinicians to be more familiar with their state legislatures and with the public agency structures. They should be familiar with the process of legislative oversight, relevant and powerful committees, and particular interests of their own representatives. Legislators and agency directors are often receptive to well-reasoned and objective presentations of the circumstances of individuals in their districts, especially when there are several organizations representing a consensus and when realistic strategies are developed for dealing with problems. As public funds diminish and their distribution becomes more controversial, more informed members of the public need to become involved in the decision-making process.

NEXT STEPS

The scientific community in general and the behavioral medicine community in particular have avoided involvement in health policy development. In the wake of the national debate on health care reform, health policy development now clearly needs informed consumers, including those who happen to be clinicians and researchers. It has become increasingly clear to health policy-makers that some of the main predictors of health status (e.g., good nutrition, adequate exercise, avoidance of initiating cigarette smoking) are largely dependent on individual choices made on a daily basis. One role of government may be to protect the public, but to what extent should government protect individuals from overeating, drinking too much, or smoking cigarettes? Where does the nation or a community choose to draw its line between protection and interference? These are core health policy questions, and they are being played out in a number of arenas in the 1990s. If health care professionals are silent on the issues on which they have expertise, others who are less well informed will be making the decisions that will affect national funding for research and services.

FURTHER READING

Edmunds, M. (1995) Policy research: Balancing rigor with relevance. *Women's Health: Research on Gender, Behavior, and Policy*, 1(1), 97–119.
Broad overview of clinical, research, and health policy issues that are likely to affect the development of the field of women's health, including key federal agencies, national policy initiatives, and methodological and technical issues for research.

Lee, P. R., & Estes, C. (Eds.). (1990). *The nation's health* (3rd ed.). Boston: Jones & Bartlett.
A key textbook in public health, health policy, and health services research, including chapters on health care delivery; the health care work force; costs, accessibility, quality, and appropriateness of care; and social issues affecting health care.

Luft, H. S. (1985). Competition and regulation. *Medical Care, 23,* 383–400.
A classic health care economics article that describes a range of public policies on cost containment; their impacts on cost, access, and quality of care; and the difficulties and limitations of evaluative research.

McGinnis, J. M. (1994). The role of behavioral research in national health policy. In S. J. Blumenthal, K. Matthews, & S. M. Weiss (Eds.), *New research frontiers in behavioral medicine: Proceedings of the National Conference* (DHHS Publication No. NIH 94-3772, pp. 217–222). Washington, DC: U.S. Government Printing Office.
The former Deputy Assistant Secretary for Health states that behavior is the central challenge for health policy, and makes recommendations about research on health and behavior.

Miller, R. H., & Luft, H. R. (1994). Managed care plan performance since 1980: A literature analysis. *Journal of the American Medical Association, 271*(19), 1512–1519.
Comprehensive analysis of research comparing utilization, expenditures, quality of care, and satisfaction of enrollees in several types of managed care and traditional health care plans.

Starr, P. (1981). *The social transformation of American medicine.* New York: Basic Books.
The author won a Pulitzer prize for this social history of the medical profession, which describes the development of U.S. health care in the context of power and social structure.

48

Accountability

Rona L. Levy

*A*ccountability was originally defined as being capable of giving a report. This definition, at least as it applies to health and mental health treatment, now carries the expanded expectation that the report given will in some way justify actions taken. Health care workers are increasingly held accountable for their work with patients. "Evidence-based health care," "empirically validated treatment," and "data-based practice" are all terms that refer to this paradigm, which is rapidly emerging as the standard for health care. Practitioners under this paradigm are now expected to utilize information-seeking skills to locate and practice interventions with empirically demonstrated effectiveness. This trend is growing in popularity in medicine, psychology, social work, and related disciplines. It is likely to have profound implications for the delivery of women's health care. For accountable practice to occur, a minimum of three conditions must be met. First, contingencies must be in place that encourage this form of practice; second, clinicians must possess the knowledge and skills required of accountable practice; finally, a data base of techniques with proven effectiveness from which clinicians can draw must exist and be accessible. These three points, and the implications of accountability for behavioral medicine with women, are discussed below.

WHY IS ACCOUNTABILITY AN ISSUE NOW?

The call for accountability in practice is not new. For decades, various methods of clinical evaluation or "empirical clinical practice" have been taught to students in such disciplines as psychology and social work. Follow-up studies of students trained in these method-ologies have generally shown, however, that these procedures (at least in their entirety) have not routinely been practiced once students graduate.

However, there is currently increased pressure for accountability in the clinical arena. This pressure is a result of the larger changes occurring throughout the United States in the administration of and reimbursement for health care services. Resources are being dispensed with an increasingly watchful eye. Third-party payers (e.g., health maintenance organizations, insurance companies) are in many ways controlling which procedures are being done, as well as how long these procedures should take. The payers exert this control through their control over reimbursement. Patients are encouraged through financial incentives to use "preferred providers," who are preferred because they provide services that are less costly to the payers. It is becoming increasingly rare for a provider to reimburse a psychologist, for example, simply for stating that he or she met with a patient. More often, the common scenario begins with a payer's requiring authorization in advance for a given number of sessions. The provider is asked to indicate the expected mode of treatment, duration of contact, and outcome. Currently, the expected mode of treatment typically stops at a category such as "individual," "group," "supportive," or "problem-focused." If current trends continue, there is every indication that the level of specificity will expand to *types* of treatment, such as "systematic desensitization," "exposure and response prevention," and "applied relaxation." It is a likely future scenario that clinicians will be encouraged to choose the procedures that cost less. These will be the procedures that take less time and, most importantly, are effective, so that return visits are not necessary. The requirement to describe interventions and possibly to choose some interventions over others may not be looked upon favorably by clinicians; nevertheless, professional survival may require these actions.

KNOWLEDGE AND SKILLS NECESSARY FOR ACCOUNTABILITY/EVIDENCE-BASED PRACTICE

Some professions have already taken the initiative to move in the direction of more accountable practice. This move is wise, because the professions may then be in a position to regulate themselves, instead of having control exerted over them by external forces perhaps less familiar with their activities. In discussing this "new" way of practicing medicine, the Evidence-Based Medicine Working Group listed the following requirements for the practice of evidence-based medicine in a 1992 report:

> These include precisely defining a patient's problem, and what information is required to resolve the problem; conducting an efficient search of the literature; selecting the best of relevant studies and applying rules of evidence to determine their validity; being able to present to colleagues in a succinct fashion the content of the article and its strengths and weaknesses; and extracting the clinical message and applying it to the patient's problem.

Recent advances in data-processing techniques, with ready access to computer literature searches, greatly facilitate this process. This group also states that traditional skills of medical training, such as a sound understanding of pathophysiology and a sensitivity to patients' emotional needs, are still necessary.

On a similar track, David Barlow, president of Division 12 (Clinical Psychology) of the American Psychological Association (APA), requested the formation of the Task Force on Promotion and Dissemination of Psychological Procedures. The purpose of this group was to educate the public, clinical psychologists, and third-party payers about effective (i.e., empirically validated) therapies. Clinicians are encouraged to judge studies as meeting criteria for effectiveness if they utilize treatment manuals and clearly specify the characteristics of the client samples. In addition, one of the following two types of research must have occurred:

1. At least two good group studies conducted by different investigators, demonstrating efficacy in one or more of the following ways: superior to pill or psychological placebo or to another treatment, and/or equivalent to an already established treatment in studies with adequate statistical power (about 30 per group).
2. A large series of single-case studies demonstrating efficacy; these studies must have used good experimental designs and must have compared the intervention to another treatment.

Both the medical and psychological groups place heavy emphasis on how training in their professions needs to be changed if this form of practice is to occur. The Evidence-Based Medicine Working Group focused on a residency training program at McMaster University. In this program, residents are trained first to critically review research studies that meet such methodological criteria as control groups, randomization, and low dropout rates, and then to select treatments that have been shown to be effective in studies meeting these criteria.

Although basic research methodology is traditionally taught to psychology students, the emphasis of APA's Division 12 task force was on encouraging training in techniques that meet the criteria outlined above. The report of the task force includes recommendations that (1) training in empirically validated treatments be considered in the accreditation of doctoral programs; (2) the APA enforce guidelines regarding efficacy of new treatment procedures taught in continuing education courses; and (3) all promotional material for APA-sponsored continuing education programs should state whether treatments are empirically validated.

AVAILABILITY OF EMPIRICALLY VALIDATED TREATMENTS

There has been an ongoing debate in the health care professions, especially psychology, as to whether sufficient evidence does in fact exist on which to base evidence-based practice. The title of a recent article frames some of this debate: "Everyone Was Wrong: There Are Lots of Replications Out There."

The APA's Division 12 has published a list of empirically validated treatments that it states meet the criteria given above. Treatments for problems of particular interest to behavioral medicine include the following: behavior modification for enuresis and encopresis; behavior therapy for headaches, irritable bowel syndrome, female orgasmic dysfunction, and male erectile dysfunction; cognitive-behavioral therapy for chronic pain; and interpersonal therapy for bulimia nervosa. The task force is careful to point out that this list is a noninclusive, beginning effort, as some treatments that meet the criteria may have been missed. Another APA Division 12 task force has subsequently published a list of manuals that are available for empirically validated treatments.

IMPLICATIONS FOR BEHAVIORAL MEDICINE FOR WOMEN

Bias has often existed in the medical treatment of women. There is a long history of women receiving different diagnoses and different treatments than men receive for the same problems. Similarly, there has been extensive bias in behavioral medicine research with women; this has occurred in all phases of the research process. Although there appears to be some evidence that this is changing, women were often not the subjects of many research studies. The excuse was typically given that their physiology (menstrual cycles, pregnancy, etc.) complicated the research. As discussed below, an alternative approach is to incorporate these phenomena into the research design. The research topics selected have also ignored many questions important to women. Moreover, procedures for obtaining informed consent to participate in research studies may not have been structured in a way to maximize obtaining women's valid preferences. For example, in a situation involving a male physician/researcher and a female patient/subject, the patient/subject may feel intimidated. Similar concerns have been raised about the choice of measurement methods, experimental design, and data analysis procedures. For example, research that includes women subjects should measure menstrual cycle variation in women, and data analysis should take the timing of each woman's cycle into account. Research in some areas of behavioral medicine with women has demonstrated the significant effect these cycles can have on symptomatology.

The move toward greater accountability can only serve to reduce these areas of bias. First, if there is increased demand for empirically validated treatments, clinicians should be encouraged to be more precise in making diagnoses and selecting treatments that match these diagnoses. Second, with greater demands for information on empirically validated treatments, it also seems reasonable to expect that more research will be conducted to match this demand. A less optimistic perspective, of course, could suggest that in these times of diminishing health care resources, women will simply receive less of the services they need—perhaps in an unbiased way, right along with men!

FURTHER READING

Evidence-Based Medicine Working Group. (1992). Evidence-based medicine. *Journal of the American Medical Association, 268*(17), 2420–2425.
Discussion article defining evidence-based medicine and its effect on outcomes, outlining its requirements, providing an example of an evidence-based medical residency program, and describing barriers to the dissemination of evidence-based medicine.

Eyde, L. D., Moreland, K. L., & Robertson, G. J. (1988). *Test user qualifications: A data-based approach to promoting good test use.* Washington, DC: American Psychological Association.
Report on the results of research studies to identify test user qualifications and behaviors, common factors of test misuse, and the development of empirically based purchaser forms.

Jayaratne, S., & Levy, R. L. (1979). *Empirical clinical practice.* New York: Columbia University Press.
One of the first texts outlining the techniques of empirically based practice, including measurement methods and single-subject design techniques.

Levy, R. L., & Richey, C. A. (1988). Measurement and research design. In E. A. Blechman & K. D. Brownell (Eds.), *Handbook of behavioral medicine for women* (pp. 421–438). New York: Pergamon Press.
Discussion chapter on methods for improving behavioral medicine research on women, including areas of topic selection, informed consent, measurement selection, and design and analysis issues.

Neuliep, J. W., & Crandall, R. (1993). Everyone was wrong: There are lots of replications out there. *Journal of Social Behavior and Personality, 8*(6), 1–8.
Uses a survey of recent articles in the reporting journal, which found a high proportion of replications, to confirm that psychology is producing an increasing number of research replications.

Sanderson, W. C., & Woody, S. (1995). *Manuals for empirically validated treatments: A project of the Task Force on Psychological Interventions.* Washington, DC: Division of Clinical Psychology, American Psychological Association (APA).

List of manuals of well-established treatments, organized alphabetically by problem area, as discussed by the Task Force on Promotion and Dissemination of Psychological Procedures (see below).

Task Force on Promotion and Dissemination of Psychological Procedures, Division of Clinical Psychology, APA. (1995). *The Clinical Psychologist, 48*(1), 3–24.

Report that defines empirically validated treatments; discusses recommendations for predoctoral, internship, and advanced training in empirically validated treatments; and describes methods for informing clinicians and the public about these methods.

49

Medical Curricula and Training

Lila A. Wallis

REASONS FOR DEVELOPING A COMPREHENSIVE CURRICULUM IN WOMEN'S HEALTH

Over the last several decades, a number of women physicians and medical school faculty members have critically examined the health care needs of their women patients and observed disparities and gaps in research, in the education and training of physicians, and in clinical practice concerning women's health. Several reasons underscore the urgent need for a comprehensive curriculum in women's health in medical schools, specialty training programs, and continuing medical education of physicians.

Differences Between Men and Women

Differences in women's health go beyond the boundaries of the reproductive tract and affect every system—cardiovascular, gastrointestinal, immune, musculoskeletal, urological, and psychological. Environmental, societal, and economic circumstances, as well as the hormonal milieu, shape the course of illness and response to treatment differently in women than in men. Gender differences in the metabolism of pharmacological agents are also well documented.

Fragmentation of Women's Care

Women's health needs are frequently lost in the gaps between different medical specialties. Whereas men are not ordinarily sent by an internist to a urologist for a routine male genitorectal exam, women are constantly being referred back and forth between gynecologists, internists, family practitioners, and various other specialists. Routine fragmentation of care is expensive, wasteful, and unjust.

Women's Morbidity/Mortality

A compelling reason for physicians to be trained and retrained in women's health is that women may suffer and die as a result of the gender bias in research and medical education. Inadequate research translates into inadequate education and training of physicians, and thus into delayed and inappropriate clinical care. Although women succumb to arteriosclerotic heart disease later in life than men do, female mortality after a myocardial infarction is higher than male mortality. Thrombolysis therapy in women is associated with more side effects, including hemorrhage, than in men. After an angioplasty, female blood vessels close off more readily than those of men. Female mortality after bypass surgery exceeds that of men. It is not known whether these gender differences are biological or whether they result from bias. Little or no research has been directed at the resolution of this question, and no research at all has been directed at possible remedies.

The Expanding Role of Women Physicians

The movement to develop a women's health curriculum is largely the result of an increase in the numbers of female medical students and female doctors. The mission of the American Medical Women's Association (AMWA) is to promote the entrance of women into the health care profession and to address concerns about women's health care. Also, the National Council on Women's Health, which is primarily composed of women in various health professions, has as its missions educating the public on women's health issues and improving communication between providers and consumers.

Gender Bias

The basic reason for the development of a women's health curriculum is to undo the damage caused by gender bias in medical education, research, and clinical practice. Gender bias is inherent in a male-dominated, male-taught discipline. Few women physicians and medical students have female professors as role models. An informal poll taken at a recent AMWA meeting disclosed that the most frequently identified female role model by the gathering of women doctors was Madame Curie—an introspective scientist, not an outgoing practitioner of medicine. The dearth of female role models has resulted in women's turning to male role models. Many women doctors have accepted gender bias as a norm or have denied its prevalence.

Failure of identification can lead to the pervasive stereotype of the woman as complainer, as someone who manifests her mental woes in physical symptoms—for example, the hysteric or the neurasthenic, about whom the physician does not have to be too concerned, because her headaches and her chest pain are "imaginary." Dysmenorrhea and premenstrual syndrome are similarly written off as "psychosomatic." This same reluctance to identify with the female patient has led to such phenomena as rough, painful, inconsiderate, uncommunicative, hurried, incompetent pelvic exams, and superficial and incompetent breast exams.

In general, a training paradigm based on male needs does not serve women patients well. Women have different prevalences and patterns of health and disease. For instance, anxiety disorders and depression are much more common in women, whereas men have at least twice the rates of antisocial personality and alcohol abuse/dependency. Conditions common to men and women frequently have different manifestations in each gender. Alcohol abuse leads most commonly to violence in men and to depression in women.

To take another example, urologists, who are almost exclusively men, have spent much of their time dealing with prostate problems. However, women have urological problems, too; these include cystitis, urethritis, the "honeymoon pyelitis," the poorly understood "interstitial cystitis," and the various forms of urinary incontinence. These problems have received less medical attention and less interest in research. One reason is that there are few female urologists to identify with the female patient. Similarly, why do mammograms continue to be painful for many women? Medical school education and physician training programs have over the centuries reflected male attitudes and interests, and many of women's health needs are left unattended or fragmented, as noted above. Individual women physicians, confronting the unmet needs of female patients, have gone on to take additional courses and informal preceptorships to fill the gaps in their training. This process has been largely haphazard, intuitive, unorganized, and guided by the individual physicians' perception of their needs.

NEW CURRICULAR INITIATIVES

In November 1990, a loosely knit Coalition on Women's Health, representing a number of medical societies and women's health consumer organizations, drafted the first Core Curriculum on Women's Health—a list of skills and knowledge that primary physicians should possess in order to meet the health needs of women. In November 1991, an ad hoc committee within the AMWA drafted a women's health curriculum. In 1992, the AMWA formulated its vision of designing and offering practicing physicians an Advanced Curriculum in Women's Health, in order to improve and integrate the care of women patients, to increase physicians' awareness of the psychosocial aspects of women's treatment, to improve the physician–patient partnership, and to increase physicians' understanding of the differences and unique qualities of women's health.

It was the consensus of physicians attending an AMWA-sponsored retreat of 17 medical specialty societies in August 1992 that a comprehensive and multidisciplinary curriculum should be developed around the life phases of the woman. The life phase structure was felt to be more "organic" and unique to women than a division by specialties, diseases, or organ systems. The curriculum was divided into five modules: early years (birth to 18), young adulthood (19–39), midlife (40–64), mature years (65–79), and advanced years (80 and beyond). Nine content areas were addressed to varying degrees in each module: sexuality and reproduction; women and society; health maintenance and wellness; violence and abuse; mental health and substance abuse; transition and changes; the patient–physician partnership; normal female physiology; and abnormal female physiology, including diagnosis and management of conditions common to each age group.

In 1994, the National Academy on Women's Health Medical Education (NAWHME), cosponsored by the AMWA and the Medical College of Pennsylvania, was organized. The mission of the NAWHME is to infuse women's health into all levels of medical education, including medical school curricula, graduate specialty training programs, and continuing medical education (CME) for physicians. The NAWHME consists of five major groups: directors of existing women's health medical education programs, educators with experience with gender-related education, representatives of advocacy groups in women's health, members of medical professional organizations concerned with women's health, and representatives of regulatory bodies. At the request of the Federated Council for Internal Medicine, the NAWHME has created a list of competencies (knowledge and skills) that an internist must possess in order to meet the health needs of a woman patient. There is now an effort to include questions about women's health on the certifying exam for boards of internal medicine, and such efforts may spread to other specialty boards as well.

MODEL TRAINING APPROACHES AND MEDICAL SCHOOL CURRICULA

Of the three levels of medical education (medical school, graduate specialty training, and postgraduate CME) that the NAWHME has targeted for promotion of information about women's health, the medical school curriculum and the graduate specialty training have been slower to change than the postgraduate CME. Medical educators have developed examples of how a traditional medical school curriculum (structured by departments) can be enriched by inclusion of knowledge specific to women's health. For instance, lactation can be included in the course on physiology; the composition of human milk can be included in the course on biochemistry and immunology; and detection of signs of domestic violence can be included in the course on physical examination.

Another approach to training in women's health is based on a conviction that women's health is multidisciplinary. For instance, a comprehensive symposium on breast cancer should involve interlocking presentations by an anatomist, a physiologist, a pathologist, a biochemist, an internist, a surgeon, a radiologist, a geneticist, a psychiatrist, and a social worker. Medical students and physicians should learn from all these specialists. Women's health is a superordinate discipline that calls for a team approach and for the integration of psychosocial information and skills with biomedical knowledge.

In addition to the systematic program in women's health at the Medical College of Pennsylvania, which runs through all 4 years of medical school, there are efforts at the University of Miami Medical School to develop women's health as a rotation slot in the third year (obligatory) and fourth year (elective). In these programs, medical students attend special lectures and clinics at both attached and free-standing women's health centers. In several other medical schools (e.g., Cornell University Medical College, University of Pennsylvania School of Medicine), electives on women's health have been organized by medical students and sometimes encouraged by their faculty advisors. These electives are very popular with men and women medical students alike, and are well attended for academic (elective) credit.

In some medical institutions (University of Pittsburgh and University of Pennsylvania School of Medicine), the departments of epidemiology have become the administrative home for the fledgling women's health programs. In New York City, the Columbia University College of Physicians and Surgeons has recently embarked on a Partnership for Women's Health, a global project coordinating research, clinical, and educational activities at all levels of medical education. The Uniformed Services University of the Health Sciences also contemplates inclusion of women's health into the curricula within the next few years. The NAWHME has published a resource guide that helps faculty members to introduce women's health in their medical schools. The resource guide includes a list of opportunities to teach women's health, samples of curricula that are available, lists of competencies in women's health, and a list of available resources.

GRADUATE AND POSTGRADUATE TRAINING

The next level of improvement in training has been the introduction of women's health into graduate education—the training of residents and fellows in various specialties. There are now approximately a dozen residencies and fellowships in women's health in the United States, and Canada based in internal medicine and in family medicine. The Office of Women's Health in the Office of the Deputy Assistant Secretary of Health of the U.S. Department of Health and Human Services is developing a directory of women's health academic programs in the United States.

At the postgraduate (CME) level, there are numerous conferences and courses in women's health targeted at physicians. The most systematic and comprehensive of these courses is the AMWA's Advanced Curriculum on Women's Health, given in 1993 and 1994; in March 1998, an updated Advanced Curriculum on Women's Health will be presented to international audiences in Florida. The interest in the CME courses is being generated by the growth of women's health centers, which have sprouted both inside and outside the traditional teaching medical centers in the aftermath of the publicity accorded to the 1990 congressional hearings.

Women's health is currently fashionable. The label attracts women patients to clinics that may be little more than gynecology clinics dressed up with mammography and bone density measurement equipment. It cannot be emphasized too strongly that women's health is a comprehensive discipline; accordingly, a woman's health clinic should be directed by a generalist (internist or family physician), with services available from a gynecologist, a psychiatrist, an exercise and nutrition specialist, a nurse, and a nurse practitioner. It is in such an environment that medical students and residents can learn, and clinicians can relearn, women's health.

FURTHER READING

Harrison, M. (1992). Women's health as a specialty: A deceptive solution. *Journal of Women's Health, 1,* 101.
A reply to Johnson (see below): Described why establishment of a specialty of women's health would be injurious to women.

Johnson, K. (1992). Women's health: Developing a new interdisciplinary specialty. *Journal of Women's Health, 1,* 95–100.
Describes why establishment of a specialty of women's health is needed.

National Academy on Women's Health Medical Education (NAWHME). (1996). *Women's health in the curriculum: A resource guide for faculty: Undergraduate, residency, and continuing education.* Compiled and edited by G. D. Donoghue with the participants of NAWHME. Philadelphia: Medical College of Pennsylvania and Hahnemann University.
Important compilation of aids and tools in teaching women's health in medical schools, graduate programs, and continuing education. Emphasizes how to make the most of the opportunities and how to overcome resistance. Also includes a list of competencies in women's health, a directory of

academic programs in women's health with sample curricula, pertinent facts, bibliography, addresses, and telephone numbers.

Symonds, A. (1980). Women's liberation: Effects on physician–patient relationship. *New York State Journal of Medicine, 80,* 211–214.
Seminal paper on changes in the physician–patient relationship (as of 1980), as well as changes still needed.

Wallis, L. A. (1982). The patient as a partner in the pelvic exam. *Female Patient, 7,* 3662–3667.
Describes the assumption of true partnership by the patient in her pelvic examination.

Wallis, L. A. (Senior Author and Editor-in-Chief). (1996). *Modern breast and pelvic examinations: A handbook for health professionals* (4th ed.). New York: National Council for Women In Medicine.
Detailed description of painless, sensitive, and competent examinations of the breast and pelvis, compatible with total emancipation of women.

Wallis, L. A., & Jacobson, J. S. (1984). The hundred years are up. *Journal of the American Medical Women's Association, 39,* 59–62.
Emphasizes that there is no excuse for the pelvic exam to be painful, insensitive, or uncomfortable.

Wallis, L. A., & Klass, P. (1990). Toward improving women's health care. *Journal of the American Medical Women's Association, 45,* 219–221.
Describes the inequality and inappropriateness of the health care provided to women.

50

Substance Abuse
and Health Care Utilization

Jacqueline Wallen

HOW SUBSTANCE ABUSE AFFECTS
WOMEN'S USE OF HEALTH CARE

Throughout most of their lives, women visit their physicians more frequently than men do. This difference is particularly marked in women between 25 and 44 years of age (the childbearing years). Women who have substance abuse problems, or who have family members with substance abuse problems, have higher rates of health care utilization than women who are not affected by substance abuse problems. That is, women who abuse alcohol or drugs use more health care services than those who do not, both for themselves and for their children; furthermore, women whose partners have substance abuse problems also have higher rates of health care utilization, even if they themselves do not abuse alcohol or drugs.

Women with substance abuse problems also have higher mortality rates than women in the general population. Frequent causes of death include suicide, accidents, cirrhosis of the liver, cardiovascular disorders, and malignancies. Though only a small minority of women with substance abuse problems ever receive specialized treatment for these problems, almost all encounter the health care system for other reasons. When women who abuse alcohol or drugs seek health care for problems related to their own or their children's health, they rarely report that they also have a substance abuse problem. They are more likely to report such symptoms as digestive problems, anxiety, insomnia, or depression. It is important for primary care physicians and other health care personnel to be aware of indicators of substance abuse in women, and to be able to make appropriate referrals for women who show signs of substance abuse.

THE RELATION OF SUBSTANCE ABUSE
TO OTHER HEALTH PROBLEMS

Alcohol and drugs may be factors in a large number of emergency room visits for accidental injuries, sexual assault, or domestic violence. Substance abuse is among the highest-ranking risk factors for suicide in women, and women who abuse alcohol and other drugs (particularly younger women) are more likely than other women to attempt suicide. According to the Office of Applied Studies of the Substance Abuse and Mental Health Services Administration, more than half of the drug-related suicide attempts seen in emergency rooms and reported to the system in 1992 were made by women, and more women than men died in drug-related suicides.

A large proportion of women who abuse alcohol or drugs have concomitant psychiatric conditions. This may be because the substance abuse results in psychiatric symptoms, such as anxiety, depression, or psychosis; or it may be because women with psychiatric conditions use alcohol or drugs to reduce painful feelings associated with their psychiatric disorders. Sometimes both processes are operating to reinforce each other. The most common psychiatric conditions in drug- and alcohol-addicted women who seek psychiatric care are anxiety disorders (including phobias and panic disorder) and mood disorders (particularly depression). Rates of substance abuse are also high in women with schizophrenia and other psychoses.

Women who seek help for obstetrical and gynecological problems have also been found to have a higher rate of substance abuse than the general female population. It is difficult to determine the extent to which such problems result from heavy alcohol or drug use, as opposed to preceding (and perhaps contributing to) substance abuse. Whatever the direction of causality, this is an important association, since substance abuse may worsen reproductive problems even if it did not originally cause them. Women with substance abuse problems are also overrepresented among women seeking help for sexual dysfunction. Again, it is difficult to distinguish sexual dysfunction caused by substance abuse from sexual dysfunction that is a result of substance abuse. Many women report that they feel less sexually inhibited after drinking, and women's use of alcohol and drugs has been found to be associated with nontraditional sexual behavior, such as premarital sex or cohabitation. The connection between sexual abuse and reduced sexual inhibition is particularly important in light of the AIDS epidemic.

Children born to substance-abusing mothers often have lower-than-normal birth-weights; as a result, they may have longer hospital stays at birth and higher-than-average hospital costs. A number of birth defects, including fetal alcohol syndrome, are also thought to be associated with maternal alcohol and drug use during pregnancy.

SCREENING AND REFERRAL
FOR SUBSTANCE ABUSE PROBLEMS

Though it is important for health care providers to be sensitive to the possibility of substance abuse problems in women using health care and to refer women appropriately for treatment, substance abuse problems are significantly underdiagnosed in health care settings. Some research suggests that physicians may be less effective in identifying substance abuse in women than in men. This reflects the fact that women, even more than men, may be reluctant to report alcohol or drug problems to their physicians.

Women substance abusers are viewed especially negatively in society and may be ashamed to identify themselves as such. In some cases they may fear losing custody of their children. Also, women who are abusing alcohol or drugs may not see this as their main problem. Instead, they may see it as a response to other problems, such as depression, stress, work conflicts, medical problems, or relationship problems, and may report those other problems to their physicians instead.

Even when women report symptoms that are strong indicators of substance abuse, or when they are admitted to the hospital for medical complications related to substance abuse (e.g., pancreatitis or a withdrawal seizure), the underlying substance abuse problem often remains undiagnosed. Physicians and other health care professionals may fail to identify substance abuse problems in women because they are reluctant to assign them a stigmatizing diagnosis. Often, however, they simply do not recognize the problem. Physicians and other health care providers typically receive very little training in how to detect substance abuse problems. Even when they suspect an underlying substance abuse problem, health care providers may refrain from discussing it because they lack knowledge about how to work with substance-abusing patients or feel that there is little that can be done to help substance abusers. Indeed, they may view substance abusers negatively and consider them difficult patients.

Because women's substance abuse patterns differ from those of men, techniques used to screen substance abuse problems in men may fail to detect problems in women. For example, a woman with a drinking problem may drink less frequently and in smaller amounts than most men; consequently, her alcoholism may go undetected by measurement tools that stress quantity and frequency of drinking. Her alcoholism may remain undetected even though moderate alcohol use in a woman can result in blood alcohol concentrations and negative health effects similar to those experienced by a male who consumed alcohol heavily, especially if she is also using or abusing a prescription drug. Most screening instruments are based on male norms and may stress negative consequences of alcohol or drug use that are more common in men than in women. Women are less likely to report behavioral consequences of alcohol and drug abuse (e.g., money problems, unsafe driving, or trouble with the police) and more apt to report psychological or interpersonal problems (e.g., depression, arguments/fights with family and friends). Such commonly used assessment tools as the Michigan Alcoholism Screening Test and the MacAndrew Alcoholism Scale, the norms for which are based primarily on male responses, may provide inconsistent and inconclusive results when used with women. The Addiction Severity Index (ASI) is another commonly used instrument that omits questions about factors that may be related to alcoholism in women, such as sexual abuse or assault, reproductive dysfunction, or sexual issues. The ASI, however, was originally developed with female as well as male subjects; therefore, it may be more reliable and valid when used with women than some of the other instruments may be, especially when it is used by a sensitive, trained interviewer familiar with women's substance abuse issues.

Problems frequently reported by substance-abusing women themselves include salience of the substance (the substance becomes more important than other aspects of life), belligerence, and health problems. Some research suggests that physicians may learn more about whether drinking or drugs constitute a problem by exploring women's feelings about their use of substances than by attempting to determine the quantity and frequency of use. It is also important to recognize that prescribed sedatives may combine with moderate amounts of alcohol to have major effects on women's health and functioning.

To help patients with substance abuse problems, health care providers must be familiar with the different kinds of treatment resources that are available. These include detoxification, rehabilitation, outpatient substance abuse treatment, medical or psychiatric hospitalization, outpatient psychiatric treatment, and peer support programs such as Alcoholics Anonymous. The appropriate referral for a woman patient with substance abuse problems depends on a number of factors, including the types of treatment options available in the community, the severity of the substance abuse problem, the presence or absence of a psychiatric disorder, previous treatment experience, motivation, family and social support, and the patient's financial and other resources. It can be helpful to suggest consultation with an addiction counselor or an addiction treatment specialist if the patient is hospitalized.

FURTHER READING

Gomberg, E. S. L. (1995). Risk factors for drinking over a woman's life span. *Alcohol Health and Research World, 18,* 220–227.
A review of factors that increase the likelihood of alcohol problems in women.

Lex, B. W. (1995). Alcohol and other drug abuse among women. *Alcohol Health and Research World, 18,* 212–219.
A discussion of health consequences of women's use of alcohol and drugs.

Miller, N. S., & Gold, M. S. (1991). Dual diagnoses: Psychiatric syndromes in alcoholism and drug addiction. *American Family Physician, 43,* 2071–2076.
A discussion of mental health correlates of alcohol and drug problems.

Office of Applied Studies. (1994). *Annual emergency room data 1992.* Rockville, MD: Substance Abuse and Mental Health Services Administration.
An annual publication that presents reasons for emergency room admissions in a national sample of hospitals.

Wilke, D. (1994). Women and alcoholism: How a male-as-norm bias affects research, assessment, and treatment. *Health and Social Work, 19,* 29–35.
A discussion of gender bias in alcoholism treatment and research.

Wilsnack, S. C. (1990). Alcohol abuse and alcoholism. Extent of the problem. In R. Engs (Ed.), *Women: Alcohol and other drugs* (pp. 17–30). Dubuque, IA: Kendall/Hunt.
A report on the epidemiology of women's alcohol and drug use.

Wilsnack, S. C., Klassen, A. D., Schur, B. E., & Wilsnack, R. W. (1991). Predicting onset and chronicity of women's problem drinking: A five-year longitudinal analysis. *American Journal of Public Health, 81,* 305–318.
A review of factors that increase the likelihood of alcohol problems in women.

51

School-Based Clinics

Mary Lou Balassone

School-based and school-linked health clinics constitute an important health care delivery mechanism for adolescents. Since the opening of the first such clinic in 1970, there has been steady growth in both the numbers and types of health and mental health services offered in these settings in the United States. Today over 230 clinics operate in school settings in 32 states. This chapter provides an overview of the needs of medically underserved female adolescents; the organization and operation of school-based clinics; the services provided, clients served, and problems seen in these clinics; and the results of evaluations of the clinics' effectiveness.

ADOLESCENTS' NEED FOR CLINICS

Data from a variety of sources suggest that adolescents' health needs are not being met. As a group, teenagers are fairly healthy; however, morbidity and mortality figures for this age group have worsened over the last 20 years. Increases in accidents, suicides, sexually transmitted diseases, pregnancies, and drug use can be traced to the increased environmental and social risks faced by teenagers. In addition, adolescents often lack access to a regular source of health care. Some teenagers have difficulty getting care because of financial difficulties and lack of insurance, but other barriers also play a role. These barriers include concerns about confidentiality, lack of knowledge about exactly where to get needed health care, lack of transportation, and having to miss school (or parents' having to miss work) to get care. For young women, concerns about privacy and parental permission often create a substantial barrier to reproductive health care.

School-based clinics were established to increase teenagers' access to primary health care and to address important social problems, such as pregnancy, school dropout, and drug use. School-based clinics offer services in a convenient and familiar setting by a staff trained to work with adolescents. There is usually no cost associated with clinic visits; transportation, parental involvement, and missed school do not pose barriers. Privacy is also better assured, since young women can use any of the clinic services (including reproductive health care) once an overall parental permission form has been signed.

Baseline surveys of students prior to opening a clinic offer clues as to the range of unmet health needs faced by adolescents. Typical among the problems cited by students in one such survey (in descending order of frequency) were general feelings of sickness; headaches, stomachaches, and backaches; stress; injuries; vision problems; weight problems; allergies; fainting; hearing problems; pregnancy, sexually transmitted diseases; and physical or sexual abuse.

CLINIC ORGANIZATION AND OPERATION

Most clinics are located on high school grounds, although some serve middle school and junior high students. A smaller number of clinics are "school-linked," meaning that the clinic provides services to a particular school's student body, but the site of the clinic is not on school grounds. Each school-based clinic has a team of health and mental health professionals who provide care. Although the makeup of this team varies, it generally includes a nurse practitioner, a part-time physician, a social worker, a health educator, and a medical assistant or receptionist. Other types of staff members, including a nutritionist, a dentist, a psychologist, and a school nurse, may also be part of the team.

As the number of school-based clinics has grown, so have the combinations of administrative sponsorship and funding supporting them. Commonly, school-based clinics are operated by public health departments, medical schools, and voluntary nonprofit organizations, with funding from a variety of private foundations (e.g., Robert Wood Johnson, Ford) and public dollars (e.g., city and county governments, federal block grants for maternal and child health). This means that administrative responsibility and medical practice liability for such a clinic reside outside the school, and the clinic operates independently of school law. One result of this arrangement is that a broader range of health services can be offered than those typically offered by a school nurse. Young women's access to reproductive health care is enhanced by this arrangement. This sponsorship relationship also requires a strong link between school administration and the clinic sponsor. Support from school personnel is integral to the successful operation of the clinic and to the clinic's receiving referrals from teachers and other members of the school staff. In addition, schools often provide in-kind support (e.g., physical space, clerical help, and supplies).

SERVICES PROVIDED BY CLINICS

Most clinics began with a focus on providing primary health care services, but a need for mental health care was soon recognized. Now both health and mental health services are typically offered. Clinics offer the following services: primary health care; diagnosis and treatment of injuries and illnesses; laboratory tests; health and nutrition education; pregnancy, contraceptive, and HIV/AIDS counseling; mental health counseling; immunizations; weight reduction programs; prenatal care; drug abuse counseling; and assessment and referral to community services. Some of the first clinics to be established focused on the need to decrease unwanted pregnancies among young women. These clinics provide access to education about contraception and pregnancy, as well as a range of gynecological services for adolescent women.

TYPES OF CLIENTS SERVED AND PROBLEMS SEEN

School-based clinics tend to serve low-income adolescents. Most teenagers served are between the ages of 14 and 19 years, and their racial and ethnic backgrounds tend to mirror those found in the community where a school is located. A majority of school-based clinics are in schools that are located in urban areas and have a large percentage of low-income, minority youths. All clinics require parental consent to enroll students for clinic use, and the rate of enrollment varies across clinics. Typically, over half of the student body enrolls; the vast majority of these (80%) actually use clinic services. Female students are more likely than males to use the clinic for both health and mental health care. Data from a variety of clinics also show a range in the amount of usage by students. Although the majority of students use the clinic fewer than 3 times a year, a substantial subgroup use it a great deal (more than 15 visits a year). In addition, young women tend to be more frequent users of school-based clinics than young men.

Data from clinics vary in terms of the reported reasons why students use clinic services. One fairly typical clinic in Washington State reported the following reasons for clinic visits in 1991 (in descending order of frequency): respiratory infection, drug or alcohol problem, dermatology concern, injury, reproductive health concern, sexually transmitted disease, nutritional deficiency, family conflict, allergy, blood disorder, depression, urinary tract infection, hypertension, gastrointestinal problem, neurological problem, sexual abuse/assault, suicide risk, and physical abuse or neglect.

EFFECTIVENESS OF CLINICS

There have been several studies of the impact of a school-based clinic on various adolescent problem behaviors (i.e., unwanted pregnancy, drug use, school dropout, sexual behavior, and contraceptive use). Unfortunately, well-designed and scientifically sound evaluations of school-based clinics have not been reported extensively in the literature. A couple of well-designed studies have found that the presence of a school-based clinic does not result in school-wide health status changes; that is, reduced pregnancy rate, fewer emergency room visits, and reduced drug use are not associated with the presence of a clinic. However, studies comparing users of clinics to nonusers have shown positive results for the adolescents who use the clinic. Increased use of contraceptives, fewer pregnancies, reduced drug use, fewer absences, and reduced dropout rates have all been reported.

Other studies have focused not only on clinic use rates among students, but on parent and student satisfaction with clinic services. In general, school-based clinics are given highly positive ratings by both students and parents. Students report receiving the help they need, finding the staff members understanding and respectful, and feeling that their privacy and confidentiality are maintained. Most clinics report that about half of the school's student body actually uses the clinic for health and mental health care, and that high-risk students tend to be more frequent users. Students also tend to report that getting health and mental health care is easier with a school-based clinic. Thus, it appears that these clinics have had substantial success in preventing and treating a range of adolescent problems. However, scarce financial resources and opposition to school-based clinics by conservative groups may make it difficult for these clinics to continue. Active community involvement and support by health care professionals can help ensure the viability of this service model for adolescent women.

FURTHER READING

Balassone, M. L., Bell, M., & Peterfreund, N. (1991). A comparison of users and nonusers of a school-based health and mental health clinic. *Journal of Adolescent Health, 12,* 240–246.
Study compares student health and mental health knowledge, behavior, and access to services for adolescents who used and did not use a school-based clinic. Presents data on the high-risk psychosocial issues reported by clinic users.

Dryfoos, J. (1988). School-based health clinics: Three years of experience. *Family Planning Perspectives, 20,* 193–200.
Provides a summary of school-based clinic programs, services, and clients across the United States. Summarizes information on the organization and funding of these clinics as well as the minimal program evaluation data available at the time.

Hyche-Williams, J., & Waszak, C. (1990). *School-based clinics: 1990.* Washington, DC: Center for Population Options.
Summarizes information on school-based clinics in operation in 1990. Information on program services, students served, funding, program structure, and organization of various clinics is provided.

Kirby, D., Resnick, M. D., Downes, B., Kocher, T., Gunderson, P., Potthoff, S., Zelterman, D., & Blum, R. W. (1993). The effects of school-based health clinics in St. Paul on school-wide birthrates. *Planning Perspectives, 25,* 12–16.
Reports on pregnancy related outcomes for the earliest school-based clinics to open in the United States. Summarizes data on birthrates before and after opening of school-based clinics in St. Paul.

Kirby, D., Waszak, C., & Ziegler, J. (1989). *An assessment of six school-based clinics: Services, impact and potential.* Washington, DC: Center for Population Options.
Book presents a vast amount of information on six school-based clinics. Chapters cover research methodology, community and clinic summaries, clinic utilization data, the impact of clinics on medical care utilization, the impact of the clinics on pregnancy prevention and risk-taking behaviors, and strategies for improving clinic services.

Kirby, D., Waszak, C., & Ziegler, J. (1991). Six school-based clinics: Their reproductive health services and impact on sexual behavior. *Family Planning Perspectives, 23,* 6–16.
Reports on the evaluation of reproductive health services in six school-based clinics. Reviews the influence of the clinics on student sexual behavior and contraceptive use.

Waszak, C., & Neidell, S. (1991). *School-based and school-linked clinics: Update 1991.* Washington, DC: Center for Population Options.
Summarizes information on school-based and school-linked clinics in operation in the United States. Information on program services, students served, and program organization is provided.

52

Worksite Nicotine Treatment

Marlene M. Maheu

*T*his chapter describes recent trends in worksite health promotion programs for women. Nicotine treatment programs are the primary examples discussed here, but many if not most of the points made are applicable to other types of health promotion programs as well.

ADVANTAGES OF WORKSITE PROGRAMS

Despite many studies examining workplace nicotine cessation and other health promotion programs, there is a distinct lack of information specifically related to meeting the diverse needs of working women. This void in the research literature is significant, because worksites have great potential to reach employed women in a familiar setting, where they congregate on a daily basis throughout their working years. The convenience of worksites is unparalleled. There is no other locale where large numbers of women spend much of their waking day. The varied composition of the work force results in programs' being accessible to many different groups simultaneously. Many worksites also address the pragmatic issue of having large rooms to accommodate large numbers of people.

Worksites offer other advantages over clinics as well. Since worksites are daily environments, learned skills (e.g., practicing relaxation techniques prior to meetings) are likely to generalize to other daily situations. A visible worksite program can provide a multitude of cues for behavior change, as well as maintenance of that change through social support. It is also important to consider organizational and environmental changes that warrant as much attention as those directed at promoting individual change. Worksite programs that are supported by management, union, or employee groups can help create acceptance and financial support for programs that may not otherwise be accessible to employees. Worksite groups provide incentives for positive, health-related behavior change. Moreover, there is a high probability that such programs will be considered a benefit by employees.

In addition, workplaces offer such advantages as efficient information dissemination through preestablished formal and informal communication channels. Preestablished hierarchies can easily be used to enforce no-smoking policies and other restrictions.

Finally, worksite health promotion is an important component of a community-wide approach and lends itself well to long-term research because of fairly stable populations at the workplace.

REPORTED FINDINGS OF WORKSITE RESEARCH

Despite the methodological problems associated with much worksite research, several findings do appear relevant. There seems to be greater overall success when programs address multiple risk factors (e.g., weight control, hypertension, exercise, smoking, etc.) rather than single risk factors (e.g., only smoking). Worksite programs making use of behavioral strategies and incentives have shown greater changes than less intensive programs, such as simple interviews or educational interventions. Research based on the theory of "stages of change" in smoking cessation has shown that women and men may use differing percentages of change processes to stop smoking successfully, but that the overall effects of these differences are equal. However, basic research is still needed on the general effects of gender on the stages, as well as how the stages are manifested in nicotine cessation.

PROGRAMMING SUGGESTIONS

Given the severity of health issues related to smoking cessation and other problem behaviors, attention to the specific issues differentiating women from one another is critical. Not only do women need to be viewed as having their own issues separate from men's; they need to be seen as a heterogeneous group with very different needs. Tailoring programs to meet these needs is the job of their health care providers. Legislators and the researchers they fund must seriously examine how women of all ages and racial/cultural groups, and with various health-related problems, can be optimally served within their own environments.

Programs for women must address such concerns as menstrual cycle effects. For instance, women who are trying to stop smoking may experience more severe withdrawal symptoms from nicotine during the premenstrual phase of their cycles. Such women may need extra support to be successful during this time, and workplaces can be especially conducive to offering this support. Child care services, flexible hours, "comp" time, and lunchtime seminars are various ways employers can address the needs of their female employees who smoke. These circumstances sometimes create "teachable moments" for women smokers. For example, new mothers may be highly motivated to quit; employers of large worksites can offer specialized classes for pregnant women and new mothers, even if these classes are small. Even self-help materials designed for pregnant women in a single brief session have been shown to be successful.

Employers can also make pharmaceutical products available for their female employees by negotiating for their coverage by company insurance carriers. In the case of smoking cessation, the most widely used medications are nicotine replacement products—nicotine gum (Nicorette) and the transdermal nicotine patch, now over the counter. All have been proven effective when prescribed and used correctly in the context of a behavioral change program. Some medical practitioners combine the use of these two products for problematic smokers. Research is also supporting the future use of a nicotine nasal spray (which mimics the fast rise time of plasma nicotine from smoking) and a nicotine inhaler (a cigarette-like nicotine product).

Other medications can be used for the successful treatment of women smokers who are allergic to nicotine replacement products, or who have a condition contraindicating their use (e.g., pregnancy, recent heart attack or stroke). Some medications can act as supplements to treat time-limited withdrawal symptoms or can be used to treat a psychiatric condition (e.g., depression). Much remains to be learned about the specific uses of various medications. For example, one study found nicotine gum to be more effective in men than in women; another study found the opposite for clonidine. Cultural and workplace factors supporting smoking abstinence and other self-care behaviors are also likely to be influential in generating gender differences. The specific composition of a worksite's employee population must be examined in detail before optimal programming can be designed for that worksite.

THE BOTTOM LINE

Accomplishing successful health care delivery at the worksite must make financial sense to employers. Programs must show a return on their investment, and programmers must be willing to provide written outcome measures to employers. In such a report, cost-effectiveness projections can be used to demonstrate direct savings for each successful graduate of a program. (Cost effectiveness estimates for worksite nicotine treatment programs range from $200 to $2,000 of savings per year, per employee.)

In a good outcome report, employers can be prompted for other ways to improve the health and welfare of their employees. Suggestions can range from including fruit, yogurt, fat-free health bars, or fruit juices in vending machines to holding health fairs in company parking lots. Health fairs involve a range of health care providers' setting up booths and offering free services and information, such as blood pressure screening, chiropractic exams, cholesterol tests, and smoking cessation materials. Employers can also be encouraged to set up small committees to support such events as the National Lung Association's "Great American Smokeout" every November. Female members of such a committee can be encouraged to choose materials that will be particularly relevant to the groups they represent (older women, women of color, pregnant women, managers, staff, etc.).

As noted earlier, worksites can maximize the impact of their efforts by offering multitargeted health care services, such as cardiovascular risk reduction programs addressing weight management, exercise, smoking, blood pressure, and cholesterol. Studies suggest that packaged services are more successful in convincing individuals to incorporate other self-care behaviors with time. The model underlying such an approach is called "harm reduction theory." This model reflects the view that individuals must be approached in a way they find useful. If they are satisfied with the services, rapport with the provider allows for the introduction of yet another self-care behavior.

UTILIZING RESOURCES OF THE FITNESS INDUSTRY AS EXTENSIONS OF THE WORKPLACE

The fitness industry has recently shown a keen interest in offering smoking cessation and other health care services. Some fitness facilities offer cardiovascular risk appraisal, stress management, and more traditional medical and psychological services. It is easier for a fitness club to provide a room to a physician or psychologist for an afternoon each week than for physicians to equip themselves with aerobic and weight training facilities. Fitness clubs usually have the largest dollar investment in preventive health care equipment, as well as the largest square footage of all preventive health care facilities. As a result, it is only reasonable to find fitness organizations recruiting employers to their facilities for "one-stop shopping" in preventive health care.

Employers can benefit from the tendency for people to establish rapport with a multiservice, multipurpose staff by encouraging employees to attend company-sponsored individual and family events at the local fitness club. Employers can easily negotiate for discounted rates and can insist that their insurance policies cover additional services offered by licensed health care providers working within the fitness facility. Whether these sites are called "wellness centers" or "gyms," centralizing services can benefit employers in a number of ways:

1. Employees gain access to services in a neutral location, close to but not at the worksite, which offers increased confidentiality.

2. Attendance at a fitness club is seen as an "elite" activity, rather than one that is easily stigmatized; this frees employees of the fear of ostracism or ridicule if an entire group of coworkers sees them walking over to the counseling office.

3. Many fitness clubs are already equipped with full-service day care services for low or no fees.

4. Some fitness clubs, such as YMCAs, offer discounted rates to new members who cannot afford the usual sign-up fees.

5. While attending a blood pressure screening, HIV testing, or cholesterol check up at a fitness facility, employees are exposed to the gym and staff, who can also be offering 10-minute tours of the facility and programs. At these times, employees can be encouraged to participate in other club activities.

6. Some fitness clubs have multiple sites throughout adjoining geographic areas. Arranging reciprocal services can allow clubs to accommodate a working mom who wants to pick up her children from school and stop in at the gym in her own neighborhood on the way home. Facility sharing is an optimal way for a mother who lives within commuting distance either to attend an aerobics class down the street from her job during a lunch break or to attend such a class in her neighborhood gym affiliate on Saturday mornings. If these facilities can also be educated about offering support groups for women who are trying to stop smoking or change other harmful behaviors, health maintenance strategies can be maximized, and costs can be kept to a minimum.

THE NEED FOR SPECIFIC RESEARCH

Researchers must be able to offer employers feasible and efficient nicotine treatment and other health promotion programs. Many areas of programming for women are still in need of empirical research. These include the following:

1. Effects of subtargeted programs directed toward the specific needs and concerns of women with differing occupations, women with various psychiatric condi-

tions (depressed vs. anxious vs. psychotic), pregnant women, younger women, alcoholic and/or drug-addicted women, older women, and other high-risk female populations.

2. Optimal worksite smoking and substance use policy formation and program implementation timelines.

3. Optimal programming of worksite and fitness facilities to meet the specific needs of various cultural and racial groups.

4. Detection of pharmacological response differences among different subgroups of women.

5. Long-term effectiveness of medication with appetite-suppressing effects and of social support for women concerned with weight gain.

6. Methods of assisting women with postpartum abstinence from nicotine and other self-care behaviors.

7. Effects of allowing former smokers to continue taking "smoke breaks," but to use the time to meet and discuss weight management or stress management techniques throughout the day.

8. The impact of lunchtime seminars (on smoking cessation, weight management, stress management, etc.).

9. Effects of offering "healthy alternatives" (e.g., fruit, fruit juices, or yogurt) in vending machines.

10. The most effective form of governmental legislation supporting worksite bans on smoking and tobacco chewing, as well as other substance use.

11. Ways of reaching to access women in managerial positions versus staff positions, and tailoring programs specifically for their respective schedules and pressures.

12. Measurement of program satisfaction in both managerial and staff groups.

13. Impact of developing "worksite steering committees" to design programs within the workplace.

14. Gender differences in the "stages of change" as related to race, culture, class, psychiatric diagnosis, and occupational subgroups.

15. Effects of targeting the worksite environment itself at the organizational and managerial levels, rather than just individuals, on the long-term effectiveness of individual programs.

FURTHER READING

Chadwick, J. H. (1982). Health behavior change at the worksite: A problem oriented analysis. In R. S. Parkinson & Associates, *Managing health promotion in the workplace: Guidelines for implementation and evaluation* (pp. 144–161). Palo Alto, CA: Mayfield.
Seminal chapter on worksite health promotion programming.

Cohen, W. S. (1985). Health promotion in the workplace. *American Psychologist, 40*(2), 213–216.
Well-organized article detailing the advantages of workplace health promotion programs.

Gilbert, D. G. (1995). Gender differences in tobacco use and effects. In C. D. Spielberger (Ed.), *Smoking: Individual differences, psychopathology, and emotion* (pp. 177–191). Washington, DC: Taylor & Francis.
Explanation of current research on the effects of smoking on emotion.

Gomel, M., Oldenburg, B., Simpson, J. M., & Owen, N. (1993). Work-site cardiovascular risk reduction: A randomized trial of health risk assessment, education, counseling, and incentives. *American Journal of Public Health, 83*(9), 1231–1238.
Explanation of how worksite nicotine treatment programming can be successfully incorporated into an overall cardiovascular risk reduction program at the worksite.

Hatsukami, D., Skoog, K., Allen, S., & Bliss, R. (1995). Gender and the effects of different doses of nicotine gum on tobacco withdrawal symptoms. *Experimental and Clinical Psychopharmacology, 3*(2), 163–173.
Examines the role of gender in nicotine replacement therapy.

Maheu, M. M. (1989). Competition/cooperation in worksite smoking cessation using nicotine gum. *Preventive Medicine, 18,* 867–876.
Article describing the use of competition to increase recruitment and success rates of worksite nicotine treatment programming.

O'Connor, E. A., Carbonari, J. P., & DiClemente, C. C. (1996). Gender and smoking cessation: A factor structure comparison of processes of change. *Journal of Consulting and Clinical Psychology, 64*(1), 130–138.
Gender-related issues and their impact upon the stages of change.

Pomerleau, C. S., Kurth, C. L., & Pomerleau, O. F. (in press). An association between binge-eating and "weight-control" smoking in women smokers. *Journal of Smoking-Related Disorders.*
Smoking and its complicated relationship to weight are examined in great detail by a group of knowledgeable and thorough researchers.

53

The Military and Health

Penny F. Pierce

> One of the lessons we've learned from Operation Desert Storm
> is the extent to which the nation accepted the significant role
> of women in the operation. Until then, there had always been
> a concern that having women involved in combat would be
> traumatic for the country.
> —*Pete Williams, spokesman for the U.S. Secretary
> of Defense*, The Washington Post, *June 16, 1991*

*I*n the United States, women in uniform were dramatically pushed to the forefront of national attention in 1990–1991, with the mass media coverage of Operations Desert Shield and Desert Storm in the Persian Gulf War. Just as women had done in previous military conflicts, they answered the call to duty and fulfilled their responsibilities as they were trained. In each branch of the service, women were involved in all aspects of the operation—driving supply trucks into Kuwait; flying helicopters, cargo planes, and reconnaissance aircraft; commanding units in combat support missions; and retaining enemy prisoners of war. It hardly escaped attention that for the first time in U.S. history women were deployed in large numbers. Indeed, Desert Storm was the largest deployment of U.S. military women to date: 40,793 women served in the Persian Gulf, where 17 lost their lives and 3 became prisoners of war. Many women left young children and served alongside their male counterparts in both traditional and nontraditional jobs, under extreme environmental conditions and against an unpredictable enemy.

The participation of U.S. women in the Gulf War has significantly changed all branches of service, where women now constitute 11% of the active-duty military and 13% of the reserve forces. Subsequent changes in the Federal Code now permit Air Force and Navy women to fly in combat aircraft, and women are being integrated into previously male-dominated Navy ships. These experiences and changes are raising an assortment of questions about women's participation in military service and the effects of wartime military service on their physical and emotional health. Research has begun to answer some of these questions, but to date more have been asked than answered. This chapter discusses two major issues: the effects of wartime stressors and the gender-specific health concerns of deployed women.

THE STRESSORS OF WARTIME MILITARY DUTY AND THEIR EFFECTS ON WOMEN

Stressors of Deployment and Wartime Service

Military service requires individuals to be physically and emotionally fit for the stressors inherent in the demands of worldwide deployment, in times of peace as well as war. The modern, voluntary U.S. force is older and more family-oriented than it has ever been in the past; this creates additional stressors during separation, particularly under uncertain and dangerous circumstances. There is little research to date describing the impact of the unique and cumulative stressors of deployment and wartime service on the physical and emotional health of military women.

The predictable stressors of deployment begin with the separation from family and friends, and the need to make arrangements for family members' well-being during an uncertain absence. Many of the arrangements focus on making legal, financial, and personal plans in the event of death or disability, since the job entails an increased threat to safety and security. Modern technological warfare provides no safe area where women can be protected behind battle lines, as the military has attempted to do in previous conflicts. Specific fears arising during Desert Storm—including the threats of chemical and biological weapons, the likelihood of Scud missile attacks, the risk of petrochemical exposure from the oil well fires of Kuwait, and fears about the environmental and cultural stressors of the Persian Gulf—raised concerns about women's participation in the war effort. Some of these fears were realized. Studies of returning women indicated that a large number reported involvement in alerts for chemical and biological attacks, received incoming fire, and witnessed the death and disfigurement of both allied and enemy troops.

We have learned from previous wars that combat exposure can have not only immediate but delayed effects, both physical and emotional. Unfortunately, there is little research concerning these delayed effects on women. Previous measures of posttraumatic stress disorder (PTSD) bear little relevance to today's combat scenario and have not had extensive use in measuring the effects of combat exposure on women. Assessments of wartime stressors need to include issues that are gender-specific and take into account the findings that women tend to report emotional distress more readily than men.

Stressors of the Work Environment

At midnight in England, when the troops were loading B-52s in the cold misty rain, you couldn't distinguish the men from the women. The women were loading and fusing the 500-pound bombs the same as the men.
—*Senator John Warner,* Money *magazine, March 18, 1991*

The military work environment involves long and unpredictable work hours, physical demands, and threats to physical safety. Particularly during wartime operations, there is little opportunity for time off to provide for physical or emotional restoration, and coping resources are soon depleted. A high-intensity work environment where women are often in the minority can create additional stressors.

Specifically, the issues of cohesion, morale, and job performance are of paramount concern as women are integrated into organizational units previously dominated by men. Women experience the social context of the work environment in unique ways that affect their levels of occupational stress, as well as their job performance and organizational commitment. To maximize unit readiness and performance, we need to identify specific job stressors that influence job distress as a determinant of the preference for military life. Once these stressors are recognized, specific interventions relevant to supervisory training or policy development may be instrumental in reducing some occupational stressors.

Stressors of Nontraditional Roles

Military women have been at the forefront of changing the norms of what has traditionally been called "women's work." As more and more women accept the opportunity to compete for positions in combat aircraft, aboard ships, and within highly technical career fields, we will have much more information about the roles that genuinely require gender-specific attributes. Until such time, women will continue to experience work-related stressors related to gender integration.

Working in a male-dominated environment increases stress among women. Such problems as gender stereotyping, sexual (and other) harassment, and social isolation have been shown to increase psychosomatic symptoms, emotional exhaustion (burnout), and diminished feelings of personal accomplishment. In recent years, researchers have begun to study the effects of nontraditional jobs on the health and well-being of service women. It has been noted, for example, that use of health services increases among women working in nontraditional roles and male-dominated work environments. Women in these nontraditional occupations visit "sick call" at a significantly higher rate than women in traditional military occupations. The rates of physical injury increase as well, because of improper training, ill-fitting equipment, and lack of attention to specific physical conditioning that may be required for specific duties. Such findings are also relevant to nonmilitary settings where women have begun to work, such as police forces and fire departments.

Social scientists have suggested that as the work role patterns of men and women converge, some of the gender differences we currently see in role quality and distress in the workplace may eventually disappear. Until that time, military women will continue to be the pioneers in expanding career opportunities and equity for all women.

GENDER-SPECIFIC CONCERNS OF MILITARY WOMEN

Women's Health Care Needs

The mobilization and deployment of large numbers of women during Desert Storm created an awareness of the need to provide for their health care at deployed locations.

Women requiring even routine gynecological attention had to be airlifted to a medical facility where such services could be provided. Such an airlift required several days and seriously disrupted these women's ability to perform their duties. As more and more women are involved in military deployments, increased attention needs to be directed toward delivering gender-specific health care at the deployed locations.

There has been little systematic, system-wide study to date of the health care needs of military women. Although women use health care resources more than men, women's health care has not been widely accessible within the military. Further work needs to be done to examine military women's preferences concerning utilization of, and satisfaction with, the health care services provided.

Health Concerns of Childbearing Women

Reproductive issues are of primary concern to young military women who have been exposed to unusual occupational and environmental stressors, such as dangerous biological and chemical agents, thermal and microwave exposure, and communicable viral and bacterial diseases. For example, large-scale epidemiological studies are needed to determine whether there are any long-term effects on the health of women and their subsequent children following service in the Middle East, where they may have received exposure to a number of noxious agents. However, it is not always known whether a woman is pregnant when exposure occurs, to what extent the exposure is dangerous at the time, or whether there is any effect on later pregnancies. It is known that the incidence of preterm birth is high among active-duty women, and the contributing factors are not fully understood. There is a need for research on the physical and mental stress of military women during pregnancy, as well as for closer monitoring of their perinatal outcomes.

Work and Family Stress

The multifaceted relationship between work in the military and family stress, and the impact of these combined stressors on women's lives, constitute a rich area for further study—particularly as military women move into more demanding work roles. For example, recent research is beginning to suggest that the relationship between women's work and family stressors has a significant impact on their physical and emotional health, and may ultimately affect their ability and willingness to remain in the military work force. Research has shown that women have a greater vulnerability to family role strain, parenting stress, and depression. Separation from families, particularly during wartime, is an unusual and sometimes extraordinary stressor for a woman caught in the competing demands of an interesting and challenging job, the needs of her children, and her concern for their welfare in her absence.

Desert Storm was dubbed the "Moms' War" by the mass media, which captured the tearful separations of mothers and children during the troop buildup in the Middle East. Reports indicate that 36,704 children were separated from either a single parent or both parents during Desert Storm. The preliminary results of our studies suggest that separation from the mothers was not a major consideration in children's adjustment following Desert Storm, but rather was a function of the amount of disruption in the children's lives when the mothers were away. This was particularly salient when a single mother placed a child in the care of extended family members or an ex-spouse. Sometimes this placement required that the child be moved to another geographical area, and thus also separated from friends, familiar surroundings, and daily routines. It is interesting to note that in a survey 4 years later, we found that the behavioral adjustment measures of the children of mothers deployed to the Middle East were no different from those of children whose mothers were deployed elsewhere. So it seems that the disruption in children's lives affected their later adjustment more directly than whether or not their mothers were deployed to a war zone. Certainly this finding does not mean that they did not experience the pain of separation or the fear that they might lose their mothers, but it is reassuring to discover that the immediate effects did not last for a prolonged period of time. Further research is necessary to determine whether the distress of maternal separation during wartime can be reduced through military-sponsored programs and interventions sensitive to the needs of children in these families.

LOOKING AHEAD: THE READJUSTMENT OF GULF WAR VETERANS

After every war, there are public and private concerns about the ability of returning troops to resume a normal life. The legacy of the Vietnam veterans continues to be a topic of great concern and ongoing research, as investigators work toward a fuller understanding of the human responses to an overwhelming life experience. Our understanding of PTSD continues to unfold as veterans age and their coping processes are either bolstered or deteriorate with time. The initial predictions concerning Gulf War veterans were that the readjustment process would be a smooth one, particularly since the allied forces experienced a quick and decisive victory, and the nation was supportive of the U.S. troops on their return. Early media reports of a mystery illness later called the "Gulf War syndrome" seemed to shatter the hope that all was well. (And, again, many families of military women experienced unusual upheaval as mothers were deployed, resulting in role reversal within the families and disruption in the children's lives.) It remains for ongoing as well as future research to tell us how female Gulf War veterans and their families will adjust over time.

> This crisis will demonstrate to people that women are an integral part of the armed forces, that we couldn't do the job without them.
> —*Lawrence Korb*, Ladies Home Journal, *December 1990*

FURTHER READING

Holm, J. (1992). *Women in the military: An unfinished revolution* (rev. ed.). Novato, CA: Presidio Press.
A revision of a female Major General's classic work on the role of women in the U.S. armed forces, from the beginning of U.S. history to the Gulf War.

Kelley, M. L., Herzog-Simmer, P. A., & Harris, M. A. (1994). Effects of military-induced separation on the parenting stress and family functioning of deploying mothers. *Military Psychology,* 6(2), 125–138.
A study examining the responses of 118 U.S. Navy deploying mothers, to identify the stress accompanying the predeployment phase and the unique challenges faced by single parents, as well as the distinctive concerns of deploying mothers.

Leiter, M. P., Clark, D., & Durup, J. (1994). Distinct models of burnout and commitment among men and women in the military. *Journal of Applied Behavioral Science, 30*(1), 63–82.
Describes the organizational and personal stressors leading to burnout in the military work environment.

Nice, D. S., & Hilton, S. (1994). Sex differences and occupational influences on health care utilization aboard U.S. Navy ships. *Military Psychology, 6*(2), 109–123.
A study to assess health care requirements of men and women aboard U.S. Navy ships.

Pierce, P. (1997). Physical and emotional health of Gulf War veteran women. *Aviation, Space, and Environmental Medicine, 68*(4), 317–321.
Provides results of a study describing the physical and emotional health of 525 women called to service during the Gulf War. Women deployed to the theater reported significantly more general as well as gender-specific health problems than women deployed elsewhere.

Pierce, P. F. (in press). Retention among Air Force women serving during Desert Shield and Desert Storm. *Military Psychology.*
Results of a study examining the influence of military service during Desert Shield and Desert Storm on women's decision to stay in or leave the military. Identifies descriptive profiles of "leavers" and "stayers," as well as the factors predicting retention.

Pierce, P. F., Vinokur, A. D., & Buck, C. L. (in press). Effects of war-induced maternal separation on children's adjustment during Desert Storm and two years later. *Journal of Applied Social Psychology.*
Describes the results of a study of the factors most predictive of children's adjustment following the deployment of Air Force mothers during Desert Storm. Multiple measures of war-induced stressors, coping resources, and children's behavioral stress response provide a useful model for describing and predicting children's adjustment following wartime separation of women from their families.

Schneider, D., & Schneider, C. J. (1992). *Sound off!: American military women speak out.* New York: Paragon House.
Provides a compelling documentation of the issues most relevant to military women and the policies affecting their military careers. Includes interviews with women serving in Operation Desert Storm.

Vinokur, A. D., Pierce, P. F., & Buck, C. L. (1997). *Work–family conflicts of women in the Air Force: Their influence on mental health and functioning.*
Manuscript submitted for publication. Reports on the findings of a study of 525 Air Force women following Desert Storm. Provides a model of work–family conflict that includes the separate effects of marital and parental roles on mental health. An analysis using the extended model demonstrated that distress level in each role (i.e., mother, wife, and soldier) and work–family conflict had independent adverse effects on mental health.

Wolfe, J., Brown, P. J., & Kelley, J. M. (1993). Reassessing war stress: Exposure and the Persian Gulf War. *Journal of Social Issues, 49*(4), 15–31.
A study of 2,344 Persian Gulf War Army veterans (2,136 males and 208 females) to investigate three major stressor categories: traditional wartime activities; nontraditional wartime events; and non-war-zone, deployment-related experiences.

54

Access to Prenatal Care

Sarah S. Brown

Prenatal care, like much of modern life, draws on an ancient and enduring idea—that pregnancy is a unique, vulnerable life stage that merits special protections and a tender touch. But it is only quite recently that care in pregnancy has become the responsibility of the medical community. Indeed, it was not until well into the 20th century in the United States that all pregnant women were urged to seek medical care and supervision in pregnancy, and it was not until 1952 that the specialty of obstetrics and gynecology was sufficiently well-defined to be able to set up its own professional college.

All pregnant women in the United States are now urged to obtain prenatal care, and to begin it as early in pregnancy as possible—preferably during the first 3 months (the first trimester) of pregnancy. The Surgeon General's goals for the year 2000, for example, include several measures of participation in prenatal care. These various goals and standards generally state that early care is better than late care, and that more care is better than less care.

In recent years there has been a move to begin prenatal care even before pregnancy, during a so-called "preconception" visit to a health professional. During this visit a woman and her partner are screened for a variety of risk factors, treated for problems known to affect the course of pregnancy, and counseled about the best health practices during the early weeks of pregnancy, when the fetus is particularly vulnerable to such behavioral and environmental threats as smoking and exposure to toxic substances.

Nonetheless, it is important to acknowledge that many questions about the precise content and exact payoff of prenatal care remain unanswered. For example, although prenatal care can take part of the credit for the steep declines in U.S. maternal mortality and morbidity in the 20th century, the impact of prenatal care on the well-being of infants has been less clear. The usefulness of prenatal care in reducing low infant birthweight in particular has remained controversial, and its role in many areas (e.g., adequacy of subsequent breast feeding) is essentially unknown. Whatever the areas of controversy, however, there has been no serious challenge yet to the notion that all pregnant women should have some degree of prenatal supervision, and that this should address a wide variety of medical, behavioral, and psychosocial issues that commonly arise during this special life stage.

CURRENT LEVELS OF PARTICIPATION IN PRENATAL CARE

Because of the deep social consensus that prenatal care is a basic health service that all pregnant women ought to have, various surveys have been developed to document the extent to which all pregnant women have access to such care. Typically, participation in prenatal care is measured in one or more of three ways: (1) the proportion of pregnant women who begin such care within the first trimester of pregnancy; (2) the proportion who begin care only in the last trimester of pregnancy or receive no care at all; and (3) the proportion who receive "adequate care," which can be measured in a variety of ways (these typically consider when care begins, as well as the number and distribution of prenatal visits over the course of the entire pregnancy in relationship to gestational age). The first two measures are most frequently used, because the data needed to compute them are readily accessible from birth certificates. The last approach, recently discussed in detail by Kotelchuk, is often considered the most comprehensive measure.

In 1993 almost 80% of pregnant women in the United States began prenatal care in the first 3 months of pregnancy—a vast improvement over the 1969 figure of 69%. Data also show that there has been some improvement in the proportion of women who begin care only at the end of pregnancy or not at all; this figure dropped from 6% in 1983 to 4.8% in 1993. The latter measure is particularly important (and the progress especially heartening), as this group is known to be at especially high risk for a poor pregnancy outcome and for difficulty in the postpartum period and beyond.

EFFORTS TO INCREASE ACCESS TO CARE

Although refinements in how best to measure participation in prenatal services continue to be made, the leaders of health policy and services have been hard at work to increase access to prenatal care. Particularly from the mid-1980s on, many states and communities have focused on the need to increase participation in prenatal care, primarily because of evidence that such care may help reduce low birthweight and therefore infant mortality. As advocacy groups have widely publicized the poor ranking of the United States in overall infant mortality as compared to many other developed and developing countries, the U.S. Congress and numerous communities have taken a variety of steps to improve access to prenatal care.

Efforts to increase access to prenatal services typically focus on one or more of the following barriers:

1. *Financial barriers to care.* These include (a) insufficient coverage of prenatal care in private health insurance plans (e.g., the imposition of waiting periods for coverage to begin); (b) limitations in the ability of the Medicaid program to enroll women promptly in the program and to link them to a care provider in a timely way; and (c) limited options for uninsured women with neither a public nor a private source of payment to obtain care.

2. *Limits on the health care system's ability to provide care.* There is insufficient capacity in the system to care for all pregnant women early in pregnancy, especially those who are uninsured or are in a Medicaid plan with limited participation by obstetricians or other trained providers of obstetrical care.

3. *Inhospitable practices in the organizations and at the sites offering prenatal care.* These include cumbersome appointment procedures; long waits in the waiting room on the day of the appointment; inadequate transportation; inadequate child care supports; communication problems; language and cultural barriers between clients and providers; and lack of easily accessible information about where to go for prenatal care.

4. *Various personal and attitudinal issues that can limit participation in prenatal care.* These include ambivalence about whether to continue the pregnancy or seek abortion; the belief that care is needed only if one feels ill; ignorance of what prenatal care actually entails; fear of medical care providers and procedures; fear that such socially and medically sanctioned behaviors as alcohol or drug abuse will be discovered; general social isolation; and other similar matters.

Particularly on behalf of poor women, the U.S. Congress and many state legislatures have repeatedly demonstrated their commitment to reducing the first type of barriers (financial) by their sustained efforts to raise the eligibility levels for pregnant women applying for Medicaid—up to 185% of the federal poverty level and beyond. In some states the eligibility expansions have been accompanied by efforts to increase the available service capacity for poor women as well. Typically this is accomplished by increasing the fees paid for prenatal care to physicians providing services to Medicaid-enrolled women, thereby increasing the numbers of physicians willing to serve such women.

Some groups, such as the New York City chapter of the March of Dimes, have also addressed the issue of "client-friendly" or "user-friendly" services. For example, groups are working to reduce the waiting times for prenatal appointments in city-run clinics and giving awards to clinic systems that treat their clients with special dignity and consideration. The elaborate case management systems that many states have developed—often for Medicaid-enrolled clients—also address the access barriers that complicated systems can often impose.

Initiatives like these may be behind the increases in early participation in prenatal care, although no research is available to document specific cause-and-effect relationships. More importantly, it is unclear how the movement toward managed care—for Medicaid-enrolled as well as privately insured women—will affect access to prenatal care. There is reason for both optimism and pessimism. With regard to Medicaid, it may be that the mandatory assignment of pregnant women to specific providers of obstetrical care will increase overall access to care; on the other hand, if the providers to whom women are assigned are inaccessible or unacceptable, access may not be enhanced at all. A number of studies are presently underway to learn more about the relationship of various managed care arrangements to access to prenatal care. Their findings are eagerly awaited.

FURTHER READING

Alexander, G. R., & Korenbrot, C. C. (1995). *The role of prenatal care in preventing low birthweight.* Los Altos, CA: Center for the Future of Children.
This summary of research on prenatal care describes the methodological problems encountered in assessing the impact of prenatal care, and concludes that we lack excellent experimentally derived data on this intervention.

Cefalo, R. C., & Moos, M. K. (135). *Preconception health care: A practical guide* (2nd ed.). St. Louis: Mosby.
This volume summarizes both the rationale for preconception care and the actual mechanics of offering such care in a clinical setting to women as well as their partners.

Institute of Medicine. (1988). *Prenatal care: Reaching mothers, reaching infants.* Washington, DC: National Academy Press.
This report describes the many barriers that women may face in seeking out prenatal care; it also profiles a wide variety of approaches to increasingly early (i.e., first-trimester) enrollment.

Kotelchuk, M. (1994). Adequacy of prenatal care utilization index: Its U.S. distribution and association with low birthweight. *American Journal of Public Health, 84*(9), 1486–1489.
This article describes several ways of quantifying the prenatal care that a pregnant woman receives, analyzes the differences among common measures, and proposes a new one.

National Academy of Social Insurance. (1995). *Perinatal care in the changing health care system.* Washington, DC: Author.
This report analyzes how the key clinical concepts presented in a 1993 report by the March of Dimes, "Towards Improving the Outcome of Pregnancy," are being affected by changes in the organization and financing of health care.

National Commission to Prevent Infant Mortality. (1987). *Death before life.* Washington, DC: Author.
This classic report issues a call for action in all sectors of U.S. life to reduce infant mortality by a variety of interventions, particularly prenatal care.

U.S. Public Health Service. (1991). *Healthy people 2000: National health promotion and disease prevention objectives* (DHHS Publication No. PHS 91-50212). Washington, DC: U.S. Government Printing Office.
These goals for the United States provide numerical benchmarks against which progress (or the absence of progress) in promoting health and preventing disease can be measured.

55

Self-Administered Interventions

David R. Black
Lisa A. Scott

*A*ccording to former U.S. Surgeon General C. Everett Koop, very well-controlled studies have shown that patients tend to choose low-tech, low-cost treatments and to be satisfied with the results. If there is one undeniable reality in health care, it is that individuals are often not seen on a face-to-face basis. Given this new reality, empowerment, personal responsibility, and choice are keys to women's health.

THE U.S. HEALTH CARE SYSTEM

The U.S. health care system is in disarray. The United States spends more for health care than any other nation, yet crude mortality and infant mortality rates in the United States are 14th and 25th, respectively, among all industrialized nations. These rates are indicative of the health status of the general population and do not provide a positive outlook for U.S. health care policy. Women typically spend more on medical and health care services for both curative and preventive purposes. Health survey data indicate that there is an excess of morbidity among women for both acute and chronic conditions. For example, women's risk of developing cardiovascular disease (CVD), which continues to be the leading cause of death for women in the United States, is on the rise, especially because of the increasing number of women smokers. CVD among women causes over 500,000 deaths annually and costs the nation approximately $43 billion per year in direct and indirect costs.

CVD and many other major health problems confronting women in U.S. society are largely the results of lifestyle behaviors and are consequently preventable. Reallocating available resources to prevent illness before its onset could reduce morbidity rates in women remarkably. Treatments or interventions should be available that are readily accessible, suitable to the presenting symptoms, and inexpensive.

Self-administered (SA) interventions constitute a promising approach to improving the accessibility and availability of health care. Before we define these interventions and review their efficacy for women, it is important to consider advances in communication technology and the implications of computerized technologies for the health care industry.

TECHNOLOGY AND PROGRAM DISSEMINATION

In a new technological era, computer and communication strategies can be combined with low-cost and effective interventions. The health care industry and service delivery may benefit from the recent and growing fusion of computer and communication technologies. Twelve years ago, a mere 1% of U.S. households had personal computers. Today, computers can be found in approximately 30% of all homes and 32 million youths below the age of 17 are computer-literate. Over 50 million personal computers, as well as thousands of software packages are currently available to help meet the challenges of daily living. Computer networks now link millions of users together to exchange scientific and technological data, as well as to share information about topics from entertainment to complex computational modeling. Computers and communication networks operate to provide "distance education," in which interactive classes are taught from one location to students in multiple sites throughout specific geographic areas.

In the future, computers may largely replace existing media, including books, videos, and musical instruments. Indeed, computers may become universal libraries, with fingertip access to a wide variety of information and data bases on all topics. This information may be presented from different perspectives in an interactive format that will increase the probability of satisfying consumers' needs and maintaining their interest and participation. Computers can be used to build and display complex relational perspectives which can greatly enhance understanding and underscore the realities related to certain choices (e.g., career decision making). The remarkable advances in communication technology provide an opportunity for improving access to health-related interventions at relatively low cost for many women.

WHAT ARE SELF-ADMINISTERED INTERVENTIONS?

SA interventions are techniques or strategies individuals can use on their own to meet certain personal health objectives. These interventions fit within a larger structure of service delivery, in which monitoring of health outcomes is used to help individuals decide whether the intervention after trial is intense enough to produce the desired result. There are two types of self-administered programs: minimal intervention (MI) and self-instruction (SI). MI has been defined as the simplest and least costly intervention that works. The essence of MI is that it involves strategies that are simple, direct, and self-applied. It may consist of verbal or interactive education or instruction that focuses on identifying specific behavior change strategies. There are no written materials, and only a modicum of professional assistance is required.

SI refers to any intervention that includes formal program materials but does not require contact with a health professional. The program may be delivered through computer, videotape, audiotape, print, or other media. What MI and SI have in common is that there may be no professional contact, aside from periodic documented progress reports in some cases. Examples of MI and SI programs applied to the problem of moderate obesity are presented in Table 55.1 to illustrate the simplicity of both interventions.

The advantages of SA interventions are (1) the capacity for "broad spectrum" dissemination; (2) the potential to reach underserved and "at-risk" populations; (3) convenience for both practitioners and patients; (4) treatment cost reductions and cost savings for both patients and providers; (5) easy reapplication to maintain progress or in cases of relapse; and (6) consumer preference for such programs, as documented by formative research. SA interventions also can be adapted to current developments and future projected advances in technology and communication.

TABLE 55.1. Examples of the Application of Self-Administered (SA) Interventions to Moderate Obesity

Minimal intervention (MI)

Advertise/announce program's start.
Invite interested individuals to return a postcard to program sponsor in order to:
- Signify interest.
- Permit inclusion on a mailing list/data base.
Provide information about losing weight safely:
- Lose weight slowly and gradually (about 1% of total body mass per week).
- Eat a nutritious, well-balanced diet that complies with the U.S. Department of Agriculture's Food Guide Pyramid.
- Increase physical activity without necessarily engaging in strenuous exercise, and reduce caloric intake, but not to less than 1,000–1,200 calories a day.
- Adhere to this adage when selecting a diet: "If you can't live with it, don't start it."
- Purchase and use a calorie counter, but above all else, practice reasonableness and safety in losing weight.
Initiate daily self-monitoring of:
- Body weight
- Caloric intake and expenditure.
Initiate graphing and note relationships among caloric intake, energy expenditure, weight regulation, and health parameters.
Secure monetary deposit to enhance commitment to complete intervention and change behavior.

Self-Instruction (SI)

Supply weight loss educational materials for home use (printed or electronic) that emphasize problem solving and a behavioral approach.
Provide:
- Assignments and quizzes.
- Problem-solving forms.
- Forms for cognitive restructuring exercises.
Continue daily self-monitoring of:
- Body weight.
- Caloric intake and expenditure.
Continue graphing and note relationships among caloric intake, energy expenditure, weight regulation, and health parameters.
Secure another monetary deposit to enhance commitment to complete intervention.

WHAT IS THE EFFICACY OF
SELF-ADMINISTERED INTERVENTIONS?

Several empirical studies attest to the efficacy of SA interventions to effect health-promotive behavior change. Some areas in which SA interventions have been applied include smoking cessation, weight management, problem drinking and alcoholism, hypertension, and physical fitness. Other areas relevant to women's health in which SA interventions have been empirically evaluated include arthritis, asthma, diabetes mellitus (Types I and II), hypercholesterolemia, insomnia, and orgasmic dysfunction. Many women find completing tasks with a modicum of professional assistance and direction empowering. Such involvement increases women's sense of self-efficacy and fosters increased personal responsibility for health changes. Assuming a more active role in one's own care thus has long-term health-promoting benefits. It is conceivable that a host of other medical problems could be addressed in a similar way, depending on the creative talents and incentives of health care providers and third-party payers.

FURTHER READING

Black, D. R., & Hultsman, J. T. (1988). The Purdue stepped approach model: A heuristic application to health counseling. *The Counseling Psychologist, 16,* 647–667.
Articulates an application of self-administered programs to health counseling and supports their efficacy.

Black, D. R., & Hultsman, J. T. (1989–1990). The Purdue stepped approach model: Sequencing community and clinical interventions to reduce cardiovascular risk factors. *International Quarterly of Community Health Education, 10,* 19–37.
Illustrates the unique utilization of self-administered programs in public health, and reviews their efficacy; their application to women's health can be inferred.

Black, D. R., Loughead, T. A., & Hadsall, R. S. (1991). Purdue stepped approach model: Application to pharmacy practice. *DICP, The Annals of Pharmacotherapy, 25,* 164–168.
Discusses intricacies of the unique application of the stepped approach model to pharmacy practice settings; the use of self-administered programs for women's health issues can be extrapolated.

Black, D. R., & Scott, L. A. (1996). *Lay Opportunities—Collaborative Outreach Screening Team (LO-COST): A model for peer health education. Peer Facilitator Quarterly, 13*(2), 29–38.
Explains how to combine the stepped approach model with a paradigm to provide peer facilitation in a cost-effective, systematic, and sequential manner. *LO-COST* offers health professionals, peer helpers, and peer participants a structure to work collaboratively as a team to enhance quality of life, increase access to services, and to reduce health delivery "costs."

Boston Women's Health Book Collective. (1992). *The new our bodies, ourselves: A book by and for women.* New York: Simon & Schuster.
Provides historical and current accounts of factors that influence the health of women and discusses what can be done to improve women's health.

Glasgow, R. E., & Rosen, G. M. (1978). Behavioral bibliotherapy: A review of self-help behavior therapy manuals. *Psychological Bulletin, 85,* 1–23.
Thoroughly reviews the efficacy of self-instructional programs.

Glasgow, R. E., & Rosen, G. M. (1982). Self-help behavior therapy manuals: Recent development and clinical usage. *Clinical Behavior Therapy Review, 1,* 1–20.
Presents further justification for applying self-instructional programs.

Rosen, G. M. (1987). Self-help treatment books and the commercialization of psychotherapy. *American Psychologist, 42,* 46–51.
Discusses issues related to the use of self-instructional programs.

Scoggin, F., Bynum, J., Stephens, G., & Calhoon, S. (1990). Efficacy of self-administered treatment programs: Meta-analytic review. *Professional Psychology: Research and Practice, 21,* 42–47.
Presents the efficacy of self-instructional programs.

56

Alternative Medicine

B. Jane Cornman

*C*all it "alternative," "complementary," "unconventional," or "holistic" medicine—all of these terms are appropriate for referring to a type of medicine that is radically different from the typical doctor–hospital–drug system of health care in the United States. The alternative medicine movement that has emerged in the last two decades owes its genesis to many individuals who took it upon themselves to investigate centuries-old, less "scientific" realms of healing used in the East and elsewhere.

Because the atomistic approach of traditional or allopathic medicine has failed to meet the health care needs of so many people in the United States, a new health-centered movement has begun. Conventional Western medical practices are seen as a "disease care" system, not a "health care" system. An emerging consumer population is dissatisfied with dependence on an increasingly expensive approach that treats problems but takes insufficient interest in preventing them. Growing interest in health- and wellness-focused practices was reflected in a 1993 *New England Journal of Medicine* article stating that in 1991, U.S. residents spent as much as $13.7 billion a year on "unconventional" health care. The NEJM article reported that over one-third of the people surveyed preferred alternative medicine over conventional methods. Alternative practices can include many modalities of treatment, such as acupuncture and acupressure, chiropractic, homeopathy, naturopathy, spiritual healing techniques, various touch therapies (e.g., massage), energetic or bioelectromagnetic therapies, and herbology.

In 1993 the Office of Alternative Medicine (OAM) was established within the National Institutes of Health (NIH) in order "to facilitate the valuation of alternative medical treatment modalities." In 1997, the OAM was designated by the World Health Organization (WHO) as a Collaborating Center in Traditional Medicine. The OAM's responsibilities will be to "promote research in complementary and alternative medicine, expand communications and information exchange among complementary alternative medicine and traditional medical research centers through electronic means and provide consultation to WHO Centers relative to complementary and alternative medicine practices and research." Apart from the OAM, other institutes funding research on alternative medicine (and sample topics of this research) include the National Heart,

Lung, and Blood Institute (e.g., transcendental meditation in the control of hypertension); the National Institute on Drug Abuse (e.g., acupuncture and treatment of substance abuse); the National Institute of Aging (e.g., Tai Chi for movement disorders in the elderly); and the Division of Cancer Prevention in National Cancer Institute (e.g., nutritional approaches to cancer prevention). Clearly, the U.S. government and the conventional medical establishment have taken notice.

BACKGROUND

Prominent leaders in Western science and medical fields are departing from the Cartesian model that has been the central paradigm since the 17th century. After Descartes proposed that mind and matter are two separate, independent realms, the atomistic approach of treating mind and body as separate entities began. By 1930 it had flourished to such an extent that U.S. residents were spending $2.8 billion on biomedical approaches to health care (3.5% of the gross national product). In 1990 they spent 235 times that, or $666.2 billion (12.2% of the gross national product). The exploding costs of traditional Western medicine have forced even the most reluctant segments of U.S. society to view alternative medicine with new interest.

Alternative medicine differs from traditional medicine in at least three main ways: It treats the whole person; it is wellness-focused; and it includes the client as an active participant in his or her health care. Alternative medicine's focus on the whole person acknowledges and respects the interaction of a person's mind, body, and spirit within the environment. They are ever-changing systems of energy that cannot be defined or understood fully if examined separately from each other. These systems are more than and different from the sum of their parts. Because of the interconnection and interdependence of these energy systems, a change experienced by one component of the system will be felt by the other components (the "ripple effect"). For example, when their spouses die, people grieve emotionally and also exhibit measurable physical changes, such as less efficient functioning of their immune systems.

Another important characteristic of alternative medicine is its dual focus on wellness and self- responsibility. Health is not merely the absence of disease, but a balance of the physical, psychological, social, and spiritual aspects of one's life. It is a dynamic state of promoting healthy functioning while preventing imbalance and illness. Wellness behaviors can include stress management, nutritional awareness, and physical fitness. These behaviors depend on clients to be active participants in their own health care. To make informed choices requires self-awareness—knowing and caring for oneself. The care provider encourages the person to examine lifestyle behaviors and to learn methods to move toward wellness and prevent illness. This changes the role of the health care practitioner from a "pill fairy"—an authority figure whom the client approaches for a prescription to "make it all better" without changing any behavior—to a caring colleague who provides information and support. The care provider acknowledges the client's right to make independent choices.

In the remainder of this chapter, I first discuss two major modalities of alternative medicine—meditation and "therapeutic touch" (TT). I then discuss infertility as an example of a mind–body problem to which alternative practices have been successfully applied.

MEDITATION: THE CORNERSTONE OF HEALING

In dramatic contrast to the "pill fairy" perspective is the belief that each person has an aspect of the self that is an inner healer capable of personal healing. This belief is shared by millions of people worldwide. Central to the belief is the practice of activating this inner healer through meditation. Meditation is the active process by which people still the distracting effects of hyperrationality—the "chattering mind." Many different methods are employed to reach this state of mental relaxation or peace of mind. Some focus on a sound, such as a word (mantra), or an image, such as a scene from nature. Others (e.g., the practitioners of hatha yoga) emphasize returning to the breath as an ever-present experience, in order to free the mind from its usual clutter of ideas. In whatever form it takes, practitioners cite concrete and dramatic health benefits.

All of the well-known major healing programs established in the United States in recent years promote meditation as the cornerstone of wellness. Jon Kabat-Zinn's program of stress reduction at the University of Massachusetts Medical Center, Dean Ornish's program to reverse heart disease, and Deepak Chopra's Ayurvedic program of "perfect health" all teach meditation to clients. The demonstrated benefits of meditation are impressive. It has been shown to lower blood pressure, pulse rate, and levels of stress hormones and cholesterol in the blood. It also enhances the immune system's resistance. By inducing a "relaxation response," it creates a state of lowered arousal in the sympathetic nervous system, and thereby reduces many symptoms caused or aggravated by stress. It may even improve memory, concentration, intelligence, and creativity.

THERAPEUTIC TOUCH

One alternative healing method that has been termed a "healing meditation" is Therapeutic Touch (TT). This is an intentionally directed process of energy exchange, during which the practitioner uses his or her hands as a focus to facilitate the healing process in the client. TT was developed over 20 years ago by Dora Kunz, a healer, and Delores Krieger, a member of New York University's nursing faculty; it has been taught to nurses all over the world. The first step in the process of TT involves centering or meditation, in order to bring the practitioner's own energy to a harmonious state. This centered state is maintained throughout the process, during which the practitioner assesses and treats the client's energy field with the goal of restoring harmony.

The most common response to TT is a state of relaxation. TT has been shown to reduce pain and anxiety and to facilitate the body's natural restorative processes. For example, TT can accelerate wound healing, reduce the pain of dysmenorrhea, and increase relaxation during labor and delivery. TT has been used with people across the lifespan, from newborns to older adults, and in a variety of settings (including hospitals, nursing homes, and home care). TT is said to be a healing experience for both the practitioner and the client.

INFERTILITY: APPLICATIONS OF ALTERNATIVE PRACTICES

Infertility affects approximately 20% of couples in the United States. Many women today have postponed childbearing until they are in their late 30s or 40s, only to be told by the traditional medical community that they now have "old eggs" and are at risk of miscarrying or not conceiving. A woman unable to conceive reexperiences profound sorrow with each monthly menstrual cycle. Medical treatment for infertility is expensive, and treatments such as *in vitro* fertilization have only a 15% success rate.

One alternative or complementary treatment that can be utilized while continuing medical treatment is the mind–body or whole-person fertility program. Although this approach has a high success rate in helping previously infertile women become pregnant, the real goal is to help women and couples heal themselves in relation to the issue of fertility and childbearing, whether or not they conceive. This program recognizes the constant "dialogue" among thoughts, feelings, attitudes, and bodily responses, and acknowledges the potential impact of this dialogue on the reproductive system. Relaxation techniques, such as biofeedback, guided imagery, and visualizations, are utilized to decrease the anxiety and frustration of the process of "trying" to conceive, and to help a woman and her partner communicate, bond with, and nurture the unborn child *in utero* once conception has occurred. Another important aspect of this program is the exploration of the emotional and physical family health history. It recognizes the powerful influence of family behavior patterns and belief systems that tend to be repeated generation after generation. Processing this history provides insight into beliefs, thoughts, and feelings about pregnancy that can affect fertility. In short, the woman and her partner are given empowering skills and experiences that can help them create a more relaxed, joyful state of being and increase their interpersonal/relationship skills. They are the active agents in their own care.

FURTHER READING

Chopra, D. (1991). *Perfect health*. New York: Harmony Books.
A guide to restoring mind–body balance through diet, exercise, meditation, and massage.

Eisenberg, D. M., Kessler, R. C., Foster, C. F., Norlock, F. E., Calkins, D. R., & Delbanco, T. L. (1993). Unconventional medicine in the United States. *New England Journal of Medicine, 328*, 246–252.
Study reporting that vast numbers of U.S. residents are utilizing unconventional medical treatments.

Gordon, J. S. (1992, May–June). How America's health care fell ill. *American Heritage*, pp. 49–65.
An explanation of and possible first steps toward, a solution to providing and paying for a modern medical system that has become wasteful, unaffordable, and unfair.

Kabat-Zinn, J. (1990). *Full catastrophe living: Using the wisdom of your body and mind to face stress, pain, and illness*. New York: Delta Books.
The program of the stress reduction clinic at the University of Massachusetts Medical Center.

Levey, J. (1994). *The fine arts of relaxation, concentration and meditation: Ancient skills for modern minds*. London: Wisdom.
A primer with clear instructions for managing reactions to stress.

MacCrae, J. (1988). *Therapeutic touch: A practical guide*. New York: Knopf.
Comprehensive, clear instruction manual for learning TT and using it as a healing technique.

Marti, J. E. (1995). *The alternative health and medicine encyclopedia*. Detroit: Visible Ink Press.
Practical guide with facts and expert opinions on a wide range of alternative health practices.

Newshan, G. (1994). Update on Office of Alternative Medicine. *Cooperative Connection, 15*(3), 6.
A report on the funding opportunities available at the national level that encourage research in alternative nursing and/or healing modalities.

Olshansky, E. F. (1992). Redefining the concepts of success and failure in infertility treatment. *NAACOG's Clinical Issues, 3*,(2), 343–346.

A guide for nurses to help individuals and couples differentiate infertility treatment failure from personal failure, and to help them shift their meanings of "infertility" and views of themselves.

Ornish, D. (1990). *Dr. Dean Ornish's program for reversing heart disease.* New York: Ballantine Books.

The program of lifestyle changes that can reverse coronary artery disease and prevent heart attacks.

Payne, N. (1995). *Language of fertility: A revolutionary mind–body program for conscious conception.* New York: Harmony Books.

Description of the whole-person fertility program's unique therapeutic approach, which honors the mind, body, and spirit in the healing process.

Villaire, M. (1997). OAM designated as WHO collaborating center in traditional medicine. *Alternative Therapies, 3*(2), 21–22.

An OAM progress report as featured in this bimonthly journal.

Wyon, Y., Lindgrew, R., Lundeberg, T., & Hammon, M. (1995). Effects of acupuncture on climacteric vasomodor symptoms: Equality of life and urinary excretion of neuropeptides among postmenopausal women. *Menopause: Journal of the North American Menopause Society, 2*(1), 3–12.

A Swedish team's report on its investigation of the benefits of acupuncture to relieve hot flashes.

Section V

BODY IMAGE
AND SUBSTANCE USE

57

Section Editor's Overview

Kelly D. Brownell

*I*n the 1988 *Handbook of Behavioral Medicine for Women,* there was a chapter on dieting, one on smoking, and one on alcoholism. It is remarkable that at that time these three chapters covered the field of excesses and deficits in lifestyle patterns, and even then, relatively little was known about these issues in women. The authors of the chapters noted glaring deficits in our knowledge about women's health and issued repeated calls for more research. Now, a decade later, it is reasonable to ask whether the field has welcomed research on women's health and whether the deficits in knowledge are being remedied. On both counts, I see cause to celebrate.

Certainly it is true that in the world of behavioral medicine, health psychology, psychosomatic medicine, and the social sciences in general, women's health has become a credible (and in some cases fashionable) topic for study. One now sees special issues of journals devoted to the topic, conferences, courses at both graduate and undergraduate levels, and specialized postdoctoral training programs. Mainstream medicine is lagging behind, but there is positive movement nonetheless. An Office on Women's Health has been established at the National Institutes of Health; there are women's health clinics in some medical settings; and courses on women's health are beginning to appear in medical school curricula.

Some of the impressive developments in women's health have come in the areas addressed by this section of the present book. Behaviors such as smoking, drinking, drug use, and diet are implicated in many of the leading causes of death. As one sees when reading the chapters, problems in these areas are not confined to men, and in some cases are more severe in women. Advances in these areas should have a major impact on public health. The work is improving in both quality and quantity, and will yield important dividends for the health and well-being of women.

One might choose many areas to use as exemplars of important strides in the field of women's health. Because the topics covered in this section are related to so many different health outcomes, such as heart disease, cancer, and diabetes, their importance is substantial. I have chosen the area of heart disease to illustrate some of the important strides the field has made, and some of the strides that must yet be made.

WOMEN, MEN, CORONARY HEART DISEASE, AND RISK FACTORS

Coronary heart disease (CHD) is an example of how a biased view can develop when a field is dominated by studies on men. CHD is one of the chronic diseases most influenced by lifestyle factors—that is, diet, physical activity, and smoking. The diseases influenced by these behaviors (e.g., diabetes, obesity) are themselves important risk factors and have a profound impact on the health and well-being of women. Yet, aside from obesity studies (in which nearly all subjects are women), the attention given to these factors in women is minute; the vast majority of studies have been done with men.

To place in a social and political context the lack of attention to disease and lifestyle in women, please consider the following. CHD is the leading cause of death in U.S. women, leading to 250,000 deaths each year. Wenger and others have noted that one in nine women aged 45–64 years has clinical evidence of CHD, and that the proportion increases to one in three women 65 years or older. The lifetime risks of various diseases in postmenopausal women are 2.8% for hip fracture, 2.8% for breast cancer, and 0.7% for endometrial cancer, but an alarming 31% for CHD. The likelihood of dying from a myocardial infarction once CHD is diagnosed is greater for women than for men; the outcome is more severe for women; and myocardial revascularization procedures result in greater morbidity and mortality in women. Consider also that 40% of all coronary events in women are fatal, and that 67% of sudden deaths in women occur in individuals with no known previous evidence of CHD.

Given these startling facts, one must be dismayed by the history of aggressive funding of studies in CHD in men and the striking absence of studies on CHD in women. A noteworthy example is the Multiple Risk Factor Intervention Trial (MRFIT). An extremely expensive trial, and a controversial one because of its negative findings, the MRFIT was an intervention trial aimed at preventing coronary morbidity and mortality in individuals with one or more of the three leading risk factors (hypertension, elevated cholesterol, and smoking). The trial began in the 1970s, and all subjects were men. It was not until the 1900s that a trial (the Women's Health Initiative) of similar consequence began with women. There has been a clear mismatch between funding and the public health significance of CHD in women and men.

The same case can be made for the coronary risk factors. One-fourth of U.S. women have elevated cholesterol (above 240 mg/dl). One-third have hypertension (i.e., their systolic blood pressure is above 140 mm Hg, their diastolic pressure is above 90 mm Hg, or they are taking antihypertensive medications). One-third of women are more than 20% above ideal body weight. A similar picture can be painted for smoking and being sedentary. In the face of these prevalence figures, it is evident that the lack of research and intervention programs for women is not only a political injustice, but also a threat to the nation's health.

THE CHANGING LANDSCAPE

CHD is but one example of a disease that is influenced by lifestyle, has a major impact on women's health, and requires much greater attention from both basic research and public health perspectives. Two decades ago, the MRFIT study—its focus on men, suggested by its very acronym—typified the lack of attention to women's health. Although the world of health care and health research is not yet entirely free of gender bias, one can point to many heartening changes. The chapters in this sections are clear examples.

The authors contributing these chapters are among the leading experts in the world in their areas, and show the rich nature of information that is produced when bright minds focus on an important problem. We can now say that a generation of researchers has been turning toward women's health as a viable and important issue. As they educate the next generation, the picture will only become more positive.

KEY ISSUES ADDRESSED IN THIS SECTION

Eating Disorders, Body Image, and Obesity

An area represented with a flourish in this section is the spectrum of eating-related problems. Chapters on anorexia nervosa, bulimia nervosa, and obesity in a book on behavioral medicine are standard, and for good reason. Anorexia nervosa and bulimia nervosa are being reported at record rates; cases are increasing in both younger and older people; and most cases occur in females. Individuals affected by these disorders, along with their friends and families, can suffer terribly. In the case of bulimia nervosa, disabling psychological and interpersonal problems are common. The same is true of anorexia nervosa, but in addition, life-threatening medical complications may be present. The mortality rate from anorexia nervosa lies somewhere between 5% and 15%.

The chapters in this section by Sokol and Gray on anorexia nervosa, by Heffernan on bulimia nervosa, and by Troop on stress and coping in eating disorders cover in splendid detail what is known about diagnosis, complications, etiology, and treatment. With regard to etiology, the chapters take us beyond the typical (and superficial) explanation—namely, that females are exposed to repeated, compelling, and damaging messages to be thin. Nearly all females in Western culture are exposed to these messages and develop what has been called "normative discontent" with body weight and shape; yet only some develop eating disorders. It is heartening to see more sophisticated formulations that examine family, psychological, and even genetic factors. Recent work examining eating disorders from a developmental perspective is likely to produce exciting new perspectives on etiology. The chapter by Troop shows the importance of understanding stress and coping in eating disorders; it focuses attention squarely on the interaction of environmental and individual-difference variables.

With the increased interest in women's health has come a great increase in the number of treatment outcome studies. The results have been impressive. With bulimia nervosa, the success rates are very high for either cognitive-behavioral therapy or interpersonal psychotherapy (see Heffernan's chapter). With these success rates, it is difficult to justify any other treatment, except perhaps for nonresponders. Anorexia nervosa does not respond as readily to treatment and often requires immediate medical attention (see Sokol and Gray's chapter). Still, comprehensive programs including cognitive-behavioral therapy, family therapy, and in some cases medication and group psychotherapy—sometimes in inpatient settings initially—offer considerable hope.

One important aspect of this section of the book is that it addresses fundamental behavioral (dieting) and cognitive (disturbances in the way shape and weight are perceived) problems associated with eating concerns. Work on dieting and body image has exploded to the forefront, and the chapters in this section by Polivy and McFarlane, by Ecklund, and by Cash show the pervasive influence of the social environment, not only on body image, but on core psychological factors such as self-esteem. When the messages are internalized, pathological dieting and exercise behaviors can result. The process by which the social environment interacts with a person's individual psychological functioning are becoming better understood—a necessary advance to improve our efforts at treatment and prevention. An example that crosses the boundary of treatment and prevention is the conceptually rich and empirically validated body image therapy described in Rosen's chapter. This work is important to the fields of both eating disorders and obesity.

Some individuals with body image disturbances attempt to shape and mold the body with diet and exercise. Others seek out a surgeon. The chapter by Pruzinsky shows the measures some individuals will take in quest of a perfect body. It also underscores the need to evaluate plastic surgery with the same rigor applied to other medical procedures, to determine whether there is sufficient improvement in health and well-being (including psychosocial functioning) to justify the risks and costs.

The chapter by Wing helps focus attention on the massive public health problem of obesity. Affecting nearly one-third of U.S. women, obesity takes an enormous toll on health and psychosocial functioning. Most treatment studies have been done with women, so there is a lively literature to draw from in treating the problem. With new treatment options entering the scene, some based on biological and genetic discoveries, it will be important to specify their effects on women.

Women and Alcohol

Traditionally considered "male" problems, alcoholism and problem drinking affect a startling number of women. The common lore that men react to stress and other emotional upheaval with substance abuse, risk taking, and acts of violence, and that women respond with psychological problems such as anxiety, depression, and eating disorders, is giving way to a more sophisticated and less biased analysis (see McCaul's chapter). This has freed the field to look at women in their own right. What has emerged is a picture suggesting the need for great concern.

The chapters by Rohsenow and Baraona, and the discussion of alcohol problems in McCaul's chapter on substance abuse and dependence, show the remarkably different views that come from examining these issues in women. Consider that women metabolize alcohol differently than men do and are affected by much lower levels of alcohol intake (Baraona); that role demands and entry into traditional male jobs may have important (and sometimes counterintuitive) effects on alcohol use patterns (Rohsenow); and that women must consider the effects on the fetus of drinking during pregnancy (Rohsenow). Rohsenow and McCaul also note other facts that point to alcohol misuse as a major issue with women (e.g., women progress more rapidly than men from the onset of heavy drinking to serious problems, including dependence). There is a desperate need for more research on risk factors and etiology in women, and, of course, on treatment and prevention. Fortunately, as Rohsenow points out, treatments specifically for women are becoming available.

Illicit Drug Use and Smoking in Women

Turning to the use of illicit drugs, we also see striking facts when the issue is examined from the perspective of women's health. In her chapter on substance abuse and dependence, McCaul notes a pattern similar to that seen in alcoholism—namely, that compared to men, women with opiate dependence show a "telescoping pattern," consisting of later onset and more rapid development of problems. Furthermore, alcohol use co-occurs with illicit drug use in significant ways. Like alcohol use, illicit drug use during pregnancy can have a very negative effect on the fetus.

Sharon Hall's chapter on the treatment of illicit drug use reveals yet another area where much more is known about men than about women. She points out that a greater stigma is attached to such drug use in women, and that this may impede women from seeking help. I can only echo Hall's plea that the field not only develop more extensive knowledge on the effects of prevailing treatments (Twelve-step programs and clinic-based programs) on women, but also test innovative treatments based on what is known about drug use patterns in women.

One of the most discouraging facts in the women's health field at present is that the prevalence of smoking in women, including adolescents, has increased dramatically since the 1950s. As a consequence, and as Husten notes in her chapter, smoking is the single most preventable cause of death in U.S. women, accounting for a staggering 140,000 deaths per year. The suffering is unspeakable, the health care costs enormous, and the entire tragedy preventable. Like the use of alcohol and illicit drugs, smoking affects the health of unborn children as well. Smoking cessation programs must be improved; prevention programs must be used widely; and perhaps with time and increased wisdom, legislators will take a step that may improve public health more than any other—ban the sales of tobacco products.

CONCLUSIONS

That patterns of lifestyle such as diet, weight control, alcohol intake, illicit drug use, and smoking, affect health is no longer new information. What is new is a burgeoning literature on these issues in women. The chapters in this section prove once again that inferring an understanding of health issues in women from studies on men creates many problems. Rates of these problems in women are of great concern and point clearly to the need for advances in theory, treatment research, studies on etiology, prevention programs, and the delivery of care. The authors have raised this banner in thoughtful, scholarly, and compelling ways. May their work inspire others as talented.

FURTHER READING

Brownell, K. D., & Fairburn, C. G. (Eds.). (1995). *Eating disorders and obesity: A comprehensive handbook*. New York: Guilford Press.
A comprehensive book with brief chapters by leaders on nearly every aspect of anorexia nervosa, bulimia nervosa, and obesity.

Wenger, N. K. (1996). Preventive coronary interventions for women. *Medicine and Science in Sports and Exercise, 28*, 3–6.
A scholarly review of what is known about the prevention of coronary heart disease in women specifically.

58

Anorexia Nervosa

Mae S. Sokol
Nicola S. Gray

O! that this too too solid flesh would melt . . .
—*William Shakespeare*, Hamlet (*Act I, scene ii*)

Anorexia nervosa (AN) is a disorder that primarily occurs in women and is characterized by a refusal to maintain adequate body weight because of an intense fear of becoming fat. Although the etiology of AN is unknown, it has been postulated that intrinsic biological alterations, dieting, psychosocial influences, and stress are among the contributing factors. Whatever the cause, once weight loss and malnutrition occur, anorexic patients appear to enter a downward spiral of malnutrition, weight loss, and dieting. Although treatment may sometimes be lengthy, recovery from this potentially devastating illness is possible—especially when the problem is caught early, and there is a good working alliance between the patient and therapist.

PREVALENCE

The prevalence of AN appears to have increased in recent decades. It is most commonly found in industrialized countries, especially in white upper- and middle-class adolescents and young adults. Studies of older adolescent and young adult women have found that 0.5–1.0% meet the full criteria for AN. This means that approximately 1,250,000 U.S. women alive today will struggle with AN at some point in their lives. There is little information about the prevalence of AN in males, but 90–95% of cases occur in females. However, AN appears to be occurring more frequently in minorities, males, and women of all ages. Assessment and treatment of male patients are similar to those of females, except for the obvious concerns about menstruation and sexuality.

DIAGNOSIS

The *Diagnostic and Statistical Manual of Mental Disorders,* fourth edition (DSM-IV), diagnostic criteria for AN are displayed in Table 58.1. As noted there, the essential features of AN are refusal to maintain a minimally normal body weight, intense fear of gaining weight, and significant disturbance in perception of body shape or size. When AN develops in an individual during childhood or early adolescence, the individual may fail to make expected weight gains (while growing in height), instead of losing weight. Postmenarcheal females with AN are amenorrheic.

CLINICAL PICTURE

Onset of AN usually occurs anywhere from prepuberty to young adulthood, most often between the ages of 10 and 30; the mean age at onset is 17 years. In some cases of AN, the onset of illness is linked with a stressful life event (e.g., moving to a new school, leaving home for college, or a traumatic event involving dating or peer relations). However, often no specific precipitating event is apparent.

Anorexics exhibit a spectrum of disordered eating behavior. Over time, individuals commonly move in and out of the different diagnostic categories of eating disorders, both clinical and subclinical. Although AN and bulimia nervosa (BN) are considered distinct disorders, there are no clear boundaries between the two conditions. Approximately 50% of AN patients binge; up to 40% induce vomiting; and many abuse laxatives and diuretics in an attempt to reduce weight. Caffeine, cigarettes, diet pills, and ipecac are other substances frequently abused to further weight loss. Anorexics may also engage in strenuous exercise in an attempt to control their weight. In addition, there is an increased

TABLE 58.1. DSM-IV Diagnostic Criteria for Anorexia Nervosa

A. Refusal to maintain body weight at or above a minimally normal weight for age and height (e.g., weight loss leading to maintenance of body weight less than 85% of that expected; or failure to make expected weight gain during period of growth, leading to body weight less than 85% of that expected).

B. Intense fear of gaining weight or becoming fat, even though underweight.

C. Disturbance in the way in which one's body weight or shape is experienced, undue influence of body weight or shape on self-evaluation, or denial of the seriousness of the current low body weight.

D. In postmenarcheal females, amenorrhea, that is, the absence of at least three consecutive menstrual cycles. (A woman is considered to have amenorrhea if her periods occur only following hormone, e.g., estrogen, administration.)

Specify type:

Restricting Type: during the current episode of Anorexia Nervosa, the person has not regularly engaged in binge-eating or purging behavior (i.e., self-induced vomiting or the misuse of laxatives, diuretics, or enemas)

Binge-Eating/Purging Type: during the current episode of Anorexia Nervosa, the person has regularly engaged in binge-eating or purging behavior (i.e., self-induced vomiting or the misuse of laxatives, diuretics, or enemas) rate of alcohol and/or illicit drug abuse in these individuals, particularly those with the purging type of AN.

ASSOCIATED FEATURES AND DISORDERS

AN has a profound negative effect on interpersonal and vocational functioning. It causes significant distress in affected individuals and their families. Although the extent to which these problems are part of AN or are caused by it is often unclear, these negative effects on functioning highlight the importance of treatment. AN patients often have significant comorbid personality disorders, depression, anxiety, and obsessive–compulsive symptomatology.

Other features sometimes associated with AN include feelings of ineffectiveness, a powerful need to control the environment, rigid thinking, little social spontaneity or initiative, and limited emotional expression.

MEDICAL COMPLICATIONS

AN in many ways parallels other "starvation states." Findings consistent with this include changes in sodium, potassium loss, and abnormal thyroid function. Decreased production of blood cells of all types is often found in association with changes in the bone marrow. Leukopenia increases susceptibility to infections. Anemia may contribute to fatigue and cognitive impairment.

Physical signs and symptoms, in addition to amenorrhea, include dry, pale skin, lanugo (fine body hair), cyanosis, and yellow pigmentation of the skin (carotenemia). The gastrointestinal side effects of AN include abdominal discomfort and constipation. Hypothermia is also a very common complaint in AN. Hypotension and dehydration often accompany moderate to severe AN. In addition, many individuals with AN exhibit bradycardia and/or arrhythmias. These can be fatal.

Young women with AN are at risk for developing osteoporosis. The usual clinical presentation of this problem is a pathological fracture—often as a consequence of a sports injury. Weakness is usually the result of muscle wasting, but may also be a side effect of electrolyte and mineral abnormalities in cases of extreme starvation.

The complexity of physiological changes in patients with AN necessitates that the treating therapist work closely with a primary care physician who is fully trained in the medical aspects of AN. In addition, since many of the physical and biochemical abnormalities revert to normal on refeeding, careful consideration should be given before extensive evaluations are done.

ETIOLOGY

No single theory fully explains the development of AN. The cause is probably multidimensional (psychological, familial, sociocultural, neuroendocrine, hypothalamic, and genetic) and different for each individual. Although no specific cause of AN has been scientifically demonstrated, certain risk factors have been identified.

Sociocultural Factors

There is an overemphasis on the link between thinness and attractiveness, especially in the upper socioeconomic classes of industrialized societies. These societies also have an abundance of palatable and high-calorie foods, and lifestyles that require low caloric expenditure. In many individuals, this leads to weight gain, body dissatisfaction, and

TABLE 58.2. Comparison of AN and BN

	AN	BN
Prevalence in young women	0.5–1.0%	1–3%
Male–female ratio	1:20	1:10
Clinical characteristics	< 85% of average expected body weight Restriction of caloric intake Binge-eating/purging type: binge eating or purging behavior Overly controlled behavior Amenorrhea	Often within normal weight range Repeated episodes of binge eating followed by inappropriate compensatory behaviors (self-induced vomiting, or the misuse of laxatives, diuretics, or enemas) Sense of lack of control
Medical complications	Lethargy, cold intolerance Hypotension, bradycardia Anemia Lanugo (fine body hair)	Electrolyte abnormalities (also seen in AN, binge-eating/purging type) Dental caries, parotitis (also seen in AN, binge-eating/purging type) Arrhythmias (also seen in AN, binge-eating/purging type)
Psychiatric comorbidity	Depression and/or anxiety disturbances Obsessive–compulsive features Rigid, controlling personality types	Mood lability depression and/or anxiety disturbances More likely to have substance abuse or dependence 30–50% have Cluster B personality disorders (predominantly Cluster B): antisocial, borderline, histrionic, and narcissistic
Treatment of choice	Weight gain, nutritional restoration Antidepressants (?)	Cognitive-behavioral therapy more effective Antidepressants (SSRIs)
Course and outcome	Highly variable Mortality is six times that of general population 13–20% mortality at 20-year follow-up	Chronic or intermittent Long-term outcome unknown
Associated neurochemical changes	Increased serotonin levels	Decreased serotonin levels

chronic dieting. Chronic dieting frequently leads to disordered eating, which seems to develop into AN only in certain vulnerable individuals. Although many blame the entertainment and advertising fields for perpetuating this overidealization of thinness, AN pathology—which involves severe physical and mental dysfunction—is only superficially related to these societal values.

Psychological Factors

A diminished sense of self-esteem may increase an individual's vulnerability to AN. Adolescence is a time for the development of autonomy and a sense of identity, and is frequently associated with self-esteem problems in young women. Perfectionism and unrealistically high standards have also been implicated as risk factors for the development of AN. Difficulties in capacity for self-soothing and mood modulation associated with neuroticism and/or mood reactivity may also have a contributory role.

The role of sexual and physical abuse in the genesis of AN and other eating disturbances has generated intense interest in recent years. However, it seems that experiencing abuse predisposes an individual to the development of any number of psychiatric disturbances. This influence is not specific to eating disorders.

Family Factors

An anorexic is often the identified patient in a family that can accurately be described as enmeshed, overprotecting, and rigid. These families often have difficulty resolving conflict. Interestingly, patients with BN generally describe their families differently than do patients with AN. Bulimics report greater neglect, rejection, and blame, and bulimics' mothers appear emotionally distant from, rather than enmeshed with, their daughters. Despite the profusion of literature in this area, the specific contribution of family dynamics to the pathogenesis of AN is not clear. Besides psychodynamics, family comorbidity, genetic contributions, stress, and social factors may influence how individuals in a family relate to each other.

Biological Factors

A genetic predisposition for the development of AN has been hypothesized. Work is currently being done to find evidence of a gene effect to substantiate this theory. AN is 6 to 10 times more prevalent among first-degree biological relatives of individuals with the disorder than it is in the general population. There is also an increased risk of mood disorders in first-degree biological relatives of individuals with AN, particularly those with the binge-eating/purging type. Other heritable factors that may be involved in the etiology of AN include a tendency toward obesity, temperamental factors such as harm avoidance, and susceptibility to mood disorders.

The hypothalamus, an area of the brain that regulates essential body functions (weight, appetite, homeostasis, and thermoregulation) may play a role in the development of AN. Neurotransmitters (chemicals that transmit messages from one brain cell to another), including serotonin, epinephrine, and dopamine, may be dysregulated in AN. Dysregulation of central nervous system serotonin pathways has been implicated in the modulation of many of the psychopathological behaviors found in both AN and BN, including obsessionality and food intake restriction, dysphoric mood, and disturbance of impulse control. According to this hypothesis, serotonin levels are elevated in AN, and decreased in BN. This serotonin hypothesis is further supported by preliminary evidence that selective serotonin reuptake inhibitors (SSRIs) are useful in the treatment of BN and possibly AN. Furthermore, serotonin dysregulation apparently persists after resolution of eating disorder symptoms.

COURSE AND OUTCOME

AN has a variable course and outcome. There may be lasting recovery after one episode of weight loss, a fluctuating pattern or illness marked by remissions and exacerbations over many years, or a rapid deterioration resulting in death. Risk factors for poor outcome include longer duration of illness, older age at onset, lower weight, vomiting and laxative abuse, poor interpersonal relationships, and multiple treatments.

There is significant morbidity and mortality associated with AN. Most studies report mortality rates of about 5% for the first 5–8 years after onset of illness; after 20 years, the death rate is 13–20%. The usual causes of death are starvation and electrolyte disturbance, but suicide is also a contributor.

TREATMENT

Obtaining effective treatment is essential in AN, because this illness rarely remits spontaneously, and intervention improves prognosis. There are two immediate goals in the treatment of AN. The first is nutritional rehabilitation; this means restoration of normal body weight and metabolic balance. The second goal is to restore normal eating patterns. The purpose of both these goals is to correct the physical and psychological sequelae of malnutrition. Longer-term goals in the treatment of AN are aimed at relapse prevention. This includes the assessment and treatment of behavioral, intrapsychic, and interpersonal problems.

Treatment usually takes place in an outpatient setting. It may include individual, group, and family therapy, as well as partial hospitalization. Psychiatric or medical hospitalization is often necessary if treatment response is unsatisfactory or medical complications develop. Ideally, a continuum of care should be available, so that patients can receive appropriate combined modalities of treatment as their symptomatology and needs change over time.

Nutritional Considerations

Healthy target weights and expected rates of weight gain need to be established for each patient. Food types and caloric intake levels should be recommended at first by a dietitian, with the eventual goal being for the patient take on these responsibilities. Liquid food supplements, nasogastric tube feedings, or parenteral alimentation may be necessary in extreme cases. These potentially life-saving interventions should only be used for as short a time as possible, until normal eating resumes.

Psychotherapy

The type of psychotherapeutic intervention chosen depends on the cognitive capacity, complexity, and needs of the individual patient and family. Useful modalities include behavioral modification, cognitive-behavioral techniques, psychoeducation, empathic support, encouragement, insight, and problem solving. The goal of cognitive-behavioral therapy is to help the patient identify the thoughts and beliefs that perpetuate the disorder, and to restore a normal pattern of eating. Interpersonal psychotherapy is also useful in the treatment of AN. This form of therapy is based on the hypothesis that interpersonal problems (i.e., loss, role conflict, role transition, individual deficits) serve to perpetuate the cycle of eating-disordered behavior. Issues such as relationships with friends and family members are explored and discussed.

Family therapy is a particularly important component of treatment for children, adolescents, and adult patients who live in the parental home. This modality is helpful when the disturbed eating behavior has been perpetuated by or has created disturbed family interactions. Group therapy and support groups can also be effective treatment modalities. A number of national organizations can provide referral and educational services:

National Association of Anorexia Nervosa and Associated Disorders (ANAD)
P.O. Box 7
Highland Park, IL 60035
(708) 831-3438

National Eating Disorders Organization (NEDO)
6655 S. Yale Ave.
Tulsa, OK 74136
(918) 481-4044

The American Anorexia/Bulimia Association Inc.
293 Central Park West, Suite 1R
New York, NY 10024
(212) 501-8351

Treatment can be complicated in patients with AN, because they often do not seek treatment on their own and deny the seriousness of the illness. Clinicians are often faced with patients brought in unwillingly by their families or friends. They frequently resist hospitalization or leave the hospital against medical advice. In treatment, they tend to focus on criticizing the eating protocol, rather than on their own problems. It is therefore important to establish a structured behavioral contract early in treatment, and not to make modifications in it. This allows the clinician and patient to work productively on developing a therapeutic alliance, and on understanding and changing deleterious thoughts, feelings, and behaviors.

Medications

Pharmacological intervention may be a useful adjunct to the treatment of AN. Antidepressants, such as tricyclics or SSRIs (e.g., fluoxetine), appear to be modestly effective in the treatment of AN. These medications have been shown to decrease bingeing and purging behaviors. Recent double-blind trials suggest that fluoxetine may help weight-recovered AN patients maintain a healthy body weight, in addition to reducing depressive and obsessive–compulsive symptomatology. It should be noted, however, that depression in AN can remit with weight gain. Also, malnourished patients are less responsive to antidepressants and more prone to their side effects.

Other medications can be used to treat the accompanying symptoms in individual patients. Anxiolytics (e.g., benzodiazepines such as alprazolam) can be used to treat comorbid anxiety, as well as the acute anxiety anorexics often experience in response to refeeding. Low doses of neuroleptics can decrease psychotic-like thinking, severe obsessionality, and anxiety; their antiemetic effect may also be helpful. Estrogen replacement may be considered when amenorrhea is present, to reduce calcium loss and osteoporosis. However, weight gain with nutritional replacement is the preferred means to correct these problems.

FURTHER READING

American Psychiatric Association. (1993). Practice guidelines for eating disorders. *American Journal of Psychiatry, 150*(2), 212–228.
A set of patient care strategies developed to assist in clinical decision making.

American Psychiatric Association. (1994). *Diagnostic and statistical manual of mental disorders* (4th ed.). Washington, DC: Author.
The section on eating disorders provides a helpful guide to clinical practice.

Andersen, A. E. (Ed.). (1990). *Males with eating disorders.* New York: Brunner/Mazel.
For professionals and the public.

Bruch H. (1978). *The golden cage: The enigma of anorexia nervosa.* Cambridge, MA: Harvard University Press.
A seminal work by a pioneer in the field.

Bruch, H. (1988). *Conversations with anorexics* (D. Czyzewski & M. Suhr, Eds.). New York: Basic Books.
Insight into the disorder by a pioneer in the field. Her last book, completed just before her death in 1984.

Fisher, M. (1992). Medical complications of anorexia and bulimia nervosa. In S. B. Friedman, M. Fisher, & S. K. Schonberg (Eds.), *Comprehensive adolescent health care* (pp. 487–503). St. Louis, MO: Quality Medical.

Halmi, K. A., Agras, W. S., Kaye, W. H., & Walsh, B. T. (1994). Evaluation of pharmacologic treatments in eating disorders. In R. F. Prien & D. S. Robinson (Eds.), *Clinical evaluation of psychotropic drugs: Principles and guidelines* (pp. 547–577). New York: Raven Press.
A good overview.

Halmi, K. A., Eckert, E., Marchi, P., Sampugnaro, V., Apple, R., & Cohen, J. (1991). Comorbidity of psychiatric diagnoses in anorexia nervosa. *Archives of General Psychiatry, 48,* 712–718.

Kaye, W. H., & Weltzin, T. E. (1991). Serotonin activity in anorexia and bulimia nervosa: Relationship to the modulation of feeding and mood. *Journal of Clinical Psychiatry, 52*(12, Suppl.), 41–48.

Kaye, W. H., Weltzin, T. E., & Hsu, L. K. G. (1993). Relationship between anorexia nervosa and obsessive and compulsive behaviors. *Psychiatric Annals, 23,* 365–373.

Kaye, W. H., Weltzin, T. E., Hsu, L. K. G., & Bulik, C. M. (1991). An open trial of fluoxetine in patients with anorexia nervosa. *Journal of Clinical Psychiatry, 52*(11), 464–471.

Keys, A., Brozek, J., Henschel, A., Mickelsen, O., & Taylor, H. L. (1950). *The biology of human starvation* (2 vols.). Minneapolis: University of Minnesota Press.

Zerbe, K. J. (1993). *The body betrayed: Women, eating disorders, and treatment.* Washington, DC: American Psychiatric Press.
A comprehensive and clearly written book that should be read by all patients, family members, significant others, and professionals.

59

Bulimia Nervosa

Karen Heffernan

*B*ulimia nervosa is characterized by recurrent episodes of binge eating and by behaviors intended to compensate for this eating and to prevent weight gain. These include self-induced vomiting or laxative misuse. It typically begins in adolescence or early adulthood, and occurs in approximately 1% to 3% of adolescent and young adult women in the general population. Bulimia nervosa appears to be more common in higher socioeconomic groups and among college women. It occurs predominantly in females, although cases do exist among males.

CLINICAL CHARACTERISTICS

Binge Eating

The American Psychiatric Association's *Diagnostic and Statistical Manual of Mental Disorders*, fourth edition (DSM-IV), defines "binge eating" as (1) eating, within a limited time period (e.g., 2 hours), an amount of food that is clearly more than most people would eat during a similar period of time and under similar circumstances; and (2) experiencing lack of control over eating during this period (e.g., feeling that the act of eating, the amount and type of food eaten cannot be controlled). Research has shown that people often use the term "binge" to describe a sense of losing control or of overeating, regardless of the amount of food actually eaten. To meet the DSM-IV binge-eating criteria for bulimia nervosa, an individual must engage in the behavior as defined by these criteria, on average, at least twice a week for 3 months.

Binge eating may be triggered by dysphoric mood, by interpersonal stressors, or by hunger or feelings of deprivation following dietary restriction. Typical binge foods tend to be desserts and snacks that are sweet or high in fat content. Despite the widespread belief that binge eating is caused by craving for carbohydrates, patients with bulimia nervosa do not consume larger amounts of carbohydrates during binge eating than other people do.

Purging

The most common method used to compensate for binge eating (to reduce either fear of weight gain or physical discomfort) is self-induced vomiting. In some cases, vomiting occurs after even small amounts of food are consumed, or becomes a goal in its own right (i.e., the individual eats in order to vomit). Other purging behaviors include the misuse of laxatives and diuretics. There is a nonpurging subtype of bulimia nervosa, in which the individual does not regularly engage in these behaviors, but instead uses fasting or excessive exercise to compensate for binge eating. Like the binge eating, the compensating behaviors must occur, on average, at least twice a week for 3 months to meet DSM-IV criteria for bulimia nervosa.

Attitudinal Disturbance

Individuals with bulimia nervosa are excessively concerned with their body shape and weight, which strongly influence their self-evaluation. There is typically a high degree of body dissatisfaction, and either a strong desire to lose weight or a fear of gaining weight. Consequently, episodes of binge eating may lead to intensified self-criticism and dysphoric mood. Most individuals with bulimia nervosa are within the normal weight range, although some may weigh slightly above average, and a history of being overweight prior to onset of the disorder is common. There is typically a pattern of dietary restriction between binges, with avoidance of foods perceived to be high in calories or likely to trigger a binge.

Medical Complications of Bulimia Nervosa

Common medical consequences of bulimia nervosa include fatigue, headaches, puffy cheeks caused by enlarged salivary glands, and dental problems caused by recurrent vomiting (which erodes tooth enamel). More serious complications include blood chemistry imbalances, which may increase the risk of kidney and heart problems.

FACTORS THAT INCREASE RISK FOR BULIMIA NERVOSA

Despite a voluminous literature of proposed theories, the etiology of bulimia nervosa is still unclear, and is likely to remain so until prospective studies investigate the putative influences suggested by retrospective and cross-sectional studies. Nonetheless, research has pointed to important elements in the development and maintenance of bulimia nervosa.

The Sociocultural Context

Research on bulimia nervosa has consistently pointed to the direct and indirect influence of sociocultural variables in its development and maintenance. Increasingly thin standards of female beauty, and the inability of most women to achieve them, are thought to contribute to widespread body dissatisfaction. It has been argued that the socialization of girls to evaluate themselves in terms of their appearance lays the groundwork for the low self-esteem and poor body image that result from failing to meet these ideals, and for efforts to close the gap through dieting and other behaviors that may lead to bulimia nervosa.

Personal and Family Weight History

Studies have indicated that individuals with bulimia nervosa are more likely to have a previous history of being overweight and to have parents with such histories. It may be that a tendency toward heavier weight prompts more intense weight control measures in these women when striving to meet culturally valued standards of thinness that their own bodies resist. Also, parents who diet are more likely than parents who do not diet to encourage dieting in their children. A recent study of the etiology of bulimia nervosa found that family dieting, along with critical comments from parents about weight, shape, or eating, made significant contributions to the risk for later bulimia nervosa.

The increased incidence of eating disorders during adolescence suggests that certain developmental transitions may play a part in their onset. In addition to the normal challenges of developing a coherent self-identity during adolescence, and increased self-consciousness and concern with how they are viewed by others, girls experience significant physical maturation during this period. This involves weight gain in the form of increased fat tissue, which moves them further away from the culture's lean physical ideal. Onset of breast development and menarche have also been found to be linked to increased dieting in high school girls.

Dieting

Dieting has been consistently implicated in the onset and maintenance of bulimia nervosa, although the nature of this relationship has yet to be elucidated. Studies have shown that chronic dieting can predispose an individual to binge eating, either through physical and psychological feelings of deprivation, or through the negative emotional state that results when the dieter feels that she has "blown it" by eating too much. This sense of deprivation and vulnerability to loss of control are viewed as part of the vicious cycle that characterizes bulimia nervosa. Once control is lost and binge eating occurs, the individual purges in an effort to "undo" the bingeing; this typically results in feelings of disgust and renewed efforts at abstinence and dieting, which set the cycle in motion once again.

However, dieting is not implicated in all cases of binge eating. Many women diet while only a minority develop eating disorders. The best evidence to date suggests that dieting interacts with as yet unidentified factors, be they psychological or biological, in precipitating an eating disorder. However, binge eating also develops in the absence of prior dieting. For example, clinical evidence suggests that negative emotional states sometimes trigger binge eating, which functions as a maladaptive form of short-term coping to reduce distress.

Individual Psychological Characteristics

Women with bulimia nervosa have been stereotyped as emotionally unstable and impulsive individuals who "lose control" not only with regard to food, but in areas ranging from substance abuse to sex. Although bulimia nervosa is associated with high rates of substance abuse and personality disorders, there is no evidence to support the existence of this stereotyped "bulimic" personality. In the absence of evidence for the premorbid existence of affective lability and impulsivity, such features are difficult to disentangle from the pattern of restraint and disinhibition that characterizes bulimia nervosa. Women with bulimia nervosa do exhibit high rates of comorbid depression (which often remits as a result of treatment for the eating disorder), have a high need for approval, and often exhibit an all-or-nothing style of thinking (in which they view food as either "good" or "bad," or themselves as either completely in or out of control).

Family Influences

Observational studies of the families of patients with bulimia nervosa have described patterns of conflict, ineffective modulation of anger and hostility, poor communication of feelings, and deficient problem solving. Hence, the risk for bulimia nervosa may be increased by self-regulation deficits stemming from such family environments. In the context of body image concerns and dieting, deficits in coping with negative affect may lead to episodes of dysregulation (binge eating) alternating with self-reproach and purging.

However, it has yet to be shown that such family patterns are pathognomonic of bulimia nervosa, or that they account for the occurrence of an eating disorder specifically, as opposed to any other psychological disorder. The importance of such patterns may lie in their role in sustaining or reinforcing certain aspects of eating disorders, which makes them a salient dimension of treatment, particularly for adolescent patients still living within the family system.

There is also a more "ordinary" influence from the family, which functions to some extent as a mediator of sociocultural values. The risk for eating disorders may be heightened if family members model weight preoccupation and dieting (as noted above), if weight is a form of evaluation and thinness is valued, and if weight is believed to be something one can and should control. Data from one study showed that girls whose mothers were more critical of their daughters' weight had elevated scores on measures of disordered eating, compared to girls whose mothers accepted their daughters' appearance.

TREATMENT OF BULIMIA NERVOSA

Although bulimia nervosa has been described as a chronic, refractory disorder characterized by high relapse rates, recent studies of specific psychological therapies have shown significant improvements that are maintained at a 1-year follow-up.

The two treatments most thoroughly studied to date are antidepressant medication and cognitive-behavioral therapy (CBT). Antidepressants (i.e., the tricyclic desipramine and the selective serotonin reuptake inhibitor fluoxetine) are more effective than a pill placebo in reducing the frequency of bingeing and purging by the end of treatment, and reduce associated depression. However, these reductions are often modest; remission rates are low; and most patients relapse when medication is withdrawn or even when they are continued on maintenance medication. Given the absence of positive long-term findings, the high dropout rate, and the reluctance of some patients to take medication, the current picture suggests that drug treatment has only limited effectiveness for bulimia nervosa.

The results with CBT are more promising. CBT for bulimia nervosa is designed to address patients' extreme attitudes about the importance of shape and weight, to replace dysfunctional dieting with more normal eating patterns, and to help patients develop skills for coping in circumstances that trigger binge eating and purging. Studies of CBT have shown significant reductions in binge eating, purging, and dieting, as well as improvements not only in attitudes about shape and weight, but in self-esteem, depression, and related areas of functioning.

Nonetheless, a sizeable proportion of patients receiving CBT fail to benefit, and others make only limited gains. Further progress toward successful treatment of bulimia nervosa will depend on increased understanding of what causes and maintains it. One study found that although CBT was more effective at the end of treatment, interpersonal psychotherapy (IPT), which explicitly did not target eating and weight issues, was equally successful at a 1-year follow-up. This study demonstrates that interpersonal issues may influence at least the maintenance of bulimia nervosa, and that improvement may result from addressing such issues alone.

FURTHER READING

American Psychiatric Association. (1994). *Diagnostic and statistical manual of mental disorders* (4th ed.). Washington, DC: Author.
Provides the official criteria for a psychiatric diagnosis of bulimia nervosa.

Fairburn, C. G., Jones, R., Peveler, R. C., Carr, S., Solomon, R., O'Connor, M. E., & Hope, R. A. (1991). Three psychological treatments for bulimia nervosa: A comparative trial. *Archives of General Psychiatry, 48,* 463–469.
A study in which CBT was shown to be more effective than behavior therapy and IPT in the treatment of bulimia nervosa.

Fairburn, C. G., Jones, R., Peveler, R. C., Hope, R. A., & O'Connor, M. E. (1993). Psychotherapy and bulimia nervosa: The long-term effects of interpersonal psychotherapy, behavior therapy, and cognitive behavior therapy for bulimia nervosa. *Archives of General Psychiatry, 50,* 419–428.
A study in which IPT was found to be as effective as CBT at a 1-year follow-up.

Fairburn, C. G., Marcus, M. D., & Wilson, G. T. (1993). Cognitive-behavioral therapy for binge eating and bulimia nervosa: A comprehensive treatment manual. In C. G. Fairburn & G. T. Wilson (Eds.), *Binge eating: Nature, assessment, and treatment* (pp. 361–404). New York: Guilford Press.
A detailed manual outlining the CBT approach to the treatment of binge eating and bulimia nervosa.

Fairburn, C. G., & Wilson, G. T. (1993). Binge eating: Definition and classification. In C. G. Fairburn & G. T. Wilson (Eds.), *Binge eating: Nature, assessment, and treatment* (pp. 3–14). New York: Guilford Press.
Presents a clear definition of binge eating and its role in eating disorders.

Hsu, L. K. G. (1990). *Eating disorders.* New York: Guilford Press.
A concise synthesis of the theoretical and clinical literature on eating disorders.

Polivy, J., & Herman, C. P. (1993). Etiology of binge eating: Psychological mechanisms. In C. G. Fairburn & G. T. Wilson (Eds.), *Binge eating: Nature, assessment, and treatment* (pp. 173–205). New York: Guilford Press.
A detailed analysis of the psychological factors and processes involved in binge eating.

Striegel-Moore, R. H., Silberstein, L. R., & Rodin, J. (1986). Toward an understanding of the risk factors for bulimia. *American Psychologist, 41,* 246–263.
A thorough review of research on risk factors for bulimia nervosa, which addresses these questions: Why women? Which women in particular? Why now?

Strober, M., & Humphrey, L. L. (1987). Familial contributions to the etiology and course of anorexia nervosa and bulimia. *International Journal of Eating Disorders, 5,* 654–659.
A review of research on family interaction and personality factors.

60

Stress and Coping in Eating Disorders

Nicholas Troop

O ver the past 30 years, there has developed a huge literature on stress and its role in psychiatric disorder, most of which uses depression (or depressive symptoms) as the dependent variable. The most important conclusion drawn from this literature is that the experience of stress, not simply the occurrence of a stressor, is of vital importance. How people perceive and cope with a stressor, and the quality of the support they receive in response, all mediate between the potentially stressful event and the subsequent experience of distress. Unfortunately, many stress measures include the contamination of subjective response; that is, they fail to separate coping response and support from the existence of a stressor. The word "coping" has become almost synonymous in colloquial use with experiencing stress, and thus coping processes are confused with outcome (e.g., "I can't cope!" = "I am stressed/depressed/anxious/unhappy/etc."). However, "coping" is actually defined as the cognitive or behavioral (especially cognitive) strategies an individual uses to reduce, manage, or tolerate situations that are perceived as taxing or exceeding his or her resources. It is a set of processes in which the environment and the individual's internal and external resources interact.

The research literature on the role of stress in eating disorders is still relatively young, despite the fact that its relevance was outlined in the earliest references to anorexia nervosa. Schmidt and colleagues reviewed the literature on stress in eating disorders and, from their own studies, reported that bulimia nervosa patients experienced more childhood adversity than restricting anorexia nervosa patients and non-eating-disordered women, but that the rates of adversity in bulimic women were comparable to those found in depressed women. In the year before onset of an eating disorder, approximately three-quarters of both anorexia nervosa and bulimia nervosa patients experienced a severe life event, compared with the same frequency in women with depression and about 40% in women with no psychiatric diagnosis. The occurrence of a stressor therefore appears to be important in the vulnerability to and onset of eating disorders.

Soukup and colleagues also found that anorexia nervosa and bulimia nervosa patients reported experiencing more stress than controls. However, as described above, experiencing more *stress* is not the same as experiencing more *stressors*; other factors, such as appraisal, coping, and support, affect such a perception. Of greater interest are the findings that patients reported less confidence in their problem-solving ability and a greater tendency to avoid confronting and sharing their problems. Other cross-sectional studies have shown similar results, that symptoms are positively related to strategies aimed at managing distressing feelings (emotion-oriented) and negatively related to strategies aimed at dealing with the problem itself (task-oriented).

Defense styles (habitual responses to stress) can be viewed as a kind of trait measure of coping. Schmidt and colleagues found that bulimia nervosa patients used less mature defenses (sublimation, humor, anticipation, and suppression) and more immature defense styles (projection, passive aggression, acting out, isolation, devaluation, autistic fantasy, denial, splitting, rationalization, and somatization) than control subjects.

All the studies cited above have used *trait* measures of coping (or defense). However, there is some debate as to how well *trait* measures of coping predict the *state* processes of coping that people actually use in response to real-life stressors. In fact, many so-called "trait" measures of coping actually seem to measure trait *appraisals*, such as the tendency to attribute negative events to internal causes (e.g., self-blame).

Two studies measuring situation specific coping are those by Neckowitz and Morrison in 1991, and by my colleagues and myself in 1994. Neckowitz and Morrison asked bulimics to complete two coping checklists—one in response to a stressful experience in an intimate relationship, and one in a nonintimate relationship. Both bulimics and controls sought more support, used more escape-avoidance, and made more positive reappraisals in response to the intimate relationship problems than in response to the nonintimate ones, as well as perceiving them to be more threatening. The only group differences were that bulimics perceived relationship difficulties (intimate and nonintimate) as more threatening and used more escape avoidance than controls. Whereas Neckowitz and Morrison nominated stressors for subjects to respond to, my colleagues and I asked anorexic, bulimic, and non-eating-disordered subjects to nominate for themselves a stressful experience which was of current concern to them. Anorexic and bulimic subjects used more avoidance than control subjects. In addition, bulimics used more wishful thinking (a form of avoidance characterized by fantasizing or hoping for a miracle) and sought less support than controls. Anorexic patients did not differ from bulimics or controls on seeking support, although there was a trend for anorexics to be lower than bulimics on wishful thinking ($p < .06$). There was no significant difference between groups on self-blame or problem-focused coping (although there was a trend toward significance in the latter). Numbers did not allow a detailed analysis of coping in response to different types of problems, but there appeared to be few differences (the only differences seemed to occur when subjects nominated psychological problems).

The studies cited above were all cross-sectional. Because coping is a set of processes, the ideal study would measure coping longitudinally. As yet, however, there have been no longitudinal studies of coping in eating disorders. Yager and colleagues compared current bulimics with women who were recovered from bulimia and those who had never suffered from an eating disorder. Current bulimics scored differently on a trait measure of coping than recovered bulimics and control subjects; that is, they scored lower on the scales assessing active coping, planning, seeking emotional support, and venting emotions. However, recovered bulimics did not differ from women who had never had an eating disorder. In the group of recovered bulimics, those who were thought to be completely recovered were more active, made more positive reinterpretations and were less (behaviorally and mentally) avoidant than those who were only behaviorally recovered. This study emphasizes the association of coping with current psychiatric status. However, because of its cross-sectional nature, it (like the other studies already mentioned) cannot shed light on the causal processes through which coping is linked with bulimia nervosa.

In their 1993 study on defense styles in eating disorder patients, Schmidt and colleagues found in bulimic patients that excessive parental control during childhood was related to less use of a mature defense style in adulthood, and that physical abuse in childhood predicted a greater use of immature defense styles. Defense styles were not related to childhood care in the anorexia nervosa group. These associations between parental care and adult defense style suggest that there may be stable differences in coping, up to and including the onset of an eating disorder; however, as Yager and colleagues demonstrate, recovery may be associated with a reduction in these coping differences.

More recently, we have found that eating disorder patients show high rates of helplessness both in childhood and in response to the specific life events that lead directly to onset of eating disorders. Furthermore, there appears to be a link between helplessness at these two time points. In particular, in response to the events that lead to onset of eating disorders, women developing anorexic symptoms show high rates of cognitive avoidance, while those developing bulimic symptoms show high rates of cognitive rumination. This latter finding is in line with laboratory studies showing that worry and mild dysphoria can disinhibit restrained eating. Although by necessity these studies were retrospective, recall was cued using semistructured interviews and ratings were based on objective behavior rather than subjective report. Despite these methodological concerns, these papers represent the only attempt so far to investigate coping before onset of eating disorders.

Coping elicited in response to a stressor is related to a series of appraisals, both of the situation itself (primary appraisal—e.g., attribution of responsibility, likely outcome, etc.) and of one's own coping resources (secondary appraisal—e.g., self-efficacy). Although there may be certain coping strategies that people prefer to use, it may also be that an appraisal style—a consistent way of interpreting the environment—is responsible for much of the consistency in apparent "coping styles." That is, appraisals such as expecting the worst or perceiving oneself as helpless (both of which may be relatively constant) affect the coping response. For example, if an individual appraises a situation as hopeless and believes that it cannot be resolved, then she is unlikely to make active attempts to solve it. Similarly, if she appraises herself as helpless, then she may also be less likely to make active attempts to solve the situation herself, although she may elicit support from others who may be able to do so. If in addition, however, she anticipates criticism from a potential support figure, then she is also not likely to seek support from that individual. To the extent that these cognitive sets are related to coping, they suggest some stable differences in coping. Although I refer to "stable differences in coping," it is not necessary to assume them to be coping *styles*. Rather, "stable differences in coping" may be attributable to trait-like cognitive sets.

Severity of eating disorder symptoms are correlated with coping when trait measures of coping are used, although my colleagues and I found no such correlations using a process measure of coping. However, similar correlations are found between coping and levels of depression, whatever type of coping measure is used. That is, active strategies (such as problem-focused coping, planning, and seeking support) are associated with lower levels of depression, and avoidance is related to higher levels of depression. This finding is not surprising; similar correlations tend to be found between coping and levels of depression, whatever the disorder under study (e.g., depressive or anxiety disorders) and whatever the population (clinical or community).

One of the most consistent findings across the studies reviewed appears to be the use of cognitive or emotional avoidance of problems. So what does this mean for the maintenance of eating disorders? Some authors take the relationship between (inadequate) coping and eating disorders as evidence to infer that an eating disorder is itself a coping strategy. If coping is defined as the strategies used to reduce, manage, or tolerate stress, then how can an eating disorder fulfill this requirement (i.e., reduce or manage stress)? To discuss the role of avoidance in bulimia nervosa, bingeing has been viewed as a way of changing mood. Clearly, if avoidance can perpetuate low mood, then it is easy to see how bingeing may be perpetuated: Continued low mood may lead to continued efforts to increase mood. However, the evidence for the mood-altering effects of food are equivocal: Bingeing may not improve mood, but may in fact lead to feelings of guilt.

Ironically, efforts to avoid certain thoughts and feelings increase the chances of having those very thoughts one is trying to avoid (the literatures on obsessive–compulsive disorder and worry show this). This increase in focus on negative thoughts and feelings leads to dysphoria. Heatherton and Baumeister propose their escape theory to account for how this then leads to bingeing. These authors suggest that this increase in dysphoria is aversive and that the individual is motivated to escape the distress. One way to do this is to narrow the focus of one's thoughts and feelings, reducing the range from complex thoughts (about the self, goals, etc.) to simple, narrow experiences such as physical states (e.g., sensory perceptions of taste, smell, and color of food, as well as perceptions of hunger). If physical sensations become the most salient focus of attention, then food may become a positive reinforcer by its sensory stimulation. Bingeing, then, is not a way of avoiding distress as such; it is the result of the strategy used to avoid the distress, which itself may be perpetuated by cognitive avoidance of problems. This view suggests that maladaptive coping simply perpetuates distress and that distress is what perpetuates the eating disorder, rather than there being a direct link between coping and specific eating disorder symptoms.

In conclusion, maladaptive coping is associated with eating disorders. However, there is little to suggest that any coping processes are specific to eating disorders rather than distress in general. The precise role of coping in the onset and maintenance of eating disorders is still not known, but future research should investigate the following more fully: (1) processes of coping in eating disorders rather than trait assessments (i.e., how people *actually* cope in response to real-life stress), with particular attention to how these processes evolve over time; and (2) the relation between coping and appraisal (it may be that the coping elicited by eating-disordered women is appropriate to the appraisals they make, in which case apparent differences in coping may be misleading, and the differences in appraisal may be of key importance). Clearly, the research on coping in eating disorders has barely begun to scratch the surface.

FURTHER READING

Heatherton, T. F., & Baumeister, R. F. (1991). Binge eating as escape from self-awareness. *Psychological Bulletin, 110,* 86–108.
An interesting and detailed discussion of the possible role of focus of attention in the maintenance of binge eating.

Neckowitz, P., & Morrison, T. L. (1991). Interactional coping strategies of normal-weight bulimic women in intimate and nonintimate stressful situations. *Psychological Reports, 69,* 1167–1175.
A study showing more similarities than dissimilarities between bulimic and nonbulimic women on a state measure of coping with stress in relationships.

Schmidt, U. H., Slone, G., Tiller, J. M., & Treasure, J. L. (1993). Childhood adversity and adult defence style in eating disorder patients: A controlled study. *British Journal of Medical Psychology, 66,* 353–362.
A study showing differences in defense styles between anorexia nervosa and bulimia nervosa patients, as well as the relation between these defense styles and parental care in childhood.

Schmidt, U. H., Tiller, J. M., & Treasure, J. L. (1993). Psychosocial factors in the origins of bulimia nervosa. *International Review of Psychiatry, 5,* 51–59.
An excellent review of environmental, individual, and social factors in the onset of bulimia nervosa.

Soukup, V. M., Beiler, M. E., & Terrell, F. (1990). Stress, coping style and problem solving ability among eating disordered inpatients. *Journal of Clinical Psychology, 46,* 592–599.
A study assessing perceived stress and coping styles, as well as confidence in problem-solving ability—an important but often overlooked variable in coping research.

Troop, N. A., Holbrey, A., Trowler, R., & Treasure, J. L. (1994). Ways of coping in women with eating disorders. *Journal of Nervous and Mental Disease, 182,* 535–540.
A study using a state measure of coping (albeit cross-sectionally) to show differences between anorexia nervosa and bulimia nervosa.

Troop, N. A., & Treasure, J. L. (1997). Setting the scene for eating disorders II: Childhood helplessness and mastery. *Psychological Medicine, 27,* 531–538.
Shows that helplessness in childhood is a vulnerability to developing eating disorders.

Troop, N. A., & Treasure, J. L. (in press). Psychosocial factors in the onset of eating disorders: Responses to life events and difficulties. *British Journal of Medical Psychology.*
Shows coping differences in response to the stressors that lead directly to onset of eating disorders may play a role in their onset.

Yager, J., Rorty, M., & Rossotto, E. (1995). Coping styles differ between recovered and nonrecovered women with bulimia nervosa but not between recovered women and non-eating-disordered control subjects. *Journal of Nervous and Mental Disease, 183,* 86–94.
The title speaks for itself.

61

Dieting, Exercise, and Body Weight

Janet Polivy
Traci L. McFarlane

HISTORICAL CONTEXT

Body weight and shape have traditionally been important indicators of attractiveness for women; in modern society, these have become the major single factors for determining women's beauty and desirability. The particular weight and shape deemed ideal have varied considerably over time. In the 17th and 18th centuries, a more rounded, curved, voluptuous shape was preferred. During the 20th century, there has been a series of shifts in preference for women's shapes. The turn-of-the-century, tubercular, ethereal ideal of women's beauty gave way to more robust, bustled forms, followed by the tubular, thin, "flapper" look of the 1920s, the more curvaceous body of the 1950s and early 1960s, and finally the increasingly emaciated fashion models emulated by women from the 1970s to the present time.

Whereas excess body weight was once a sign of affluence, indicating that the person had plenty to eat, in current prosperous Western societies thinness has become the status symbol for women. The association of body weight and social class is much stronger for women than for men, and appears to reflect the influence of upward and downward mobility for women of slimmer or fatter physiques, respectively. More successful men generally have thinner wives, and fat is generally derogated and reviled in the middle and upper classes of the Western world.

Since the late 1960s, the ideal female body size has been getting smaller and less rounded. Coupled with the fact that the actual weight and size of the female population have been increasing over this same time period, this shrinking ideal has put increasing pressure on women to become ever thinner. Women are confronted with an onslaught of messages from the mass media indicating that beauty, success, happiness, and self-worth are all predicated on achieving this slender body shape. Moreover, these messages imply that women can and should change their bodies to correspond to prevailing fashions, just as they would change their skirt length. Unfortunately, this is not the case. In fact, very few women are physiologically capable of being as thin as the ideal that media images portray (or, for that matter, of achieving whatever "ideal" shape is imposed upon them by the fashion of their day). Throughout history women have gone to great lengths to comply with these physical ideals, forcing themselves to suffer uncomfortable and dangerous corsets, high-heeled shoes, cosmetic surgery, fad diets, and punishing exercise regimens. This has had a variety of implications for women's health and well-being.

DRAWBACKS OF DIETING

The societal demand that women be thin forces the vast majority of women, who are not thin but are merely normal-weight or even fat, to try to become thinner. (It is interesting that one of the main arguments touted to convince women to lose weight is the insistence that fatness is unhealthy. The evidence for this has been drastically overstated, and such data as do exist suggest that the persons for whom overweight is potentially a health hazard are predominantly men, not women!) The only routes available to women to achieve such a slender body are surgery, dieting, or exercise. Surgery, including gastric stapling or bypass and liposuction, appears to bring with it at least as many health hazards as it is supposed to cure. All surgeries for weight reduction have risks, including mortality rates of 3–5%, and none guarantee that any weight or fat lost will not be regained. For many, this is exactly what happens.

Dieting is the preferred route to a slimmer body for women (men appear more likely to choose to exercise when they want to lose weight), and large-scale surveys since the 1960s all indicate that the majority of women have at least tried dieting to lose weight. Women's heightened desire for thinness has spawned a proliferation of weight loss techniques, books, programs, and aids, as well as chronic caloric restriction or dieting to promote weight loss. It should be noted that the concern with weight loss is evident even among preteenage females. Since the 1970s, dieting in order to lose weight has become widespread and statistically normal among young women in Western society. Women tend to see themselves as being too fat, and believe dieting to be the solution to this "problem" of overweight. And dieting, as often as not, does work initially; most diets produce some weight loss in the short term. Unfortunately, there is no proven effective means of long-term weight loss (lasting 5 years or longer).

In fact, for many, dieting actually leads to weight gain in the long term; changes in levels of galanin and neuropeptide Y occur when fat intake is reduced, and these in turn influence insulin levels and response, producing metabolic shifts that promote fat intake and storage. Thus both overweight and normal-weight women frequently find that dieting makes them fatter. This may help to explain the increase in levels of overweight in Western society over the last decade or two, concomitant with the obsessive concern of society with dieting and weight loss.

In addition to the physiological changes accompanying dieting, there are changes in eating patterns associated with restricting one's food intake. Dieting entails eating less than one wants to eat or usually eats, so that one loses weight. This means ignoring the body's hunger signals, and eating on the basis of externally derived cognitive cues or regimens. Ignoring hunger often means disrupting normal caloric regulation, to the point that one loses touch with internal signals not only of hunger, but of satiety as well. Chronic dieters (often called "restrained eaters" in the eating literature) are prone to overeating and even binge eating in a variety of situations, including times when they have broken their diets or even simply expect to do so; when they feel any strong positive or negative emotion, particularly ego-threatening anxiety; when they have had alcoholic beverages to drink; and when they spend time sitting and thinking about or smelling attractive food. Laboratory studies have documented increased eating in all these situations for chronic dieters or restrained eaters as compared to nondieters. This sort of overeating in the face of almost any provocation or threat to the diet may contribute to the increasing weight reported by many dieters over time, and may help account for the repeatedly observed fact that individuals who describe themselves as chronic dieters or restrained eaters do not lose weight when followed over time.

More importantly, chronic, on-again-off-again dieting or diet–binge cycles are associated with increased emotionality and changes in cognitive functioning. Dieters appear to be more focused than nondieters on food and weight, according to cognitive tasks such as the Stroop color-naming test (at least under some conditions) and to memory tasks. Restrained eating is also associated with lower self-esteem and increased neuroticism, possibly because of the frustration and dysphoria of repeated failures at attempts at long-term weight loss. Most disturbingly, according to Polivy and Herman, dieting has been implicated as a precipitant of anorexia nervosa and bulimia nervosa in susceptible individuals.

Dieters are also vulnerable to media images of thin body shapes and diet messages. Studies of college females show that they indicate that they would like to have a smaller physique than they currently possess, and that the physique they choose as ideal is thinner than the one that males consider most attractive. It is generally assumed that this female preference for ultraslim bodies is influenced by the media, which have portrayed increasingly slender female bodies as most attractive over the last two decades. The number of diet and exercise advertisements has been growing steadily for the last 30 years, and there are now magazines entirely devoted to advice on dieting and reshaping the body. One study by Anderson and DiDomenico found that women's magazines contained 10.5 times more advertisements and articles promoting weight loss than a comparable sample of men's magazines contained. Interestingly, this ratio approximates the sex ratio for eating disorders. These images of unrealistically thin or "toned" women illustrate the myth that it is possible for all women to reshape their bodies—a myth that produces feelings of failure and frustration in women confronted with these images they cannot attain. It has been shown that women report feeling more depression, stress, guilt, shame, insecurity, and body dissatisfaction when they are exposed to thin models than when they see average-sized models or no models at all. Other research, such as that by Heatherton, Herman, and Polivy, has shown that dieters increase their food intake when their self-image is threatened; a study by Stice and colleagues found similar increased eating in dieters exposed to diet commercials while watching a movie. Thus it is possible that the very articles and advertisements written to encourage food restriction and smaller body sizes may instead produce increased eating and weight gain in this vulnerable (i.e., dieting) segment of the female population.

DRAWBACKS OF EXERCISE

Exercise is the other major avenue being offered as a means to achieve the ideal thin body shape. This focus on exercise as a weight loss or body-sculpting technique has several negative ramifications. For one thing, exercise is not a good weight loss method, because it does not produce large changes in weight unless the individual spends hours each day in vigorous activity (which is unrealistic and unhealthy for most people). Second, this focus changes people's use of and motivation to exercise from simple enjoyment, or an attempt to improve health, fitness, and well-being, to an attempt to reshape their bodies for reasons of attractiveness and appearance. Because exercise replaces fat with muscle, and muscle weighs more than fat, weight does not decrease very much or very rapidly even when the exercise is having a beneficial physical effect. But because the beneficial effects of exercise, such as improved cardiovascular fitness, are not measurable on the bathroom scale, and are not necessarily manifested in sculpted or toned muscles in a particular body region, many people mistakenly abandon exercise as unsuccessful.

The problem is in using weight or appearance as the measure of success. It is this focus on superficial appearances that encourage many males (and increasing numbers of females) to abuse steroids in order to achieve the desired appearance, while sacrificing health. Similarly, there have been increasing reports of exercise addiction or abuse, such that individuals continue to exercise even when they are injured or when the exercise is clearly interfering with their health, happiness, and well-being in other spheres of life. It thus seems that using either diet or exercise as a means to control and manipulate appearance, rather than in response to bodily feedback indicating health and comfort, backfires.

CONCLUSIONS

Pressure to look a certain way has led to abuses of the female body throughout history. One would think that our more self-aware society would be somewhat immune to this sort of social demand to conform to useless, crippling, and unrealistic expectations about how women "should" look, but apparently it is not. Women's health and well-being appear to be worth less than their attractiveness and appearance. The current emphasis on thinness has encouraged women to mistreat their bodies through inappropriate dieting and exercise regimens. The outcome of this appears to have been an increase in weight and fatness over the last 15 years or so, as well as escalating problems with food, eating, and self-acceptance for women. The more women try to control their bodies from without, the more out of control they appear to become within.

FURTHER READING

Andersen, A. E., & DiDomenico, L. (1992). Diet vs. shape content of popular male and female magazines: A dose–response relationship to the incidence of eating disorders? *International Journal of Eating Disorders, 11,* 283–287.
A sample of popular magazines was surveyed, and it was found that the magazines most often read by women contained 10.5 times more advertisements and articles promoting weight loss than the magazines most often read by men did.

Ernsberger, P., & Haskew, P. (1987). Health implications of obesity: An alternative view. *Journal of Obesity and Weight Regulation, 6,* 55–137.

This general review of the literature concerning body weight and health consequences arrives at the unorthodox conclusion that obesity is not itself a significant health risk.

Heatherton, T. F., Herman, C. P., & Polivy, J. (1991). Effects of physical threat and ego threat on eating behavior. *Journal of Personality and Social Psychology, 60,* 138–143.

This experiment demonstrated that chronic dieters significantly increased their food intake when they were exposed to a task that threatened their self-image; however, their consumption was not significantly altered by a task that threatened their physical well-being.

Heatherton, T. F., Polivy, J., & Herman, C. P. (1991). Restraint, weight loss and variability of body weight. *Journal of Abnormal Psychology, 100,* 78–83.

After subjects were weighed daily for a 6-week period, it was shown that neither restrained nor unrestrained eaters lost a significant amount of weight, and that restraint was a better predictor of weight fluctuation than relative body weight.

Leibowitz, S. F. (1995). Brain peptides and obesity: Pharmacologic treatment. *Obesity Research, 3,* 573–589.

This review focuses on two hypothalamic peptide systems, neuropeptide Y and galanin; it illustrates how the brain operates through different mechanisms to control the body's nutrient stores.

Polivy, J. (1994). Physical activity, fitness, and compulsive behaviors. In C. Bouchard, R. J. Shephard, & T. Stephens (Eds.), *Physical activity, fitness, and health* (pp. 884–895). Champaign–Urbana, IL: Human Kinetics.

This review examines evidence on exercise that becomes out of control or compulsive, and compares this to problems such as eating disorders.

Polivy, J., Garner, D. M., & Garfinkel, P. E. (1986). Thinness and social behavior. In C. P. Herman, M. P. Zanna, & E. T. Higgins (Eds.), *The Ontario Symposium: Vol. 3. Physical appearance, stigma, and social behavior* (pp. 89–112). Hillsdale, NJ: Erlbaum.

The authors review and discuss the societal shifts toward a preference for thin female body shapes, and the effects of this on eating and psychopathology in women.

Polivy, J., & Herman, C. P. (1987). Diagnosis and treatment of normal eating. *Journal of Consulting and Clinical Psychology, 55,* 635–644.

This article argues that dieting has become the norm (or normal eating), but is itself pathogenic.

Stice, E., Schupak-Neuberg, E., Shaw, H. E., & Stein, R. I. (1994). Relation of media exposure to eating disorder symptomatology: An examination of mediating mechanisms. *Journal of Abnormal Psychology, 103,* 836–840.

In data from 238 female students, structural equation modeling revealed a direct effect of mass media exposure on eating disorder symptoms.

Stice, E., & Shaw, H. E. (1994). Adverse effects of the media-portrayed thin ideal on women and linkages to bulimic symptomatology. *Journal of Social and Clinical Psychology, 13,* 233–308.

In this experiment, women who were exposed to magazine pictures of very thin models reported greater negative affect (i.e., depression, guilt) than control subjects, and these negative feelings also predicted bulimic symptomatology.

62

Social Physique Anxiety

Robert C. Eklund

N ot only have the benefits of exercise and physical activity for health and well-being been well documented, but there is a generalized awareness of these benefits in the lay population. Nonetheless, adherence to exercise programs is disturbingly low, and only a minority of the adult population is sufficiently active to attain or maintain desirable levels of physical fitness. Paradoxically, it has also been noted that some individuals have embraced exercise with a fervor that can only be characterized as obsessive even to the point of undermining well-being.

SELF-PRESENTATION

"Self-presentation" refers to the processes by which individuals monitor and attempt to control the impressions others may form. The basic premise is that people engage in selective presentation and omission of aspects of the self in social encounters, both to create desired impressions and to avoid undesired impressions. The physical self plays a prominent role in the current Western cultural ethos, and thus must play an important role in exercise motivation. Self-presentational processes are clearly operating when desires to improve or maintain physical appearance through exercise, or to construct a certain social identity or image (such as being fit or athletic), are considered. People exercise to improve their health and well-being, to lose weight, and to improve their appearance. Some investigators have argued that self-presentational motives also underlie health motives, since being healthier also enhances one's image for others.

Nevertheless, physique-related perceptions may also stimulate protective self-presentational behaviors, or may deter individuals from being active when they have concerns about being negatively evaluated while exercising. Thus, despite an interest in exercising to improve physical appearance, to lose weight, or even to improve health and well-being, people's exercise behaviors may be constrained by fears of engendering physique-related negative evaluation. For example, concerns about being observed and evaluated by others have been identified as the most influential factors limiting the willingness of overweight female exercisers to exercise in public or to attend exercise studios. Indeed, one would be hard pressed to ignore the extremely lean aesthetic ideal propagated in virtually all segments of public life or, particularly for women, to misunderstand the self-presentational consequences of flaunting any significant deviance from this standard. Hence, perceptions of threat (real or imagined) in this regard seem likely to influence motivated behavior in exercise settings.

SOCIAL PHYSIQUE ANXIETY

A central construct in much of the recent self-presentational research on exercise behaviors has been "social physique anxiety" (SPA). "Social anxiety" is an affective consequence that may be experienced when people doubt their ability to make desired impressions on others but when doubt their ability to do so. SPA is the specific form of social anxiety associated with concerns that one's body may be negatively evaluated. Given the current cultural ethos, the important role that physical appearance plays in self-esteem, and the well-documented and widespread incidence of body dissatisfaction, it is intuitively reasonable to expect that physique-related self-presentational anxiety should be salient.

Research on SPA and exercise is only in its preliminary stages. Nonetheless, results from initial investigations have been promising, and considerable research is now in progress to more fully explore the utility of self-presentational perspectives for understanding exercise behavior. Most research exploring associations between SPA and exercise published to date has been conducted with young adult (college-age) women. Unfortunately, the examination of exercise and SPA in age groups beyond young adulthood has been limited to a single training study with middle-aged adults.

CORRELATES OF SOCIAL PHYSIQUE ANXIETY

SPA has been found to correlate with a number of psychosocial variables logically associated with evaluative concerns among young adult women, including measures of global self-esteem and body esteem, fear of negative evaluation, weight dissatisfaction, body dissatisfaction, and body cathexis; it has also been linked with perceptions of physical competence among adolescent female gymnasts. High-SPA women have also been found to experience more stress during physical fitness examinations and to report more negative thoughts about their bodies during the examinations. Finally, a variety of physical characteristics correlate with SPA, including weight, height, and percentage of body fat among young adult women, and hip, abdomen, and waist circumferences and percentage of body fat among middle-aged adults (aged 45–64 years).

SOCIAL PHYSIQUE ANXIETY, GENDER, AND AGE

As previously mentioned, exploration of SPA has largely been conducted among young adult women. Some tentative comments can, however, be made in regard to males and other age groups. Perhaps not surprisingly, given gender-related cultural expectations, females have been consistently found to be significantly higher in SPA than males in both young adult and middle-aged populations. Examination of age cohorts within a middle-aged sample (45–64 years) has given some indication that SPA decreases with age for both men and women. Unfortunately, it appears that high SPA is not solely the province of young women, given the observation that "younger" middle-aged women (between the ages of 45 and 54), in particular, suffer from substantially greater SPA than normative samples of adolescent and young adult females. It may be that a salient motive to appear physically attractive, combined with doubts about the ability to so (probably influenced or exacerbated by an awareness of the cultural aesthetic ideal), increases the potential for SPA among females in this age group. In any case, the fact that levels of SPA are higher among "younger" middle-aged women may be a cause for public health concern.

SOCIAL PHYSIQUE ANXIETY AND MOTIVES FOR EXERCISE

Consistent with theoretical predictions, empirical evidence reveals SPA to be significantly associated with the importance individuals assign to self-presentational motives for exercise. Specifically, the importance of motives for exercise related to the development or maintenance of easily observable physical qualities, including exercising for body tone, weight control, and physical attractiveness, appears to be positively associated with SPA. Furthermore, associations between SPA and self-presentational motives for exercise appear to be independent of body composition; that is, these associations are robust even when considered in the context of objective measures of body fat. Hence, associations between SPA and self-presentational reasons for exercise cannot be simply attributed to some rational health-related need to reduce fat. Although motives for engaging in exercise that are largely independent of self-presentation (e.g., exercising for fitness, mood enhancement, enjoyment) are salient among women, they do not appear to be significantly associated with SPA.

SOCIAL PHYSIQUE ANXIETY AND EXERCISE BEHAVIOR

Preliminary evidence suggests that in the absence of consideration of social context, there is no relationship between SPA and the frequency or duration of women's exercise. In other words, dispositional anxiety associated with physique evaluation is not independently a sufficient index of the propensity to exercise. It does appear, however, that SPA interacts with social context in shaping exercise behaviors. For example, evidence suggests that SPA is associated with attendance at specific exercise programs (a particular social context), and that high-SPA women are more likely to engage in exercise in private settings.

SOCIAL PHYSIQUE ANXIETY AND ATTITUDES TOWARD EXERCISE SETTINGS

Attitudes toward exercise settings may be suggestive of how SPA interacts with social context to shape exercise behaviors, and recent studies I have conducted with Crawford have explored associations between SPA and the favorability of attitudes toward exercise settings emphasizing or deemphasizing physique salience. In these investigations, physique salience in an aerobics dance setting was manipulated in two otherwise identical videotapes by clothing exercisers in physique-revealing aerobics fashion attire in one instance, and loose-fitting shorts and T-shirts in the other. Undergraduate women responded to questions indicative of favorability of attitudes toward the settings after viewing each of the two tapes. In the first investigation, attitudes were more favorable toward the less revealing shorts and T-shirts setting. Furthermore, patterns of association revealed that higher-SPA women had less favorable attitudes toward the setting emphasizing the physique (i.e., aerobics fashion attire) and more favorable attitudes toward the same setting when the physique was deemphasized by loose T-shirts and shorts. As would be expected upon consideration of evaluative potential relative to the body, SPA was most strongly (and negatively) associated with the favorability of attitudes toward the exercise setting emphasizing the physique. SPA was a better predictor of favorability of attitudes toward the exercise settings than were other self-perception variables (e.g., weight dissatisfaction and body dissatisfaction) in those analyses.

Our second investigation provided indications that the relationship between SPA and social context in shaping attitudes toward exercise settings may be mediated or moderated by factors such as participatory or educational experience, or other personal characteristics. Specifically, we were unable to replicate previous findings with a sample of physically active women from physical education classes, who were normatively low in weight dissatisfaction and percentage of body fat, but not notably low in SPA. Despite the absence of association between attitudes toward the settings and SPA, significant (albeit modest) correlations, in expected directions, were observed between SPA and personal preferences for loose-fitting and tight-fitting exercise clothing. These correlations were robust when body composition was controlled for. Further research is needed to explore factors that may lead to desensitization or selective disinhibition for situations saturated with potential for evaluation of the physique.

SOCIAL PHYSIQUE ANXIETY AND SOCIAL CONTEXTUAL FACTORS

Preliminary exploration of aspects of the exercise social context (beyond physique salience) from a self-presentational perspective has also been revealing. These initial efforts suggest that SPA is associated with preferences in class composition (e.g., fitness level relative to that of other class participants, presence of males in class) and the relative desirability of spectators in exercise settings. Once again, it appears that these associations are robust when body composition is controlled for.

First, it appears that young adult women on average have a modest preference for exercising in classes where other members are obviously in "worse shape," and a modest dislike of classes where other members are obviously in "better shape." Not surprisingly, given the potential for negative evaluation, the disinclination for participating with people in "better shape" tends to be most pronounced among individuals higher in SPA. SPA does not, however, appear to be systematically associated with preferences for classes where other class members are in "worse shape." Apparently, perceptions of self-presentational threat are attenuated when one is in better shape than other class members, and this accounts for the absence of any systematic association with SPA.

Second, the contextual salience of males participating in aerobics classes appears to vary systematically among women differing in SPA. Overall, the extent of awareness of and preference for males in aerobics dance classes appears to be rather moderate; young adult women reveal no particularly strong sentiment one way or the other. However, the awareness of and preference for males in the exercise setting are systematically associated with SPA. Specifically, women high in SPA tend to be less amenable to coed classes and more aware of the presence of members of the opposite sex attending classes. Hence it appears that the presence of males does stimulate perceptions of evaluative threat relative to the physique, at least among women prone to such concerns.

Third, as aerobic dance participants can attest, interested or curious spectators will accumulate to observe if they are given the opportunity, and these onlookers do appear to influence the social context of exercise settings. Young adult women, on average, do not tend to indicate any particular affinity for aerobics class spectators. Women highest in SPA tend to find the presence of spectators the least desirable. The tendency to be concerned about physique evaluation in the presence of spectators was found to be independent of body composition, and hence is not simply a matter of degree of fatness. It seems safe to say that onlookers are not particularly welcome—particularly among those with the greatest concerns about having their bodies evaluated negatively.

THE EFFECTS OF EXERCISE
ON SOCIAL PHYSIQUE ANXIETY

Indirect evidence suggests that experienced exercisers are lower in SPA than inexperienced exercisers on average. Evidence from a recent study with middle-aged adults (aged 45–64 years) also supports this conjecture. A relatively low-impact 20-week exercise program of moderate intensity (e.g., brisk walking) was found to produce significant reductions in SPA. This reduction was more prevalent for women than for men, and for younger than for older subjects. Furthermore, changes in social-psychological variables (e.g., physical self-efficacy and positive outcome expectations) were associated with reductions in SPA, and these associations were robust even when the influence of gender and of changes in physical parameters (e.g., body fat, weight, and body circumferences) was controlled. Hence it appears that exercise may well have anxiolytic effects on physique-related self-presentational concerns.

FURTHER READING

Bain, L. L., Wilson, T., & Chaikind, E. (1989). Participant perceptions of exercise programs for overweight women. *Research Quarterly for Exercise and Sport, 60,* 134–143.
This qualitative investigation revealed the significant impact of self-presentational concerns upon overweight women's willingness to exercise.

Crawford, S., & Eklund, R. C. (1994). Social physique anxiety, reasons for exercise, and attitudes toward exercise settings. *Journal of Sport and Exercise Psychology, 16,* 70–82.
This investigation explored SPA as a motivating and demotivating influence for exercise behavior among college-age women.

Eklund, R. C., & Crawford, S. (1994). Active women, social physique anxiety, and exercise. *Journal of Sport and Exercise Psychology, 16,* 431–448.
This investigation examined associations between SPA on the one hand and social-contextual features of aerobic dance settings, motives for exercise participation, and attitudes toward aerobic dance settings on the other.

Eklund, R. C., Mack, D., & Hart, E. (1996). Factorial validity of the Social Physique Anxiety Scale for Females. *Journal of Sport and Exercise Psychology, 18,* 281–295.
This study of the Social Physique Anxiety Scale with 760 young women revealed the existence of the complementary subcomponents of SPA of "Negative Physique Evaluation Concerns" and "Physique Presentation Comfort."

Eklund, R. C., Kelley, B., & Wilson, P. (1997). The Social Physique Anxiety Scale: Men, women, and the effects of modifying item-2. *Journal of Sport and Exercise Psychology, 19,* 188–196.
This brief report clarifies the measurement properties of the Social Physique Anxiety Scale for use with males and females, and evaluates previously recommended modifications to item-2.

Hart, E. A., Leary, M. R., & Rejeski, W. J. (1989). The measurement of social physique anxiety. *Journal of Sport and Exercise Psychology, 11,* 94–104.
The report of initial validation studies for the Social Physique Anxiety Scale.

McAuley, E., Bane, S. M., & Mihalko, S. L. (1995). Exercise in middle-aged adults: Self-efficacy and self-presentational outcomes. *Preventive Medicine, 24,* 319–328.
This study with middle-aged adults revealed that exercise-related reductions in SPA were mediated by physiological and psychological changes.

McAuley, E., Bane, S. M., Rudolph, D. L., & Lox, C. L. (1995). Physique anxiety and exercise in middle-aged adults. *Journal of Gerontology: Psychological Sciences, 50B,* 229–235.
This study with middle-aged adults revealed that females and subjects between 45 and 54 years of age were significantly more physique anxious than older counterparts, and that participation in a 20-week aerobic exercise program reduced SPA.

McAuley, E., & Burman, G. (1993). The Social Physique Anxiety Scale: Construct validity in adolescent females. *Medicine and Science in Sports and Exercise, 65,* 1049–1053.
This construct validity study with adolescent competitive gymnasts revealed inverse relationships between aspects of physical efficacy and social physique anxiety.

Rodin, J. (1992). *Body traps.* New York: William Morrow.
This book examines the current cultural ethos regarding the body and its consequences among women.

63

Negative Body Image

James C. Rosen

Although most practitioners who work with women are aware that negative body image can be an important problem, how to help people to change the way they view their appearance can seem mysterious. Fortunately, body image can change even when physical appearance does not change. The purpose of this chapter is to provide practical guidelines for changing negative and promoting positive body images in women.

WHAT IS NEGATIVE BODY IMAGE?

Unlike normal concerns about physical appearance, a "negative body image" implies a preoccupation that is excessively time-consuming, is distressing, and interferes with activities. To place importance on physical appearance or to be self-conscious at times is not unusual. A negative body image, by contrast, implies that *too* much attention is given to appearance in self-evaluation. A devotion to exercise or fashion that takes a great deal of time may seem extreme. However, a negative body image implies that lengthy fitness or beauty routines are accompanied by worrying about appearance and are more like compulsions than like healthy, pleasurable pursuits.

WHO HAS NEGATIVE BODY IMAGE?

Although the boundary between normal and abnormal concerns about appearance is difficult to specify, there are two diagnostic categories that accommodate persons with body image disorder. Body dysmorphic disorder is an excessive concern with an imaginary, or at most a minor, defect in appearance. Whereas body dysmorphic disorder can center on any aspect of appearance, persons with eating disorders typically are more concerned about body size and shape. Negative body image in anorexia nervosa and bulimia nervosa is important, because it is the most common precipitant of dieting and the most difficult feature of these disorders for the patients to overcome. Seldom is a woman with an eating disorder able to eliminate abnormal eating and dieting behavior permanently without coming to terms with her physical appearance.

Body image problems are also common in overweight, physically ill, and physically injured persons (e.g., persons who have had a mastectomy, stoma, or amputation). Although these persons may not imagine their appearance defects or the resulting social prejudice, they still can exhibit a problem that deserves intervention if their concern becomes unnecessarily distressing or interfering. In addition, negative body image occurs with some frequency in persons seeking cosmetic surgery or dentistry and in dermatology patients. Concern about appearance is a common issue for pregnant women as well. In total, probably close to 10% of women suffer from significant body image problems.

A COGNITIVE-BEHAVIORAL APPROACH TO OVERCOMING NEGATIVE BODY IMAGE: SUGGESTIONS FOR THE THERAPIST

Several controlled clinical trials of interventions for body image have been conducted. Cognitive-behavioral body image therapy administered in 8 weeks or less is effective in producing positive body image change in college women and clinical samples of overweight women and women with body dysmorphic disorder. To date, no other form of therapy, psychological or pharmacological, has been tested systematically. Suggestions for conducting this type of therapy follow.

Changing the Patient's Attitudes toward Therapy

In appearance-conscious U.S. society, people are taught that if they want to feel better about their appearance, they should lose weight, exercise, or have cosmetic surgery. In other words, they should eliminate or correct the defect. Consequently, it is difficult for most patients at first to imagine how they could view themselves differently at the end of a psychological therapy if the offending appearance feature is still present. Nothing, they might argue, could convince them that they look good when they know, or the rest of society tells them, that they look bad. Another typical concern is that self-acceptance will cause a loss of self-control and a worse problem, as if disliking oneself is necessary to remain in control.

To deal with a patient's initial skepticism about therapy, it is important to provide information about the concept of body image and the goals of treatment. Make it clear at the beginning that although the patient is free to pursue beauty remedies on her own, therapy is designed to change body image, not appearance. Explain that body image is a psychological construct, and that because it is subjective, it can be independent of actual appearance. Use examples, preferably from the patient's own experience, to demonstrate that losing weight or other beauty remedies may not change self-image. Aside from any physical "problem," a person can have habits that interfere with her functioning. The goal of therapy will not necessarily be for her to like her appearance, but to tolerate it and to eliminate self-defeating behavioral tendencies. It can help to reassure the patient that most participants in body image therapy change, regardless of the severity of their defects, and do not give up healthy beauty and fitness routines or gain weight.

Changing Body Image Thoughts and Assumptions

Ask the patient to keep a diary of body image experiences, dividing them into an A-B-C sequence: (1) *Activating* events (the situations and triggers for physical self-consciousness or body dissatisfaction), (2) *Beliefs* (thoughts about the situation or self), and (3) *Consequences* in her emotional and behavioral reactions.

Negative Body Talk

Much time can be spent dwelling on repetitive, intrusive thoughts of body dissatisfaction. This negative body talk, such as "My thighs are really disgusting; they make me look like a fat slob," must change. The patient must be helped to construct more objective, neutral, or sensory self-descriptions that are believable and not emotionally loaded self-criticisms. For example, she might practice calling her thighs "smooth" and "muscular" rather than "thunder thighs." She should practice this neutral body talk regularly, especially when reminded of her appearance. When she slips into negative body talk, she can distract herself by repeating the more forgiving description. It does not matter whether she likes what she sees. The point is to eliminate the negative body talk that causes distress.

Self-Defeating Thoughts and Assumptions

Using her diary, help the patient examine the effect of negative body on other thoughts or assumptions about her appearance. For example, ask: "What was upsetting about your *thunder thighs* in that situation? What did you imagine people were thinking when they saw you?" A frequent thought pattern is the following: "I look bad; people notice and care about my appearance; they judge me negatively as a person. Therefore, my appearance proves something negative about me (e.g., I'm unlovable, foolish, lazy, weak, unfeminine, immoral, etc.)." Another common assumption, as Cash has noted, is this: "If I could look just as I wish, my life would be much happier. If people knew how I really look, they would like me less. My appearance is responsible for much of what has happened to me in my life. The only way I could ever like my looks would be to change how I look."

Now change the patient's body image diary from an A-B-C to an A-B-C-D-E format. The D section will be the place for her to write *Disputing* thoughts to correct self-defeating beliefs. The E section is for the positive *Effects* of corrective thinking. Instruct her to write the disputing thought and practice it in anticipation of and during situations that trigger body dissatisfaction: "I'm not weak-willed. I'm competent. People think I am a smart dresser." Settle on thoughts that are reasonable, and encourage her to practice them until they become familiar and believable. Ask the patient to notice the positive emotional effects of these experiences.

At first, concentrate on beliefs that are somewhat less convincing (they will be easier to modify), and then progress to firm convictions. For example, a patient may be willing to question whether strangers care so much about her appearance, but she may be convinced that her husband wants to leave her because of her weight. The latter *seems* more justified, because a husband should be more invested in his wife's appearance than strangers. Do not argue with the patient about whether the supposed defect really exists.

To construct disputing thoughts, help the patient evaluate the evidence for and against the belief. For instance, she should take stock of comments on her appearance that people actually make, rather than what she *thinks* people might think. She should reflect on abilities and personal traits other than appearance. Ask questions that will encourage her to examine her assumptions: "How important are your looks compared to other characteristics? What would happen if you looked different? Is there anything other than looking different you would have to do in order to make that happen, or would looking different be all that is necessary? If you didn't hide your looks, what do you imagine would happen? Have you ever tested that prediction? Are there other explanations for events that have happened besides your appearance? Has changing your looks always led to feeling better about your appearance? Are you really capable of changing your appearance the way you wish? Is the problem your body or your body image?"

Overweight patients and others with objective physical disadvantages may be confronted with discrimination. Realistic thoughts about these encounters should not be discounted. However, help the patient learn more self-enhancing ways to respond. The patient should be discouraged from looking for defects to explain negative attitudes from other people. Help her realize that discrimination results from stereotypes (usually erroneous) about an entire segment of society, rather than accurate perceptions of an individual. Stereotypes might influence initial encounters, but they have little influence in established relationships. Discourage self-blame for appearance and uncritical acceptance of negative stereotypes.

Changing Body Image Behaviors

To feel more confident, the patient must begin to act more confident. The following exercises and suggestions have been found to be helpful.

The Mirror Exercise

Before the patient faces more challenging situations, first encourage her to develop some comfort with viewing herself in the private. She should list her body areas or attributes in order from most satisfying to most distressing. Using a full-length mirror, and starting with the most satisfying area, she should view each body area for a full minute. As she feels comfortable with each body area, she should proceed to the next item on the list. Be prepared to spend up to several weeks of daily practice on this exercise. Ultimately, she should carry out the exercise without clothes. Remind her that she does not need to like what she sees, but she must refrain from negative body talk and build tolerance for imperfections.

Facing Avoided Situations

Avoiding situations, styles of dress, or activities may prevent a patient from coming to terms with her appearance. She can liberate herself from these inhibitions and be inoculated against self-consciousness. Plan a strategy of gradual exposure to things she avoids because of negative body image feelings. A patient of mine who was overly self-conscious about her "chubby cheeks" and fleshy upper shoulders took the following step-by-step actions: She wore her hair pulled back rather than combed over her face;

she applied rouge to her cheeks; she wore a blouse with a scooped collar instead of a turtleneck; and finally, with the lights on, she let her husband give her a neck massage.

Body Checking and Excessive Grooming

A patient who constantly checks her appearance in mirrors can perpetuate distressing body image feelings, and one who changes her clothes over and over before going out can be exasperating to herself and others. It is important to identify these self-defeating habits and to set limits on them. For instance, if your patient is an excessive clothes changer, allow her only two changes before leaving for work. Limit her to 45 minutes for the entire grooming regimen. She should also stop asking people for reassurance (e.g., "Does it look like I've lost weight?"). Teach her to refrain from inspecting skin blemishes in the mirror. Reduce checking by starting with the easiest habits to break. If she weighs herself after every meal, in the morning, and at night, she might start by avoiding the scale at night. Ask her, "What are the consequences of eliminating or limiting your rituals?" A patient usually discovers that the outcomes she fears do not materialize. For example, avoiding the scale for a few days will *not* make her gain weight.

Accepting Compliments

Modesty is a virtue, but a patient should beware of rejecting compliments. Because other people can be more objective, and usually more positive, about her appearance, it is desirable for her to listen to positive feedback and incorporate it into her self-image. Help her to plan in advance how she will respond to compliments. If her inclination is to reject compliments, she should replace "Oh, you can't mean that; I really look terrible today," with "Thanks, it *is* a new hairstyle," and repeat the comment silently in order to remember it.

Comparing

When a person dislikes something about her appearance, it is natural for her to compare the offending area to that of other people. It is easy for her to become preoccupied with these comparisons, and they are often biased toward people whom she considers more perfect-looking. Identify and reduce such self-defeating comparisons. For example, one patient decided to stop buying fashion magazines. She also changed her normal position in an aerobics class to the front so that she would not compare herself with "better-looking" classmates. And, finally, she stopped verbalizing such comparisons as "How do you stay so thin?" or "I wish I had your color!" Another patient focused on other women's smiles rather than their physiques. Still another tried to appreciate beauty in women ("What a lovely figure she has"), instead of dwelling on hostile, jealous thoughts ("I can't stand these skinny women").

CONCLUSIONS

Good health and fitness practices, and pleasing styles of dress and makeup, can help people look younger and more attractive. But for some individuals, looking better to the outside world is not enough. In addition, many people have less-than-perfect appearances that cannot be remedied with weight loss, cosmetics, or surgery. The psychological methods described above can be successful with women who vary widely in age, education, and physical appearance. Not only is body image change possible; it is essential for individuals who struggle with these issues.

FURTHER READING

Cash, T. F. (1995). *What do you see when you look in the mirror?: Helping yourself to a positive body image.* New York: Bantam Books.
A body image therapy program written for the consumer in a self-help format. It can be used by itself or as a companion to psychotherapy.

Cash, T. F., & Pruzinsky, T. (Eds.). (1990). *Body images: Development, deviance, and change.* New York: Guilford Press.
Covers the entire field of body image and its manifestation in different clinical populations.

Rosen, J. C. (1995). The nature of body dysmorphic disorder and treatment with cognitive behavior therapy. *Cognitive and Behavioral Practice, 2,* 143–166.
Details on the clinical presentation of severe body image disorder and its diagnosis and treatment.

64

The Emergence of
Negative Body Images

Thomas F. Cash

Body image attitudes consist of self-perceptions, cognitions, affects, and behaviors pertaining to one's physical attributes. As a prominent facet of self-concept, body image bears a moderate relationship to self-esteem and to the occurrence of eating disturbances, depression, social anxiety, and sexual difficulties.

Although much of the literature on body image consists of studies of college students and eating-disordered patients, large-sample surveys of body image were conducted in *Psychology Today* magazine in 1972, 1985, and 1996. Both men's and women's body images became more negative over this 24-year period. A representative survey of 803 adult U.S. women I conducted with Henry in 1993 (and published in 1995) indicated substantial levels of body dissatisfaction. As summarized in Table 64.1, nearly half of the women reported globally negative evaluations of their appearance.

In several respects, women possess more dysfunctional body image attitudes than do men. The greatest gender differences pertain to women's affect-laden concerns about their shape and weight, particularly fears about being or becoming fat, which foster widespread dieting. Moreover, cognitive and behavioral investments in appearance are clearly greater for women than for men. These gender differences in body image occur across the lifespan, and the adolescent years may be notably associated with stronger investment in appearance and a more negative body image.

THE DEVELOPMENT OF A NEGATIVE BODY IMAGE

The causal factors in the emergence of a dysfunctional body image may be divided into two basic categories. First are the historical causes in a person's background that shape the acquisition of particular body image attitudes. Second are the proximal influences in the present that direct the flow of body image experiences in everyday life.

TABLE 64.1. Percentages of U.S. Women Dissatisfied and Not Actively Satisfied with Their Overall Appearance and with Specific Physical Attributes

Physical area/attribute	Percentage dissatisfied	Percentage dissatisfied or neutral[a]
Global appearance evaluation	47.9	59.5
Specific attribute		
Face	11.7	30.4
Height	13.4	30.4
Hair	16.3	28.0
Upper torso	25.1	47.3
Muscle tone	36.9	63.9
Weight	46.0	63.3
Lower torso	47.4	64.2
Mid torso	51.0	69.8

Note. Adapted from Cash and Henry (1995). Copyright 1995 by Plenum Publishing Corporation. Adapted by permission.
[a]Includes dissatisfied respondents (ratings of 1 or 2), as well as those indicating "neither satisfied nor dissatisfied" (rating of 3) on the survey's 1–5 response scale.

Historical Determinants

One's sense of self is rooted in the experience of embodiment. The body is the boundary that separates a person from all that is not the person—from the outside world. Humans, like certain other higher primates, have the capacity for self-awareness. By 2 years of age, most children can recognize their bodily selves in the mirror. Increasingly, this physical reality becomes a self-representation. Body image takes shape as preschoolers internalize the messages and aesthetic standards of society and then judge themselves against them. In this way, children develop conceptions of what is good (how one *should* look) and what is bad (how one should *not* look)—with respect to height, weight, muscularity, hair color, and even the style or brand name of clothing. From childhood on, people not only evaluate their appearance in terms of how well it matches the "shoulds," but also appraise their self-worth on the basis of these standards.

Western culture teaches that thinness for women and muscularity for men are socially desirable. Unlike earlier periods, recent decades have heralded a thinner, not-so-curvaceous body type as the standard of feminine beauty. Fashion models, film stars, and beauty pageant contestants have become thinner, even as the female population has become heavier. Liposuction has emerged as one of the most frequently performed cosmetic surgeries. Recent societal messages stress not only that women must be slender but also that they must be well toned, and the primary motives of women's exercise regimens are weight and appearance management. Furthermore, as body image experiences often mirror the cultural context, intercultural and racial/ethnic diversity has been observed in body satisfaction. For example, African-American women have more favorable attitudes toward their physical appearance, even at heavier body weights, than do European-American and Hispanic women.

Various researchers have examined people's physical standards for the other gender and the accuracy of people's assumptions concerning these ideals. Evidence attests to distorted beliefs about what the other gender truly finds most attractive. People seem to equate others' standards with their own personal ideals, though others' expectations are seldom as extreme or as stringently held. For example, men are often more appreciative of a heavier female body type than women believe men are. Nor do men idealize blonde beauty and large breasts to the degree that women think. Similarly, women do not necessarily hold the narrow standards of male attractiveness that men assume women hold.

The process of socialization about the meaning of human bodily appearance goes beyond media messages. Families also model values pertaining to physical appearance. Parents who spend considerable time and effort perfecting their children's appearance are modeling the attitude that good looks are essential to acceptance in the "outside world." Recent research suggests that growing up with a mother who stresses and disparages her own looks may adversely affect a daughter's sense of body acceptance. Moreover, growing up with a sibling who is doted on for being attractive may lead to implicit social comparisons that diminish one's own body satisfaction.

Recurrent teasing or criticism about appearance during one's youth can have an enduring effect on body image. Indeed, appearance is the most common content of social teasing in childhood. In several surveys of college women, approximately 70% revealed that earlier in their lives they had been repeatedly teased or criticized about some aspect(s) of their appearance, especially facial features and weight. Among these women, nearly half said that this occurred moderately to very often; it came especially frequently from peers during the middle childhood to early teen years. Almost half reported having an unappealing, appearance-referential nickname—"Dumbo," "Carrot Top," "Bubble Butt," "Pizza Face," "Stick." Moreover, nearly three-fourths indicated that these experiences had marred their body image development. In fact, more frequent and upsetting teasing and criticism were significantly associated with greater body discontent and distress later on, in young adulthood.

Changes in one's appearance are a natural part of aging and development. People have control over some aspects of their appearance, and can make choices (e.g., a new haircut or hair style) that either can enhance body image *or* can lead to a gnawing concern about ruined looks. Other aspects are beyond one's control, the results of heredity or life's misfortunes. For example, being a "fat kid" often entails social apathy and antipathy, which may contribute to a sense of physical unacceptability that may persist despite subsequent weight loss. Body image difficulties may also result from traumatic disfigurements of appearance, such as severe facial injuries or mastectomy, or from more gradual appearance-altering conditions, such as "normal" hereditary hair loss.

Puberty brings dramatic changes in appearance. It can also bring an intense preoccupation with these changes and with how they will be perceived by others. The timing of physical maturation can be critical to the emotional meaning that adolescents attach to their changing bodies. Girls whose breasts and hips develop earlier than those of their peers may receive unwanted attention and become self-conscious. Rather than welcoming their new shape as a sign of emergent womanhood, many girls view it as unappealing fat and an impetus to diet. However commonplace facial acne may be during adolescence, it too can pose problems of self-consciousness and body image despair. Teenagers' sense of acceptability—whether they expect to be popular, especially in dating—revolves around how they *believe* their looks are regarded by their peers.

Another source of influence on body image development pertains to certain moderating personality traits. Perhaps most salient is the extent to which persons are "appearance-schematic." Such individuals define much of their selfhood in terms of their physical attributes, and their perceptions of events are often colored by assumptions about their appearance. Public self-consciousness, which is an attentional disposition to view oneself as an audience, can potentiate self-scrutiny and preoccupation with one's appearance.

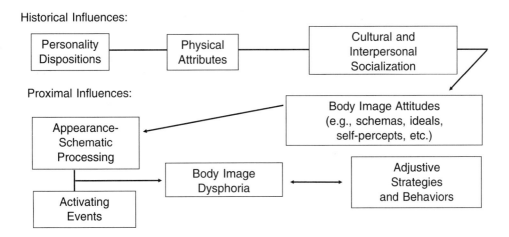

Historical Influences:

Proximal Influences:

FIGURE 64.1. Causal factors in development of a negative body image.

Self-esteem and social confidence are also crucial moderator variables. The child, adolescent, or adult who has acquired a positive sense of self is less vulnerable to societal "shoulds" or assaults on his or her physical worth. Finally, my own recent research suggests that women who have acquired more traditional values and expectations about gender roles in male–female relations are especially dysfunctionally invested in their looks.

Proximal Determinants

Cultural socialization, interpersonal experiences, physical traits and changes, and personality factors serve as predisposing causes of positive or negative body image attitudes. How these attitudes affect day-to-day body experiences depend upon precipitating, cognitive mediational, and maintaining factors. Figure 64.1 summarizes these proximal causal influences, as well as historical ones.

From my perspective, specific contextual events serve to activate schema-driven processing of information about and self-appraisals of one's body and appearance. The activating events typically involve body exposure, social scrutiny, social comparison processes, wearing certain clothing, looking in the mirror, eating, weighing, exercising, or some unwanted change in appearance. The self-evaluations draw upon extant body image attitudes and upon discrepancies between self-perceived and idealized physical characteristics. Implicit or explicit "internal dialogues" (i.e., automatic thoughts, interpretations, and conclusions) reflect habitual and faulty patterns of reasoning via the commission of specific cognitive errors (e.g., dichotomous thinking, selective abstraction, arbitrary inference, etc.). These cognitions potentiate various body image affects, which in turn motivate adjustive, emotion-regulating actions. Among the "defensive" actions are situational avoidance, appearance-concealing behaviors, compulsive appearance-correcting rituals, social reassurance seeking, and compensatory behaviors. These patterns function as negatively reinforced, maintaining causes to the extent that they enable the person to escape, reduce, or regulate dysphoric experiences.

SCIENCE, SOCIETY, AND SOLUTIONS

Body image concerns continue to be prevalent among U.S. women. Unfortunately, there is little scientific evidence that the recent economic, occupational, and political gains of women in the United States have brought improvements in their body images; appearance pressures have not lessened. Many feminist writers regard macrosocietal changes as necessary to remedy the sexist victimization of women by the mass media and by the beauty and fashion industries. Other scholars emphasize the psychoeducational empowerment of women (and men) to resist such forces and to enhance body acceptance. The needs for social change, preventative education, and effective therapies certainly remain crucial. In a previous chapter of this volume, Rosen describes guidelines for cognitive-behavioral body image therapy, and notes the utility of this therapy for a range of body-dissatisfied populations. Structured cognitive-behavioral programs, even when largely self-administered, are efficacious in the promotion of positive body image changes.

FURTHER READING

Berscheid, E., Walster, E., & Bohrnstedt, G. (1973). The happy American body: A survey report. *Psychology Today, 7*(11), 119–131.
Presents findings of the 1972 magazine survey.

Cash, T. F. (1991). *Body image therapy: A program for self-directed change.* New York: Guilford Press.
An audiocassette program to guide clients and therapists in promoting body image change.

Cash, T. F. (1995). *What do you see when you look in the mirror?: Helping yourself to a positive body image.* New York: Bantam Books.
An eight-step self-help program based on cognitive-behavioral principles and procedures.

Cash, T. F. (1997). *The body image workbook.* Oakland, CA: New Harbinger Publications.
The eight-step cognitive-behavioral program in a workbook format.

Cash, T. F., Ancis, J. R., & Strachan, M. D. (1997). Gender attitudes, feminist identity, and body images among college women. *Sex Roles, 36,* 433–447.
An examination of the relationship of gender role and body image attitudes.

Cash, T. F., & Deagle, E. A. (1997). The nature and extent of body image disturbances in anorexia nervosa and bulimia nervosa: A meta-analysis. *International Journal of Eating Disorders, 22,* 107–125.
A quantitative review of the literature on body image and eating disorders.

Cash, T. F., & Grant, J. R. (1996). Cognitive-behavioral treatment of body-image disturbances. In V. Van Hasselt & M. Hersen (Eds.), *Sourcebook of psychological treatment manuals for adult disorders* (pp. 567–614). New York: Plenum Press.
Details cognitive-behavioral body image therapy for clinicians.

Cash, T. F., & Henry, P. (1995). Women's body images: The results of a national survey in the U.S.A. *Sex Roles, 33,* 19–28.
A survey of how U.S. women feel about their bodies.

Cash, T. F., & Pruzinsky, T. (Eds.). (1990). *Body images: Development, deviance, and change.* New York: Guilford Press.
A documentation of theory and research on body image.

Cash, T. F., Winstead, B. A., & Janda, L. H. (1986). The great American shape-up: Body image survey report. *Psychology Today, 20*(4), 30–37.
Presents findings of the 1985 magazine survey.

Freedman, R. (1986). *Beauty bound.* Lexington, MA: Lexington Books.
A feminist perspective on the historical and cultural forces pertaining to women's appearance.

Garner, D. M. (1997). The 1997 body image survey results. *Psychology Today, 30*(1), 30–44, 75–80, 84.
Presents findings of the 1996 magazine survey.

Jackson, L. A. (1992). *Physical appearance and gender: Sociobiological and sociocultural perspectives.* Albany: State University of New York Press.
A review of research on the psychology of appearance.

Rodin, J. (1992). *Body traps.* New York: Morrow.
A very readable book on the pitfalls and excesses of beauty, dieting, and exercise.

65

Breast Implants

Thomas Pruzinsky

Women facing decisions regarding breast implant surgery are understandably looking for definite answers about the safety of these medical devices. Unfortunately, no such answers currently exist. There is considerable divergence in scientific and medical opinion on breast implant safety. Therefore, although I present some general conclusions, in this very brief chapter it is impossible to provide a thorough review of the many complicated methodological considerations regarding breast implant safety.

HEALTH-RELATED CONCERNS

In 1992 the U.S. Food and Drug Administration (FDA) imposed a moratorium on the use of silicone-gel-filled breast implants for solely cosmetic purposes, because, according to Kessler, "Thirty years after silicone breast implants appeared on the market, the list of unanswered questions remains long." Consequently, these devices are only available to women undergoing breast reconstruction surgery after mastectomy.

The complexity of evaluating the relative health risks of breast implants is influenced by many variables. Different types of implants (e.g., silicone-gel-filled, double-lumen, and polyurethane-coated) are associated with varying levels of risk, but these can be difficult to determine. Similarly the level of risk associated with saline-filled implants (which are constructed of silicone materials and filled with a saline solution) is also unknown, but is assumed to be less.

Table 65.1 lists some risks associated with silicone-gel-filled breast implants. In this limited review, I focus on the risk of capsular contracture, and on the possible associations of breast implants with autoimmune disease and cancer.

Capsular Contracture

"Capsular contracture," the most frequently reported problem in breast implant surgery, refers to the tightening and squeezing of the scar tissue that forms around breast implants. Capsular contracture can result in unnatural firmness, pain, breast sensitivity, and implant malposition. Treatment may consist of open capsulotomy (surgical release of the capsule)

TABLE 65.1. Potential Risks of Silicone-Gel-Filled Breast Implants

Breast-specific risks

Capsular contracture; gel bleed; breakage/rupture of implant with leakage
Calcium deposits in tissue surrounding implant
Granulomas
Changes in the nipple and breast sensation
Silicone in breast milk and/or problems with nursing

Potential systemic problems

Autoimmune disease
Cancer-related concerns
   Interference with tumor detection
   Increased incidence of cancer
Birth defects

Note. This list is not exhaustive. Rather, it is included to illustrate the potential range of health risks associated with breast implants. No attempt to record the exact incidence of these problems has been made. Not included are the risks associated with most surgical procedures, including the potential for infection, hematoma, poor wound healing, necrosis, or potential problems from anesthesia.

or closed capsulotomy (wherein the physician squeezes the breast to break the capsule). Closed capsulotomy can result in implant rupture. Implant rupture (e.g., through closed capsulotomy, other trauma, preimplantation damage, insertion of needle biopsy, etc.) and gel bleed (i.e., microscopic leakage of silicone in intact implants) probably leads to increased silicone gel migration beyond the capsule to other body sites. However, the degree to which migration of silicone increases the probability of a negative health impact is unclear.

Autoimmune Disease

The potential health risk receiving the greatest attention from the medical (and legal) community is the possibility of increased risk for autoimmune disease (e.g., rheumatoid arthritis, scleroderma, and lupus). The concern for this possible connection resulted from a series of case reports. Larger-scale investigations, such as those by Gabriel and colleagues and by Sanchez-Guerrero and colleagues, have not found such an association. However, according to Gabriel et al., their results "cannot be considered definitive proof of the absence of an association between breast implants and connective tissue disease." Currently, several large studies that will add to our understanding are being conducted. However, even when these methodologically improved studies are complete, uncertainty regarding the risk and benefit of implants is likely to remain.

Cancer

Current data have not yet revealed any definite association between breast implants and breast cancer. However, breast implants can interfere with mammography. All women with breast implants undergoing mammography should seek out professionals with experience in evaluating breast implant patients.

SURGICAL REMOVAL OF BREAST IMPLANTS

In response to concerns about health risks, many women have chosen to undergo breast implant removal. Indications for implant removal include breast pain, implant rupture, and patient or physician concern regarding the etiology of some physical symptoms. In 1994, surgeons certified by the American Society for Plastic and Reconstructive Surgeons (ASPRS) treated over 37,000 women for "explantation" (i.e., implant removal).

Empirical data regarding women who choose to have their implants removed are limited. According to a study by Slavin and Goldwyn, in one series of 46 patients requesting explantation, "fear of the possible harmful consequences of the silicone implants . . . was the most common reason for requesting removal." Another study by Wells and colleagues of 52 women requesting implant removal who also had rheumatological symptoms reported that the majority (67%) of these women initially underwent implantation for aesthetic reasons, with the remaining undergoing breast reconstruction after breast cancer. At the time of explantation, as a group, these 52 patients were mildly depressed (Beck Depression Inventory average scores of 15) and reported elevations on all scales of the Brief Symptom Inventory (with highest elevations on the Somatization and Obsessive–Compulsive scales). As a group, these women also reported a significant number of rheumatological symptoms, with the most common being fatigue, muscle pain, general stiffness, and painful joints. The investigators note that this study could have been influenced by sampling bias and should be interpreted with caution. They also explicitly note that there is no causal connection regarding the etiology of the psychological and physical symptoms.

Of the more than 37,000 patients treated by ASPRS surgeons in 1994 for explantation, approximately 28,500 had undergone implantation for cosmetic breast augmentation. According to the ASPRS, of those patients having implants removed, 74% were for "physical symptoms related to implant such as capsular contracture," 15% for "physical symptoms the patient believed related to implant," and 11% for "fear alone."

Many of these patients had their implants replaced with saline-filled implants (59%) or had no replacement (32%). A particularly poignant negative result of explantation is the fact that these women, who were concerned enough about their appearance to undergo breast surgery in the first place, would inevitably have been left with some residual breast deformity if they chose not to have their implants replaced. The psychological effect of such residual disfigurement has yet to be studied.

The ASPRS also reported that over 9,000 patients who had previously undergone breast reconstruction with breast implants chose to undergo explantation in 1994. The reported reasons for removal for 80% of these woman were for "physical symptoms related to implant such as capsular contracture," 15% for symptoms believed by the patients to be related to the implants, and 59% for fear alone. According to the ASPRS, of these 9,000-plus patients, 38% chose not to have any replacement and 52% chose replacement with saline-filled implants. Again, it will remain for future research to determine the relative rates of satisfaction with these decisions.

SATISFACTION WITH SURGERY

Prior to the 1992 FDA moratorium on breast implants, the majority of women (about 80%) undergoing breast surgery with silicone-gel-filled breast implants were doing so for breast augmentation. Consistent documentation of high levels of patient satisfaction (over 80%) existed for this operation, according to the ASPRS.

With the current scientific debate regarding the safety of breast implants, it can no longer be assumed that the same high rates of patient satisfaction will be maintained. A study by Handel and colleagues conducted near the time of the FDA hearings found a lower rate of patient satisfaction than that usually reported (61% satisfaction). The psychological efficacy of saline-filled breast implants or other methods of breast augmentation (e.g., using autologous tissue) will need to be evaluated in the future.

Research on the psychological impact of breast reconstruction prior to the breast implant moratorium can be generally summarized by concluding that the vast majority of women who underwent breast reconstruction were satisfied with the surgical outcomes. However, for many reasons, large numbers of women chose not to undergo breast reconstruction, even prior to the increased concern regarding the health effects of implants.

In 1994, almost 26,000 women whose surgeons were board-certified by ASPRS underwent breast reconstruction. Of these, 21% underwent reconstruction with implants. The largest number of women chose saline-filled implants, though some chose the gel-filled or the double-lumen implants. The other patients chose methods of breast reconstruction that involved using the patients' own tissue for the reconstruction, including TRAM (pedicle), latissimus dorsi, or microsurgical free flaps. Generally, procedures using autologous tissue require more extensive surgery, result in additional residual scarring (from the tissue donor site), are more expensive, and require greater surgical expertise than procedures using breast implants. The question of whether there are measurable psychological differences when different forms of breast reconstruction are used (i.e., autologous tissue vs. implants) is unclear. It remains for future research to determine whether the rates or degree of satisfaction with reconstruction will change as more women choose alternative reconstruction methods.

CONCLUSION: INFORMED CONSENT
AND BREAST SURGERY

An informed decision to undergo any operation is based on the individual's subjective evaluation of the expected benefits of the operation (to psychological or physical functioning), weighed against the surgical risks (to health and well-being) and costs (e.g., monetary and time). Inherent in providing informed consent for breast implant surgery are the basic principles that each woman is an individual with her own subjective evaluation of risks and benefits, and that her right to decide what to do with her body is sacrosanct.

However, women currently making decisions about breast surgery must sort through a great deal of conflicting, complicated, and often confusing information and scientific data regarding the safety of breast implants. Also of great concern is that the perceived credibility of plastic surgeons, who often are the most likely sources of information regarding risk, has been seriously questioned and undermined by some. The difficulty in sorting through information is clearly evident in the burgeoning empirical documentation of the profound effect of the mass media on women's perceptions of the risks of breast implants. The challenges in providing informed consent are especially difficult, in light of the extremely complex methodological considerations in evaluating risk (e.g., determining and defining the specific diseases that may result from silicone), and the fact that new studies and debates regarding the adequacy of these studies are constantly going on. Finally, these decisions are made even more difficult by the often complex financial implications associated with the massive amount of litigation currently being pursued with respect to breast implants.

FURTHER READING

American Society for Plastic and Reconstructive Surgeons (ASPRS). (1995). *Breast surgery statistics.* Arlington Heights, IL: Author.
An informative survey providing critical information on trends in the type and number of surgical procedures performed by board certified plastic surgeons.

Duffy, M. J., & Woods, J. E. (1994). Health risks of failed silicone gel breast implants: A 30-year clinical experience. *Plastic and Reconstructive Surgery, 94,* 295–299.
A retrospective analysis of the health status of 200 women who had undergone secondary breast implant surgery (i.e., reoperation), 65 of whom had failed or deteriorating silicone-gel-filled breast implants.

Gabriel, S. E., O'Fallon, M. W., Kurland, L. T., Beard, C. M., Woods, J. E., & Melton, L. J. (1994). Risk of connective-tissue diseases and other disorders after breast implantation. *New England Journal of Medicine, 330,* 1697–1702.
A retrospective investigation of 749 women who had undergone breast implantation; it "found no association between breast implants and the connective tissue diseases" and other disorders.

Handel, N., Wellisch, D., Silverstein, M. J., Jensen, J. A., & Waisman, E. (1993). Knowledge, concern, and satisfaction among augmentation mammaplasty patients. *Annals of Plastic Surgery, 30,* 13–20.
An evaluation of 85 patients who had undergone breast augmentation, to assess level of satisfaction with surgical outcome and knowledge of (as well as concern about) reported risks associated with breast implants.

Kessler, D. A. (1992). The basis for the FDA's decision on breast implants. *New England Journal of Medicine, 326,* 1713–1715.
A statement from the director of the FDA regarding the rationale for imposing a moratorium on the sale of silicone-gel-filled breast implants.

Sanchez-Guerrero, J., Colditz, G. A., Karlson, E. W., Hunter, D. J., Speizer, F. E., & Liang, M. H. (1995). Silicone breast implants and the risk of connective-tissue diseases and symptoms. *New England Journal of Medicine, 332,* 1666–1670.
A cohort study of 87,501 patients, which identified 516 with connective tissue disease and 1,183 with breast implants, but "did not find an association between silicone breast implants and connective tissue diseases."

Slavin, S. A., & Goldwyn, R. M. (1995). Silicone gel implant explantation: Reasons, results, and admonitions. *Plastic and Reconstructive Surgery, 95,* 63–69.
A report of a series of 46 women who underwent silicone gel implant removal, and an analysis of the medical challenges in treatment and medical decision making.

Wells, K. E., Roberts, C., Daniels, S. M., Kearney, R. E., & Cox, C. E. (1995). Psychological and rheumatic symptoms of women requesting silicone breast implant removal. *Annals of Plastic Surgery, 34,* 572–577.
Standardized psychological tests (the Beck Depression Inventory and the Brief Symptom Inventory) were utilized to assess the psychological symptoms of 52 women requesting removal of silicone-gel-filled breast implants; scores were found to be related to patients' reports of rheumatic symptoms.

66

Obesity

Rena R. Wing

Obesity is a major health problem for women. It is a highly prevalent condition that has been associated with increased risk of disease and mortality, and unfortunately is extremely difficult to treat. The purpose of this chapter is to address some of the recent findings in the field of obesity, with a specific focus on gender differences and on aspects of obesity unique to women.

PREVALENCE OF OBESITY IN WOMEN

Data from the third National Health and Nutrition Examination Survey (NHANES III) show that the prevalence of obesity is increasing in the United States. Over one-third of U.S. adults are now overweight (defined as a body mass index [BMI; weight/height^2] of greater than 27.8 in men and greater than 27.3 in women). The prevalence of obesity is somewhat greater in women than in men: 35% of women, as opposed to 31% of men, are overweight. The rates of obesity are far greater in certain subgroups of women, with obesity occurring in almost 50% of non-Hispanic black women and Mexican-American women.

HEALTH CONSEQUENCES OF OBESITY AND WEIGHT GAIN

Obesity in women increases the risk of coronary heart disease (CHD), diabetes, hypertension, and certain forms of cancer (cancers of the cervix, breast, ovary, gallbladder, and endometrium). Although the negative health consequences of obesity are related to the degree of obesity, recent data suggest that even slight elevations in body weight can increase the risk of CHD in women. The current guidelines for weight suggest that a BMI of 21–27 is desirable; however, the lowest risk of CHD observed in this recent study was in women with a BMI of < 21. Women with a BMI of 25–29 had twice the risk of

CHD as women with a BMI of < 21, and those with a BMI of > 29 had even greater risk. Moreover, there is a very clear tendency for women (and men) to gain weight as they age. Such weight gain also appears to increase the risk of CHD. The lowest risk of disease is seen in those women who are lean at age 18 and do not lose or gain more than 10 pounds over their adult lives.

ATTEMPTS TO LOSE WEIGHT

Women also are about twice as likely as men to report being on a diet to lose weight. In those who are overweight, about two-thirds of women report being on a diet, compared to about 50% of men; in those who are of normal weight, 50% of women and 20% of men report being on a diet. However, despite the differences in the frequency of dieting, men and women report using similar approaches to weight loss, with about half of each gender using diet plus exercise as their approach to modifying their body weight.

SUCCESS OF WEIGHT LOSS EFFORTS

The largest literature on weight loss outcome comes from the study of behavior modification. A review of this research by Wadden showed that between 1970 and 1990, there was a marked improvement in the initial weight losses achieved in behavioral weight control programs. Whereas the average patient entering a behavioral program in 1970 lost about 10 pounds, by 1990 this had increased to about 20 pounds. More recent studies (1990–1995) have average weight losses of 21.3 pounds.

One factor responsible for the improvement in outcome has been the lengthening of the typical treatment program. Initially, behavioral programs usually lasted about 10 weeks; they have since been increased to 20–24 weeks, and some investigators are even trying year-long programs. Another factor related to the improved outcome may be that programs have treated heavier patients with more weight to lose. Men tend to lose more weight than women, in part because they are heavier at baseline.

Unfortunately, however, there has been less improvement in the area of maintenance of weight loss. Recent research studies usually follow patients for 1 year after treatment. During this year, patients regain about one-third of the weight they have lost. The limited data on this issue suggest that women may maintain their weight losses better than men. Although weight losses of 10–20 pounds will not bring most patients to ideal body weight or produce BMI levels of < 21, these modest weight losses have been shown to have a positive effect on blood pressure, lipids, and glucose and insulin levels. In fact, recent recommendations focus on helping overweight individuals lose 10% of their initial weight and then maintain their loss, since even weight losses of this magnitude appear to have a positive effect on health parameters.

In my recent study with Dr. R. W. Jeffery, we reported that men experience greater reductions in lipids, blood pressure, and waist-to-hip ratio with weight loss than women. However, most of this gender difference appears to derive from the fact that men have higher CHD risk factors than women at the start of treatment. When adjustments are made for these baseline differences and for the magnitude of weight loss, the data suggest that men and women benefit equally from weight loss.

STRATEGIES TO IMPROVE WEIGHT LOSS OUTCOME

The treatment approach that is most strongly associated with successful maintenance of weight loss is the combination of diet and exercise. Correlational studies consistently show that individuals who report changing their exercise level, as well as their diet, have the best long-term maintenance of weight loss. Similar data come from randomized controlled studies comparing diet alone, exercise alone, and the combination. Subjects who are treated with diet plus exercise maintain their weight losses the best; they also show the greatest improvements in lipids, fitness, and other health-related parameters.

Another factor that has been shown to improve outcome is continuing contact with the patient. Treatment programs that start with weekly sessions for about 6 months, and then continue to see patients every other week for the next year, produce better results than programs where monthly or less frequent contact is utilized during the maintenance phase. Phone and mail contact can also improve maintenance of weight loss.

Very-low-calorie diets (diets of < 800 calories/day, often consumed as a liquid formula) have been shown to improve initial weight losses, but do not improve maintenance. Other approaches to structuring the diet for patients, by actually providing subjects with the food they should eat or giving out menus and meal plans as a way to help patients learn how to develop healthier eating, seem to have some benefit for patients. Recent studies suggest that focusing on both calorie and fat restriction may be the most effective dietary approach for long-term weight control.

OVERWEIGHT WOMEN WITH BINGE-EATING DISORDER

Another approach to improving treatment outcome is to identify subgroups of the obese population who may require specialized intervention. One such subgroup may be overweight women who report severe problems with binge eating. It has been suggested that about one-third of participants in behavioral weight control programs meet criteria for binge-eating disorder (BED), a recently identified syndrome characterized by regular binge eating and feelings of loss of control, but without compensatory purging or strict dieting. BED appears to occur more commonly in women than in men, both in community samples and in those entering treatment. Patients with BED, compared to equally overweight individuals without BED, report excessive concern about shape and weight, more depressive symptomatology, and greater psychiatric symptomatology in general. Thus it has been suggested that these patients may benefit from a treatment program that emphasizes modification of binge eating per se and changes in abnormal thoughts about shape and weight.

There is some evidence that obese binge eaters do less well in standard weight loss programs than obese individuals who do not binge, with the two groups losing comparable amounts of weight initially, but the binger eaters regaining faster. Recent studies, however, have questioned this. At present, it remains unclear whether obese binge eaters would do best in a program that targets their binge eating directly, a program that focuses on their obesity, or a program that targets obesity and binge eating at the same time.

IDENTIFYING KEY TIMES FOR WEIGHT GAIN PREVENTION EFFORTS IN WOMEN

Given the difficulty of treating obesity, there has also been recent interest in trying to prevent this condition by intervening at times when weight gain commonly occurs. Two such times have been identified for women—namely, pregnancy and the time of menopause.

Women are most likely to experience major weight gains (> 30 pounds over 10 years) during their young adult years (ages 25–34). This weight gain is associated with getting married and may also be related to pregnancy. Cross-sectional studies provide little evidence that pregnancy is associated with obesity. Women with no, one, two, or three children have similar BMIs; it is only when women have had more than three births that increased rates of obesity are observed. Moreover, studies following women through pregnancy show that on average women will return to within 0–3 pounds of their prepregnancy weights within 1 year after pregnancy. However, these data hide a fair amount of diversity among women. Although women on average do not retain weight after pregnancy, about 25% of women will retain 10 pounds or more 1 year after a pregnancy. Women who gain large amounts of weight during pregnancy are most likely to retain large amounts of weight. Moreover, black women are more likely than whites to retain significant amounts of weight after pregnancy.

A second time when women may be especially vulnerable to obesity is during the period surrounding menopause. Data from the Healthy Women Study, a prospective study of 540 healthy women who have been followed through the menopause, suggest that women gain about 1 pound per year between the ages of 45 and 55. This weight gain appears to be attributable to aging, rather than to menopause per se. Women who gain the most weight during the menopause period have the greatest worsening in CHD risk factors. The amount of weight gained was not related to the baseline weight of the women, but did appear to be greater in black women than in white women. However, the strongest predictor of magnitude of weight gain was change in physical activity; those women who had the greatest increases in physical activity gained the least weight.

These findings suggest two time periods when women may be vulnerable to weight gain. Further research is needed to determine whether these periods can be used to help prevent the development of obesity in women.

FURTHER READING

French, S. A., & Jeffery, R. W. (1994). Consequences of dieting to lose weight: Effects on physical and mental health. *Health Psychology, 13,* 195–212.
Dieting occurs very frequently in women, but has few adverse nutritional or psychological effects.

Keppel, K. G., & Taffel, S. M. (1993). Pregnancy-related weight gain and retention: Implications of the 1990 Institute of Medicine guidelines. *American Journal of Public Health, 83,* 1100–1103.
Amount of weight gain during pregnancy is positively associated with weight retention 10–18 months post pregnancy.

Kuczmarski, R. J., Flegal, K. M., Campbell, S. M., & Johnson, C. L. (1994). Increasing prevalence of overweight among U.S. adults: The National Health and Nutrition Examination Surveys, 1960 to 1991. *Journal of the American Medical Association, 272,* 205–211.

These surveys show that the prevalence of obesity is increasing and that, as of 1991, one out of every three U.S. adults is overweight.

Marcus, M. D. (1993). Binge eating in obesity. In C. G. Fairburn & G. T. Wilson (Eds.), *Binge eating: Nature, assessment, and treatment* (pp. 77–96). New York: Guilford Press.
Binge eating affects large numbers of obese patients entering weight control programs; these individuals may require specialized treatments.

Pronk, N. P., & Wing, R. R. (1994). Physical activity and long-term maintenance of weight loss. *Obesity Research, 2,* 587–599.
This review of randomized, controlled studies and correlational data shows that physical activity is the strongest determinant of long-term weight loss.

Wadden, T. A. (1993). The treatment of obesity: An overview. In A. J. Stunkard & T. A. Wadden (Eds.), *Obesity: Theory and therapy* (pp. 197-218). New York: Raven Press.
This review of the history of behavioral treatments of obesity examines the progress made in this field.

Willett, W. C., Manson, J. E., Stampfer, M. J., Colditz, G. A., Rosner, B., Spiezer, F. E., & Hennekens, C. H. (1995). Weight, weight change, and coronary heart disease in women. *Journal of the American Medical Association, 273,* 461–465.
This study shows that obesity is strongly associated with CHD in women.

Williamson, D. F., Kahn, H. S., Remington, P. L., & Anda, R. F. (1990). The 10-year incidence of overweight and major weight gain in US adults. *Archives of Internal Medicine, 150,* 665–672.
Major weight gains occur most frequently in young adults, and are seen more often in women than in men.

Wing, R. R., & Jeffery, R. W. (1995). Effect of modest weight loss on changes in cardiovascular risk factors: Are there differences between men and women or between weight loss and maintenance? *International Journal of Obesity, 19,* 67–73.
Men show greater initial improvements in CHD risk factors with weight loss, but women show better long-term effects.

Wing, R. R., Matthews, K. A., Kuller, L. H., Meilahn, E. N., & Plantinga, P. L. (1991). Weight gain at the time of menopause. *Archives of Internal Medicine, 151,* 97–102.
Women gain weight at the time of menopause, more because of aging than because of menopause per se.

67

Alcoholism

Damaris J. Rohsenow

Although the term "alcoholism" has no specific definition, it usually refers to continued use of alcohol in spite of significant problems resulting from such use. These problems include needing markedly more alcohol to produce the same effects (tolerance), having withdrawal or drinking to avoid withdrawal, drinking more than intended, unsuccessfully trying to reduce or quit drinking, spending considerable amounts of time seeking alcohol, giving up or decreasing important activities, or having persistent physical or psychological problems. The terms "alcoholism" and "alcohol dependence" generally refer to a greater degree of severity than do the terms "problem drinking" and "alcohol abuse." In the late 1980s, about 4.6 million women in the United States had alcohol abuse or dependence.

SOME FACTORS AFFECTING DEVELOPMENT OF ALCOHOLISM

Genetic factors have recently been found to play about as strong a role in alcoholism for women as for men. The heritability for women is in the 50–60% range, suggesting that genetic factors play a strong role, but that environmental factors also have a strong role. Some earlier studies also suggested that major depression and alcoholism may run in some of the same families. In many families with alcoholic men, the nonalcoholic women have a higher risk of being diagnosed with major depression. Similarly, women alcoholics are more likely than men to have been diagnosed with depressive disorder as well, whereas men are more likely to have an additional diagnosis of antisocial personality disorder. (Since alcohol intoxication and withdrawal both increase depressive states, it is important to realize that a diagnosis of depression cannot be validly made for an alcoholic until after 3 weeks of sobriety.)

Women who later develop alcohol abuse have their first drink about 3 years earlier than women who do not develop alcohol abuse, and also drink with family members at a younger age. Earlier studies found that women started excessive drinking later in life than men did, but that their problems progressed more rapidly, so that they entered treatment at about the same age as men. More recently, no gender differences are being found in the age at which excessive drinking starts. Although younger women report more alcohol-related problems, alcohol dependence is greatest among women aged 35–49.

Stress, particularly stress resulting from role overload (having to handle both work and family responsibilities), used to be believed to increase alcoholism or heavy drinking among women. However, the opposite seems to be the case. Women who are married are less likely to be heavy drinkers than are single or cohabiting women, and women who are both married and working outside the home are even less likely to drink heavily. Role deprivation seems to be more of a problem; single women with no stable jobs are at more risk. Furthermore, a study in which women recorded their levels of daily stress over time found that the women drank less during high-stress weeks than during low-stress weeks. This seemed to be moderated by coping style, with women who used problem-focused coping drinking less than women with less effective coping styles.

Women in traditionally male jobs tend to drink more heavily than women in jobs that traditionally employ more women. This does not seem to result from increased stress or any role confusion, however. Rather, since the men in these jobs tend to drink more than women, (1) there may be more opportunities to drink; (2) the women may be drinking more to imitate higher-status colleagues; and (3) the women may be expressing their power or equality with the men by matching the men's drinking level. When women are married or cohabiting, their drinking levels tend to match those of their partners. When problem-drinking women divorce, their drinking and their drinking-related problems decrease significantly, particularly if their ex-partners were heavy drinkers or the relationships were sexually dysfunctional.

Sexual abuse or dysfunction may predispose many women to alcohol abuse. About 40% of a sample of adult women, and about 75% of a sample of adolescent women enrolled in inpatient alcohol abuse treatment, had a history of childhood sexual abuse, as compared to about 4% of the adult men. Childhood sexual abuse involving contact shows a stronger relationship to problematic consequences and to alcohol dependence symptoms than does abuse without direct contact. Among adult women, the strongest predictor of continued problem drinking in 1 year was reported sexual dysfunction 10 years earlier. Heavy drinking may be used to self-medicate some of the issues resulting from the sexual abuse or dysfunction. Some women may use alcohol to overcome aversion to unpleasant sexual contact with their partners.

CONSEQUENCES OF PROLONGED DRINKING

Women have been shown to be more seriously affected by chronic heavy drinking than are men. Women drink less on the average than men, but require less alcohol per kilogram of body weight than men to reach the same peak blood alcohol level and same level of impairment. (For a fuller discussion of male–female differences in alcohol metabolism, see Baraona's chapter in this volume.) Moreover, women alcoholics generally experience more medical problems related to their drinking than do men. This is especially true for liver disease, stroke, breast cancer, and osteoporosis. The risk for hemorrhagic stroke is particularly elevated in women alcoholics who have also used oral contraceptives. Fewer years of heavy drinking occur for women than for men before the first incidence of fatty liver, hypertension, obesity, malnutrition, and gastrointestinal hemorrhage. Alcohol abuse also decreases fertility, increases amenorrhea, increases ovarian pathology, and results in earlier menopause. The rate of mortality is 50–100% higher for alcoholic women than for alcoholic men. Death is frequently caused by suicide, accidents, violence, liver cirrhosis, and cardiovascular problems.

Although a minority of children of women who drink heavily during pregnancy show the full fetal alcohol syndrome (it occurs more often among poor women, in whom malnutrition may also be implicated), various abnormalities falling short of the full fetal alcohol syndrome may occur among children if their mothers consume even moderate amounts of alcohol during gestation. Moreover, during breast feeding, a small amount of alcohol can pass through the milk. Infants have been found to suck harder, receive less milk, and sleep more poorly when their mothers have consumed an alcoholic drink. Alcohol in the milk also impairs the transfer of immunities to the child.

RECOVERING FROM ALCOHOLISM
AND PROBLEM DRINKING

One study reinterviewed in 1991 a group of women problem drinkers identified in 1981. About one-third continued to have the same level of problems; about one-third had decreased their number of alcohol problems; and about one-third no longer had drinking-related problems. In a study of men and women who had recovered from alcohol problems without formal treatment, women were more likely than men to have become nonabstinent nonproblem drinkers, and men were more likely to have chosen abstinence as their means of resolving their alcohol problems.

Women are more likely than men to seek treatment through non-alcohol-specific settings, particularly mental health settings. The social stigma of alcoholism is greater for women and may be a barrier to their using substance abuse treatment programs. Also, lack of child care is a serious barrier to treatment for many alcoholic women. However, the proportion of women who are alcoholics in treatment for alcoholism (25%) is similar to the proportion of alcoholics in the general population who are women (30%).

Women are more likely to seek treatment because of alcohol-related problems with their health and families, whereas men more often seek treatment because of job and legal problems. Women more often abuse other legal medications in addition to alcohol, particularly sedatives, tranquilizers, and stimulants. Dealing with this medication abuse is an important treatment issue, not only because of the increased risk of death that the alcohol–drug combination poses, but because such women may replace alcohol abuse with increased medication abuse.

Little research has compared the effectiveness of specific different treatment methods or components for women. In general, women do as well in most treatment settings as men of comparable demographic characteristics and degree of alcoholism do. A few differences in treatment response were found in two patient–treatment matching studies. Women did better in terms of drinking outcomes in programs with low peer group orientation; group therapy sessions resulted in worse outcomes for women; and lectures and films resulted in better outcomes for women. For men, the opposite was true in each case. Since the majority of peers and group members in treatment programs are men, it was possible that this could account for the decreased effectiveness of the group or peer approaches in these two studies. However, in one of these same studies, treatment outcome was better for women in the facility with fewer other women clients (the opposite was true for men). This study was not adequately controlled, but it provides some preliminary information that may have implications for treatment choices.

Because of concerns about the predominance of men in self-help groups, a moderator-led self-help group for women was started in 1976: Women for Sobriety. Another concern was that issues such as the emphasis on powerlessness in Alcoholics Anonymous may be counterproductive for women, as many women need a greater sense of empowerment. This organization focuses on helping women to achieve a sense of competence, to take charge of their lives, and not to dwell on the past or on negative cognitions.

CONCLUSIONS

Women's health is seriously affected by prolonged heavy alcohol use. On the whole, women and men benefit about equally from alcoholism treatment; however, barriers to women's entering treatment remain concerns and need further research. In addition to child care issues, women's fear that being labeled with an alcohol problem will cause their children to be removed from their care is a serious concern. Financial resources may be more limited for many women as well. In particular, women without stable jobs are more likely to be alcoholic and less likely to have access to employer-paid insurance or alcoholism treatment. More research is also needed to identify the aspects of treatment that are most favorable to improving treatment outcome for women.

FURTHER READING

Blume, S. B. (1986). Women and alcohol. *Journal of the American Medical Association, 256,* 1467–1470.
A summary of the research-based knowledge of alcohol use and alcoholism among women.

Breslin, F. C., O'Keefe, M. K., Burred, L., Ratliff-Crain, J., & Baum, A. (1995). The effects of stress and coping on daily alcohol use in women. *Addictive Behaviors, 20,* 141–147.
An empirical study of several factors influencing drinking.

Kendler, K. S., Heath, A. C., Neale, M. C., Kessler, R. C., & Eaves, L. J. (1992). A population-based twin study of alcoholism in women. *Journal of the American Medical Association, 268,* 1877–1882.
A recent empirical study of genetic factors in women's alcoholism.

McCrady, B. S., & Delaney, S. I. (1995). Self-help groups. In R. K. Hester & W. R. Miller (Eds.), *Handbook of alcoholism treatment approaches: Effective alternatives* (pp. 160–175). Needham Heights, MA: Allyn & Bacon.
Includes a brief description of the group Women for Sobriety.

National Institute on Alcohol Abuse and Alcoholism. (1990, October). Alcohol and women. *Alcohol Alert,* No. 10.
A succinct summary of the research-based knowledge of alcohol use and alcoholism among women.

Sokolow, L., Welte, J., Hynes, G., & Lyons, J. (1980). Treatment-related differences between female and male alcoholics. *Journal of Addictions and Health, 1,* 43–56.
A study of gender differences in treatment outcomes, based on treatment program characteristics.

Weisner, C., & Schmidt, L. (1992). Gender disparities in treatment for alcohol problems. *Journal of the American Medical Association, 268,* 1872–1876.
A study of the settings women choose for treatment of alcohol abuse.

Wilsnack, S. C., & Wilsnack, R. W. (1993). Epidemiological research on women's drinking: Recent progress and directions for the 1990s. In E. S. L. Gomberg & T. D. Nirenberg (Eds.), *Women and substance abuse* (pp. 62–99). Norwood, NJ: Ablex.
A description of the changes seen in factors affecting women's drinking between 1981 and 1991.

68

Alcohol Metabolism

Enrique Baraona

*T*he traditional predominance of alcoholism and alcohol-related pathology in the male gender has led most researchers to focus their attention on alcoholic men. However, even though problem drinking in women still occurs at less than half the rate of that in men, the male–female differences in drinking have become smaller than they were a generation ago—a fact that appears to relate primarily to drinking by young women. Moreover, despite greater barriers to women's seeking treatment (particularly the problems of child care), the interval between the onset of drinking-related problems and entry into treatment is shorter in women than in men, reflecting the greater impact of alcoholism in the female gender.

Indeed, it is well recognized that women are more vulnerable than men to alcohol-related problems, with a higher death rate and greater percentage of suicides, alcohol-related accidents, circulatory disorders, and cirrhosis of the liver. Women develop brain, heart, muscle, and liver damage upon shorter and less intense exposure to alcohol (ethanol or ethyl alcohol). The average cirrhogenic dose of alcohol, as well as the threshold amount, is also lower in women than in men: A daily alcohol intake of 40–60 grams in men, but only 20 grams in women, resulted in a statistically significant increase in the incidence of cirrhosis in one well-nourished population. There is evidence as well that the progression to more severe liver disease is accelerated in women. In addition, alcohol abuse has a specific impact on the female reproductive system, resulting in menstrual disorders, infertility, fetal alcohol syndrome, and a probable increase in risk for breast cancer. Thus, contemporary women are experiencing the double burden of an increase in alcohol consumption and an enhanced vulnerability to its adverse effects.

The mechanisms by which the female gender potentiates alcohol-induced damage have just begun to be unraveled. Several mechanisms could contribute to the increased vulnerability of women to alcoholic injury: (1) an enhanced bioavailability of ethanol; (2) an increased rate of ethanol metabolism and generation of toxic products; and (3) a less efficient metabolic compensation for some alterations produced by ethanol.

GENDER DIFFERENCES IN THE BIOAVAILABILITY OF ETHANOL

Most of the physiological and metabolic effects of ethanol, as well as its secondary toxicity, are dependent upon the concentrations reached at its site of action. Blood and tissue alcohol concentrations are affected by the dose, its volume of distribution, and its rate of breakdown (metabolism).

Differences in the Distribution of Alcohol in the Body

Women develop higher blood ethanol concentrations than men after an equivalent oral dose, even when their differences in body weight are corrected for. The volume in which alcohol dissolves is similar to that of total body water. The volume of distribution of ethanol is smaller in women than in men, because of a smaller water content at the expense of a greater contribution of fat. As a consequence, the dilution of the same amount of alcohol in a smaller volume of water should increase its concentration. However, the largest sex-related differences in blood ethanol concentrations were observed after oral administration. After intravenous infusion, the volume of distribution for ethanol was found to be only 12% larger in normal men than in normal women, which did not result in significant differences in blood levels when the alcohol was given by this route. This suggested that additional factors may contribute to the much higher differences in blood alcohol levels observed after oral consumption, since the volume of distribution for ethanol should not be affected by the route of alcohol administration. The apparently much higher volume of distribution reported after an oral alcohol dose can probably be attributed to an overestimation, resulting from the assumption that the entire dose of ethanol reaches the systemic circulation and is distributed in the body water.

Differences in the First-Pass Metabolism of Ethanol

The administration of the same alcohol dose (per kilogram of body weight) via the intravenous route produces larger areas under the curve of blood alcohol concentrations than when the dose is taken by the oral route. It was found that this difference was significantly smaller in women than in men (see Figure 68.1). Although confirming these findings, other studies emphasized a confounding effect of age: They found significantly elevated blood ethanol concentrations in younger nonalcoholic women as compared to younger nonalcoholic men, whereas these results were reversed in subjects over 50 years of age. Another confounding factor was chronic alcohol abuse: In alcoholic men, the differences between intravenously and orally produced areas under the curve were significantly smaller than in nonalcoholic men. This effect of alcoholism was markedly exaggerated in women, whose blood alcohol curves after oral consumption were indistinguishable from those produced by infusion of the ethanol dose into the vein. These findings suggested that a higher fraction of the orally consumed alcohol reaches the blood in women than in men, at least in younger age groups. This was subsequently confirmed when the quantity of alcohol reaching the circulation was calculated from the blood levels by applying the Michaelis–Menten kinetics of ethanol elimination.

My colleagues' and my research has indicated that only a fraction of the dose of imbibed ethanol reaches the systemic blood. This incomplete bioavailability of the orally consumed alcohol has been shown to result from the breaking down of part of the alcohol during its transit through the stomach and the liver before it reaches the systemic blood

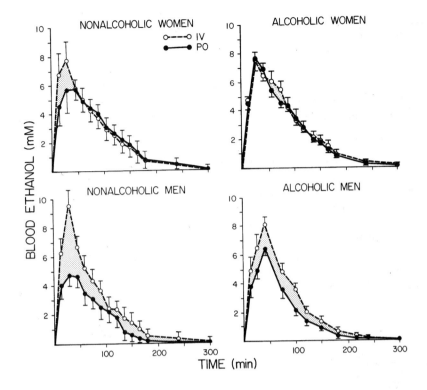

FIGURE 68.1. Effects of gender and chronic alcohol abuse on blood ethanol concentrations. Ethanol was administered orally (solid lines) or intravenously (dashed lines) in a moderate dose (0.3 grams per kilogram of body weight). The shaded area represents the difference between the curves for the two routes of administration. From Frezza et al. (1990). Copyright 1990 by the Massachusetts Medical Society. Reprinted by permission.

("first-pass metabolism"). Although it is generally recognized that the bulk of ethanol metabolism occurs in the liver, extrahepatic metabolism also occurs. The capacity of the stomach to metabolize ethanol was previously recognized and related to the presence of alcohol dehydrogenase (ADH) in the stomach. The quantitative contribution of the stomach and the liver to this first-pass metabolism has been a matter of debate. Levitt has argued that the smaller blood levels after oral consumption are attributable merely to gastrointestinal absorption's occurring at a slower rate than infusion, and thereby increasing the contribution of hepatic first-pass metabolism. However, Gentry, Lieber, and I have shown that the hepatic extraction of ethanol is maximal at concentrations much lower than those produced by clinically relevant doses of alcohol. Moreover, after the rate of infusion is adjusted to be similar to that of absorption, the first-pass metabolism of alcohol is minimized when ethanol is administered by routes bypassing the stomach. A similar effect is observed in patients in whom most or all of the stomach has been removed for therapeutic reasons. Conversely, the first-pass metabolism persists when the liver is bypassed (by diverting the blood normally entering this organ to a distal vein). It is therefore our opinion that, except for doses resulting in very small ethanol concentrations (less than 10 mg/dl), most of the first-pass metabolism of alcohol occurs in the stomach.

It has been estimated that approximately one-fourth to one-third of a moderate dose of alcohol (0.3 gram per kilogram of body weight) undergoes first-pass metabolism, does not reach the systemic blood, and therefore does not contribute to the concentrations of alcohol in blood. The two major determinants of the magnitude of this first-pass metabolism are the activity of ethanol-metabolizing systems in the stomach and the duration of the exposure of those systems to optimal ethanol concentrations, which is in turn determined mainly by the rate of gastric emptying.

Role of Gastric Alcohol Dehydrogenase

The effects of gender (as well as those of age and alcoholism) on first-pass metabolism are associated with a parallel change of ADH activity in endoscopic samples of the gastric mucosa (see Figure 68.2). The immunohistochemical demonstration of ADH (the principal enzyme involved in ethanol oxidation) in the stomach has attracted the attention of most researchers to this enzyme. The interest has been further increased by the characterization of an ADH isoenzyme (named sigma ADH), encoded by a gene (*ADH7*) that is expressed in the upper digestive tract (including the stomach), but not in the liver.

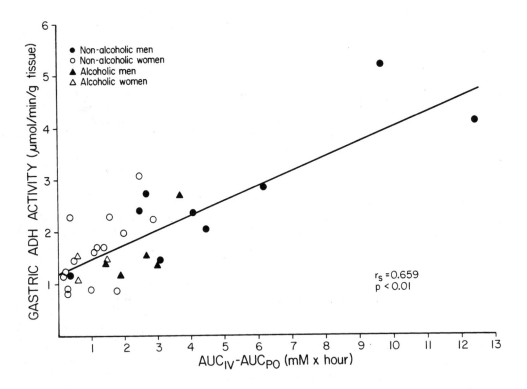

FIGURE 68.2. Correlation between the activity of gastric alcohol dehydrogenase (ADH) and the differences in areas under the curve (AUC) of blood ethanol concentrations produced by intravenous (AUC_{IV}) and peroral (AUC_{PO}) administration of ethanol (0.3 gram per kilogram of body weight); r_s denotes the Spearman's correlation coefficient. From Frezza et al. (1990). Copyright 1990 by the Massachusetts Medical Society. Reprinted by permission.

Moreover, some ADH isoenzymes with very small affinity for ethanol may become operative at the high concentrations prevailing in the gastric lumen during alcohol consumption. It has been argued that the ADH activity of the stomach, measured *in vitro*, is too small to account for the first-pass metabolism of ethanol. However, isolated cells from the gastric epithelium metabolize ethanol in amounts sufficient to account for the first-pass metabolism indicating either that the *in vitro* measurements of ADH activity underestimate the activity *in vivo*, or that other enzyme systems contribute to the gastric metabolism of ethanol. Catalase, which can also oxidize ethanol, has been found in the gastric mucosa, and inhibitors of this enzyme have been shown to decrease the first-pass metabolism of ethanol in some species.

Role of Gastric Emptying of Ethanol

In addition to the activity of the enzymes involved in gastric ethanol metabolism, the rate of gastric emptying is a major factor in determining the magnitude of the first-pass metabolism. This metabolism is markedly decreased by fasting, which accelerates the gastric emptying of ethanol. In addition, fasting decreases ethanol oxidation in the liver. As a consequence of the changes in both the gastric and hepatic metabolism of ethanol, the blood concentrations are considerably higher when alcohol is consumed in the fasted than in the fed state. Moreover, ethanol by itself has an inhibitory effect on the rate of gastric emptying, particularly when the alcohol is given at concentrations commonly encountered in alcoholic beverages. Thus, the first-pass metabolism is substantial with 10% or higher ethanol, and minimal with 4% ethanol.

The best-recognized gender difference in gastric emptying is that this activity is diminished during the luteal phase of the menstrual cycle and in pregnancy, which are characterized by high estradiol and progesterone levels. The increased blood levels in women were observed during the luteal phase of the menstrual cycle; therefore, the differences in blood alcohol levels may have actually been attenuated by the menstrual changes in gastric emptying.

Role of Dose and Modality of Alcohol Consumption

The amount of alcohol undergoing first-pass metabolism is not affected by the dose of alcohol. Therefore, as the dose of alcohol is increased, the contribution of the first-pass metabolism to the blood alcohol level becomes progressively smaller. Thus, the effect of first-pass metabolism becomes more difficult to detect when a large alcohol dose is given as a bolus. Conversely, the effects of single small doses become cumulative after repetitive drinking, which is the more common modality of alcohol intake by social drinkers and even by alcoholics. Therefore, the differences in the bioavailability of the imbibed alcohol may become considerable in a long-term drinking situation.

GENDER DIFFERENCES IN HEPATIC METABOLISM OF ETHANOL

Women differ from men not only in terms of gastric ethanol metabolism. When effects of first-pass metabolism are minimized or canceled out with large alcohol doses administered in the fasted state or by the intravenous route, some investigators have found that women eliminate alcohol more rapidly from the blood than men do. The more convincing differences have been obtained when the genetic variabilities in ethanol elimination are reduced by comparing natural siblings rather than subjects taken at random, or when the dose is adjusted to compensate for the gender differences in the volume of alcohol distribution. Thus, the female liver not only is exposed to higher alcohol levels after oral consumption, but also metabolizes ethanol at a faster rate. Most of the deleterious effects of ethanol on the liver have been linked to its metabolism, which leads to the production of potentially toxic products such as acetaldehyde. In keeping with this possibility, the blood levels of acetaldehyde have been found to be higher in women than in men consuming the same dose of ethanol. A similar combination of decreased gastric first-pass metabolism with enhanced hepatic metabolism of alcohol develops after chronic alcohol consumption, and may be an important factor in the development of alcoholic liver injury.

GENDER DIFFERENCES IN THE METABOLIC RESPONSES TO ETHANOL

The possibility that women may differ from men in their metabolic responses to the derangements induced by ethanol has been less fully explored. Some supportive evidence has been gathered at early and late stages of alcoholic liver injury. For instance, one of the earliest effects of alcohol consumption is a decrease in the capacity of the liver mitochondria to oxidize fatty acids; the accumulation of fatty acids can be deleterious, unless it is prevented by their esterification and the development of accessory pathways for their oxidation. This compensatory response has been shown to be more efficient in ethanol-fed male than female rats, with a threefold greater accumulation of nonesterified fatty acids in the females. Preliminary findings suggest that similar gender differences may pertain to human subjects.

At later stages of alcoholic liver injury, the higher incidence and poorer long-term prognosis of alcoholic hepatitis (a severe form of liver inflammation) in women than in men have been attributed, at least in part, to a more intense autoimmune response in the female gender, as suggested by higher autoantibody titers in the serum.

CONCLUSIONS

Women are particularly vulnerable to both the acute and the chronic deleterious effects of alcohol consumption. Awareness of this fact may induce women to resist social pressures to consume as much alcohol as men. Women develop higher blood alcohol levels than men do, with a corresponding aggravation of associated psychomotor impairments. This can be attributed to an increase in alcohol bioavailability, and to the distribution of the dose in a smaller volume because of the usual smaller contribution of water to women's body weight.

Also in terms of alcohol-induced pathology, alcohol consumption that may be considered moderate and innocuous in men is not necessarily so in women. This gender difference is now being recognized in guidelines for "moderate drinking," which is defined as less than two drinks per day in men, but only one drink per day in women. Enhanced hepatic alcohol metabolism and differences in the metabolic responses to the injurious effects of alcohol on the liver may also contribute to the propensity of women to develop alcoholic liver injury with less alcohol consumption than men. Therefore, efforts to diagnose and rehabilitate alcoholic women should be particularly intensified.

FURTHER READING

Frezza, M., DiPadova, C., Pozzato, G., Terpin, M., Baraona, E., & Lieber, C. S. (1990). High blood alcohol levels in women: The role of decreased gastric alcohol dehydrogenase activity and first-pass metabolism. *New England Journal of Medicine, 322,* 95–99.
Principal study indicating the role of first-pass metabolism and gastric ADH activity on the gender differences in blood alcohol levels after consumption of ethanol.

Gavaler, J. S. (1982). Sex-related differences in ethanol-induced liver disease: Artifactual or real? *Alcoholism: Clinical and Experimental Research, 6,* 186–196.
Critical review of the initial studies reporting a difference between males and females in susceptibility to ethanol-induced liver disease.

Gentry, R. T., Baraona, E., & Lieber, C. S. (1994). Agonist: Gastric first-pass metabolism of alcohol. *Journal of Laboratory and Clinical Medicine, 123,* 21–26.
Part of a debate on the respective contribution of the stomach and the liver to the first-pass metabolism of ethanol.

Gomberg, E. S. L. (1993). Gender issues. In M. Galanter (Ed.), *Recent developments in alcoholism: Vol. 11. Ten years of progress* (pp. 95–107). New York: Plenum Press.
A discussion of the consequences of problem drinking and alcoholism in women—interpersonal, legal, occupational, and medical.

Krasner, N., Davis, M., Portmann, B., & Williams, R. (1977). Changing pattern of alcoholic liver disease in Great Britain: Relation to sex and sign of autoimmunity. *British Medical Journal, i,* 1497–1500.
Study supporting the possibility that the severity and poor prognosis of alcoholic hepatitis in women may be related to an enhanced autoimmune response.

Levitt, M. D. (1994). Antagonist: The case against first-pass metabolism of ethanol in the stomach. *Journal of Laboratory and Clinical Medicine, 123,* 28–31.
The other part of the debate on the stomach's and liver's respective contribution to the first pass metabolism of alcohol.

Lieber, C. S. (1993). Women and alcohol: Gender differences in metabolism and susceptibility. In E. S. Gomberg & T. D. Nirenberg (Eds.), *Women and substance abuse* (pp. 1–17). Norwood, NJ: Ablex.
More detailed information on some of the issues discussed in the present chapter.

National Institute on Alcohol Abuse and Alcoholism. (1990, October). Alcohol and women. *Alcohol Alert,* No. 10.
Concise but well-referenced information on the drinking problems affecting women.

Van Thiel, D. H., Tarter, R. E., Rosenblum, E., & Gavaler, J. S. (1989). Ethanol, its metabolism and gonadal effects: Does sex make a difference? *Advances in Alcohol and Substance Abuse, 7,* 131–169.
Thorough review of gonadal effects of alcohol and their possible impact on the gender differences in ethanol metabolism.

69

Drug Abuse

Mary E. McCaul

*H*istorically, addictions to alcohol and illicit drugs have been considered male problems. Men are more likely than women to develop substance abuse and dependence, and men predominate among admissions to substance abuse treatment programs. However, in recent years there has been growing research on and treatment efforts for substance-misusing women. This chapter provides a brief overview of four areas: the etiology of substance abuse and dependence in women; the prevalence of alcohol and illicit drug use and misuse by women; demographic characteristics of substance-using and -misusing women; and biopsychosocial correlates of substance abuse and dependence among women.

ETIOLOGY OF SUBSTANCE ABUSE
AND DEPENDENCE IN WOMEN

Research has provided clear evidence of a genetic vulnerability to alcohol and drug dependence in men and, more recently, women with a family history of alcoholism. For example, adoption studies confirm the elevated risk for alcoholism in biological sons and daughters of alcoholics. Across studies, male and female adoptees with a family history of alcoholism are 2.4 and 2.8 times more likely to develop alcoholism, respectively, than male and female adoptees without such a family history. Similarly, twin studies have found a significantly higher co-occurrence of alcoholism in male and female monozygotic twins (who are genetically identical) than in dizygotic twins (who on average share half of their genes). These results suggest an important genetic influence on the development of the disorder. When the relative contribution of genetic and environmental factors to alcoholism risk is examined, genetic factors are found to exert a moderate to strong influence on development of alcohol dependence for men and women; specifically, heritability estimates typically exceed 50% for both genders. There is also emerging evidence for the importance of genetic factors in the development of opiate and tranquilizer use.

414

In contrast to the evidence of comparable genetic risk for alcoholism in men and women, gender differences have been observed in reported motives for substance use. For example, among adolescents, girls score higher on coping motives for substance use, whereas boys score higher on social pressure and self-confidence. Similarly, adult men who have been treated for alcoholism report drinking to increase sociability, whereas treated women are more likely to report drinking because of negative mood and marital conflicts. When alcoholic women in treatment were compared with age-matched nonalcoholic control women, the two groups did not differ in their reports of the number of traumatic and painful early life events; however, alcoholic women were more likely to report stronger negative affective responses to the life events.

Finally, in an important U.S. national study of women's drinking conducted in the 1980s, three factors predicted the development of problem drinking: young age, cohabitation, and use of other drugs. There is also growing evidence for the important role of childhood sexual abuse as a predictor of drinking problems among adult women; abuse as a correlate of alcoholism is further discussed below.

PREVALENCE OF SUBSTANCE USE AND MISUSE IN WOMEN

Alcohol

Alcohol use is normative in the U.S. adult population. The 1993 National Household Survey on Drug Abuse reported that 88% of males and 80% of females had used alcohol in their lifetimes. Recent alcohol use was also widespread, with 72% of men and 62% of women reporting alcohol use in the last year, and 57% of men and 42% of women reporting use in the last month. However, regular consumption of alcohol was acknowledged by only a small proportion of women; for example, 13% of women reported drinking alcohol once a week or more.

It is estimated that 14% of the U.S. population will experience symptoms of alcoholism in their lifetimes. Rates of alcohol abuse or dependence are considerably lower for women than for men; approximately 4% of U.S. women will experience the symptoms of these disorders. Women begin alcohol use at a later age and present for treatment after a shorter duration of use, suggesting a more rapid development or "telescoping" of alcohol-related problems in women. Although women appear to be potentially more vulnerable than men to the physical effects of excessive alcohol use, men appear to experience higher rates of social and legal problems associated with their alcohol misuse.

Illicit Drugs

Although clearly not as widespread as alcohol use, illicit drug use is still fairly common in the United States. Overall, 42% of men and 32% of women in the National Household Survey reported a lifetime history of illicit drug use (i.e., marijuana, cocaine [including crack], opiates, inhalants, and hallucinogens, as well as sedatives, tranquilizers, and analgesics used nonmedically). During the preceding year, 14% of men and 10% of women reported use of an illicit drug; use in the past month was reported by 7% of men and 4% of women.

Whereas the lifetime prevalence of alcohol abuse and dependence is significantly higher in males than in females, gender differences in drug abuse and dependence are not as striking, with approximately 7% of males and 5% of females experiencing these disorders during their lifetimes. Among those reporting illicit drug abuse, rates of alcoholism are also strikingly high; for example, 84% of those reporting cocaine abuse also met criteria for alcohol abuse at some time in their lives. At present, abuse of multiple drugs (including alcohol) is the most common presenting complaint reported by persons entering substance abuse treatment. As has been noted for the development of alcohol problems in women, there is evidence that women with opiate dependence also experience a "telescoping" of their disorder, with a later onset, more rapid development of problems, and more rapid presentation for treatment as compared with opiate-dependent men.

Whereas men are more likely to report recent use and misuse of marijuana, cocaine, inhalants, and hallucinogens, women report somewhat higher rates of recent nonmedical use and misuse of sedatives and tranquilizers, and comparable rates of nonmedical analgesic misuse. One recent study examined gender differences in the relative risk among drug users for development of drug dependence. For six out of eight illicit drug classes, male and female drug users were at comparable lifetime risk for development of drug dependence. For example, slightly more than 22% of heroin users progressed to develop symptoms of drug dependence, regardless of gender. Comparable rates for men and women were also observed for cocaine, analgesics, hallucinogens, and inhalants. For marijuana, male users were somewhat more likely to become dependent, and for sedatives and tranquilizers, female users were more likely than male users to develop dependence. Thus, although there was substantial overlap in risk of dependence development among male and female users, several interesting differences in dependence risk emerged.

Intravenous (IV) use represents the most extreme method of drug self-administration, with 1.4% of the general population reporting lifetime use of this method. Men are roughly three times more likely than women to report IV drug use. Similarly, women are less likely than men to report needle sharing in high-risk situations (e.g., "shooting galleries").

Drug abuse is also a significant problem among pregnant women. It has been estimated that 11–20% of pregnant women in the United States have a problematic pattern of illicit drug use. Cocaine abuse has been found to account for up to half of these cases, with the prevalence of cocaine abuse estimated at between 5% and 17%. These figures probably represent an underestimation of the problem, because of social and psychological pressures to deny substance use during pregnancy, as well as the illegal nature of much of this drug use. In addition to cocaine, alcohol and marijuana are often detected in the toxicology screens of pregnant women. As in the larger population of drug abusers, polydrug abuse is frequently observed among pregnant women who use drugs.

DEMOGRAPHIC CHARACTERISTICS OF SUBSTANCE-USING AND -MISUSING WOMEN

Age

Recent substance use and misuse peak in young women and then decline with increasing age. In the National Household Survey, 55% of young women (18–34 years old) reported alcohol use in the last month, as compared with 40% of women aged 35 or older. This same age-related pattern was observed for 1-year prevalence rates of alcohol abuse or dependence. Specifically, 10% of women aged 18–29 reported symptoms of alcohol abuse or dependence, as compared with 4% of women aged 30–44, 2% aged 45–64, and only

0.4% of women aged 65 or older. Importantly, rates of alcohol abuse and dependence were more similar in younger men and women than in middle-aged and older men and women, suggesting a converging of rates over age cohorts.

Illicit drug use demonstrates an age-related pattern similar to that of alcohol use (i.e., use peaks among young adults and then declines with age). Rates of illicit drug use in the National Household Survey were especially high for 18- to 25-year-olds, with 31% of men and 22% of women in this age range reporting illicit drug use during the preceding year. A similar pattern was found within individual drug classes. For example, regular cocaine use (once a month or more) was reported by 1% of women aged 18–25, 0.4% of women aged 26–34, and 0.3% of women aged 35 or older.

Race/Ethnicity

Overall, white women (84%) were more likely to report any alcohol consumption than either black women (72%) or Hispanic women (68%) in the National Household Survey. These racial/ethnic differences among women were even more pronounced for recent alcohol consumption: 46% of white women reported alcohol use during the past month, compared with 30% of black women and 33% of Hispanic women. Similarly, 14% of white women report drinking once a week or more, whereas only 8% of Hispanic and 10% of black women reported drinking this often. There is evidence that among women who drink, black and white women drink similar amounts of alcohol, although black women experience considerably higher rates of alcohol-related morbidity and mortality.

In the National Household Survey, lifetime prevalence of illicit drug use was somewhat higher in white women (35%) than in black women (27%) or Hispanic women (24%). However, rates of recent drug use were fairly similar across these racial groups, with approximately 9% of women reporting illicit drug use in the past year. Within drug classes, racial/ethnic differences emerged. For example, white women were somewhat more likely than Hispanic or black women to report recent sedative and tranquilizer use. In contrast, black women were more likely to report recent crack use than white or Hispanic women; 0.7% of black women, 0.3% of Hispanic women, and 0.1% of white women reported crack use during the past year.

Marital Status

Women who have never married or are divorced or separated are more likely to drink heavily than women who are married. It also appears that when women drink with their male partners, the amount and duration of women's drinking conform to those of their partners. Thus, women whose male partners drink frequently are more likely to report drinking problems themselves than are women whose partners are nondrinkers or occasional drinkers. In contrast, there is evidence that women whose husbands experience drinking problems are more likely to be abstinent or light drinkers than women whose husbands drink regularly but not problematically. A similar influence of male partners occurs for drug use; that is, women are at increased risk for heavy drug use or abuse/dependence if their male sexual partners are regular drug users.

Educational and Occupational Status

Alcohol abstinence is associated with attainment of less than a high school education for both white and black women. Slightly more than half of women with less than a high school education abstain from alcohol use. Conversely, the higher a woman's educational achievement, the heavier her self-reported alcohol use. Women who work outside the home are more likely to be drinkers than women who are unemployed, full-time homemakers, or retired (see Rohsenow's chapter in this volume for a fuller discussion of women, work, and alcoholism). Finally, heavier drinking is correlated with higher income for women.

BIOPSYCHOSOCIAL CORRELATES OF SUBSTANCE ABUSE AND DEPENDENCE AMONG WOMEN

Various biopsychosocial differences have been found between substance-misusing women and men. Women with substance abuse or dependence experience more medical problems than do either women without these disorders or men with them. For example, menstrual disturbances, hysterectomy and/or oophorectomy, abortions, and miscarriages occur more frequently in chronic alcoholic women than in age-matched controls. Also, alcoholic women are at increased risk of early-onset liver and brain damage, relative to alcoholic men. One factor in this increased alcohol toxicity in women is their reduced first-pass gastric metabolism of alcohol (see Baraona's chapter for further details). Drug use is the most significant risk factor for HIV infection among women. Among women, approximately 50% of AIDS cases have resulted from IV drug use by the women themselves, and an additional 20% from IV drug use by their sexual partners.

Women with substance use disorders are also at elevated risk for psychiatric problems, particularly mood disorders. A significantly higher proportion of alcoholic women (40%) than of nonalcoholic women (8%) report a history of suicide attempts. Alcoholic women experience low self-esteem and self-concept as well. Female substance abusers tend to be more socially isolated than male substance abusers, to have fewer friends and fewer romantic relationships, and to report feeling more lonely. Finally, alcoholic women report exceptionally high rates of childhood sexual abuse. One recent study found that 66% of women in alcoholism treatment had experienced childhood sexual abuse, as compared with 35% in a random household sample of women. Even more striking differences were observed in the more extreme forms of childhood abuse and violence, with 47% of alcoholic women reporting sexual penetration by the abuser, compared with 9% of the household sample.

One-third to one-half of substance-misusing women report living with substance-misusing partners. An even larger proportion of women who are IV drug users report sexual activity with men who also use these drugs. For example, 83% of female methadone patients in one clinic reported having had sex with active IV drug users. These relationship patterns have important implications for physical and sexual abuse risk, since alcohol and drug misuse are overrepresented in cases of spousal abuse. Finally, substance use by women themselves increases their risk of becoming victims of violence. Women are at elevated risk for assault when they and/or their sexual partners are intoxicated (typically with alcohol). Such risk appears to be particularly increased during pregnancy.

CONCLUSIONS

Clearly, substance abuse and dependence are important and widespread health concerns for women. As they do with men, genetic factors appear to play an important role in the development of substance use disorders by women with a family history of alcoholism. In contrast to men, women who misuse substances may be more heavily influenced by intrapersonal factors than by interpersonal influences. Women who experience alcohol or drug abuse or dependence are at increased risk for a variety of harmful medical, psychiatric, and psychosocial consequences, which can facilitate case identification and which must be addressed in comprehensive treatment systems. It is critically important for the welfare of individual women, their children, their families, and society at large that we direct increased research and clinical resources to this understudied and underserved population.

FURTHER READING

Blume, S. (1986). Women and alcohol: A review. *Journal of the American Medical Association, 256,* 1467–1470.
This landmark article provides a comprehensive review of the early literature on alcohol metabolism, medical complications, diagnosis, and treatment of alcoholism in women.

Day, N. L., Cottreau, C. M., & Richardson, G. A. (1993). The epidemiology of alcohol, marijuana and cocaine use among women of childbearing age and pregnant women. *Clinical Obstetrics and Gynecology, 36,* 232–245.
This article reviews rates and correlates of alcohol, marijuana, and cocaine use for women of childbearing age, with special emphasis on pregnant women.

Gomberg, E. S. L. (1993). Women and alcohol: Use and abuse. *Journal of Nervous and Mental Disease, 181,* 211–219.
This paper reviews etiological factors for alcohol problems in women, changes in alcohol consumption patterns over time, and differences in social attitudes toward female versus male intoxication.

Lex, B. (1991). Some gender differences in alcohol and polysubstance users. *Health Psychology, 10,* 121–132.
This article provides a broad spectrum of information about biological, psychological, and sociocultural aspects of substance use as it affects women.

Miller, B., Downs, W., & Testa, M. (1993). Interrelationships between victimization experiences and women's alcohol use. *Journal of Studies on Alcohol* (Suppl. 11), 109–117.
This paper examines relationships between childhood physical and/or sexual victimization and the development of alcohol-related problems among women, controlling for treatment condition and family background variables.

Ross, H. (1989). Alcohol and drug abuse in treated alcoholics: A comparison of men and women. *Alcoholism: Clinical and Experimental Research, 13,* 810–816.
The prevalence of individual alcohol and drug symptoms, patterns of abuse, and different drug disorders were compared in male and female substance abuse treatment patients.

Substance Abuse and Mental Health Services Administration. (1994). *National Household Survey on Drug Abuse: Population estimates, 1993* (DHHS Publication No. SMA 94-3017). Washington, DC: U.S. Government Printing Office.
This publication presents prevalence of use of illegal drugs, prescription drugs used nonmedically, alcohol, and tobacco products as a function of age, gender, and race for a U.S. household sample of persons 12 years old and older.

Wilsnack, R. W. (1995). Drinking and problem drinking in U.S. women: Patterns and recent trends. *Recent Developments in Alcoholism, 12,* 29–60.
This comprehensive review article examines changes in the prevalence of and risk factors for heavy alcohol consumption and drinking-related problems in women over the last two decades.

70

Drug Abuse Treatment

Sharon Hall

*T*his chapter discusses interventions available for drug use problems, patients, with an emphasis on how these modalities specifically affect women. In addition, issues that span specific interventions and that are especially important for women are discussed. This chapter emphasizes illicit drugs, especially opioids and cocaine, the two most common illicit drugs in the 1990s.

AVAILABLE INTERVENTIONS

Self-Help Groups: The Twelve-Step Model

The first, and most pervasive, type of intervention involves self-help groups. Cocaine Anonymous (CA) and Narcotics Anonymous (NA) are offshoots of Alcoholics Anonymous (AA). AA began as a mutual support group of alcoholics, founded early in the 20th century by two men. Like AA, CA and NA are based on the Twelve-Step philosophy. Underlying this philosophy is the premise that drug addiction, like alcoholism, is a progressive disease, and that complete abstinence from all psychoactive drugs is necessary to prevent progression of the disease. The Twelve-Steps involve a series of behaviors and changes in beliefs that include turning one's life over to a higher power, being honest and straightforward, and redressing wrongs that have been done to others as a result of the drug use. Like AA meetings, CA and NA meetings are open to anyone. The leadership and membership of these groups have been predominantly male, however, and some commentators have raised concerns that women do not feel welcome or are not able to speak freely in groups that consist predominantly of men. Although Twelve-Step groups are widespread, it is difficult to assess their efficacy, because these organizations do not traditionally encourage research. Twelve-Step traditions and beliefs are integrated into many drug treatment programs.

As noted above, the Twelve-Step models emphasize the concept of a "higher power" as crucial to recovery from drug addiction. Many potential participants find these religious overtones unacceptable. Because of this, self-help groups that do not rely on Twelve-Step concepts have developed, and these may be open to users of illicit drugs. Such groups may be an option for those seeking help who live in larger towns and in metropolitan areas, but they are not nearly so prevalent as traditional Twelve-Step groups.

Psychological Treatments

The second most common drug treatment modality is provision of services by a psychologist, social worker, or other mental health professional; the precise services provided are based on eclectic psychological models. Often these models include combinations of translations of Twelve-Step philosophy, adaptations of psychodynamic models, and adaptations of behavioral and cognitive-behavioral models. Urine monitoring for illicit drugs is often involved.

Much of the more sophisticated psychotherapy research in treatment for drug use problems is based on cognitive behavioral interventions. Nevertheless, it is rare to find programs that are based solely on cognitive-behavioral principles. One exception is the community reinforcement approach (CRA) for cocaine users; this is an adaptation of earlier work with alcoholics. CRA programs have two components. One is a voucher-based reinforcement system, in which patients earn vouchers that can be exchanged for various socially acceptable reinforcers, which are chosen in collaboration with a counselor. The voucher component is buttressed by a behaviorally based psychotherapy program that includes family and individual counseling. This model, with its intrinsic ability to modify the treatment program to the preferences of the individual, would seem particularly useful to women; the reinforcers women choose may well be different from those selected by men, and may in fact be crucial to the maintenance of abstinence. For example, the availability of 1 hour of child care as a voucher-selected reinforcer may make the difference between treatment attendance and dropout for a poor woman who is undergoing a crisis.

Medication

The most common medication for drug addiction treatment is methadone treatment for opioid dependence. This involves prolonged use of methadone, a synthetic opioid, in the place of heroin or other opioids. The underlying model varies. Some assume that methadone is useful because of a metabolic dysregulation resulting from prolonged opioid use. Others suggest that the primary advantage of methadone over heroin is its legality. As a legal replacement, methadone helps to remove the patient from the dangerous and unhealthy lifestyle inherent in opioid use, and therefore increases the probability that the user will develop a more productive life. There has also been interest in buprenorphine, a partial opioid agonist that can be used much like methadone as a maintenance drug, but, properly administered, does not have the strongly agonist properties of methadone. It is possible that this medication will replace methadone as the primary maintenance drug for opioid addicts.

There has been a great deal of interest in the use of antidepressant medications that increase dopamine availability in the central nervous system to treat cocaine withdrawal and cocaine craving. This is based on the "dopamine depletion hypothesis," which assumes that cocaine craving and relapse are attributable to lowered dopamine levels as a result of cocaine use. No dopaminergic drug has clearly proven useful, however.

Other medications may be used to treat illicit drug users as adjuncts to psychological treatment. For example, non-dependence-producing medications such as diphenhydramine may be prescribed to facilitate sleep.

SPECIAL ISSUES FOR WOMEN IN DRUG TREATMENT

Psychological and Physical Trauma and Posttraumatic Stress Disorder

Recent studies indicate a high level of trauma and posttraumatic stress disorder (PTSD) among drug treatment patients, especially cocaine users. There is some suggestion that the level of trauma among women drug treatment patients, and the possibility of PTSD, are higher in women than men. Women in drug abuse treatment programs may be at excessive risk of PTSD as a result of both childhood and adult trauma. The trauma experienced may have been psychological, physical, or sexual assault. Drug treatment providers should assess patients for the possibility of trauma during intake interviews, and staff members should be trained to make appropriate referrals when necessary. The topic should be revisited later in treatment, when a therapeutic alliance has been established

The Drug Treatment Culture

Men have a higher probability of using illicit drugs than do women. Treatment systems tend to reflect their patient populations; as a result, the drug treatment culture has traditionally not been very sensitive to the needs of women or to their lifestyles. For example, until very recently it was a rare treatment program that provided child care; most still do not. Yet many women in drug treatment programs have children or grandchildren under their care, and the inability to find care for these children while they attend treatment may be a significant barrier. Also, professionals have only recently recognized that female patients with drug use problems are often physically abused, and need to find shelter for themselves and their children.

Women drug treatment patients often do not control other resources that would allow them to become engaged in intensive drug treatment. For example, a woman may not have a car, or the only car in the family may be needed by the sole breadwinner, which she is not.

Also, clinicians have informally noted that drug use patterns in women are closely linked to and dependent upon the significant others with whom they live. Despite this, efforts to involve partners of women with drug use problems in treatment are not common. When such attempts are made, they may be met with active resistance or violence directed toward the patients.

Lack of Research

There is a lack of research targeted at the problem of women drug treatment patients. For example, we know that women metabolize alcohol differently from men, but little is known about gender differences in the metabolism of illicit drugs. Specialized treatments for women have not been reported widely in the literature, or evaluated. Clinically, it appears that women may benefit from an array of services, including same-sex groups and specialized legal and vocational services; again, however, research is needed.

AIDS Risk and HIV Transmission

Acquisition of HIV disease is a risk of illicit drug use for both men and women. Many women entering drug treatment maintain a lifestyle that includes prostitution and "sex for drugs," and are at high risk for becoming HIV-positive. Either HIV screening or referral to appropriate screening clinics at entrance to treatment is essential, as is postscreening counseling. Special groups to assist women in dealing with issues related to HIV and sexuality are important. It is not unusual for women patients to report that their requests for condom use by their partners were met by violence directed at them for making the requests. Support and suggestions from the group members and leaders to deal with such situations are important, and should include discussion of "safe" and "safer" techniques.

Stigma

Illicit drug users are stigmatized in Western culture. Unlike chronic medical disorders, such as hypertension, diabetes, and chronic lung disease, drug addiction is viewed as a self-inflicted disorder. It is seen as a moral issue, a disorder of will, rather than a health problem. Perhaps because traditional stereotypes view women as more moral than men, and as the guardians of culture and home, women with drug use problems are more sternly and negatively regarded by society than men with such problems are. Relatives and friends may actively discourage treatment for women because of the stigma of illicit drug use. Abandonment by a woman's partner is not unusual.

Nowhere is this perception more obvious than in the case of pregnant women who use illicit drugs. Such women have been viewed as child abusers. The punitive attitude of society toward the pregnant drug user is counterproductive. Many pregnant women do not seek drug use treatment because they fear negative that consequences for themselves will ensue if their drug use is uncovered during pregnancy, or that their children will be taken from them after birth. Despite years of research, the precise effects of use of illicit drugs on the fetus are not entirely clear. The lifestyle often accompanying illicit drug use exposes a woman and her fetus to other unhealthy influences, including poor nutrition, insufficient rest, inadequate access to health care, and stress. In addition, cigarette smoking and alcohol use—both known to have deleterious effects on pregnancy and infant health—are more prevalent in illicit drug users, and their effects cannot be separated from those of illicit drugs.

FURTHER READING

Carroll, K. M., Rounsaville, B. J., Gordon, L. T., Nick, C., Jatlow, P., Bisighini, R. M., & Gawin, F. H. (1994). Psychotherapy and pharmacotherapy for ambulatory cocaine abusers. *Archives of General Psychiatry, 27*, 177–187.
Well-designed study of desipramine and cognitive-behavioral therapy for cocaine abusers.

Hall, S. M., Clark, H. W., & Sees, K. L. (1995). Drug abuse, drug treatment and public policy. In W. K. Bickel & R. J. De Grandpre (Eds.), *Drug policy and human nature: Psychological*

perspectives on the control, prevention, and treatment of illicit drug use. New York: Plenum Press.
Book chapter discussing the effects of culture and social perception on treatment of illicit drug use.

Higgins, S. T., Budney, A. J., Bickel, W. K., Hughes, J. R., Foerg, F., & Badger, G. (1993). Achieving cocaine abstinence with a behavioral approach. *American Journal of Psychiatry, 152*(5), 763–769.
Controlled study of CRA for cocaine users.

Lowinson, J. H., Ruiz, P., Millman, R. B., & Langrod, J. G. (Eds.). (1992). *Substance abuse: A comprehensive textbook* (2nd ed.). Baltimore: Williams & Wilkins.
Good general resource.

Schatzberg, A. F., & Nemeroff, C. B. (1995). *Textbook of psychopharmacology.* Washington, DC: American Psychiatric Press.
Readable overview; for the nonpharmacologist.

U.S. Public Health Services. (1994). *Practice approaches in the treatment of women who abuse alcohol and other drugs.* Rockville, MD: U.S. Department of Health and Human Services.
Clinical resource.

71

Cigarette Smoking

Corinne G. Husten

Cigarette smoking is the leading preventable cause of death among women in the United States. Cigarettes cause more deaths among women than do AIDS, automobile accidents, alcohol use, drug use, fires, homicides, and suicides combined. More than 150,000 women die each year from smoking-related diseases; most of these deaths are from heart disease, lung cancer, and chronic lung diseases. Lung cancer now kills more U.S. women than breast cancer does (Figure 71.1). Although the lung cancer death rate for men is leveling off, the rate for women continues to increase.

Cigarette smoking also causes reproductive health problems among women, such as having a low-birthweight infant. Smoking during pregnancy is also associated with miscarriages, premature delivery, respiratory problems in newborns, and infant deaths—including deaths from sudden infant death syndrome (SIDS). Smoking is also associated with early menopause among women and with infertility among both women and men. Finally, exposure to environmental tobacco smoke (ETS) causes lung cancer in women and lung infections, middle-ear disease, decreased lung function, and asthma attacks in children. Exposure to ETS may also increase an infant's risk for SIDS.

This chapter presents the trends in cigarette smoking among U.S. women. Trends in the use of other forms of tobacco are not presented, because cigarette smoking is the main form of tobacco used by women.

TRENDS IN CIGARETTE SMOKING
AMONG ADULT WOMEN IN GENERAL

Cigarette smoking was rare at the beginning of the 20th century. The most common form of tobacco was chewing tobacco, which was used primarily by men. The rise in cigarette use in the early 1900s was made possible by the development of safety matches and the automatic cigarette-making machine. The initial increase in cigarette use occurred among men: In a national survey, 18% of women and 52% of men smoked in 1935. After 1940,

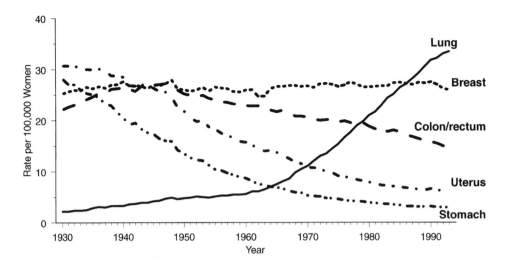

FIGURE 71.1. Cancer death rates among women, by cancer site—United States, 1930–1993. Data from the American Cancer Society.

however, cigarette smoking among women increased. In 1965, 34% of women and 52% of men smoked. For men, cigarette smoking peaked in the 1950s, but it did not peak for women until the 1960s. The smoking rate for women remained fairly stable throughout the 1970s, but then decreased between 1983 and 1994 (Figure 71.2). Although women (23%) still smoked at a lower rate than men (28%) in 1994, the gap had narrowed considerably over the decades.

In 1994, smoking rates were highest for women who were American Indians and Alaska Natives (33%). Rates were comparable for black women (22%) and white women

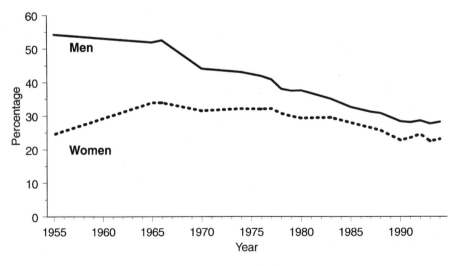

FIGURE 71.2. Percentage of adults aged ≥ 18 years who are current cigarette smokers, by sex—United States, 1955–1994. Data from Current Population Survey (1955): National Health Interview Surveys (1965–1994).

(25%); the rates were lowest for Hispanic women (15%) and Asian and Pacific Islander women (8%). The rate was highest for women aged 25–44 years (28%) and lowest among women 65 years of age and older (11%). Women with a high school education (27%) or less (26%) were more likely to smoke than were women who had completed college (10%). Women were less likely than men to be heavy smokers (25 or more cigarettes per day), and white women were more likely than black or Hispanic women to be heavy smokers.

TRENDS IN SMOKING AMONG ADOLESCENT GIRLS AND YOUNG WOMEN

In 1996, 22% of high school senior girls smoked daily. Cigarette smoking among high school senior girls decreased from 40% in 1977 to 26% in 1992; it then increased to 32% in 1996 (Figure 71.3). In recent years, cigarette smoking also increased dramatically among 10th grade girls (from 21% in 1991 to 31% in 1996) and among 8th grade girls (from 13% in 1991 to 21% in 1996). Although girls were more likely than boys to be daily smokers from 1976 through 1987, girls and boys smoked at the same rate from 1988 to 1996.

Cigarette smoking among black high school senior girls decreased dramatically from 25% in 1976 to 4% in 1996 (Figure 71.4). In contrast, smoking among white high school senior girls declined only slightly from 30% in 1976 to 27% in 1996. The more rapid decrease in smoking among black adolescents is now being seen among young black women (aged 18–24 years) as well. Overall, smoking rates increased in the early 1980s among young women aged 18–24 years, especially the less educated, making this group a cause for concern. Between 1983 and 1993, however, the smoking rate among these women declined.

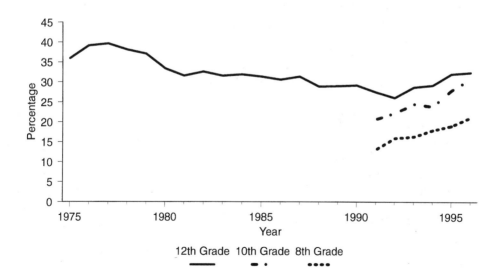

FIGURE 71.3. Current cigarette smoking among girls by grade in school—United States, 1975–1996. Data from the University of Michigan, Monitoring the Future Study.

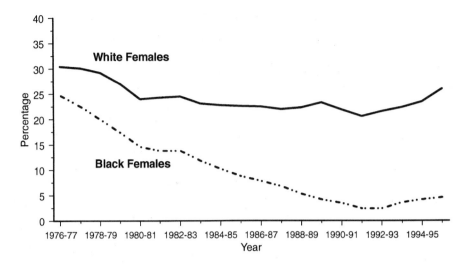

FIGURE 71.4. Percentage of female high school seniors who are daily smokers by race—United States, 1977–1996. Data from the University of Michigan, Monitoring the Future Study.

TRENDS IN SMOKING AMONG WOMEN OF REPRODUCTIVE AGE

In 1994, 27% of women aged 18–44 years smoked cigarettes. Patterns of smoking among these women are similar to those among adult women: American Indian and Alaska Native women were most likely to smoke, and Asian and Pacific Islander women were the least likely.

It is estimated that in 1995, 14% of pregnant women smoked during their pregnancy. Seventy percent of women who quit smoking during pregnancy start again within 1 year after giving birth. Women with 9–11 years of education (26%) were most likely to smoke during pregnancy.

QUITTING BEHAVIOR AMONG WOMEN

Among those who have ever smoked cigarettes, men are more likely than women to have quit (51% vs. 46% in 1994). These statistics have sometimes been interpreted to mean that women have a harder time quitting smoking than men do. However, men are more likely than women to use pipes, cigars, or smokeless tobacco when they stop smoking cigarettes. If other tobacco use is taken into account, the difference in quitting between men and women is small. Also, between 1965 and 1994, the trend in quitting was similar for women and men. White and Hispanic women who had ever smoked were more likely to have quit than black women. Women who had completed college were the most likely to have quit smoking.

NICOTINE ADDICTION AMONG WOMEN

In a recent survey, 80% of girls and women who smoked reported at least one indicator of nicotine addiction: feeling dependent on cigarettes; needing more cigarettes to get the same effect; feeling unable to cut down on their smoking, even though they tried; or feeling sick when they cut down on their smoking. Girls and young women were as likely as older women to report these indicators of nicotine addiction. Even light smokers (fewer than six cigarettes per day) reported indicators of nicotine dependence: 56% of girls and women who were light smokers reported at least one indicator of nicotine dependence.

Ninety-three percent of females under age 22 who smoked daily reported at least one symptom of nicotine withdrawal (feeling sad, blue, and depressed; difficulty concentrating; hunger; restlessness; irritability or craving cigarettes) when they tried to quit. Even among light smokers, 80% reported at least one symptom of nicotine withdrawal.

CONCLUSIONS

One public health goal in the United States is to reduce smoking among adults to 15% by the year 2000; however, this goal will probably not be met for women. In addition, smoking among certain groups of women (such as American Indian and Alaska Native women) is high and not decreasing. Seventy-three percent of women who smoke cigarettes want to stop completely. Women and men are equally likely to try to stop smoking, and they are equally likely to succeed. Easy access to cessation services, including treatment for nicotine addiction, is essential for progress in decreasing smoking rates among women. In addition, public policies (e.g., higher taxes on cigarettes and restrictions on smoking in public places) can encourage women to try to quit and may help them stay abstinent.

Another U.S. public health goal is that no more than 15% of young people become regular smokers by age 20. However, smoking among adolescent girls has been increasing in the 1990s; in 1996, smoking rates among white high school senior girls were higher than in any of the previous 16 years. Finally, young women, even light smokers, often report symptoms of nicotine dependence; in fact, they are as likely as older women to report indicators of dependence.

Greater efforts to prevent girls from starting to smoke are essential. Measures such as restrictions on advertising and promotion that appeal to girls, smoking prevention media messages that target girls, restricted access by minors to cigarettes, higher cigarette taxes, restrictions on smoking in public places, school education programs, and community interventions can all help achieve this goal. Cessation services must also be available to adolescents.

Smoking is a critically important issue for women. The fact that more U.S. women die from lung cancer than from breast cancer each year shows that women have indeed "come a long way, baby" with regard to their smoking behavior. We need a greater awareness that cigarette smoking takes a great toll on the health of women, and that smoking has truly become a women's issue. A comprehensive tobacco prevention and control strategy—one that includes individual interventions, as well as policy and community interventions—could accelerate the decline in smoking among women and significantly decrease illness and death among women in the United States.

FURTHER READING

Centers for Disease Control and Prevention. (1997). Smoking-attributable mortality and years of potential life lost—United States, 1984. *Morbidity and Mortality Weekly Reports, 46,* 444–451.
Summarizes the numbers of deaths from various diseases that are attributable to cigarette smoking.

Centers for Disease Control and Prevention. (1993). Mortality trends for selected smoking-related cancers and breast cancer—United States, 1950–1990. *Morbidity and Mortality Weekly Reports, 42,* 857, 863–866.
Summarizes trends in lung cancer and breast cancer mortality in the United States.

Centers for Disease Control and Prevention. (1995). Indicators of nicotine addiction among women—United States, 1991–1992. *Morbidity and Mortality Weekly Reports, 44,* 102–105.
Summarizes the prevalence of indicators of nicotine dependence among adolescent and adult women.

Environmental Protection Agency. (1993). *Respiratory health effects of passive smoking: Lung cancer and other disorders. The report of the U.S. Environmental Protection Agency* (Smoking and Tobacco Control Monograph No. 4, DHHS Publication No. NIH 93-3605). Bethesda, MD: U.S. Department of Health and Human Services, National Institutes of Health, National Cancer Institute.
Summarizes the effects of environmental tobacco smoke on health.

Floyd, R. L., Rimer, B. K., Giovino, G. A., Mullen, P. D., & Sullivan, S. E. (1993). A review of smoking in pregnancy: Effects on pregnancy outcomes and cessation efforts. *Annual Review of Public Health, 14,* 379–411.
Reviews information about cigarette smoking during pregnancy.

Husten, C. G., Chrismon, J. H., & Reddy, M. N. (1996). Trends and effects of cigarette smoking among girls and women in the United States, 1965–1993. *Journal of the American Medical Women's Association, 51*(1 & 2), 11–18.
Summarizes the patterns of cigarette use by girls and women in the United States.

Klonoff-Cohen, H. S., Edelstein, S. L., Lefkowitz, E. S., Srinivasan, I. P., Kaegi, D., Change, J. C., & Wiley, K. J. (1995). The effect of passive smoking and tobacco exposure through breast milk on sudden infant death syndrome. *Journal of American Medical Association, 273*(10), 795–798.
Describes the impact of cigarette smoking during and after pregnancy on risk for SIDS.

Lynch, B. S., & Bonnie, R. J. (Eds.). (1994). *Growing up tobacco free: Preventing nicotine addiction in children and youths.* Washington, DC: National Academy Press.
Discusses nicotine addiction among youths and how to prevent it.

National Cancer Institute. (1991). *Strategies to control tobacco use in the United States: A blueprint for public health action in the 1990's* (Smoking and Tobacco Control Monograph No. 1, DHHS Publication No. NIH 92-3316). Bethesda, MD: U.S. Department of Health and Human Services, National Institutes of Health, National Cancer Institute.
Describes individual and community interventions to reduce tobacco use in the United States.

Orleans, C. T., & Slade, J. (Eds.). (1993). *Nicotine addiction: Principles and management.* New York: Oxford University Press.
A comprehensive clinical text on tobacco dependence.

U.S. Department of Health and Human Services. (1990). *The health benefits of smoking cessation.* (DHHS Publication No. CDC 90-8416). Rockville, MD: U.S. Department of Health and Human Services, Centers for Disease Control and Prevention, Office on Smoking and Health.
Summarizes the health problems that result from smoking, and the benefits of quitting.

Section VI

SEXUALITY AND REPRODUCTION

72

Section Editor's Overview

Elizabeth L. Williams

*I*t is undeniable that women have benefited from increased research on their unique needs. It is now recognized that gender-specific assessments of risk factors for heart disease (e.g., exercise and stress) are more accurate than nominally gender-free assessments that are male-based. Gender-specific health interventions to decrease smoking, hypercholesterolemia, and hypertension take into account women's different physiology and psychology.

Still, the field of women's health has the potential to overemphasize women's differences from men. This is particularly the case with respect to sexuality and reproductive issues. Women share a host of health concerns with men. What aspects of women's health are fundamentally "human health" with a female guise? There is the additional concern that the field of women's health has embraced mainly women's diseases. Breast cancer is widely regarded as a legitimate women's health issue, for example, whereas breastfeeding is not.

With the explosion of interest in women's health have come new challenges. Major interests include promoting the sharing of information from diverse areas, providing women with accurate information that will facilitate informed decision making, reducing the number of conflicting health messages women receive, and lessening the barriers women experience in assessing coordinated health care.

Nineteen authors from diverse fields were asked to contribute to this section, which explores linkages between women's sexuality and reproduction on the one hand, and physical and mental health on the other.

SEXUAL FUNCTIONING

Morokoff reviews normal sexual functioning, possible problems in sexual functioning, and interventions to improve sexual functioning. Sexual stereotyping and cultural expectations, as well as neuroendocrine factors, are shown to affect women's sexual behavior. Changes in sexual functioning through the life stages are the net effects of changing roles, physiology, and personality.

SEXUAL AND REPRODUCTIVE ENDOCRINOLOGY

Warren and Solidum review the endocrine basis of puberty and menstruation, and discuss the interaction between behavior and neurophysiology. Rather than being at the mercy of fluctuating hormones, women's behavior is shown to reflect a complex interaction between physiological substrate and psychology. The menstrual cycle is a cause of certain behaviors that are carried out in a particular cultural milieu, as well as an effect of hormonal change. Anorexia nervosa is an excellent example of the mind's and body's interacting via hypothalamic integration; other examples are also provided.

PREMENSTRUAL DISORDERS

McFarlane questions the existence of premenstrual disorders. Do certain phenomena that have been observed to occur in a certain temporal relationship to menses have any causal connection? She asks not only whether the symptoms lumped together as premenstrual syndrome (PMS) are related to women's reproductive systems, but whether they are related uniquely to women. As in all areas relating to women's health, there is a need for greater collaboration among the diverse investigators working in this field. McFarlane proposes a more stringent definition of the PMS phenomenon, in order to permit comparison of studies; the inclusion of men as study subjects; and a search for other cycles that may be relevant. Finally, she provides a fresh look at what constitutes a "placebo effect," and suggests that the benefit some women receive from nonmedical interventions (so-called "placebos") indicates a possible nonmedical etiology for at least some of their symptoms.

GYNECOLOGICAL PAIN

Wilkie and Schmidt illustrate the limits of the traditional dichotomous model that asks, "Is it physiological or psychological?" More helpful is an approach that seeks to integrate what we know about both the physical and psychological dimensions of pain. Focusing on chronic pelvic pain (CPP), they point out the limitations of studies to date, particularly the difficulty in deciding which comes first—the CPP or the psychopathology with which it is often associated. Or are they both the common manifestation of another phenomenon (e.g., stress)? Ways to use operant conditioning, relaxation, and cognitive strategies for coping with chronic pain are discussed, with the caveat that there have been few adequately controlled trials of these interventions.

SEXUAL ABUSE

Laws explores the links between sexual abuse and physician visits for such problems as CPP, headaches, sleep disturbances, gastrointestinal problems, and vaginal discharge.

Survivors of sexual abuse are less likely to seek regular gynecological care than are women with no history of abuse, and yet they are at higher risk of STDs and unwanted pregnancies because of their riskier sexual behavior. The associations between sexual abuse and eating disorders, substance abuse/dependence, and health care seeking are also discussed, and possible mechanisms are explored. How to identify survivors of sexual abuse in various settings is unknown, as is how to tailor care when this history is known. Effective approaches are needed in fields as diverse as eating disorders, substance use treatment, chronic pain, STDs, and family planning.

PREGNANCY AND CHILDBIRTH

Pregnancy is influenced by a host of factors. Like menarche and menopause, it heralds a major life transition. Dunkel-Schetter and Lobel explore the possible contributions of three psychosocial variables—psychological stress, physical strain, and social relationships—and call for a multidisciplinary approach to studying ways to identify women at high risk for negative outcomes and providing effective interventions. That birth outcomes such as length of labor, medication use, and mode of delivery have been shown in randomized trials to be favorably influenced by the presence of a labor companion argues for a powerful psychosocial contribution to what has been approached as a primarily medical problem. (In addition, what accounts for the fact that Hispanic women in the United States are among the least likely to receive prenatal care, but have the lowest rate of low-birthweight babies? Why are African-American women who receive prenatal care still at higher risk of having low-birthweight infants, compared to white women of the same educational and economic strata?) Perhaps the medical components of prenatal care are incidental, and the psychosocial dimensions are the ones that are effective in improving pregnancy outcomes. Even in environments where the prenatal care is anonymous and the emphasis on social support is low, women receiving prenatal care may have heightened perceptions of their own competence or preparedness that decrease their stress during pregnancy or labor and favorably influence their outcomes.

PREGNANCY IN WOMEN WITH DISABILITIES

Rogers argues that if pregnant women without disabilities would benefit from more comprehensive, more coordinated prenatal care, this is doubly the case for women with disabilities. Women with disabilities experience discrimination from health care providers, who may assume that women with disabilities are not sexual beings, or that in any event they should not reproduce. Some women with disabilities are at increased risk of infertility, yet are less likely to receive assistance in conceiving because of such "disablist" attitudes. Pregnancy-related care for women with disabilities, as for all women, is needlessly compartmentalized, and too often the pregnant state deprives women of relevant expertise. Hyperglycemia and high blood pressure during pregnancy, for example, too often are viewed as totally distinct from the same phenomena occurring in the nonpregnant human. Expertise in rehabilitative medicine is highly relevant to many of the problems encountered by pregnant women with disabilities. Yet the pregnant woman is too frequently seen as the exclusive domain of the obstetrician or midwife.

Pregnant women with disabilities are different from pregnant women without disabilities in some respects, but alike in others. More information is needed on the pregnancy-related problems associated with particular disabilities and ways to solve them. Rogers suggests a number of approaches to increasing our knowledge base and facilitating innovative approaches.

POSTPARTUM DEPRESSION

As McFarlane has done with PMS, Gotlib questions whether postpartum depression exists as a distinct phenomenon. He reminds us that simply because an event such as depression is observed to follow a change in a woman's reproductive or hormonal status, this does not mean that there is a causal relationship. Most phenomena in a woman's life between menarche and menopause qualify as either premenstrual, menstrual, or postmenstrual. Gotlib points out that the rates and symptoms of postpartum depression are equivalent to those of nonpostpartum depression among women of childbearing age. As with PMS, not only is it uncertain that postpartum depression is related to women's reproductive cycles; it is unclear that it is uniquely female. More research, with a clearer definition of postpartum depression and a broader search for risk factors, is needed in this area. Perhaps giving birth is merely a marker for stress.

BREASTFEEDING

The reproductive cycle does not end physiologically with birth, Lawrence points out, but rather with lactation. During pregnancy, breasts undergo rapid changes in preparation for breastfeeding, and approximately 8 pounds of the weight gained is to provide energy stores for breastfeeding. Women's bodies are thus prepared hormonally and anatomically to breastfeed their young. Yet little more than 50% of U.S. mothers breastfeed for any length of time. The reasons are diverse, but most mothers are denied the information that would permit them to make an informed decision regarding how to feed their infants.

Lawrence reviews the many medical benefits of breastfeeding for the child as well as for the mother. Many of these benefits are lifelong, including a reduced risk of diabetes, certain bowel diseases, and cancers for the child who breastfeeds, and a reduced risk of ovarian cancer and premenopausal breast cancer for the mother. A dose–response relationship has been shown for total months of breastfeeding and reduced risk of premenopausal breast cancer. Lactation may also assist in lowering women's risk of heart disease, the leading cause of death for women in the United States, by increasing the "good" cholesterol (high-density lipoprotein) during breastfeeding and by lowering the risk of chronic diseases associated with obesity (e.g., adult-onset diabetes and hypertension) through greater postpartum weight loss. Unfortunately, many pregnant women base their choice on misinformation regarding the health- or sexuality-related effects of breastfeeding. (It should also be noted that one of the reasons women choose not to breastfeed is a history of being sexually abused. Those caring for mothers and babies must be sensitive to this possibility and not insist that every mother "at least give it a try.")

Among mothers who do start out with breastfeeding, a major reason for quitting is poor coordination of care. A mother may give up trying to reconcile the conflicting advice from her own doctor, the baby's doctor, the night nurse, the day nurse, the lactation consultant, and the peer counselor, as well as from family members and friends. Women who do breastfeed deserve accurate information regarding what to expect at each stage, access to competent health providers when problems occur, and a coordinated approach to solving problems that takes into account the symbiotic relationship of mother and baby. Breastfeeding mothers also benefit from coordination among the different providers of care, including those in the arenas of family planning, sexually transmitted diseases (STDs), and mental health.

CONTRACEPTION BY THE LACTATIONAL AMENORRHEA METHOD

The lactational amenorrhea method (LAM) of family planning or child spacing has been demonstrated to provide 99.6% protection against pregnancy. As Labbok notes in her chapter, it is an attractive alternative to many women who do not like the side effects or inconvenience of other contraceptive methods. Yet few pregnant women or breastfeeding mothers in the United States receive accurate information regarding the LAM. As with the decision to breastfeed, women deserve full information on which to base their choice of child-spacing method, and support for this choice from the various members of their health care team.

CONTRACEPTION

In her chapter, Ballagh discusses methods of contraception (other than the LAM) that are currently available in the United States. In decreasing order of effectiveness, these include permanent and reversible sterilization methods; estrogen-containing oral contraceptives and the progesterone-releasing intrauterine device; traditional (male) condoms and progestin-only contraceptives; and female barrier methods, fertility awareness also called the "rhythm method"), and withdrawal. Ballagh emphasizes that better use of existing contraception methods and selection of more effective methods could have a major impact on rates of unwanted pregnancy in the United States.

ABORTION

Adler and Smith stress that therapeutic abortion is not a simple matter: It involves a number of parties (the pregnant women, her partner and family, her health care provider, and society at large) and a wide range of issues (biomedical, religious, moral, psychological, legal, and social factors). They also note that responses to abortion are reactions not merely to the procedure itself, but to the entire experience of having an unwanted pregnancy. Nevertheless, in their review of research on the risks and consequences of abortion, they find that the medical risks are considerably lower than those of childbirth, and that the period of greatest psychological distress is prior to the procedure; after abortion, positive emotions predominate over negative ones. Risk factors for negative psychological sequelae include poor prior mental health, termination of pregnancy for medical indications (e.g., problems with the developing fetus as determined by genetic screening), and lack of support within a woman's personal context. Although considerable controversy has centered around adolescents' ability to make decisions concerning abortion, it appears that adolescents' reasoning about abortion is similar to that of adults, and that most adolescents do consult adults before making a decision. Adler and Smith note the need for continuing efforts to identify factors that contribute to negative responses to abortion, to provide support to women who are at risk for such responses, and to prevent unwanted pregnancies so that fewer abortions will be necessary.

REPRODUCTIVE TECHNOLOGIES

Giudice explains the common causes of infertility, the tests that can be done to diagnose the cause of infertility, and the technologies available to assist women experiencing infertility. Although research on the physical aspects of infertility has been copious, relatively little attention has been given to the attendant psychological issues. As in many areas of medicine, advanced reproductive technologies have created unique psychological dilemmas. To decrease the prevalence of infertility, greater collaboration is needed among experts in STD prevention, family planning, substance abuse prevention, and other areas. To promote informed decision making about artificial reproductive technologies, women need clear information as to what options exist. They need attention to the nontechnological, nonphysical aspects of their infertility as well. (As an afterthought, one wonders how the experience of infertility, whatever the outcome, affects women's health subsequently. Are infertile women less likely to seek regular gynecological care because of a more conflicted view of their sexual organs? Do they perceive themselves as less healthy and seek more health care generally, as perhaps survivors of sexual abuse do?

MENOPAUSE

The experience of menopause is influenced by what has come before (e.g., women who smoke are more likely to enter menopause earlier), and the decisions that are made during menopause potentially affect the rest of a woman's life. Menopause marks an acceleration in osteoporosis, the beginning of women's catching up with men in terms of risk of cardiovascular disease, and a change in the psychological and physiological climate of sexual relations. O'Hanlan discusses the health-promoting choices available to women that may ameliorate annoying symptoms of menopause, as well as counter the increased risks of cardiovascular disease, breast cancer, and osteoporosis that occur in the postmenopausal years. Information is provided that will assist women in making an informed choice regarding hormone replacement therapy—another area where women often receive conflicting advice.

SEXUALITY AND AGING

Sexual activity decreases with age in U.S. society. Are women fulfilling a widely heralded cultural expectation, or responding to the hormonal and physical changes accompanying aging? Zeiss explores the interplay of diseases that are more common with aging (e.g., diabetes) and sexuality. Physical impairment of a woman or her partner can dramatically affect her sexuality, oftentimes in excess of what can be accounted for by the medical problem alone. Even in the absence of disease, older women may perceive themselves as less sexually desirable. Expectations may become self-fulfilling prophecies. Among women who have had a mastectomy or other surgery, decreased stamina may be less important than altered body image. An interdisciplinary approach to sexual dysfunction in older women, and rejection of the false biomedical–psychogenic dichotomy, are encouraged.

CONCLUSIONS

There has been an explosion of knowledge in fields affecting women's sexuality and reproductive capability (e.g., infertility and menopause). Still, there is much that is unknown, particularly in such areas as pregnancy in women with disabilities, where the need for more research has been relatively underacknowledged.

A common theme in this section is the need to empower women consumers of health care through providing information that will permit informed decision making. Too often, women are insufficiently informed regarding available choices. This is true of contraception, abortion, birth, infant-feeding methods, sexual functioning, and menopause.

Women are barraged with a confusing array of conflicting messages. Alcohol lowers the risk of heart disease, but it raises the risk of breast cancer. Interventions to treat a reproductive or sexual issue may have a negative impact on another aspect of a woman's health. Some of the drugs used to treat infertility, for example, may cure infertility but raise the risk of ovarian cancer. Losing weight may lower a woman's risk of hypertension or diabetes, but may raise her risk of osteoporosis.

Women of all ages should benefit from the streamlining and integrating of health services. Whether an alcoholic in need of detoxification, a pregnant woman with no prenatal care, a lesbian with vaginitis, or a middle-aged adult with a family history of premature coronary artery disease, the individual woman of any age needs coordinated care. Too often, services are fragmented.

Finally, there is an understandable bias toward medical interventions in the medical community—the prescription of drugs rather than behavior change. Yet, as most of the authors in this section point out, a woman's well-being can be enhanced significantly by health-promoting behaviors and psychosocial support.

FURTHER READING

Williams, E. L., & Hammer, L. D. (1995). Breastfeeding attitudes and knowledge of pediatricians in training. *American Journal of Preventive Medicine, 11*, 26–33.

Williams, E. L., Winkleby, M. A., & Fortmann, S. P. (1993). Changes in coronary heart disease risk factors in the 1980's: Evidence of a male–female crossover effect with age. *American Journal of Epidemiology, 137*, 1056–1067.

73

Sexual Functioning

Patricia J. Morokoff

*T*here are a number of important topics for health and mental health practitioners with respect to women's sexuality. These include (1) normal sexual functioning in women, especially related to age and reproductive life cycle events; (2) antecedents of sexual difficulties in women; and (3) assessment and interventions to address sexual problems and to prevent sexually transmitted diseases (STDs) and sexual victimization.

The context of women's sexuality includes gender expectations, ethnic and cultural expectations, reproductive life stages, interpersonal relationships, individual history (including history of sexual victimization), medical status, and intrapersonal characteristics. A conceptualization of normal sexual functioning must take such factors into account, and any assessment or treatment intervention needs to be conceptualized in the context of these factors.

NORMAL SEXUALITY IN WOMEN

Before examining the question of what causes sexual problems, it is important to conceptualize what is normal for women. It is now clear that women enjoy sex as much as men do. In a meta-analysis of studies on gender differences in sexuality, Oliver and Hyde found no gender difference in sexual satisfaction. This supports other research, which has demonstrated no differences in self-reported arousal between men and women. Some significant gender differences were found by Oliver and Hyde, however, especially in incidence of masturbation and attitudes toward casual premarital sex, and to a lesser extent in incidence and frequency of intercourse, sexual permissiveness (men were more permissive and engaged in more sexual behaviors), and some other sexual behaviors.

Sexual Disorders, Satisfaction, and Assertiveness

In order to look at the question of what is normal, I first present evidence concerning the frequency of various sexual experiences in women. The experiences examined constitute what we believe are important aspects of sexuality, such as sexual satisfaction, the presence of positive physiological responses, the absence of pain and anxiety, and the ability to be autonomous in sexual decision making. The best evidence comes from studies of women in the general population—that is, not women who sought treatment for sexual problems. It should be noted that large-scale studies in which formal diagnostic criteria for sexual dysfunctions are applied to nonclinical populations have not been conducted, so highest-quality data are not available concerning frequency of dysfunctions.

Sexual disorders are prevalent in women. A study conducted by Rosen, Taylor, Leiblum, and Bachmann of 329 women at a gynecological clinic revealed that about a quarter of women indicated dissatisfaction with their sexual relationships. Questions were asked to shed light on the specific nature of sexual problems. Lack of pleasure was the most commonly endorsed problem (61% of women said they had problems at least some of the time), followed by difficulty experiencing orgasm (58%), feelings of anxiety or inhibition (50%), difficulty with lubrication (43%), and lack of pleasure (20%). Substantially fewer women had always experienced these problems, but 9% of women reported always having problems with lubrication, and the same percentage reported always having a problem experiencing orgasm. Elsewhere (Morokoff, 1993), I have reviewed literature on the prevalence of arousal disorders in women. Estimates ranged from 12% of women diagnosed with an arousal phase disorder, to 48% of a sample of normal women who indicated "difficulty getting excited."

Another aspect of sexuality typically considered important for positive sexual functioning is autonomy in sexual decision making. In order to protect themselves from unwanted pregnancy and STDs, women must be able to enter into decisions concerning sexual behaviors such as condom use. Osmond et al. however, found that one-third of women in their sample of women at risk for HIV/AIDS had no voice in decisions with partners concerning condoms. Women were asked to indicate who made condom decisions, indicating "self," "partner," "both," or "never discussed." One-third of women endorsed either "partner" or "never discussed." In this study it was found that when women did not have a voice in decision making about condoms, they were seldom used.

These data indicate that many women in Western society are dissatisfied with their sexual relationships, and that the specific components we think signal a positive sexual relationship (including both sexual response and sexual assertiveness) are in many cases lacking. It is thus statistically normal for women to have a variety of dissatisfying experiences during sexual relationships, and to have partners make decisions for them concerning sexual practices.

Reproductive Life Stages and Aging

The experiences of menarche, menstrual cycling, pregnancy, the postpartum period, lactation, perimenopause, and menopause, with their physiological/hormonal components as well as psychosocial expectations, have significant effects of women's sexuality. I have reviewed research on the relationship of these life events to women's sexual arousal (Morokoff, 1993). Sexual feelings vary across the menstrual cycle. Peaks in sexual activity have been reported at various cycle phase points, including the midfollicular phase and premenstrual phases. Various explanations have been posed for these findings, including changes in feelings of well-being across the cycle, fluctuations in testosterone levels (evidence suggests that sexual functioning is more related to testosterone than estrogen), or increased pelvic congestion and edema prior to menstruation.

Sexual feelings during pregnancy appear to be a complex combination of psychosocial and physiological changes. Especially during the first trimester, feelings of physical well-being may be diminished by morning sickness or anxieties concerning the pregnancy. Overall, women's sexual enjoyment appears to decline during pregnancy, although there are some indications that this trend is partially reversed during the second trimester. Numerous factors may influence sexual feelings, including the large changes in pregnancy hormones; increased vaginal vasocongestion, edema, and the pressure of the fetus; physical symptoms of discomfort, such as morning sickness; anxieties over how sex may harm the baby; fears about sexual attractiveness; and many other concerns.

Multiple factors continue to affect sexual functioning during the postpartum period, especially if the mother is breastfeeding her baby. An important lactation hormone, prolactin, may also play a role in inhibiting sexual response. Prolactin is released during the postpartum period, especially during breastfeeding. In addition, estrogen levels remain low for a variable length of time after parturition. The length of time before normal cycling resumes appears related to length of full-time breastfeeding. Although estrogen levels during normal cycling do not appear to be related to sexual response, the estrogen deprivation characteristic of the early postpartum period has consequences for sexual functioning. Specifically, research has demonstrated that estrogen deprivation results in thinning of the vaginal mucosa and vaginal atrophy, as well as less vaginal fluid. These phenomena can lead to vaginal discomfort or dyspareunia during intercourse. Such discomfort may have a domino effect on other aspects of sexual functioning, leading to less sexual arousal, diminished desire for sex, and less satisfaction. In addition to physiological changes, a myriad of other factors can have a negative impact on sexuality during the postpartum period. Lack of sleep, stress associated with care of the newborn, stress associated with the transition to motherhood, episiotomy pain, and the partner's pressure to resume sex earlier than desired as well as other conflicts between partners, may all lead to a lower level of sexual enjoyment.

A well-established body of research, which I have reviewed elsewhere (Morokoff, 1993), demonstrates that sexuality declines in both women and men with aging. Specifically, with age people engage in less sexual behavior. Vaginal vasocongestion was found to develop more slowly in older women than in younger women. The rate and amount of vaginal lubrication were both diminished. Menopause itself appears to have a negative effect on sexuality, apart from the general effects of aging. Research indicates that menopausal status is associated with decreased frequency of sexual activity, decreased sexual desire, decreased frequency of orgasm, and decreased vaginal lubrication. These decreases may be related to hormonal changes that accompany menopause; research indicates that the most likely hormonal cause of such changes is declining testosterone rather than estrogen. (The topic of sexuality and aging is discussed in more detail in Zeiss's chapter of this volume.)

ANTECEDENTS OF SEXUAL DIFFICULTIES IN WOMEN

Cultural Factors Related to Gender

Gender roles for sexuality prescribe that women be sexually passive and at the same time act as sexual gatekeepers. This means that women are traditionally expected not to take the sexual initiative, as well as to prevent unwanted sexual activities from occurring.

Sexual stereotypes in Western culture suggest that men have a stronger sex drive than women and therefore are expected to desire sex more frequently. It is considered appropriate for men to initiate sex as often as they would like, and to try to get partners to engage in desired sexual activities. It is the traditional obligation of female partners both to provide sexual satisfaction to partners and to set limits on inappropriate sexual behaviors requested by partners. This set of norms is consistent with rape myths indicating that it is a woman's fault if she is raped: It is her fault in the context of the expectation that women must set limits on inappropriate sexual behaviors. However, women may lack the ability to set these limits for multiple reasons. If women accommodate men, rather than asserting their rights to sexual decision making concerning such factors as the frequency of sexual activity, the timing of sexual activity, and the specific behaviors to be engaged in, then it is not surprising if women are dissatisfied with sex and do not experience the emotional and physiological responses they would like.

Sexual Trauma

Childhood sexual abuse (CSA) is a serious and common problem, with prevalence estimates ranging from 15% to 33%, in part depending on how CSA is defined, according to Polusny and Follette. The chapter by Laws in this volume discusses the relation of CSA to various health and mental health problems; it is now established that CSA is related to adult sexual functioning as well. The clearest findings are with respect to frequency and number of sexual relationships and age of first intercourse. A number of investigations reviewed by Polusny and Follette reveal that women with sexual abuse histories change partners more frequently, engage in sexual activities with casual acquaintances more, have more short-term sexual relationships, engage in voluntary sexual intercourse at an earlier age and have more sexual partners than do women without such histories. These behaviors are significant because they put women at risk for HIV and other STDs, as well as unplanned pregnancies. In fact, research conducted by Wyatt, Guthrie, and Notgrass revealed that women who were abused in childhood and again as adults had a significantly higher rate of unintended and aborted pregnancies than other women. Furthermore, among women involved in commercial sex, a high rate had sexual abuse histories. For example, Zierler et al. found that female CSA survivors were almost three times more likely than their nonabused peers to report a history of prostitution. In addition, they found that women with CSA histories had a higher rate of HIV infection.

Research evidence is less clear with respect to specific effects of CSA on sexual satisfaction and dysfunctions—in part because, as discussed above, base rates for these phenomena are extremely high in the general population. Nevertheless, a number of studies reviewed by Polusny and Follette did report significantly greater dissatisfaction or incidence of dysfunction among CSA survivors than among nonabused peers.

Finally, CSA has been shown to be related to revictimization experiences. According to Polusny and Follette, "Overall, sexually abused females reported significantly more negative adult experiences, including sexual assault, physical assault, and force used in adult relationships than did nonabused women." The particularly good study conducted by Wyatt et al. found that almost half of women who had been sexually victimized before the age of 18 reported abuse in adulthood. Women who were sexually abused during childhood were 2.4 times more likely to be revictimized as adults.

Relationships

Feelings toward a partner at the time of a sexual experience are an important determinant of satisfaction with that experience. If a woman engages in sex with a partner at a time when she desires sex, her feelings and potential sexual enjoyment will be different than if she engages in sex only to please her partner or if she is experiencing resentment or other negative emotions. Beck and Bozman conducted a laboratory study of the effects of anger and anxiety on sexual desire in women and men. Participants listened to audiotapes depicting an initial sexual contact between a man and woman who had been dating for several months. Anger-evoking statements, anxiety-evoking statements, or neutral statements were embedded in the narrative for each of these conditions. Sexual desire was measured continuously by lever rating, and participants were asked to indicate at any point whether they would have terminated the sexual encounter. The researchers found that for women, both anger and anxiety significantly reduced desire for sex, compared to a control condition. Significantly more women than men indicated that they would have terminated the encounter during the anger condition. These findings demonstrate that health and mental health practitioners need to pay close attention to the quality of relationship in evaluating the causes of sexual problems. Clearly, couples in which physical abuse or sexual coercion is present can be expected to have impaired sexual relationships.

ASSESSMENT AND INTERVENTIONS FOR SEXUAL PROBLEMS IN WOMEN

The most important assessment technique currently available for assessing sexual functioning is the structured interview. Many sources are currently available to suggest specific questions to be followed in taking a sexual history. No standardized paper-and-pencil questionnaires have been well accepted as measures of specific aspects of sexual functioning in women or men.

The brief directed treatment of sexual problems in women has been used for over 30 years. This approach has proved very successful in helping women who do not experience orgasm to do so. Brief directed therapy has also been used with many other sexual problems, such as desire disorder, arousal disorder, or vaginismus for women, but treatment success for these difficulties is variable. Lack of success with treatment of sexual desire problems, for example, may relate to the fact the treatments have not adequately conceptualized CSA or relational aspects of the presenting problem and included measures to address these problems. Furthermore, the traditional brief intervention for treatment of sexual problems includes structured sexual assignments, which may be subtly coercive to women who have difficulty asserting themselves sexually.

Interventions have also been developed to train women in sexual assertiveness. The need for such interventions is highlighted by the risk of STD transmission through unprotected sexual activity with a risky partner. The life-threatening nature of HIV exposure has lent urgency to the need for health and mental health professionals to teach women methods for protecting themselves sexually. The possibility of increasing condom use and other safer sex behaviors in women was demonstrated by Kelly and colleagues' report of an intervention with inner-city women. A four-session intervention that included detailed information about HIV risk, role plays of initiating discussion of AIDS concerns and condom use, and role plays of declining sex from men whose risk history was unknown was compared to a control intervention. Results showed that the intervention was successful in increasing condom use from 26% of the time to 56%, whereas no change was demonstrated by the control group.

There are difficulties in teaching sexual assertiveness, however, as other studies reporting negative results have shown. This is probably because training in sexual assertiveness goes against many deeply ingrained cultural norms for women's behavior, as discussed above.

CONCLUSIONS

Health and mental health professionals need to be aware of women's capacity for healthful and satisfying sexual relationships, as well as how sexuality is affected by life stage. They also need to be aware of the prevalence of sexual problems women experience. Assessment and interventions to modify women's sexual behaviors or responses must take into account the multiplicity of factors that influence sexual functioning. Women need accurate information concerning their sexual functioning across the lifespan, information concerning behaviors that put them at risk for HIV and other STDs, and steps they can take to enjoy sex safely.

FURTHER READING

Beck, J. G., & Bozman, A. W. (1995). Gender differences in sexual desire: The effects of anger and anxiety. *Archives of Sexual Behavior, 24,* 595–612.
Laboratory study examining the effects of anger and anxiety on sexual desire in men and women.

Kelly, J. A., Murphy, D. A., Washington, C. D., Wilson, T. S., Koob, J. J., Davis, D. R., Ledezma, G., & Davantes, B. (1994). Effects of HIV/AIDS prevention groups for high-risk women in urban primary health care clinics. *American Journal of Public Health, 84,* 1918–1922.
Landmark intervention study to increase safer sexual behavior in women.

Morokoff, P. J. (1993). Female sexual arousal disorder. In W. O'Donohue & J. H. Geer (Eds.), *Handbook of sexual dysfunctions: Assessment and treatment.* Boston: Allyn & Bacon.
Thorough review of literature on sexual arousal in women, with a focus on sexuality across the reproductive lifespan.

O'Donohue, W., & Geer, J. H. (Eds.). (1993). *Handbook of sexual dysfunctions.* Boston: Allyn & Bacon.
Comprehensive volume on many aspects of assessment and treatment of sexual dysfunctions.

Oliver, M. B., & Hyde, J. S. (1993). Gender differences in sexuality: A meta-analysis. *Psychological Bulletin, 114,* 29–51.
First meta-analytic review of gender differences in sexuality.

Osmond, M. W., Wambach, K. G., Harrison, D. F., Byers, J., Levine, P., Imershein, A., & Quadagno, D. M. (1993). The multiple jeopardy of race, class, and gender for AIDS risk among women. *Gender and Society, 7,* 99–120.
Empirical study examining factor of gender, race, and class with respect to condom use in women.

Polusny, M. A., & Follette, V. M. (1995). Long-term correlates of child sexual abuse: Theory and review of the empirical literature. *Applied and Preventive Psychology, 4,* 143–166.
Thorough review of literature on consequences of child sexual abuse.

Risen, C. (1995). A guide to taking a sexual history. *Psychiatric Clinics of North America, 18,* 39–52.
Current approaches to sexual history taking.

Rosen, R. C., Taylor, J. F., Leiblum, S. R., & Bachmann, G. (1993). Prevalence of sexual dysfunctions in women. *Journal of Sex and Marital Therapy, 19,* 171–188.
Provides current information on prevalence of sexual dysfunctions in women from the general population.

Wyatt, G. E., Guthrie, D., & Notgrass, C. M. (1992). Differential effects of women's child sexual abuse and subsequent sexual revictimization. *Journal of Consulting and Clinical Psychology, 60,* 167–173.
Important paper on effects of sexual revictimization in African-American and European-American women.

Zierler, S., Feingold, L., Laufer, D., Velentgas, P., Kantrowitz-Gordon, I., & Mayer, K. (1991). Adult survivors of childhood sexual abuse and subsequent risk of HIV infection. *American Journal of Public Health, 81,* 572–575.
Important study documenting the increased risk for HIV infection in women with childhood sexual abuse histories.

74

Reproductive Endocrinology

Michelle P. Warren
Arneli A. Solidum

*I*t is now well established that sexual development and reproduction are mainly regulated by the hypothalamic–pituitary–ovarian (H-P-O) axis. The discovery of the gonadotropin-releasing hormone (GnRH) pulse generator has contributed a great deal to our understanding of the role of the hypothalamus in the neurohumoral modulation of these processes. Although the mechanisms of this modulation are at present still unclear, evidence is mounting that adaptive measures toward preservation of life take precedence over "perpetuation of the species."

THE HYPOTHALAMIC–PITUITARY–OVARIAN AXIS

An intact H-P-O axis is necessary for normal sexual maturity, cyclicity, and reproductive capability. Understanding this complex endocrine system is fundamental to properly approaching and managing the wide spectrum of clinical problems that may be encountered.

The hypothalamus is a complicated gland that integrates endocrine, vegetative, and neuropsychiatric functions. It is connected to higher centers of the brain and to the pituitary gland (Figure 74.1), and is the final endocrine pathway for many systems. It receives input from other brain regions, such as the temporal lobe and brainstem. The nerve bundles that connect the hypothalamus to the higher centers include the median forebrain bundle, which connects the hypothalamus to the higher sensory and motor areas of the cerebral cortex; the dorsal longitudinal cortex, which sends messages concerning satiety and digestion back to the body; the mamillo-thalamic tract, which is involved in emotional responses; and the fornix, which connects the hypothalamus with memory centers in the limbic system (Barchas, Akil, Elliott, Holman, & Watson, 1978; Krieger, 1980). There are probably other connections, but these are not well understood. Input from the central nervous system is also mediated by chemical transmitters. Thus,

447

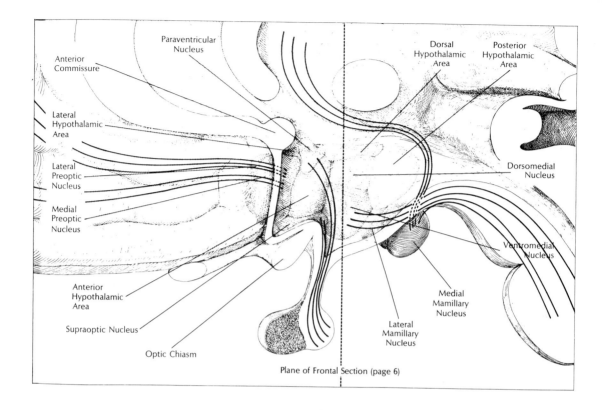

FIGURE 74.1. Major nuclear center of the hypothalamus and its interconnections with the remainder of the central nervous system. From Warren (1988). Copyright 1988 by E. A. Blechman. Reprinted by permission.

there appear to be direct neural connections as well as chemical transmissions of signals to the hypothalamus.

The pituitary gland hangs from the hypothalamus by means of a stalk consisting of a delicate network of blood vessels and nerves (see Figure 74.1). The blood vessels originate at a vascular area in the medial central area of the hypothalamus, and carry hormones from here to the anterior pituitary gland. They constitute the pituitary portal system, and it is through this system that GnRH from the median basal hypothalamus (MBH) reaches its target cells—the gonadotropes. The nerve channels represent mostly axons, terminals, or nerve bodies that originate in the hypothalamus and travel down the stalk bundle directly into the posterior pituitary. These neurosecretory tracts carry hypothalamic hormones to the pituitary, where they are stored.

GnRH stimulates the production of the gonadotropins luteinizing hormone (LH) and follicle-stimulating hormone (FSH) by gonadotropes in the anterior pituitary gland. It is released by the GnRH pulse generator neurons in a pulsatile manner, normally every 60–90 minutes. This periodicity, in turn, dictates the episodic secretion of gonadotropins. The resulting pulses of LH and FSH throughout the day are necessary for normal development of the ovarian follicles, which secrete the sex hormones responsible for cyclicity. Any aberration from this physiologic set point can give rise to menstrual cycle abnormalities, as discussed in more detail later.

PUBERTY

Neuroendocrine Mechanisms

The H-P-O axis is fully developed at birth. In very early infancy, gonadotropins (particularly FSH) are secreted in large amounts, and levels remain relatively high throughout the first 2 years of life (Schwartz, 1995). This is followed by a progressive decline that is attributed to a central inhibitory modulation probably exerted by hypothalamic beta-endorphin and dopamine (Figure 74.2). This inhibition is suggested by findings that women with functional hypothalmic amenorrhea have demonstrated increases in LH secretion following blockade of these receptors by their respective antagonists, naloxone and metoclopramide (Quigley, Sheenan, Casper, & Yen, 1980; Khoury, Reame, Kelch, & Marshall, 1987).

The onset of puberty is characterized by an increase in the pulsatile release of GnRH that initially occurs during sleep (Figure 74.3). This sleep-entrained amplification of GnRH pulsatility is critical to the activation of pituitary–ovarian function (Boyar et al., 1974). What triggers the release of inhibitory control over GnRH secretion at this particular stage of development, however, is still unknown.

With time, the secretory response of LH to GnRH increases progressively, until by late puberty it occurs approximately every 90 minutes. FSH levels are also higher initially, but then plateau as puberty progresses (Schwartz, 1995).

Finally, as noted above, increasing levels of LH and FSH associated with a normal pulsatile secretion promote the development of ovarian follicles; these eventually secrete the sex hormones responsible for the physical changes of puberty.

Physical Changes of Puberty

The normal episodic secretion of LH and FSH promotes ovarian secretion of estradiol, and to some extent androgens, the male hormones. The role of these hormones in the physical changes at puberty has been defined, as has the role of adrenal androgens that surface at the same time. Thelarche (the beginning of breast development), for example, is related to ovarian estrogen, whereas pubarche (the beginning of body hair growth) is related to adrenal androgen. In the normal situation, these two pubertal events occur within the same 4- to 5-year span (Warren et al., 1975). On the other hand, the relationship of psychological functioning to physical maturity has not yet been specified, so that it is difficult to evaluate which behavior relates to which hormone.

Very specific events are related to estrogen secretion. Primarily, it determines the onset of thelarche, which is the first sign of puberty in the majority of girls. Other clinical indices of estrogen secretion are body fat distribution, bone maturation, vaginal cell cornification, cervical mucus, proliferative endometrium present on biopsy, withdrawal bleeding after administration of progesterone, and plasma estradiol measurement.

Adrenarche and thelarche precede menarche by several years. Synchronization of the H-P-O axis then takes place over a period of 1–2 years, giving rise to ovulatory menstrual cycles, which signify the completion of puberty.

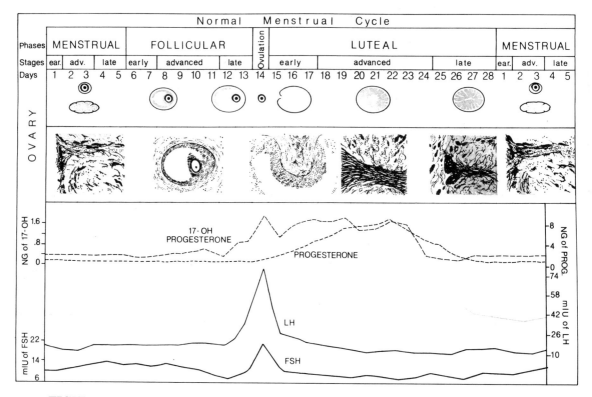

FIGURE 74.2. Schematic representation of the normal menstrual cycle and the interactions between ovary and pituitary. From Warren (1988). Copyright 1988 by E. A. Blechman. Reprinted by permission.

THE NORMAL MENSTRUAL CYCLE

Once a woman reaches full reproductive maturity, a cyclical pattern of hormonal secretion creates the normal menstrual cycle (Figure 74.3). It is the result of the integration of hormones secreted by the hypothalamus, the pituitary, and the ovary. As noted earlier, LH and FSH stimulate specialized areas in the ovary, called follicles. The follicle consists of the central ovum or egg, surrounded by one or more layers of supporting cells. Thses cells secrete hormones and other substances, some of which are unidentified.

A woman is born with all the follicles she will ever have, usually about 400,000. The majority will never develop, or if development starts, they will quickly regress and become atretic while a dominant follicle takes over. During her reproductive years, a woman will release about 400 mature follicles. The mechanisms for the development of the dominant or mature follicle are not understood.

The follicle develops under the influence of FSH and, to some extent, LH. The ratio of these two hormones is important. It is the developing follicle that makes estrogen—in particular, estradiol. When it is large and fully mature, a large increase in estrogen sets off a peak in LH and FSH, and ovulation occurs, which involves rupture of the ovum from the dominant follicle.

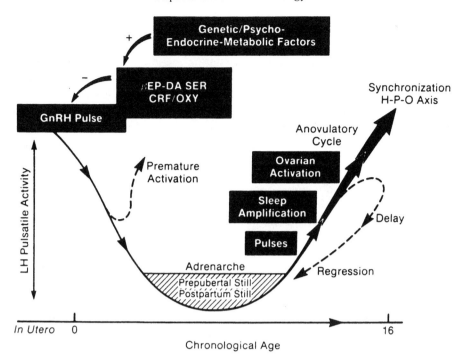

FIGURE 74.3. Diagrammatic display of the U-shaped curve relating the time-compressed neuroendocrine events of puberty. The prepubertal restraint of GnRH and LH pulses, putatively because of the expression of hypothalamic inhibitors or modulators such as beta-endorphil (B-EP), dopamine (DA), serotonin (SER), corticotropin-releasing factor (CRF), and oxytocin (OXY), is depicted. The final synchronization of the H-P-O axis in generating ovulatory cycles follows a sequence of decline of inhibitory mechanisms, initiation of GnRH and LH pulsatile activity, and sleep-entrained amplification. The time course of these events is determined by genetic, nutritional, psychological, and social-environmental factors. Interruptions of this sequence of events occur in several clinical abnormalities, as exemplified by premature activation in central precocious puberty and delay or regression to prepubertal state in patients with anorexia nervosa. From Yen (1993). Copyright 1993 by W. B. Saunders, Inc. Reprinted by permission.

The high concentration of LH occurs approximately 12–36 hours before ovulation and helps divide the menstrual cycle into the follicular and the luteal phases. During the luteal phase, the follicle from which the ovum was extruded changes into a temporary endocrine organ known as the corpus luteum. The corpus luteum secretes several hormones, including progesterone, which helps prepare the lining of the uterus for implantation should the egg be fertilized. In the absence of fertilization, the endometrial lining that developed is shed off during menstruation, and a new cycle begins.

If fertilization of the ovum occurs, the corpus luteum continues to synthesize and secrete steroid hormones that maintain pregnancy for the first 4–6 weeks. It is aided by another hormone, human chorionic gonadotropin (hCG), that is biologically very similar to LH. hCG is secreted by cells in the conceptus that are destined to become the placenta. It is present throughout pregnancy and its concentration is 10-fold higher in the first trimester. The function of hCG in other parts of pregnancy is unknown.

CLINICAL MODELS OF HYPOTHALAMIC REGULATION

Any aberration from the normal in the neurohumoral signals transmitted along the H-P-O axis can result in menstrual cycle disorders. Centrally, the hypothalamus is now considered to be responsible for a wide spectrum of menstrual abnormalities, which may range from a prolonged follicular phase or a shortened luteal phase to amenorrhea (complete cessation of menses). The underlying mechanism is hypothalamic regulation of metabolic, neural, and humoral signals from higher centers. This regulation is carried out by the GnRH pulse generator.

The GnRH pulse generator is a loose network of neurons within the arcuate nucleus of the MBH and the preoptic area of the anterior hypothalamus. These neurons exhibit a rhythmic pattern of electrical activity that occurs approximately every 60–90 minutes. This rhythmicity is responsible for the pulsatile release of GnRH, and consequently, LH and FSH, as mentioned earlier. Recent studies, however, have showed that GnRH pulse generator activity is diminished in conditions where a hypometabolic state or a negative energy balance exists. A decrease in pulse amplitude and frequency is seen, resulting in a suboptimal release of GnRH and therefore, understimulation of the gonadotropes.

The hypothalamic mechanism that dictates GnRH pulse generator activity is still unclear. Studies on the new polypeptide hormone leptin, however, may lead to a better understanding of the metabolic regulation in relation to reproductive functions.

Leptin is secreted by fat cells in response to nutritional factors. It induces satiety and down-regulates eating behavior in association with increased fat mass. Serum levels are reduced significantly in women who have a low body fat percentage or those who are below their ideal body weight. These women usually have menstrual irregularities as well.

Because receptors for leptin are present in the hypothalamus and granulosa cells of the ovary, it is possible that leptin is part of a metabolic–endocrine axis that regulates reproductive function during periods of caloric deprivation.

Amenorrhea without a clinically demonstrable organic cause is very common in young women. It is referred to as "functional hypothalamic amenorrhea" because the disorder seems to be a physiological adaptive response to certain physical and metabolic stressors, and thus is usually reversible.

Functional hypothalamic amenorrhea is seen in women with eating disorders, especially anorexia nervosa; in the presence of weight loss and dieting; and during periods of unusual stress or excessive physical activity. It is characterized by low to normal gonadotropin levels, and is attributed to diminished activity of the GnRH pulse generator.

Anorexia Nervosa

Anorexia nervosa is a syndrome presenting with amenorrhea, weight loss, and behavioral changes. The menstrual cycle stops, and signs of hypothalamic dysfunction develop, which are usually reversed with refeeding and weight gain. The clinical signs and symptoms of this disease appear to be related to food restriction. Thus, the syndrome is predominantly one of starvation.

Interesting endocrine changes occur in anorexia nervosa, particularly with reference to the reproductive system. There is a deficiency in the secretion of gonadotropins (LH and FSH, but especially LH) from the anterior pituitary. When one examines the 24-hour secretion of LH, there is a lack of the normal episodic variations of gonadotropin levels; instead, reversion to a prepubertal pattern with low baseline 24-hour secretion is seen. Occasionally, anorectics demonstrate another type of immature gonadotropin secretion:

nocturnal spurting, a pattern that is usually only seen in early puberty. Severely ill anorectics challenged with GnRH show a prepubertal pattern of response (Warren et al., 1975): The FSH response remains greater than the LH response, even near normal weight. The reversion to a prepubertal state is interesting, in view of the perceptual problems that develop in this illness.

Bulimia Nervosa

Bulimia nervosa is characterized by recurrent episodes of binge eating followed by purging through artificial means (induced vomiting, laxative abuse, or diuretic abuse). The patients are usually older than those with anorexia nervosa, but they may have a history of previous anorectic behavior as well. Since this binge–purge behavior is often carried out in secret, and the weight may remain within normal range, a high index of suspicion and particular attention to the associated physical findings are important for the diagnosis. Often, a history of other impulsive behavior (alcohol or drug abuse, stealing, promiscuity) may be elicited. Physical findings may include swollen parotid glands, tooth decay, positive Chvostek or Trousseau sign, "chipmunk" jowls, and hypercarotenemia. There may be cramps of the hands and feet (from metabolic alkalosis secondary to vomiting), and the decrease in ionized calcium may lead to tetanic seizures.

Bulimics also present with menstrual irregularities, but the dysfunction is less severe than that encountered in anorexia nervosa. They may have anovulatory cycles with normal estrogen secretion, or functional hypothalamic amenorrhea with low to normal gonadotropin levels.

Weight Loss and Dieting

Weight loss and dieting can also result in menstrual abnormalities, ranging from prolongation of the follicular phase or a shortening of the luteal phase to prolonged amenorrhea (Pirke, Schweiger, Lemmel, Krieg, & Berger, 1985; Schweiger, 1991). These women are generally healthy and without a distorted body image, but a history of recent dieting and weight loss is usually present. Physical exam may reveal body weight to be 10–12% below the ideal, especially among those who are amenorrheic. Pulse rate and blood pressure may also be low. If prolonged amenorrhea is present, LH and FSH may be low to normal, but generally with a more marked suppression of LH. Estrogen levels are low, and the patient may not respond to Provera (Warren, 1996).

The type of diet may also affect menstrual and reproductive functions. A vegetarian diet, for example, is associated with a higher-than-expected incidence of reproductive disorders and anovulation (Pirke, Schweiger, Laessle, Dicknaut, & Waechtler, 1986); depressed LH and estrogen levels have also been documented (Hill, Garbaczewski, Haley, & Wynder, 1984). A high-fiber vegetarian diet may affect estrogen levels by increasing fecal estrogen excretion in a bulky stool and preventing a normal enterohepatic circulation (Goldin et al., 1982).

Similar menstrual abnormalities may also occur in women who are of normal weight but have high "restrained eating" scores. These women do not exhibit the psychological features associated with eating disorders, but when tested with standardized scales, they exhibit high scores that reflect dieting behavior (Warren et al., 1994). The menstrual problems associated with weight loss and dieting are usually reversed with weight gain or normalization of eating behavior. But amenorrhea may persist for as long as a year after weight is regained and osteoporosis has been described, which does not appear to be reversible with estrogen–progesterone therapy (Klibanski, Biller, Schoenfeld, Herzog, & Saxe, 1995).

Exercise-Related Amenorrhea

The reproductive dysfunction that occurs with exercise training alone is usually subtle and presents as irregular cycles with prolonged follicular, or inadequate luteal phases (Prior, 1987; Bullen et al., 1985; Shangold, Freeman, Thysen, & Gatz, 1979). This can be magnified, however, in the presence of weight loss, with patients weighing 10–12% below the ideal at greatest risk. Exercise-related amenorrhea may represent the extreme end of the spectrum of menstrual dysfunctions. The pathogenesis is now considered to be multifactorial, and may include low weight or weight loss, eating disorders, inadequate caloric intake that is unable to meet energy demands (energy drain), stress, genetic predisposition, or an inherent H-P-O susceptibility that is reflected in the high incidence of delayed menarche and nulliparity (DeSouza & Metzger, 1991).

The menstrual irregularities are also related to the type of sport or physical activity engaged in, and the age at which this has started. Amenorrhea is more frequent among women who engage in high-intensity endurance exercise (e.g., marathon runners) and those who have to maintain a certain degree of leanness (e.g., ballet dancers, gymnasts, and figure skaters). When training starts before menarche, this event is delayed by about 3 years, and the incidence of secondary amenorrhea or chronic anovulation later in life is higher (Yen, 1993). These menstrual problems, however, can usually be reversed with a decrease in exercise.

The neuroendocrine mechanisms behind the development of exercise-related amenorrhea are still unclear. But there is evidence showing a central inhibition of GnRH release. The 24-hour urinary cortisol concentrations are elevated in athletic women. These data suggest that, with equal exercise intensity, athletes with amenorrhea have elevated levels of cortisol throughout the 24-hour circadian rhythm, whereas athletes with cyclic menses exhibit hypercortisolism only during the early morning hours. This relative hypersecretion of cortisol is accompanied by a normal circadian rhythm of adrenocorticotropic hormone and blunted responses to hCRH in both groups of athletic women (Loucks, Mortola, Girton, & Yen, 1989).

Reduced levels of thyroid hormones (free T_4, free T_3, and total T_4) with normal thyroid-stimulating hormone have also been observed (Myerson et al., 1991). This apparent hypothyroidism may represent an adaptive mechanism toward energy conservation in the face of increased metabolic demands with no corresponding increase in caloric intake.

Psychogenic Amenorrhea

Functional hypothalamic amenorrhea may result from social-environmental stress of sufficient intensity and duration. The underlying mechanism is again impairment in GnRH secretion; this is most probably modulated through increased central opioidergic and dopaminergic activities, as seen prior to onset of puberty. In severe cases when few quasipulses of LH are present, ovarian steroidogenic activity virtually ceases, as reflected by markedly reduced levels of estradiol, androstenedione, and testosterone. In contrast, patients with modest LH pulses have a substantial degree of ovarian secretion of estradiol and normal levels of androgens (Yen, 1993).

SUMMARY

The hypothalamus is clearly emerging as the central regulatory entity that is responsible for ensuring the normal physiologic functioning of the human body. It integrates neuroendocrine and metabolic signals; it then effects appropriate responses through the H-P-O, hypothalamic–pituitary–adrenal, and hypothalamic–pituitary–thyroid axes that are geared primarily toward maintenance of life-giving processes. Reproductive function is temporarily "turned off" by diminished frequency and/or amplitude of the GnRH pulse generator.

FURTHER READING

Barchas, J. D., Akil, A., Elliott, G. R., Holman, R. B., & Watson, S. J. (1978). Behavioral neurochemistry: Neuroregulators and behavioral states. *Science, 100,* 964.

Boyar, R. M., Katz, J., Finkelstein, J. W., Kapen, S., Weiner, H., Weitzman, E. D., & Hellman, L. (1974). Anorexia nervosa: Immaturity of the 24-hour luteinizing hormone secretory pattern. *New England Journal of Medicine, 291,* 861–865.

Bullen, B. A., Skrinar, G. S., Beitins, I. Z., von Mering, G., Turnbull, B. A., & McArthur, J. W. (1985). Induction of menstrual disorders by strenuous exercise in untrained women. *New England Journal of Medicine, 312,* 1349–1353.

DeSouza, M. J., & Metzger, D. A. (1991). Reproductive dysfunction in amenorrheic athletes and anorexic patients: A review. *Medicine and Science in Sports and Exercise, 23,* 995–1007.

Fritz, M. A., & Speroff, L. (1983). Current concepts of the endocrine characteristics of normal menstrual function: The key to diagnosis and management of menstrual disorders. *Clinical Obstetrics and Gynecology, 26,* 647–689.

Goldin, B. R., Adlercreutz, H., Gorbach, S. L., Woods, M. N., Dwyer, D. T., Conlon, T., Bohn, & Gershoff, S. N. (1982). Estrogen excretion patterns and plasma levels in vegetarian and omnivorous women. *New England Journal of Medicine, 307,* 1542–1547.

Hill, P., Garbaczewski, B. S., Haley, N., & Wynder, E. L. (1984). Diet and follicular development. *American Journal of Clinical Nutrition, 39,* 771–777.

Khoury, S. A., Reame, N. E., Kelch, R. P., & Marshall, J. C. (1987). Diurnal patterns of pulsatile luteinizing hormone secretion in hypothalamic amenorrhea: Reproducibility and responses to opiate blockade and an alpha2-adrenergic agonist. *Journal of Clinical Endocrinology and Metabolism, 64,* 755–762.

Klibanski, A., Biller, B. M. K., Schoenfeld, D. A., Herzog, D. B., & Saxe, V. C. (1995). The effects of estrogen administration on trabecular bone loss in young women with anorexia nervosa. *Journal of Clinical Endocrinology and Metabolism, 80,* 898–904.

Krieger, D. T. (1980). The hypothalamus and neuroendocrinology. In D. T. Krieger & J. C. Hughes (Eds.), *Neuroendocrinology* (pp. 3–13). New York: HP.

Loucks, A. B., Mortola, J. F., Girton, L., and Yen, S. S. C. (1989) Alterations in the hypothalamic-pituitary-ovarian and the hypothalamic-pituitary-adrenal axes in athletic women. *Journal of Clinical Endocrinology and Metabolism, 68,* 402–411.

Marshall, J. C., & Kelch, R. P. (1979). Low dose pulsatile gonadotropin-releasing hormone in anorexia nervosa: A model of human pubertal development. *Journal of Clinical Endocrinology and Metabolism, 49,* 712–718.

Myerson, M., Gutin, B., Warren, M. P., May, M., Contento, I., Lee, M., Pi-Sunyer, F. S., Pierson, R. N., & Brooks-Gunn, J. (1991). Resting metabolic rate and energy balance in amenorrheic and eumenorrheic runners. *Medicine and Science in Sports and Exercise, 23*(1), 15–22.

Pirke, K. M., Schweiger, U., Laessle, R. G., Dickhaut, B., & Waechtler, M. (1986). Dieting influences the menstrual cycle: Vegetarian versus nonvegetarian diet. *Fertility and Sterility, 46,* 1083–1088.

Pirke, K. M., Schweiger, U., Lemmel, W., Krieg, J. C., & Berger, M. (1985). The influence of dieting on the menstrual cycle of healthy young women. *Journal of Clinical Endocrinology and Metabolism, 60,* 1174–1179.

Prior, J. C. (1987). Physical exercise and the neuroendocrine control of reproduction. *Baillieres Clinical Endocrinology Metabolism, 1*(2), 299–317.

Quigley, M. E., Sheehan, K. L., Casper, R. F., & Yen, S. S. C. (1980). Evidence for increased dopaminergic and opioid activity in patients with hypothalamic hypogonadotropic amenorrhea. *Journal of Clinical Endocrinology and Metabolism, 50,* 949–954.

Schwartz, I. D. (1995). Puberty in girls: Normal or delayed? *Contemporary Adolescent Gynecology, 1,* 4–14.

Schweiger, U. (1991). Menstrual function and luteal-phase deficiency in relation to weight changes and dieting. *Clinical Obstetrics and Gynecology, 34,* 191–197.

Shangold, M. M., Freeman, R., Thysen, B., & Gatz, M. (1979). The relationship between long-distance running, plasma progesterone, and luteal phase length. *Fertility and Sterility, 31,* 130–133.

Warren, M. P. (1988). Reproductive endocrinology. In E. A. Blechman & K. D. Brownell (Eds.), *Handbook of behavioral medicine for women* (pp. 63–69). Elmsford, NY: Pergamon Press.

Warren, M. P. (1996). Evaluation of secondary amenorrhea [Clinical Review 77]. *Journal of Clinical Endocrinology and Metabolism, 81*(2), 437–442.

Warren, M. P., Holderness, C. C., Lesobre, V., Tzen, R., Vossoughian, R., & Brooks-Gunn, J. (1994). Hypothalamic amenorrhea and hidden nutritional insults. *Journal of the Society for Gynecologic Investigation, 1,* 84–88.

Warren, M. P., Jewelewicz, R., Dyrenfurth, I., Ans, R., Khalaf, S., & Vande Wiele, R. L. (1975). The significance of weight loss in the evaluation of pituitary response to LH-RH in women with secondary amenorrhea. *Journal of Clinical Endocrinology and Metabolism, 40,* 601–611.

Yen, S. S. C. (1993). Female hypogonadotropic hypogonadism: Hypothalamic amenorrhea syndrome. *Endocrinology and Metabolism Clinics of North America, 22*(1), 20–58.

75

Premenstrual Disorders

Jessica Motherwell McFarlane

T he purpose of this chapter is to give a brief overview of some methodological issues in premenstrual syndrome (PMS) research, diagnosis, and treatment. After outlining some broad issues in PMS research, I discuss the need for more descriptive and varied research. Then I summarize essential and other important criteria for research design, methodology, and diagnosis. Finally, I reevaluate the "placebo effect" in PMS treatment studies, in order to suggest possibilities for future research.

AN OVERVIEW OF THE PREMENSTRUAL
SYNDROME RESEARCH FIELD

PMS is commonly believed to be some women's experience of negative moods, cognitions, and physical experiences in the premenstrual phase, and subsequent relief from distress shortly after onset of menstruation. In fact, PMS has been referred to in western culture for 60 years, and has been researched for 40 of those years by clinicians and others (see, e.g., Richardson's 1995 study). After four decades, the investigation, diagnosis, and treatment of PMS *should* be maturing past their infancy and moving on to constitute a substantive, well-founded discipline. There is no doubt that the quantity of PMS articles is substantive; still, in spite of the tremendous quantity of time generously given by participants in PMS research projects (not to mention the considerable time and expense of the researchers and their staffs) the PMS discipline is having trouble standing solidly on its own two feet and moving forward, with one step advancing upon another.

I believe that one reason for this impaired development is some researchers' lack of attention to choosing methods, instruments, and treatments that allow for the inclusion of a combination of social, cultural, psychological, biological, and other contexts. The literature abounds with traditional empirical studies based on the medical model. Although this medical model may be appropriate for the study of other apparently biological phenomena, it appears after hundreds of studies and decades of work—which show no treatment to be significantly more effective than a placebo—that the medical model alone is a poor choice of model for understanding PMS.

All too often, the motivation for PMS research begins with a new pharmaceutical or behavioral treatment. Next, some researchers focus on psychological avenues or physiological or biochemical pathways that may, in theory, be dysfunctional premenstrually and amenable to the proposed treatment. Then more research is designed around proving or disproving the treatment's effectiveness. There is a flaw in this theory- and research-driven research paradigm in the current stage of the PMS field, however.

THE NEED FOR MORE DESCRIPTIVE AND VARIED WORK

In a 1995 paper, Walker reminds us that before we begin to *explain* PMS, we must first adequately *describe* women's experiences in detail. Adequate description includes methods and instruments that allow women to describe their whole experience: both positive and negative moods; premenstrual as well as all other menstrual phases; menstrual as well as other cycles; subjective and objective experiences; common and unique experiences in relation to those of older women, within and across cultures; common and unique experiences in relation to men's experiences and so on. There has not yet been sufficient research on describing healthy cyclicity; without finishing such preliminary work on women's and men's healthy experiences, we cannot expect to place PMS and other unhealthy experiences of cyclicity in their true context.

For example, my colleagues and I have found that some women and men (randomly assigned to pseudomenstrual cycles) may experience nonpremenstrual cyclical changes that are similar in severity and frequency to PMS when diagnoses for all cycles are made by strict criteria. We developed a method for assessing whether a particular phase of the menstrual or lunar cycle or day of the week, as assessed daily over several months, is unusually positive or negative in relation to that particular individual's normal range for that measure (e.g., mood pleasantness). Most men and women did experience cyclicity, but stereotypical cyclicity was rare (e.g., PMS, "blue Mondays"). How does the possibility of significant negative—and positive—nonpremenstrual cycles (e.g., negative midcycle phase, negative Tuesdays, etc.) affect progress in PMS research?

First, by carefully describing the nature of emotional and physical cyclicity in general, we may discover that PMS, instead of being a unique phenomenon, is one of several possible ways in which both women and men may feel distressed by their cyclicity. If we acknowledged the possibility that PMS is not a unique cyclical distresser we would have to seriously reconsider the inclusion in an appendix to the fourth edition of the *Diagnostic and Statistical Manual of Mental Disorders* (DSM-IV) of the proposed diagnostic category "premenstrual dysphoric disorder" (PDD). If women can experience distress, diagnosable by conservative criteria, in nonpremenstrual phases, and if both women and men can experience negative day-of-the-week cycles, also diagnosed with strict criteria, what could be the rationale for not recognizing and validating these kinds of cycles along with PMS? What would make PMS a psychiatric disorder and other cycles not?

(As an aside, because of the failure to provide rigorous scientific evidence demonstrating that some women's premenstrual experiences constitute a psychiatric disorder, I believe that the inclusion of PDD in DSM-IV—even in an appendix—is premature. Therefore, I refer to women's distressing premenstrual experiences as PMS and avoid the use of PDD, unless I am specifically referring to the psychiatric investigation of this phenomenon. I am more comfortable with the label PMS because many women in Western culture, both with and without PMS, readily understand and use this label in casual conversation. I doubt that women frequently used "late luteal phase dysphoric disorder" [an earlier psychiatric term] as a natural way to describe their experiences, and I suspect they are not likely to adopt PDD readily now. Unfortunately, women's natural language to describe their premenstrual experiences prior to the medical community's invention of PMS as a label is difficult to know. Since the PMS label has such wide acceptance in everyday usage, however, it has, in essence, become part of many western women's natural language to describe their premenstrual experiences; thus it seems most respectful to let women choose their own language for their experiences, and not to invent new psychiatric terms unnecessarily.)

Second, if research teams conducting sound descriptive studies consistently found the existence of not only conservatively diagnosed premenstrual but also nonpremenstrual cyclicity, PDD theorists would have to account for how PDD is qualitatively different from other, nonpremenstrual cycles. Currently, the concept that premenstrual cyclicity is qualitatively distinct from the rest of the menstrual cycle and uniquely distressing for women has gone virtually unchallenged. Without having met this descriptive challenge and refined their theories to account for how PDD is distinct from negative nonpremenstrual cycles, theorists may be missing crucial social, cultural, psychological, and biological variables that could result in significant advances in our current understanding of PMS.

Finally, it is possible that premenstrual cyclicity is qualitatively distinct and deserving of special diagnostic and research status. Without having completed the preliminary descriptive work on the nature of menstrual, day-of-week, and other cyclicity; however, researchers and diagnosticians are at a loss to provide women who are distressed by their premenstrual experiences with sound answers to their questions about what specifically is happening to them and how their experiences differ from the norm.

ESSENTIAL AND OTHER IMPORTANT CRITERIA FOR PREMENSTRUAL SYNDROME RESEARCH AND DIAGNOSIS

In this section, I briefly outline criteria for rigorous, descriptive scientific study and diagnosis of PMS. The purpose of this section is to provide readers with a checklist to use when designing their own or critiquing others' work. Ideally, however, women who say they have PMS should not only ask scientists and clinicians for guidance, but should get together to develop their own set of standards, in order to increase qualitative and quantitative rigor in PMS work. Many researchers are already using excellent and rigorous scientific methods appropriate for the study of PMS. It is hoped that most if not all who publish in the PMS field will adopt these methods where appropriate.

A detailed description of the rationale for each criterion is beyond the scope of this brief chapter. Readers are directed to my 1994 paper with Williams and to other PMS reviews for further discussion. Criteria that I refer to as "essential" are those that, if not included or addressed in some way, would result in a serious weakness or even a "fatal flaw" in the research design. Other criteria, which I refer to as "important," are necessary in general if significant strides are to be made in PMS research. Since it is often necessary to economize because of limited research funds, however, it may be necessary for researchers to compromise on some aspects of comprehensiveness and limit the scope of their work. Not including the "important" criteria does not necessarily lead to a weakness in design, though it may limit the generalizability of a study.

Essential Criteria for Research and Diagnosis

The following criteria are essential for PMS research; those that apply to diagnosis as well are marked with asterisks. First, participants should be "blind" to the menstrual purpose of the research. Participants who know the researcher's menstrual interest will often show PMS patterns, whereas those unaware of the purpose will show such patterns far less often. Second (*), measures should include equal numbers of negative and positive items. Measures with predominantly negative items provide a biased view of participants' experience. In addition, since positive experiences mixed with negative ones in the premenstrual phase may provide evidence that would contradict a diagnosis of PMS, positive items are necessary. Third (*), participants' reports must not be retrospective, because retrospective reports are more likely to elicit stereotypical PMS patterns that do not match day-to-day reports. Fourth (*), data should be collected at even and frequent intervals (e.g., daily) across the menstrual cycle. In addition to frequent data collection, data should be considered from every phase of the menstrual cycle. For example, some researchers and clinicians have considered data from only the premenstrual phase in comparison with one other phase (usually the follicular, i.e., postmenstrual phase) when diagnosing PMS. A flaw in this two-phase method of diagnosis is that if a phase not considered by the researcher (e.g., menstrual, midcycle, or postmidcycle phases) should happen to be more negative than the premenstrual phase, then a PMS diagnosis would be misleading. In addition to the risk of inaccurate diagnosis, the failure to consider data from across the entire menstrual cycle may prevent the discovery of significant nonpremenstrual cyclicity. PMS may thus be reified, and a chance to advance the understanding of human cyclicity may be missed.

Important Criteria for Research and Diagnosis

The following are important criteria to include in PMS research; again, those that apply to diagnosis as well are marked with asterisks. First (*), in order to increase reliability of PMS research and diagnosis, data should be collected over a minimum of two and preferably three or more cycles. The inclusion of two or more menstrual cycles helps correct for the possibility of diagnosing PMS in women who have only an occasional unusually negative premenstrual phase.

Second, both women and men should be studied. In Western culture, women are stereotypically believed to be more emotional and men more stable. When men are studied as closely as women in PMS research, however, there is evidence that emotional cyclicity may not be unique to women.

Third, researchers should use an older community sample, as there is evidence that emotional distress over the menstrual cycle may increase with age. In addition, it is preferable to choose participants from a variety of cultures. The PMS concept may vary significantly from culture to culture.

Fourth (*) and finally, in addition to premenstrual cyclicity, other cycles (e.g., day-of-the-week, lunar, and seasonal cycles) should be studied and compared in severity and frequency with premenstrual cyclicity. It also would be interesting to study social cycles—for example, monthly and biweekly paycheck schedules.

A Reevaluation of the Placebo Effect

In this section, I reconsider the commonly found "placebo effect," in which placebos are often found to be as effective as proposed medical PMS treatments. For example, placebos have been found to be 60% effective, on average (range 19–88%), in treating PMS symptoms. In the traditional medical research paradigm, a placebo effect is a sign that a proposed treatment is ineffective or has failed. I have heard one clinician refer to the placebo effect as a "dummy effect" in front of a woman participating in a double-blind, placebo-controlled study. Although many may never refer to a placebo as a "dummy," I wonder whether some researchers have felt a sense of failure when their proposed treatment was no more effective than a placebo, as is the case almost universally in PMS research. I would like to reevaluate the "placebo effect" briefly, because I believe it is a fruitful source of inspiration for future research.

If there is one finding that has been consistently obtained in PMS research over the last few decades, it is that placebo treatments do help a significant numbers of women. If the number of women who benefited from placebo PMS treatments over this time period were totaled, the sum would be impressive indeed. Possibly in the past, women who experienced relief on placebo treatments were viewed as "suggestive" or considered not to be true PMS sufferers if their symptoms could be ameliorated by placebo. Only if the PMS placebo results are subjected to a strict medical model lens, however, can these highly consistent placebo results be construed as therapy or treatment "failures."

If we broaden the lens to include the whole scope of what a woman gains when she receives placebo treatment, we see that we may have already found important components of an effective treatment for PMS. First, a woman in a PMS study is typically interviewed by an interested and often sympathetic professional or staff member. The fact that someone is asking her for her side of the story, and is willing to listen to often private details of her menstrual and other experiences, may be very comforting and therapeutic for a woman in a placebo-controlled trial.

Second, a woman who participates in a PMS study may be providing daily data—a process that may remind her that someone with status is interested in her daily life and experiences. If she feels misunderstood or unimportant in the lives of her significant others, this daily recognition may provide additional therapy.

Third, and perhaps the main motivation for a woman to join a PMS study, is the hope that an expert may help her find and treat the source of her distress. It is well known in psychotherapeutic contexts that a sense of hope that things will change for the better is vital for resolution and a sense of well-being. To the extent that the experience of PMS may include a woman's sense of isolation, confusion over what she is experiencing, and hopelessness, a "placebo" treatment may contain therapeutic interventions that are indeed important and somewhat effective. There are doubtless other aspects of a "placebo" PMS treatment that provide effective therapeutic benefits for women. Perhaps one reason for the lack of more significant strides in the PMS field is that the partial successes of the "placebo effect" have been considered experimental failures. A thorough reframing and reexamination of the "placebo" results therefore would be beneficial for advancing our understanding of PMS.

THE FUTURE OF PREMENSTRUAL SYNDROME RESEARCH

In this chapter, I have made a plea for more qualitative, descriptive works in the study not only of PMS, but of all forms of psychological, biological, and social cyclicity in women and men. Methodologies that allow for the detailed data collection described above are by definition more time-consuming and expensive than traditional medical research paradigms. Researchers and granting agencies must be prepared to pay this cost in time and funds, however, if we are to see significant strides in the understanding of PMS in the future. In the present-day tight economy, research funds are more difficult to obtain. Nevertheless, high priority should be given to funding research that is designed to include rigorous methodologies as outlined above, as well as to combine social, cultural, psychological, and/or biological perspectives. Also, it is possible that many researchers already have in their archives menstrual data that may be analyzed for other cycles, thus adding to the PMS literature and economizing on participant effort and research expense. Finally, another important avenue for the advancement of our understanding of PMS is the reframing and reevaluation of "placebo" results. Perhaps the substantive numbers of studies with significant "placebo effects" have held some clues to the future of PMS after all.

FURTHER READING

American Psychiatric Association. (1994). *Diagnostic and statistical manual of mental disorders.* Washington, DC: Author.
This manual includes the proposed diagnostic category of PDD.

McFarlane, J. M., & Williams, T. M. (1994). Placing premenstrual syndrome in perspective. *Psychology of Women Quarterly, 18,* 339–373.
This article provides a thorough review of the PMS literature up to 1994, and is useful in directing the reader to several other references used in the preparation of this chapter.

Reid, R. L., & Yen, S. S. C. (1981). Premenstrual syndrome. *American Journal of Obstetrics and Gynecology, 139,* 85–104.
This article provides an in-depth review of medical treatments and biomedical theories of PMS.

Rossi, A. S., & Rossi, P. E. (1977). Body time and social time: Mood patterns by menstrual cycle phase and day of week. *Social Science Research, 6,* 273–308.
This research is one of the earliest and best examples of the inclusion of other cycles in PMS research.

76

Gynecological Pain

Alcuin Wilkie
Ulrike Schmidt

SOME CONCEPTUAL PITFALLS

Several conceptual pitfalls need to be pointed out to readers before they can safely get to grips with this topic. The first of these pitfalls is contained in the title of our chapter. "Gynecological" refers to the vulva, vagina, uterus, fallopian tubes, and ovaries—the female reproductive organs. Painful stimulation of these organs is usually not felt in the organs themselves, but is "referred" to other locations on the surface of the body supplied by the nerves that originate from the same segment of the spinal cord supplying the relevant organs. Thus a woman with an ectopic pregnancy in her left fallopian tube will experience excruciating pain over her left lower abdomen. Painful stimulation of both the gastrointestinal tract and the urinary tract may also give rise to pain in the same referred areas. Pain felt in the lower abdomen and perineum (the area between the anus and the vulva) is most sensibly described as "pelvic pain," which indicates where the pain is felt rather than making an assumption as to where it originates.

The second pitfall to avoid is the compulsion to search for a physical cause for the pain at the exclusion of all else. What is true of pain generally is also true of pelvic pain: There is not always a linear relationship between injury or disease and pain. Thus an ovarian tumor will rarely give rise to pain before a very advanced stage, and a fifth of fertile, pain-free women undergoing sterilization have endometriosis. These two examples show that disease may exist without pain. The converse is also true: In women referred for investigation of pelvic pain, it is common not to find evidence of any physical cause (this may be related in part to insufficient sensitivity of current methods of investigation). Furthermore, in one case report, surgical removal of the bladder, uterus, ovaries, and fallopian tubes in four women with long-standing pelvic pain was not followed by any resolution of pain—a situation possibly analogous to phantom limb pain in amputees. Because pain can exist without injury or disease and vice versa, it is clear that in some women the disease that exists may not be responsible for the pain.

The third and final pitfall we wish to point out is believing that doctors and psychologists have an understanding of pelvic pain. What doctors and psychologists have studied have been almost exclusively highly selected samples of women referred to gynecologists for investigation of pelvic pain. In many cases, the samples are further selected by referral from gynecologists to specialist pelvic pain clinics. It is therefore impossible to make informed comments on pelvic pain in community samples. By the time of referral to a specialist clinic, pelvic pain will almost always have lasted longer than 6 months; such pain is called "chronic pelvic pain" (CPP).

Bearing in mind these pitfalls, in this chapter we review the evidence regarding the relationship between CPP and psychological distress; we describe a psychosomatic condition that has been proposed as the basis of previously unexplained CPP; and we discuss the psychological treatment strategies that are being effectively used in the management of CPP.

THE RELATIONSHIP OF CHRONIC PELVIC PAIN AND PSYCHOLOGICAL DISTRESS

A number of studies have found women with CPP to have higher levels of psychopathology than either other gynecological patients without pain or normal controls. One study divided women with CPP into those with a positive and those with a negative laparoscopy result. The group with no abnormalities on laparoscopy had higher scores on a measure of neuroticism. However, the same researchers later conducted a further study in which laparoscopy-negative and laparoscopy-positive patients were matched for chronicity. There was no evidence in this second study to suggest that the women without observable pelvic pathology were more neurotic, anxious, or depressed than those with observable pathology. What is not clear is how much of this psychological distress is secondary to the chronic pain and how much is related to preexisting psychosocial maladjustment or coping styles, which may make some women more likely to seek medical help for physical symptoms.

The Role of Sexual and Physical Abuse in the Pain's Etiology

Over the last 10 years, there has been much interest in the relationship between sexual abuse (particularly in childhood) and CPP, in the hope of finding a specific explanatory factor for CPP. There are considerable methodological problems in the study of sexual abuse: how the abuse is ascertained, how it is defined, what age range is covered, and what comparison groups are chosen. So it is perhaps not surprising that studies addressing this topic in CPP have come to conflicting conclusions, with some finding CPP patients to have higher rates of sexual abuse than either normal controls or controls with other pain problems, and other studies finding no difference between these groups.

The relationship between physical abuse and CPP has also been studied. One study found CPP patients to have had more childhood physical abuse than either patients with other pain problems or normal controls, whereas another study found higher rates in CPP than in normal controls, but no difference compared to other pain patients. This suggests a nonspecific link between childhood physical abuse and the subsequent development of chronic pain. Several studies have demonstrated a variety of related coping mechanisms in women who have been subjects of childhood sexual and physical abuse—namely, somatization, dissociation, and amplification of symptoms. These women also report less perceived life control. One way of interpreting these findings is that abuse in childhood leads to difficulties with acknowledging and seeking help for emotional trauma, and to a tendency to gain adult attention through the safe domain of physical symptoms. (The links between childhood sexual abuse and a variety of physical symptoms, including CPP, are discussed by Laws in her chapter of this volume.)

An interesting community-based study compared women currently in physically abusive relationships with controls without abusive relationships, and demonstrated significantly higher rates of consultation for pelvic pain and significantly more frequent histories of pelvic pain in the abused group.

Psychological Consequences of the Pain

A great deal more has been written about abnormal antecedents of CPP than about normal, healthy women who develop pelvic pain and become depressed and anxious. This may be partly because those women who get better are never seen by a psychologist, whereas by the time previously normal women are assessed by a psychologist, the psychological abnormalities resulting from the pain are so ingrained that it is difficult to get a clear picture of the women's premorbid personality and functioning. The clearest evidence of the psychological effects of pain is the marked drop in high levels of anxiety in a group of women with CPP, following treatment and reduction in pain levels. It is interesting to note that in this study pain patients were compared with infertility patients, and that levels of anxiety were abnormally high in the pain patients but were close to normal levels in the infertility patients. It may be that high levels of anxiety are related to feelings of uncertainty in pain sufferers, and worries regarding interminability of pain have been clearly identified in women with CPP.

STRESS-MEDIATED PELVIC CONGESTION: A MODEL FOR CHRONIC PELVIC PAIN

An interesting model for CPP has been proposed. It parallels models for such conditions as asthma, eczema, peptic ulceration, and irritable bowel syndrome, in which there are direct relationships between stress and bodily symptoms. Within this model, psychological stress mediates hormonal changes in the hypothalamus, leading to an increase in the amount of estrogen secreted by the ovaries. This locally dilates the veins within the pelvis, resulting in pooling of blood, hypoxemia, local tissue damage, and release of pain-producing substances.

PSYCHOLOGICAL ASPECTS OF TREATMENT

The traditional medical model of treatment in CPP has been upward referral from general practitioner to gynecologist to pelvic pain specialist, who then carries out a number of investigations (including ultrasound, pelvic venography, and laparoscopy), followed by various drug and surgical treatments. If at the end of this process no improvement is made, a referral may well be made to a psychiatrist. This model of management has the double disadvantage of tending to reinforce a belief system that pain is entirely physically based, and depriving the patient of the benefits of psychological pain management. There is now clear evidence of the benefits of an integrated approach to the management of CPP, which from the moment of referral plays equal attention to somatic, psychological, dietary, environmental, and physiotherapeutic factors. When compared with the traditional method of treatment, this integrated approach has led to significant improvements in pain parameters at a 1-year follow-up. Furthermore, in the integrated model, laparoscopy is not routinely used and is not felt to play any important role in pain management.

SPECIFIC TREATMENT STRATEGIES

In the management of chronic pain in general, claims have been made for the effectiveness of a number of psychological techniques, including operant conditioning, relaxation, cognitive strategies, biofeedback, and hypnosis. The use of antidepressants has also been advocated. However, there have been few adequately controlled trials of these interventions with chronic pain generally, and even fewer with CPP specifically.

Operant Conditioning

The use of operant conditioning techniques is based on the theory that in chronic pain, behaviors such as inactivity, bed rest, speaking about pain symptoms, and analgesic usage have developed separate reinforcers from the pain itself—notably, attention from family members and avoidance of responsibilities. The aim of operant conditioning techniques is to decrease the frequency of "ill" behaviors and to increase the frequency of "well" behaviors by altering the reinforcers; reduction in pain intensity is not an aim.

Relaxation

The beneficial effects of relaxation were initially thought to be mediated through decreasing muscle tension. However, it is now more commonly believed that the major benefit of relaxation is cognitive, in that its practice distracts the sufferer from attending to unpleasant pain stimuli and increases the sufferer's feelings of mastery and control over pain.

Cognitive Strategies

Cognitive therapy can be used both in treating the anxiety and depression that accompany pain, and also specifically for coping with pain. The following coping mechanisms have been advocated: imaginative inattention (ignoring the pain by imagining a pleasant scenario incompatible with pain, such as swimming with dolphins in a tropical sea), imaginative transformation of pain (reinterpreting the pain as a lesser sensation, such as tingling or aching), imaginative transformation of context (imagining that the pain is the result of some courageous exploit, such as running a marathon), diversion of attention to external events (counting or describing objects around oneself), diversion of attention to internal events (performing mental arithmetic or reciting poetry), and somatization (focusing on the painful area in a detached manner, and describing the pain as though it belonged to someone else).

One study compared two different behavioral interventions with a minimal-intervention control. The two active treatments were (1) cognitive-behavioral stress management plus relaxation training, and (2) "pain analysis," which involved close monitoring of the pain and its antecedents and consequences, with the aim of identifying patterns associated with pain and teaching alternative strategies for coping with it. At a 6-month follow-up, both treatment groups did significantly better on a variety of outcome measures than the minimal-intervention group. A further study assessed the interaction between a hormonal treatment, medroxyprogesterone acetate (MPA), and brief cognitive-behavioral treatments (six sessions). Immediately following treatment, MPA with or without psychotherapy had similar results, and both MPA groups were superior to placebo; at a 9-month follow-up, however, the MPA-plus-psychotherapy group maintained its gains, whereas the MPA-only group fared much less well.

CONCLUSIONS

The problem of CPP poses a challenge to clinicians and researchers alike. More research is needed to disentangle the complex web of psychological antecedents and consequences of this condition. It is quite clear that women with CPP are not helped by a rigid categorization into those with or without observable organic pathology. A multidisciplinary approach to assessment and treatment—one that takes physical, psychological, and social factors into account from the beginning—is essential.

FURTHER READING

Baskin, L. S., Tanagho, E. A. (1992). Pelvic pain without pelvic organs. *Journal of Urology, 147,* 683–686.

Beard, R. W., Gangar, K., & Pearce, S. (1994). Chronic gynaecological pain. In P. D. Wall & K. Melzack (Eds.), *Textbook of pain* (pp. 597–614). Edinburgh: Churchill Livingstone.
This chapter provides a good overview of the topic, with particular emphasis on the physical aspects.

Farquhar, C. M., Rogers, S., Franks, S., Pearce, S., Wadsworth, J., & Beard, R. W. (1989). A randomized controlled trial of medroxyprogesterone acetate and psychotherapy for the treatment of pelvic congestion. *British Journal of Obstetrics and Gynaecology, 7,* 1152–1162.

Fry, R. P., Crisp, A. H., & Beard, R.W. (1991). Patients' illness models in chronic pelvic pain. *Psychotherapy and Psychosomatics, 55,* 158–163.

Fry, R. P., Crisp, A. H., Beard, R. W., & McGuigan, S. (1993). Psychosocial aspects of chronic pelvic pain, with special reference to sexual abuse: A study of 164 women. *Postgraduate Medical Journal, 69,* 566–574.

Hodgkiss, A. D., Sufraz, R., & Watson, J. P. (1994). Psychiatric morbidity and illness behaviour in women with chronic pelvic pain. *Journal of Psychosomatic Research, 38,* 3–9.

Kames, L. D., Rapkin, A. J., Naliboff, B. D., Afifi, S., & Ferrer-Brechner, T. (1990). Effectiveness of an interdisciplinary pain management program for the treatment of chronic pelvic pain. *Pain, 41,* 41–46.

Melzack, R., & Wall, P. D. (1988). *The challenge of pain.* London: Penguin.
A classic, highly readable text on the general topic of pain, broken down into the following four sections: The puzzle of pain; the physiology of pain; theories of pain; and the control of pain.

Pearce, S. (1986). *A psychological investigation of chronic pelvic pain in women.* Unpublished doctoral dissertation, University of London.

Pearce, S., & Beard, R. W. (1990). Chronic pelvic pain in women. In C. Bass (Ed.), *Somatization: Physical symptoms and psychological illness* (pp. 259–275). Oxford: Blackwell Scientific.

This chapter reviews the relationship between chronic pelvic pain and psychological treatment and presents a psychophysiological model which explains the causes of chronic pelvic pain and recommends appropriate treatment.

Peters, A. A., Van Dorst, E., Jellis, B., Van Zuuren, E., Hermans, J., & Trimbos, J. B. (1991). A randomized clinical trial to compare two different approaches in women with chronic pelvic pain. *Obstetrics and Gynecology, 77,* 740–744.

This controlled study demonstrates clear benefits of an integrated approach versus the traditional approach, to the treatment of chronic pelvic pain, with significant differences in pain measures one year after starting treatment.

Rapkin, A. J., Kames, L. D., Darke, L. L., Stampler, F. M., & Naliboff, B. D. (1990). History of physical and sexual abuse in women with chronic pelvic pain. *Obstetrics and Gynecology, 76,* 92–96.

Reiter, R. C., Shakerin, L. R., Gambone, J. C., & Milburn, A. K. (1991). Correlation between sexual abuse and somatization in women with somatic and nonsomatic chronic pelvic pain. *American Journal of Obstetrics and Gynecology, 165,* 104–109.

Schei, B. (1990). Psychosocial factors in pelvic pain: A controlled study of women living in physically abusive relationships. *Acta Obstetrica Gynecologica Scandinavica, 69,* 67–71.

This community-based study demonstrates significant differences between women currently living in abusive relationships and controls in terms of history and pelvic pain and consultation for pelvic pain.

Stout, A. L., Steege, J. F., Dodson, W. C., & Hughes, C. L. (1991). Relationship of laparoscopic findings to self-report of pelvic pain. *American Journal of Obstetrics and Gynecology, 164,* 73–79.

This study demonstrates the lack of a consistent relationship between physical disease detected laparoscopically and women's reports of pain.

Stovall, T. G., Ling, F. W., & Crawford, D. A. (1990). Hysterectomy for chronic pelvic pain of presumed uterine etiology. *Obstetrics and Gynecology, 75,* 676–679.

Toomey, T. C., Hernandez, J. T., Gittelman, D. F., & Hulka, J. F. (1993). Relationship of sexual and physical abuse to pain and psychological assessment variables in chronic pelvic pain patients. *Pain, 53,* 105–109.

Walker, E. A., Katon, W. J., Hansom, J., Harrop-Griffiths, J., Holm, L., Jones, M. L., Hickock, L., & Jemelka, R. P. (1992). Medical and psychiatric symptoms in women with childhood sexual abuse. *Psychosomatic Medicine, 54,* 658–664.

Walker, E. A., Katon, W. J., Neraas, K., Jemelka, R. P., & Massoth, D. (1992). Dissociation in women with chronic pelvic pain. *American Journal of Psychiatry, 149,* 534–537.

This controlled study demonstrates a significantly greater use of dissociation as a defense mechanism in women with chronic pelvic pain.

Walker, E. A., Sullivan, M. D., & Stenchever, M. A. (1993). Use of antidepressants in the management of women with chronic pelvic pain. *Obstetric and Gynecological Clinics of North America, 20,* 743–751.

Walling, M. K., O'Hara, M. W., Reiter, R. C., Milburn, A. K., Lilly, G., & Vincent, S. D. (1994). Abuse history and chronic pain in women: II. A multivariate analysis of abuse and psychological morbidity. *Obstetrics and Gynecology, 84,* 200–206.

This study demonstrates a higher lifetime prevalence of major sexual abuse in women with chronic pelvic pain, but makes the proviso that more rigorous studies are needed to clarify the exact nature of the interrelationship between adult and child physical and sexual abuse, pain in general, and chronic pelvic pain.

Walling, M. K., Reiter, R. C., O'Hara, M. W., Milburn, A. K., Lilly, G., & Vincent, S. D. (1994). Abuse history and chronic pain in women: I. Prevalences of sexual abuse and physical abuse. *Obstetrics and Gynecology, 84,* 193–199.

This study demonstrates a higher lifetime prevalence of major sexual abuse in women with chronic pelvic pain, but makes the proviso that more rigorous studies are needed to clarify the exact nature of the interrelationship between adult and child physical and sexual abuse, pain in general, and chronic pelvic pain.

77

Sexual Abuse

Ami Laws

Adverse psychological consequences of sexual abuse, including anxiety, depression, and dissociative disorders, have been recognized for some time; however, only recently has attention been focused on possible long-term medical consequences of such abuse. This chapter reviews empirical data linking a history of sexual abuse to various medical problems and symptoms in women.

SEXUAL ABUSE PREVALENCE

Numerous surveys of the prevalence of sexual abuse in childhood, determined by women's retrospective reports, have been conducted. The ascertained prevalence in these surveys is highly dependent on the research methods used; therefore, the true prevalence of sexual abuse of girls in the United States remains unclear. However, one rigorously conducted survey by Russell, using what are possibly optimal methods, showed it to be as high as 28% for contact abuse before the age of 14. Results of a national survey of rape prevalence showed that 13% of women reported a lifetime history of forced sexual penetration; 62% of the reported rapes occurred before the victim was 18 years of age. Sexual abuse of girls and women therefore appears to be fairly common in the United States.

Despite this, only recently has research been directed to understanding possible long-term physical health consequences of sexual abuse. These long-term medical symptoms and problems can be understood in part as extensions, or in some cases amplifications, of acute responses to sexual abuse. These were first defined by Burgess and Holmstrom, who described a number of somatic symptoms in survivors of rape: skeletal muscle tension, resulting in headaches, fatigue, and sleep pattern disturbances; gastrointestinal irritability, with stomach pains, nausea, and lack of appetite; and genitourinary disturbances, including vaginal discharge, itching, burning on urination, and generalized genitourinary pain.

SEXUAL ABUSE AND CHRONIC PAIN

Studies of women with chronic pain syndromes show that a substantial portion of them have a history of sexual and/or physical abuse. The pain syndrome most closely linked to sexual abuse is chronic pelvic pain. (This link is also discussed by Wilkie and Schmidt in their chapter on gynecological pain.) One well-controlled study of outpatient women by Walker and colleagues showed that 64% of women with chronic pelvic pain had a history of sexual abuse in childhood, compared to 23% of a control group. Forty-eight percent of the pelvic pain patients reported sexual abuse after the age of 14, compared to 13% of the control group. The women with pelvic pain also reported a number of other somatic symptoms, including abdominal pain, nausea, painful or irregular menses, dizziness, weakness, shortness of breath, and being "sickly" during their entire lives.

Other types of chronic pain have also been linked to sexual abuse history, including abdominal pain, headache, backache, and chronic diffuse muscle pains or fibromyalgia. The link between these types of chronic pain and sexual abuse has not yet been well defined, but some possible mechanisms are discussed below.

SEXUAL ABUSE AND GASTROINTESTINAL DISORDERS

Relations of sexual abuse to functional bowel disorders were demonstrated convincingly in a study by Drossman and colleagues of outpatients at a university gastroenterology clinic. Among 206 consecutive women patients, those with functional bowel disorders (including irritable bowel syndrome, chronic nonulcer dyspepsia, and chronic abdominal pain) were twice as likely to have a history of rape or incest as a control group of women with organic bowel disorders (including Crohn's disease, ulcerative colitis, and peptic ulcer disease). Women with sexual abuse history were also far more likely than nonabused women to report pelvic pain, fatigue, headache, back and chest pain, and shortness of breath, as well as to have had more lifetime surgeries. These associations suggest a broad pattern of somatization, rather than a specific link of sexual abuse to gastrointestinal disorders. Scarinci and colleagues' study replicating these findings also explored possible mechanisms for the associations and is discussed below.

SEXUAL ABUSE AND GYNECOLOGICAL PROBLEMS

In addition to the association of sexual abuse with chronic pelvic pain, discussed above, sexual abuse has a much broader impact on sexual and gynecological health. Women victims of sexual abuse are less likely to engage in health maintenance behaviors and wellness checks. For example, they are less likely to get regular gynecological exams and Pap smears, possibly because of the discomfort or vulnerability that is anticipated to be part of such exams. This puts abused women at greater risk for undiagnosed and hence untreated gynecological problems, including sexually transmitted diseases and malignancies.

Women with a history of sexual abuse are also more likely than nonabused women to engage in risky sexual practices, including having sex with strangers and multiple sexual partners. These activities put abused women at higher risk for sexually transmitted diseases and for unwanted pregnancies. Finally, women who have been victims of sexual abuse report a number of sexual and reproductive symptoms more often, including painful menstruation, irregular menstrual periods, excessive menstrual bleeding, burning with urination, painful intercourse, and lack of sexual pleasure.

These associations of sexual abuse with sexual and gynecological problems seem understandable in the context of traumatic sexualization that accompanies abuse. Women who have experienced loss of control, helplessness, degradation, and/or physical pain during sexual abuse might be expected to experience anxiety and hypervigilance with respect to their sexual and reproductive functions.

SEXUAL ABUSE AND EATING DISORDERS

Despite numerous studies relating sexual abuse history to disordered eating behaviors, these associations remain controversial. Clinical and population-based surveys have fairly consistently shown relationships of sexual abuse to anorexia nervosa, bulimia nervosa, and obesity. The associations may be stronger for bulimia nervosa and binge eating than for anorexia nervosa, but this is not yet definitively known. These demonstrated associations may be confounded, however, by the fact that family dynamics play an important role in the development of eating disorders. Dysfunctional families may set the stage for both sexual abuse and the development of eating disorders, and the abuse may not necessarily be an etiological factor. For example, one study that examined both sexual abuse and family variables showed an interaction of parental reliability with sexual abuse. That is, sexually abused women with unreliable parents were more likely to have high eating disorder scores than abused women with reliable parents. Another study by Hastings and Kern, which examined sexual abuse and family environment, found that abuse and environment appeared to have an additive effect on the probability of developing bulimia nervosa.

In summary, sexual abuse history is common among women with anorexia nervosa, bulimia nervosa, and obesity, but it is as yet unclear whether the relationship is etiological. Nevertheless, for eating-disordered women who do have a history of sexual abuse, addressing the abuse in the context of therapy is appropriate.

SEXUAL ABUSE AND SUBSTANCE ABUSE/DEPENDENCE

Population-based and clinical surveys have shown increases in drug and alcohol abuse or dependence among women with a history of sexual abuse. Although it has been argued that this can be explained by the fact that substance misuse may predispose women to being sexually abused, the onset of the substance misuse is far more likely to follow than to precede sexual abuse. Furthermore, the younger a woman was when the sexual abuse began, the more likely the woman is to develop problems with alcohol or drugs.

Sexually abused women are also more likely than nonabused women to use prescription tranquilizers and pain medications. Finally, one study showed that women with a sexual abuse history are more likely to smoke than women without such a history.

Problems with use or overuse of prescription and nonprescription agents including alcohol, tobacco, and illicit drugs, put sexually abused women at further risk for adverse health consequences.

SEXUAL ABUSE AND HEALTH CARE SEEKING

Studies examining health care utilization show that women with a history of sexual abuse are more likely to seek medical care than women without such a history. This is understandable, given the number and chronicity of symptoms experienced by these women. Women with an abuse history and chronic somatic symptoms are more likely to seek multiple consultations from numerous caregivers; more likely to undergo surgery, including hysterectomy; and more likely to use pain medications and tranquilizers. They are also more likely than nonabused women to rate their health as poor and to report physical disability.

POSSIBLE MECHANISMS RELATING SEXUAL ABUSE TO MEDICAL PROBLEMS AND SYMPTOMS

There are a number of possible explanations for the associations of sexual abuse with chronic medical symptoms and problems, and some have already been discussed. Sexual abuse can be construed as a stressful life event, and stress is known to be associated with poorer physical health and with physical symptoms. Women who have been sexually abused are at risk for developing depression, which can be associated with poorer subjective health. Abused women also commonly experience anxiety as a result of the trauma, which can result in a decreased ability to cope with common medical problems and symptoms, increased help seeking, increased sensitivity to pain, and amplification of somatic symptoms.

Each of these possible mechanisms can encompass the range of medical symptoms and problems associated with a history of sexual abuse. In fact, as pointed out above, women with such a history do commonly present for medical attention with multiple somatic complaints and other problems, such as eating-disordered behavior and/or substance use problems.

Scarinci and colleagues, exploring the basis for relations of sexual abuse to chronic medical symptoms, used sensory decision theory methods in an attempt to distinguish abused from nonabused patients with chronic gastrointestinal disorders. They found that women with a history of abuse had significantly lower pain thresholds than nonabused women. The abused women also reported more functional disability, more psychiatric problems, and more somatic symptoms than nonabused women. They were more likely to blame themselves for their pain, and they tended to have more maladaptive pain coping strategies. The interplay of these factors was proposed to account for the increased somatic symptoms, greater physical disability, and increased health care seeking among abused women. In this model, psychosocial stressors and psychiatric disturbances play important roles in the development and maintenance of chronic medical symptoms. This would suggest that future interventions with sexually abused women presenting with multiple medical complaints might address possible psychiatric problems and psychosocial stressors early in the course of diagnosis and treatment.

CONCLUSIONS

Sexual abuse of women is associated with a number of chronic medical problems and symptoms and with increased health care seeking. Future research should investigate appropriate treatment strategies for this group of patients.

FURTHER READING

Burgess, A. W., & Holmstrom, L. L. (1974). Rape trauma syndrome. *American Journal of Psychiatry, 131,* 981–986.
This is a classic study of physical and emotional symptoms that women experience following rape.

Drossman, D. A., Leserman, J., Nachman, G., Li, Z., Gluck, H., Toomey, T. C., & Mitchell, C. M. (1990). Sexual and physical abuse in women with functional or organic gastrointestinal disorders. *Annals of Internal Medicine, 113,* 828–833.
This was the first controlled study showing an association of sexual abuse with functional gastrointestinal disorders.

Hastings, T., & Kern J. M. (1994). Relationships between bulimia, childhood sexual abuse, and family environment. *International Journal of Eating Disorders, 15,* 103–111.
This study showed that sexual abuse and family environment appeared to combine in an additive manner, contributing to bulimia.

Kilpatrick, D. G., & Edmunds, C. N. (1992). *Rape in America: A report to the nation.* Arlington, VA: National Victim Center.
This is the definitive national prevalence study of rape. The authors estimated that one out of every eight adult women has been the victim of forcible rape in her lifetime.

Laws, A. (1993). Does a history of sexual abuse in childhood play a role in women's medical problems?: A review. *Journal of Women's Health, 2,* 165–172.
This review covers literature to date showing associations of sexual abuse history to medical problems in women.

Russell, D. E. H. (1983). The incidence and prevalence of intrafamilial and extrafamilial sexual abuse of female children. *Child Abuse and Neglect, 7,* 133–146.
This classic article used rigorous research methods to study prevalence of childhood sexual abuse.

Scarinci, I. C., McDonald-Haile, J., Bradley, L. A., & Richter, J. E. (1994). Altered pain perception and psychosocial features among women with gastrointestinal disorders and history of abuse: A preliminary model. *American Journal of Medicine, 97,* 108–118.
This study explores mechanisms for the association of sexual abuse with functional gastrointestinal disorders.

Smolak, L., Levine, M. P., & Sullins, E. (1990). Are child sexual experiences related to eating-disordered attitudes and behaviors in a college sample? *International Journal of Eating Disorders, 9,* 167–178.
This study showed that the significant relations between history of childhood sexual abuse and eating disorder symptoms were moderated by parental qualities.

Walker, E. A., Katon, W., Harrop-Griffiths, J., Holm, L., Russo, J., & Hickok, L. R. (1988). Relationship of chronic pelvic pain to psychiatric diagnoses and childhood sexual abuse. *American Journal of Psychiatry, 145,* 75–80.

78

Pregnancy and Childbirth

Christine Dunkel-Schetter
Marci Lobel

Relative to other topics in behavioral medicine concerning women, pregnancy is unique. Millions of women experience it every year, requiring extensive prenatal health care services; yet pregnancy is not a disease. And, in contrast to many other health-related experiences, pregnancy lasts a finite and predictable amount of time—approximately 9 months. Nonetheless, all pregnancies involve some degree of physical and psychological challenge, and in the case of first births, the period of life transition can last considerably longer than the time of gestation.

In the majority of cases, pregnancy is uncomplicated and proceeds smoothly to a delivery of a healthy infant. However, in a sizeable minority of cases, any number of complications can arise; these require more extensive medical observation and tests, and pose difficulties for the mother and fetus. For women whose medical complications are most severe, possible adverse outcomes include fetal demise, infant mortality, and infant morbidity. These adverse outcomes are sufficiently frequent in the United States and many other parts of the world as to warrant special research and prevention efforts. Such efforts, aimed at improving the outcomes of pregnancy for as many women as possible, have been mounted in the last decade by the World Health Organization and by several government agencies in the United States.

Thus, pregnancy has important public health implications for significant proportions of the large population of women around the world who experience it. Finally, pregnancy by its very nature is at the intersection of many biopsychosocial systems. A woman's social context, affective state, and behavior interact with her biological state in numerous and important ways during pregnancy, birth, and the postpartum period. It is for these reasons that we have been engaged in research on psychosocial processes in pregnancy and birth for a number of years.

GENERAL MODELS

For the past 25 years, there has been increased scientific interest in psychological and sociocultural factors during pregnancy. Understanding the experience of pregnancy for women of diverse backgrounds and resources provides promising avenues for predicting various outcomes of pregnancy, and possibly for intervening to improve them. For example, maternal psychosocial factors such as stress may influence any or several of the following endpoints: (1) maternal physiological, medical, and psychosocial states during pregnancy; (2) fetal behavior or states; (3) maternal and infant outcomes at birth (labor and delivery); (4) maternal postpartum condition; and (5) infant outcomes during early and later development.

A general model of psychosocial processes in pregnancy includes prenatal risk factors, mediating processes, and outcomes. Specific birth outcomes that have received the most attention are low birthweight (less than 2,500 grams); preterm labor and delivery (delivery at earlier than 37 weeks' gestation); labor complications (such as failure to progress); neonatal and infant complications (respiratory, cardiac, infection); and maternal postpartum depression (moderate to severe). Psychosocial risk factors that have received the greatest share of attention are psychosocial stress, employment and work strain, social support, and health behaviors. Mediating processes of interest include physiological ones (e.g., neuroendocrine and immune system processes) and behavioral ones (e.g., substance use, prenatal care utilization).

Despite the fact that this area of research is relatively new, it is already too large and too complex to summarize briefly. Therefore, we focus mainly on the three most commonly studied psychosocial risk factors (psychological stress, physical strain, social support) and on two specific and interrelated birth outcomes (preterm delivery, low birthweight). For information about a broader range of topics, we refer readers to recent reviews cited at the end of this chapter.

PSYCHOLOGICAL STRESS

Research on psychological stress and birth outcomes has grown remarkably in the past decade. Although other concepts (e.g., state anxiety or generalized distress) are occasionally considered, stress is most often conceptualized and measured as the negative impact of major life events. Current research indicates continuing and growing evidence for significant effects of prenatal life event stress, anxiety, or distress on preterm delivery and on fetal growth retardation—both of which contribute to low birthweight. Results from recent prospective and case–control studies indicate that women who experience high levels of stress during pregnancy are more likely to deliver low-birthweight or preterm infants, even after the effects of other factors such as smoking and medical risk are accounted for. For example, a study of approximately 5,500 Danish women found that preterm delivery was almost twice as common in those experiencing high stress in the 30th week of their pregnancy, independent of the medical condition and education of the women, and after smoking was controlled for.

Animal studies, particularly studies of nonhuman primates, are even more conclusive regarding the role of prenatal environmental stress in adverse birth outcomes. These studies are generally experimental in design, involving one group that is exposed to stress and another that is not. For example, researchers at the University of Wisconsin have examined the effects of stress on pregnant rhesus and squirrel monkeys. One recent study found that infant monkeys born to mothers exposed to mild stress throughout pregnancy had lower birthweights and showed signs of delayed neuromotor development. Similar results have been shown in infant monkeys exposed to repeated stress *in utero*, but not for those exposed to stress only once during midpregnancy. Thus, these and other nonhuman primate studies point to a key role for chronic (as opposed to acute) stress in producing adverse outcomes. There are also indications in human research that chronic stress is more influential than acute stress in terms of risk for low birthweight and its precursors, although investigators have not completely tested this issue. One reason is that it is very difficult to distinguish acute and chronic forms of stress at the human level, because they are frequently linked. For example, acute stressors often lead to chronic sequelae, and chronic stressful conditions may contribute to the occurrence of acute events or may be punctuated by them.

An important issue, with implications for the mechanisms whereby stress exerts effects on preterm delivery or fetal growth, is the timing of stress in pregnancy. Speculation and some preliminary evidence suggest that stress late in pregnancy is more deleterious than early prenatal stress, but the issue of the timing of stress has not been well investigated in human studies as yet. One hypothesis is that an accumulation of stress above certain threshold levels poses a risk of preterm labor and delivery via neuroendocrine changes that lead to early or excess uterine activity (an "accumulation-to-threshold" theory). Another hypothesis suggests that stress has steady detrimental effects, much like a drippy faucet, via adverse influence on health behaviors or other mediators that foster healthy fetal growth (a "dose–response" theory). For example, stress has been associated with greater substance use, poorer diet, and lower utilization of prenatal care, all of which are important to birth outcomes. A third hypothesis involves critical periods in pregnancy, such as the first trimester for fetal organ development, or the third trimester for early labor (a "critical-intervals" or "vulnerable-intervals" theory). Such vulnerable periods can be linked to physiological processes taking place in each trimester that may be affected differentially by stress. At present, insufficient evidence exists to indicate whether these hypotheses are valid or invalid. However, prenatal stress may have multiple effects that operate selectively in different groups of women with different medical risk factors or psychosocial profiles. Prenatal stress may also pose a variety of risks simultaneously for women who experience the highest levels of stress.

PHYSICAL STRAIN

In addition to the strong interest during the last decade in the effects of psychological stress in pregnancy, attention has also been focused on employment and work-related variables as possible prenatal risk factors. Past research on employment per se has been equivocal with respect to risk for adverse birth outcomes. This is not surprising if one considers the large variability in type and duration of work, in physical strain at work, and in other variables, each of which may operate differentially with respect to birth outcome.

Psychological stress research is pertinent to understanding work-related stress, because measures of life events, anxiety, or general distress reflect stress at work in addition to stress in other life domains. However, it is possible to distinguish physical strain from these forms of psychological stress. "Physical strain" or "exertion" refers to physical effort or activity in general, or to specific straining behaviors such as prolonged standing or heavy lifting. Research on physical exertion in general, or on specific behaviors during pregnancy, has also been inconsistent, but studies that focus on combinations of specific physical activities show more consistent results. For example, higher rates of low birthweight and preterm delivery have been found in employed women who do more standing, carrying, and other effortful activities. In one study of over 4,000 pregnant women, those whose work involved daily standing and walking for more than 5 hours were three times as likely to have a preterm delivery.

Although research on physical exertion or strain has developed from inquiries into effects of employment in pregnancy, it should not be considered exclusively among women in the labor force. Household and child care responsibilities performed by women not employed for pay are frequently strenuous. A recent study evaluated a sample of over 200 women, both employed and nonemployed, and found that extent of standing, lifting, bending, and getting up and down in the second trimester was associated with lower birthweight, even after demographic factors, medical risk, and substance use were controlled for. These effects held for nonemployed as well as employed women.

How does physical strain influence birth outcome? Fatigue associated with physical activities is thought to be one important mediator of the effects of physical strain on birth outcomes. Explanations for these effects also include the effects of physical activity on cardiovascular and neuroendocrine functioning. However, physical exercise undertaken voluntarily for fitness or pleasure does not appear to be associated with adverse birth outcomes, at least for women who are at low risk and are physically fit prior to pregnancy. The degree of choice in one's physical activities, the ability to refrain from or reduce them on occasions (and altogether at some point in pregnancy if one wishes), and other aspects of physical exercise seem to differentiate it from physical strain. The adverse effects of physical strain shown in some studies may also be attributable to the psychologically stressful nature of activities that involve exertion, rather than to exertion per se, since strain and stress often occur together. Thus, psychological stress must be controlled for in studies of physical strain, in order for investigators to be certain that the effects are from physical strain or exertion specifically. Very little research to date has considered this important issue.

Finally, there is some evidence that modifications in conditions of employment or daily activities can reduce risk of preterm delivery in women at risk. Studies in Europe and the United States suggest that sick leave or bed rest, when medically indicated, may be beneficial for reducing preterm delivery and low birthweight. These studies are consistent with the premise that physical activity may pose risk under some conditions, but unfortunately they do not clarify what conditions specifically. Does rest relieve physical strain, alleviate psychological stress, or lead to other effects (e.g., an increase in social support)? We need further information regarding the specific benefits of interventions to fully clarify these issues.

SOCIAL RELATIONSHIPS

Research on social relationships in connection with pregnancy and birth is multifaceted. The term "social relationships" is used here to incorporate the study of social integration (the existence of spouse, family, friends); social network (size, composition, and interaction with others); and social support (availability and receipt of assistance and comfort, especially in times of stress). Research on social relationships and pregnancy outcomes has concentrated on three issues. First, correlational studies have examined the effects of prenatal social support, integration, or networks on birth outcomes, often in conjunction with research on prenatal stress. Inconsistencies in definition and measures of social support and in outcome variables make it difficult to summarize conclusions from this research. However, it appears that some types and sources of social support are associated with better pregnancy outcomes. Tangible assistance (e.g., helping with tasks or providing items needed to live) and emotional support (e.g., comfort, affection, or listening) appear most likely to be beneficial; in contrast, the benefits of informational support depend more on who is the provider and the context in which information is offered. In addition, different subgroups of women appear to respond differently to social support. For example, social support effects have varied with ethnicity, socioeconomic status, age, and levels of stress in past research. In general, groups with the greatest need for social support appear to benefit most.

A second area of research on social relationships in pregnancy is intervention research that has examined the effects of providing prenatal support (often in combination with other resources) on outcomes at birth and postpartum. Interventions most often involve home visits by midwives, nurses, or social workers, who provide a blend of emotional, informational, and instrumental assistance. Such interventions are usually delivered to women deemed vulnerable because of medical or social conditions. Results have been uneven but sometimes promising. For example, Oakley and her colleagues randomly assigned British working-class women with prior low-birthweight infants to an intervention or control group. Midwives visited intervention women three times during pregnancy and called them often; women in the comparison group did not receive the intervention. Women in the intervention group subsequently had larger babies, fewer preterm labors, and experienced other benefits. Results of intervention research appear to differ by subgroups of women, as do results of correlational support and birth outcome research. For example, one investigation found that the benefits of an intervention were limited to African-American women at high risk and did not occur in two other ethnic groups studied. Other studies suggest that young mothers are especially helped by supportive interventions. Despite these encouraging findings, flaws in methods of the vast majority of studies weaken the conclusions that can be drawn from this line of research. Furthermore, research has not clarified which elements of intervention are most effective and for whom.

Finally, both correlational and experimental studies have examined the effects of having a labor companion and of getting support during labor on labor and delivery outcomes. The presence of a supportive person during birth seems to have a consistently positive effect on birth outcomes. Randomized trials in the United States and other countries have shown that both emotional and informational support have beneficial effects on length of labor, medication use, birth complications, and even on type of delivery (i.e., cesarean section vs. vaginal delivery). It should be noted that the labor coach need not be a close relation to the woman in labor. Strong positive effects are observed even when women are assisted in labor by strangers. Of the three bodies of research on social support and birth outcomes reviewed, that on the effects of social support during labor and delivery is the most definitive, and also the most consistent across cultural and ethnic groups.

INDIVIDUAL CHARACTERISTICS

Our conclusions thus far have not fully addressed various individual factors that must be considered in connection with psychological stress, physical exertion, and social relationships in pregnancy. These are a woman's age, ethnicity, socioeconomic status, parity (i.e., having had a prior birth experience), and medical risk status. Special issues arise when one is considering psychosocial risk factors in pregnant teens; women of ethnic minority background or low socioeconomic status; primaparas (i.e., women giving birth for the first time); and women with a history of chronic disease, gynecological problems, or complications in the current pregnancy.

Unfortunately, these individual factors all pose increased risk and they often co-occur. An understanding of psychosocial risks and resources in pregnancy requires careful attention to interactions and intervening processes involving these variables. For example, studies by our group and others of low-income African-American women have shown that a higher risk of low birthweight can be partially accounted for by higher rates of psychological stress. Moreover, our research has shown that the association of prenatal stress to birthweight and preterm delivery is stronger in women with existing medical risk conditions than women without such conditions. The bulk of our work has focused on pregnancies in low-income, ethnic minority women which has sensitized us to the intricacies of understanding psychosocial processes in a sociocultural context.

CONCLUSION

In this chapter, we have reviewed evidence that suggests that prenatal stress, physical strain, and social support influence important birth outcomes such as low birthweight and preterm delivery. This research has also raised a number of issues. We highlight three important questions here: (1) what are the behavioral and physiological mechanisms that account for the effects of these psychosocial variables on birth outcomes? (2) are there different effects for chronic versus acute conditions occurring in pregnancy? And might there be critical prenatal periods of heightened sensitivity to stress, strain, or support? (3) are some groups of women more sensitive or vulnerable to the effects of prenatal psychosocial variables? Previous research has not fully addressed these issues, which we believe are critical to improving our understanding of psychosocial processes in pregnancy.

National statistics indicate that American women suffer among the highest rates of low birthweight births and infant mortality of any industrialized nation, and disadvantaged women in the United States experience disproportionate rates of adverse birth outcomes. Given the social, financial, health, and health-care consequences of this public health problem, researchers must continue to examine the many factors that contribute to it. Sufficient evidence has now accumulated to implicate specific psychosocial conditions as risks and benefits to pregnant women. Therefore, we must now focus our attention on screening for psychosocial risk factors, on targeting the vulnerable pregnant women who can be assisted, and on determining how to intervene to enhance the psychosocial conditions in the lives of these women. This work will require the expertise of many disciplines including psychology, medicine, nursing, social welfare, and public health. In sum, the needs of women and their children can best be met by interdisciplinary research and programmatic efforts reflecting the biopsychosocial nature of pregnancy and birth.

FURTHER READING

Berendes, H., Klessel, S., & Yaffe, S. (Eds.). (1991). *Advances in the prevention of low birthweight.* Washington, DC: National Center for Education in Maternal and Child Health.
Series of state-of-the-art papers on issues in prevention of low birthweight including an excellent discussion by Brooks-Gunn on support and stress during pregnancy and a useful review on social support intervention research in pregnancy by Elbourne and Oakley.

Dunkel-Schetter, C., Sagrestano, L. M., Feldman, P., & Killingsworth, C. (1996). Social support and pregnancy: A comprehensive review focusing on ethnicity and culture. In G. R. Pierce, B. R. Sarason, & I. G. Sarason (Eds.), *The handbook of social support and the family.* New York: Plenum.
An up-to-date review of research on (1) social support and birth outcomes including correlational, prenatal intervention, and labor support studies, and on (2) support in pregnancy and emotions and behavior during pregnancy followed by a discussion of culture and ethnicity emphasizing Latinas and how these factors influence social support in pregnancy.

Hedegaard, M., Henriksen, T. B., Sabroe, S., & Secher, N. J. (1993). Psychological distress in pregnancy and preterm delivery. *British Medical Journal, 307,* 234–239.
Study showing that higher levels of emotional distress late in pregnancy, but not in midpregnancy, were associated with an increased likelihood of preterm delivery in a large sample of Danish women.

Henriksen, T. B., Hedegaard, M., Secher, N. J., & Wilcox, A. J. (1995). Standing at work and preterm delivery (1995). *British Journal of Obstetrics and Gynaecology, 102,* 198–206.
Study of 4,000 Danish women found that those who stood or walked at work more than 5 hours per day in the second trimester of pregnancy had a higher incidence of preterm delivery compared to those who worked in pregnancy but stood or walked less.

Institute of Medicine. (1985). *Preventing low birthweight.* Washington, DC: National Academy Press.
An excellent review of risk factors, both established ones and promising ones.

Lobel, M. (1994). Conceptualizations, measurement, and effects of prenatal maternal stress on birth outcomes. *Journal of Behavioral Medicine, 17,* 225-272.
One of the most recent and rigorous reviews focused specifically on stress and anxiety in pregnancy and effects on birth outcomes.

McAnarney, E. R., & Stevens-Simon, C. (1990). Maternal psychological stress/depression and low birth weight: Is there a relationship? *AJDC, 144,* 789–792.
Review on stress and depression as risk factors for low birthweight that focuses on mechanisms.

Molfese, V. J. (1989). *Perinatal risk and infant development: Assessment and prediction.* New York: Guilford Press.
Book providing in-depth treatment of the issues of perinatal risk assessment and the problems in this area.

Norbeck, J. S., & Anderson, N. J. (1989). Psychosocial predictors of pregnancy outcomes in low-income black, Hispanic, and white women. *Nursing Research, 38,* 204–209.
Study reporting that associations of stress, support, and anxiety to birth outcomes differ in ethnic groups. Urban black, white, and Hispanic women in San Francisco were studied.

Oakley, A., Rajan, L., & Grant, A. (1990). Social support and pregnancy outcome. *British Journal of Obstetrics and Gynaecology, 97,* 155–162.
Intervention study providing social support to women at risk and showing positive effects on outcomes.

Schneider, M. L., & Coe, C. L. (1993). Repeated social stress during pregnancy impairs neuromotor development of the primate infant. *Journal of Developmental and Behavioral Pediatrics, 14,* 81–87.

Comparison of infant monkeys born to (1) mothers exposed to mild stress throughout pregnancy, (2) mothers exposed to one stress episode in midpregnancy, and (3) undisturbed mothers, showing the first group had infants who had significantly poorer motor abilities, impaired balance, and other neuromotor problems.

Woo, G. (1995). *Strain in daily activities during pregnancy: Associations of physical exertion, psychological demand, and personal control with birth outcomes.* Unpublished doctoral dissertation, University of California, Los Angeles.

A controlled prospective study of 215 African-American, white, and Hispanic pregnant women, both employed and nonemployed, examining the influence of physical exertion and psychosocial demands in daily activities on gestational age and birthweight adjusted for gestational age. Physical exertion late in pregnancy was associated with lower birthweight after controlling for demographics, medical risk, and substance use.

79

Pregnancy in Women with Disabilities

Judith G. Rogers

This chapter explores the problems of researching the issues pertaining to pregnancy in women with disabilities. Historically, women with disabilities have been discouraged from becoming parents. However, with the recent disability rights movement, more people with disabilities are knowing successful disabled parents and are learning that they have an ability and a right to be parents. Thus they are choosing to be so. Because disabled women have been discouraged from becoming parents, there is little information on disability and pregnancy, and the information is difficult to find.

In 1980, I started research on my book, *Mother to Be: A Guide to Pregnancy and Birth for Women with Disabilities*. I interviewed 36 women who represented 14 different disabilities and who had had a total of 62 pregnancies. Each woman was successful not only in becoming pregnant, but also in carrying a child to term.

Collecting the material for this book reinforced my belief that there has been a long-standing bias against parenthood for people with disabilities. Society wants to discourage disabled women from becoming pregnant, and thus to avoid the problem of parenting with a disability. For example, health care professionals, genetic counselors,and society at large all send messages implying that it is unacceptable for a disabled person to have a baby.

My work at Through the Looking Glass—a national research and training center in Berkeley, California, that focuses on parenting with a disability—has reinforced my perception that this prejudice continues to be a disturbing trend. This discrimination will continue until society accepts parents with disabilities. As women with disabilities become aware of the availability of adaptive parenting equipment such as that developed by Through the Looking Glass, the demand for services by women with disabilities will continue to grow.

These illustrations indicate the importance of analyzing biases about women with disabilities, in order to help deliver better health care. Studying pregnancy, labor, and delivery in women with disabilities will not only help provide new treatment options for these women, but may also help other women as well.

WHY WE HAVE A LACK OF RESEARCH DATA

Because the numbers of research studies are small, and the disabilities diverse, most medical personnel are still uninformed about disabled women and pregnancy. Many physicians never see such women in their practice. Therefore, a pregnant woman with a disability will rarely find a practitioner who has any knowledge of the interactions of her specific disability and pregnancy. Moreover, there are few community agencies that can provide information to such a pregnant woman.

There is very little hard evidence on pregnancy and disability. Most of the existing case studies of pregnancy and disability focus on only a few people (fewer than 20). Indeed, most reports consist of an individual physician's account of a single pregnancy with a disabled mother, or anecdotal reports by disabled mothers of their nonmedical perceptions of pregnancy. These personal anecdotal records are often of first pregnancies. Some studies are retrospective, with the inherent problems of accurate recall.

An additional factor is the predominant focus on women with acquired disabilities, such as spinal cord injuries. These are often women who are currently receiving medical services related to their disabilities. For women with disabilities of a longer duration, particularly those congenital or having an early onset (e.g., polio or cerebral palsy), it is very difficult to find any studies.

Larger studies are beginning to be done on women with acquired disabilities. Jackson found that recruiting 474 women with disabilities to participate in one study required the collaboration of 10 regional spinal cord injury centers over a period of 3 years. She studied pre- and postinjury pregnancies and compared the differences. However, in this study of 474 women, only 66 women (14%) had 101 combined postinjury pregnancies (Jackson, 1995).

HOW WE CAN GET FACTS

There are many different strategies for addressing the problems of isolation and lack of coordinated information.

Setting Up a Data Base

A centralized resource center is essential to creating an avenue for finding information and collecting data. Individual medical providers have trouble finding the information that *does* exist, whether it concerns pregnancy related discomforts or doing a pelvic exam for women with specific disabilities. The disabled community has similar difficulties accessing information.

Interlinking Medical Disciplines

An unusual aspect of dealing with a disabled pregnant woman is that more than one medical specialist must be consulted. Unfortunately, at the present time there is very little collaboration between rehabilitation medicine and obstetrics and gynecology. This collaboration is also important for designing research because the two disciplines may be looking at different variables.

Identifying Disabled Women for Studies

Independent adult women with disabilities who are parents can be difficult to find for research studies. They may want to remain anonymous for a variety of reason; some may have some fear that society judges their parenting more harshly than nondisabled mothers. Medical researchers cannot easily identify a single pool of women who are conveniently collected in one medical facility. Identification may be problematic if a significant amount of time has passed since the onset of the disability and if the disabled women requires only minimal medical intervention.

When the disabled mother is successful at integrating in "normal society" she becomes culturally invisible. The disability culture is vast and varied. This culture operates through an extensive tightly woven network. Since this network is based more on social than organizational ties, its members are largely hidden.

An additional problem is that a number of women are not diagnosed with their disabilities prior to their pregnancies. This population is rarely studied, since the disability label is applied post-pregnancy even though the symptoms and effects were present before the pregnancy. Some women, particularly women with systemic lupus erythematosus, may not receive a disability diagnosis until after several miscarriages.

RESEARCH ISSUES

Disability as a Changing Variable

For some women with disabilities, the disability effects may make it hard to separate the disability from the pregnancy. For example, is a bladder infection a natural interaction between pregnancy and disability, or is it just a pregnancy discomfort?

For women with identified long-term disabilities the answer may be clear. But for women with changing disabilities or disabilities of a newer onset, there may be no easy assessment.

Severity of Disability as a Significant Factor

There seems to be more of a relationship between the degree of disability than the kinds. For example, women who had similar levels of functioning prior to pregnancy experienced similar problems during pregnancy. Because this requires comparing different disabilities, it is harder to study the impact of pregnancy on disability.

Physicians' Attitudes

Among the major barriers to answering the questions that need to be asked are physicians' attitudes. Many physicians have deeply entrenched beliefs about pregnancy and birthing. If physicians think that they already know the answers, then they won't even ask the questions. Most research on the pregnancy was done by nondisabled men.

Since men cannot experience pregnancy or labor, they may not have posed the right questions. The following sections are where I have seen discrepancies between commonly held beliefs and actual events.

Hormones

We need to compare disabled and nondisabled women in terms of hormonal effects on pregnancy. All women experience many side effects related to hormonal shifts during pregnancy. Since hormones affect many systems during pregnancy, research in this area can have an impact for both nondisabled and disabled women.

Respiratory Issues

Discrepancies exist in several areas of the study of pregnancy-related discomforts, and those also need to be researched. One of these areas is that of problems in the pulmonary system, my interviews produced some evidence that contradicts current beliefs. Current medical belief is that women with post-polio syndrome will experience increased respiratory problems. In fact, one interviewee with post-polio syndrome found that her breathing improved, because her baby acted like a corset. By contrast, I know a woman who did not have a known disability, but who had severe respiratory problems during pregnancy. This kind of unpredictability suggests this subject area needs further investigations.

Bladder Infections

One concern and assumption in the medical field is that during pregnancy a bladder infection can readily lead to a kidney infection. Even though women with spinal cord dysfunction commonly have bladder infections, it was a rare occurrence, however, for the women I interviewed to have had a bladder infection lead to a kidney infection. The question can be posed, then, why do some women with bladder infections progress to a kidney infection while others do not. The same question may be applied to pregnant women without disabilities. An answer to this question would benefit treatment and prevention for all women.

Pushing during Labor

There is inconsistency between scientific belief and medical practice regarding women's ability to push during childbirth. Medical professionals are taught that the uterus is a muscle, but they are not taught that it, like all muscles, can fatigue during labor. I became aware of this discrepancy during my own labors. This discovery was reinforced while I was doing research on my book: more evidence the uterus functions like other muscles. Any woman with or without a disability, who has been in labor for 20 hours, will find the second stage of labor difficult. I believe this is due to the uterus tiring. In many circumstances, the medical staff have made the woman feel incompetent or that she is an ineffectual pusher. Although doctors know that the uterus is a muscle, they seem to ignore the fact that this muscle can tire. Instead of allowing time for the uterus to recuperate, the medical establishment would prefer to use medical intervention; cesarean sections, use of forceps or suction, and pitocin drips.

Women with high spinal cord injuries do not have the ability to push because they lack innervation to the abdominal muscles. However, I found that some women with high spinal cord injuries were able to deliver their babies vaginally without medical intervention. If the medical field could treat a uterus like a muscle, fatigued from strenuous activity, and allow it to rest, it might affect medical interventions during labor. These experiences point to research that is needed to determine how long a uterus can work before exhaustion.

Blood Volume

An increase in blood volume is a natural outcome of pregnancy. It had been hypothesized without much evidence that women with spinal cord dysfunction would have skin breakdown during pregnancy, because of the extra weight gain. This hypothesis does not seem to have been researched, but was derived from "some sort of logic." Yet the evidence from our book provides some indications that the increased volume of blood during pregnancy may help prevent decubiti (pressure sores). For example, one interviewee with spina bifida had experienced continual decubiti on her foot except during her pregnancy.

Other variables that may affect skin conditions and outcome should also be studied. Diet, for instance, is a factor that may also contribute to good skin health. One of the women interviewed had poor nutrition during her pregnancy and developed a decubitus.

One theory about the cause of edema during pregnancy is that increased blood volume and lack of exercise are responsible. However, some of the interviewees, who were less active than women without disabilities, did not experience the pregnancy side effect of edema. Because it is also thought that increased blood supply and reduced activity level compound the normal pregnancy-related problems with venous return, one would have expected disabled women to have thrombophlebitis during pregnancy. Only one of the women I interviewed developed thrombophlebitis. This woman, whose disability was spinal cord injury, had this problem both before and during pregnancy. This is another example of how studying pregnant women with disabilities may expose the discrepancies between beliefs and reality.

Anesthesia and Cesarean Section

We do not know what effect anesthesia has on women with different disabilities.

In the treatment of heart problems, the medical profession has learned that treatment needed to be different for women than for men. In the case of using anesthesia (epidural or spinal), the medical profession still assumes that the same standards used for nondisabled women apply to disabled women. I believe different standards may be needed and there is no existing research to guide the medical profession. At Through the Looking Glass where I work, I have received calls from disabled women seeking information concerning recovery from the use of edpidural or spinal anesthesia during labor. For example, a year later, one woman still has not recovered her ability to walk after delivery in which an epidural was used. Research is needed on the use of epidural or spinal anesthesia on disabled women.

Some women with disabilities have respiratory problems secondary to their disabilities, as noted above. Since it is known that general anesthesia can compromise respiration, physicians need to know which disabilities have an associated risk. It is unknown how regional anesthesia interacts with certain disabilities. This lack of information may result in poor medical care. Doing unnecessary cesareans may be more debilitating than we think. For example, a woman with a progressive disability had a cesarean with her first pregnancy, but 8 years later with her next pregnancy, she was able to deliver vaginally with a speedier recovery.

Another example illustrates the prevailing attitude in the medical field that surgery is easier than labor. An interviewee with spinal muscular atrophy was given general anesthesia for her cesarean. These doctors thought that laboring would be to hard on her system, but ignored the possible complications of the general anesthesia for the respiratory system and the musculoskeletal system.

ADDITIONAL RESEARCH AREAS

Another potential result of studying pregnancy in disabled women could be the discovery of possible treatments for certain disabilities. My interviews and the literature of the multiple sclerosis and rheumatoid arthritis societies have documented that some women with either multiple sclerosis or rheumatoid arthritis, have had remissions or exacerbation's during pregnancy. In order to add to the information around treatment of these disabilities it may be helpful to learn the causes of the remissions or exacerbations.

CONCLUSION

There are two major reasons for the lack of research in the area of pregnancy and disability: (1) the small number of pregnant disabled women, and (2) the lack of awareness that discrepancies exist between medical beliefs and actuality.

FURTHER READING

Jackson, A. B. (1996). Pregnancy and delivery. In D. M. Krotoski, M. A. Nosek, & M. A. Turk (Eds.), Women with physical disabilities: Achieving and maintaining health and well-being (pp. 91–99). Baltimore: Brookes.
This chapter describes a study that compared the pregnancies of women prior to and after their spinal cord injuries.

Rogers, J. G., & Matsumura, M. (1991). *Mother to be: A guide to pregnancy and birth for women with disabilities.* New York: Demos.
This book describes positive and negative effects of pregnancy on disability.

80

Postpartum Depression

Ian H. Gotlib

$\mathcal{A}$lthough childbirth is a time of great happiness for many families, it also represents a period of change and disruption. At an interpersonal level, pregnancy and childbirth are marked by dramatic changes in the marital relationships, family and social roles, and daily routines of the family members. Psychiatric illness in a mother at this time can be one of the most devastating events for the mother and the family. It can interfere with the bonding and attachment process, and with the mother's learning and execution of effective infant caretaking and parenting skills. Moreover, recent research has documented that the consequences for a young child of having a depressed mother can be most serious.

The presumed association in women between the birth of a child and depression has long been recognized in what has come to be called "postpartum depression." Despite all that has been written on this topic, however, considerable controversy remains as to the definition and, indeed, the existence of postpartum depression as a unique disorder. There are a number of reasons for this state of uncertainty. One major difficulty is that there is little consensus as to what constitutes postpartum depression. Many studies of postpartum depression, for example, have used vaguely stated, poorly defined, or inadequate criteria to assess and diagnose depression. Moreover, investigators have often blurred the distinctions among a range of postpartum dysphoric mood states that differ significantly in terms of their severity. Consequently, there is considerable variability among studies with respect to the criteria used in operationally defining the disorder. Postpartum depression has been defined variously in terms of elevated self-report depression scores, the presence of selected symptoms of depression, a psychiatric diagnosis, or the fact that a woman was seen in psychiatric treatment or received psychotropic medication.

The purpose of this chapter is to present current information about postpartum depression. I first discuss definitional issues regarding postpartum depression, and then present information concerning the clinical features and symptom patterns associated with this disorder. Following this discussion, I present data concerning the incidence and prevalence of postpartum depression, and examine factors that have been found to increase women's risk for developing an episode of postpartum depression. Finally, I conclude the chapter by examining the impact of postpartum depression on the functioning of the women themselves and of their infants and young children.

WHAT IS POSTPARTUM DEPRESSION?

Unfortunately, as noted above, there is little consensus concerning what constitutes postpartum depression. Contemporary theorists and researchers in this area of study suggest that it is useful to distinguish among three types of postpartum depressive states: (1) "postpartum blues," a transient mood disturbance characterized by tearfulness, feelings of dysphoria, and emotional lability; (2) "postpartum psychosis," characterized by delusions and hallucinations, and generally believed to be similar to nonpuerperal psychotic disorders; and (3) "postpartum depression," characterized by sadness, loss of interest in daily activities, and various symptoms of clinically significant depression.

Although the focus of this chapter is on postpartum depression (the third type of postpartum depressive state), it is important to comment briefly on the nature of the other two depressive states. The postpartum blues state is a common phenomenon, affecting between 40% and 85% of women after childbirth. It involves a transient alteration in mood, beginning on the third or fourth postpartum day and usually lasting 2–4 days. During this period the new mother is characterized by tearfulness, irritability, and anxiety. Although many investigators believe that the postpartum blues are of biological origin, given the considerable hormonal and biochemical changes that occur during this early postpartum period, the results of empirical research to date have been equivocal. Nevertheless, the postpartum blues mood state is generally considered a normal part of postpartum adjustment, and in fact most women recover fully without formal treatment.

Postpartum psychosis is a much more severe and much rarer disorder, typically occurring within the first 2–4 weeks after delivery. Prevalence rates of postpartum psychosis have been estimated at between 1 and 3 per 1,000 births, and several studies have demonstrated that the majority of postpartum psychotic episodes occur within the first month after delivery. Most investigators believe that postpartum psychoses are not distinct from psychoses occurring at other times in a woman's life. Primiparous women (i.e., women having their first child) appear to be at higher risk for developing postpartum psychosis than are multiparous women, as are women with a personal or family history of psychopathology, particularly bipolar depression.

In contrast to the postpartum blues and postpartum psychosis, postpartum depression is a disorder that is comparable to a major affective disorder as defined in U.S. and international psychiatric diagnostic systems. Thus, women experiencing postpartum depression report sad mood or loss of interest in daily activities, in addition to such additional symptoms of depression as fatigue, loss of appetite, sleep disturbance, guilt, concentration difficulties, and decrease in self-esteem. Furthermore, these symptoms often last for 6 months or longer. In the remainder of this chapter, I examine the prevalence and incidence of postpartum depression, risk factors for this disorder, and the effects of postpartum depression on women and their children.

HOW PREVALENT IS POSTPARTUM DEPRESSION?

Prevalence is a measure of how many cases of postpartum depression exist at any particular point in time. Early studies reported that the prevalence of postpartum depression is quite extensive. For example, investigators who relied on self-report measures provided prevalence estimates for postpartum depression ranging up to 40% of all childbearing women. More recently, however, researchers have begun to use more stringent structured interviews and standardized diagnostic criteria to define postpartum depression. These criteria typically involve the presence of significant symptoms of depression in the postpartum period that persist for more than 2 weeks and interfere in some way with social functioning. Studies using such criteria provide a relatively consistent picture of the prevalence of clinical depression in the postpartum period, and obtain rates between 3% and 12%. It is critical to note that these rates of postpartum depression are not significantly higher than rates of clinical depression in the community among nonpregnant women of similar ages. Moreover, a number of studies have also found no differences in the specific symptom patterns exhibited by childbearing and nonchildbearing depressed women. Although the importance of postpartum depression should not be minimized, this equivalence of rates and symptoms of postpartum and nonpostpartum depression clearly calls into question the uniqueness of postpartum depression as a distinct psychiatric disorder.

WHAT FACTORS PREDICT POSTPARTUM DEPRESSION?

Although there is a reasonably large theoretical and empirical literature concerning predictors of nonpuerperal depression, analogous theory and research in postpartum depression have lagged behind. Recently, however, several investigators have identified factors and variables that appear to be associated with the occurrence of postpartum depression. Interestingly, and consistent with the findings presented earlier concerning the equivalence of postpartum and nonpostpartum depression, these typically are variables that have also been associated with the development of nonpostpartum depression. For example, one of the strongest predictors of postpartum depression is a history of depression. In this context, three related points are noteworthy. First, women who have had previous episodes of depression are at increased risk for the development of postpartum depression—and, indeed, for the development of depression in the face of any significant life stressor. Second, women with a family history of psychiatric disorder have also been found to be at elevated risk for developing an episode of postpartum depression. Finally, women who experience significant depression or anxiety during pregnancy are also likely to experience depression during the postpartum period. In fact, for many women who are diagnosed with postpartum depression, a detailed clinical interview will reveal that the depression began in pregnancy and continued after the delivery. In general, therefore, the level of a woman's psychological or emotional adjustment before and during pregnancy is a powerful predictor of her functioning during pregnancy.

The other relatively consistent predictor of postpartum depression is the quality of a woman's interpersonal relationships. Although some studies have implicated a lack of support from persons other than the spouse in the onset of postpartum depression, the majority of investigations have suggested more specifically that a lack of spousal support and the presence of marital conflict may be more strongly associated with this disorder. Moreover, the results of several studies indicate that poor marital relationships may not be a consequence of postpartum depression, but often precede the depression. For example, investigators in England found that postpartum depressed women who had also experienced significant life events during or shortly following pregnancy were 10 times more likely than were nondepressed women to report that they received no help from their husbands. Again, however, it is important to note that similar findings have been reported with respect to depression occurring in nonchildbearing women.

A final interpersonal factor that has been implicated in the onset of postpartum depression is the quality of a woman's relationship with her own parents during her childhood. In fact, in our large study of postpartum depression, women's perceptions during pregnancy of the level of caring they perceived from their parents during their first 16 years was the single strongest predictor of the subsequent onset of postpartum depression. Women who perceived low-quality early parenting were almost six times more likely to develop an episode of postpartum depression than were women who perceived their parents as highly caring. Finally, it is important to note here that although a number of biological factors have been examined with respect to their role in the etiology of postpartum depression, these studies have yielded primarily negative results, and there is no strong or consistent evidence that biological or gynecological/obstetrical factors are involved in the onset of this disorder.

CONSEQUENCES OF POSTPARTUM DEPRESSION

A number of investigators have now examined the long-term consequences of postpartum depression, both for the women themselves and for their marital relationships and children. It is clear that a significant proportion of women with postpartum depression will experience another clinically significant episode of depression within the next 5 years. For example, some researchers have found that as many as 80% of women who experienced postpartum depression reported additional depressive episodes over the following 42 months. Moreover, the marital relationships of women who experienced postpartum depression were characterized as less satisfying 4–5 years later than were the marital relationships of women who did not experience postpartum depression. It is likely, of course, that the adverse factors that increase women's risk for postpartum depression are simply continuing to operate, and leave them vulnerable to further episodes of depression.

A growing literature is also now examining the behavior of depressed women interacting with their infants during the postpartum period, as well as the short- and longer-term impact of postpartum depression on the infants' functioning. Although nonpostpartum depressed women have been found to be deficient in their parenting skills with older children, depression during the postpartum period may be especially critical, because mothers are likely to be the primary caregivers of their infants. Moreover, it is likely that depression during the postpartum period can interfere with the infants' mastery of developmentally salient tasks.

The results of a number of investigations indicate that postpartum depressed women engage in more problematic behaviors with their infants than do nondepressed women. Postpartum depressed mothers have been found to gaze less often at their infants, and seem to be less ready to interact with them. Postpartum depressed mothers have also been found to be less active, less playful, less affectionate, and less engaging with their infants. In fact, some studies have found postpartum depressed mothers to be explicitly angry and negative in interactions with their infants. Perhaps not surprisingly, infants of postpartum depressed mothers have been found to exhibit a variety of difficulties. Compared with infants of nondepressed mothers, infants of postpartum depressed mothers have been observed to be more drowsy or fussy, to be less relaxed or content, to cry more frequently, to show higher rates of insecure attachment, and to obtain lower scores on the Bayley Scales of Infant Development. Unfortunately, these difficulties have been found to persist at 4-year follow-up assessments.

CONCLUSIONS

Postpartum depression is a serious emotional disorder that affects 3–12% of women. It is characterized by sad mood and/or a loss of interest in daily activities, as well as a number of other symptoms of depression. A personal or family history of depression significantly elevates a woman's risk for postpartum depression, as does an unsatisfying early relationship with parents. Postpartum depression represents a vulnerability for experiencing further depressive episodes, although this vulnerability may result from the continued presence of various risk factors. This disorder often adversely affects both women and their children. Finally, there is little evidence to suggest that postpartum depression is different in any significant way from depressions occurring at other times in the life course.

FURTHER READING

Carro, M. G., Grant, K. E., Gotlib, I. H., & Compas, B. E. (1993). Postpartum depression and child development: An investigation of mothers and fathers as sources of risk and resilience. *Development and Psychopathology, 5, 567–579.*
A study examining the effects of both maternal and paternal depressive symptoms on the psychosocial and emotional functioning of the children.

Gotlib, I. H., Whiffen, V. E., Mount, J. H., Milne, K., & Cordy, N. I. (1989). Prevalence rates and demographic characteristics associated with depression in pregnancy and the postpartum. *Journal of Consulting and Clinical Psychology, 57, 269–274.*
A scientific article that documents prevalence rates and demographic variables associated with depression occurring during pregnancy and following birth.

Gotlib, I. H., Whiffen, V. E., Wallace, P. M., & Mount, J. H. (1991). A prospective investigation of postpartum depression: Factors involved in onset and recovery. *Journal of Abnormal Psychology, 100, 122–132.*
An article examining demographic and psychosocial factors that predict the onset of postpartum depression, as well as recovery from an episode of depression occurring during pregnancy.

Kruckman, L., & Asmann-Finch, C. (1986). *Postpartum depression: A research guide and international bibliography.* New York: Garland Press.
An annotated listing of published articles discussing postpartum depression.

O'Hara, M. W., Schlechte, J. A., Lewis, D. A., & Varner, M. W. (1991). Controlled prospective study of postpartum mood disorders: Psychological, environmental, and hormonal variables. *Journal of Abnormal Psychology, 100, 63–73.*
An article examining a variety of factors associated with the onset of postpartum depression.

Wallace, P. M., & Gotlib, I. H. (1990). Marital adjustment during the transition to parenthood: Stability and predictors of change. *Journal of Marriage and the Family, 52,* 21–29.
A study examining predictors of, and changes in, marital satisfaction before and after the birth of a child.

Whiffen, V. E., & Gotlib, I. H. (1989). Infants of postpartum depressed mothers: Temperament and cognitive status. *Journal of Abnormal Psychology, 98,* 274–279.
An article examining the temperament and cognitive functioning of 2-month-old infants of mothers who had experienced an episode of postpartum depression.

Whiffen, V. E., & Gotlib, I. H. (1993). A comparison of postpartum and nonpostpartum depression: Clinical presentation, psychiatric history, and psychosocial functioning. *Journal of Consulting and Clinical Psychology, 61,* 485–494.
A paper examining differences in phenomenology and family history between depression occurring during the postpartum period and depression occurring in nonpregnant women.

81

Breastfeeding

Ruth A. Lawrence

Since the mid-20th century, infant feeding has involved a choice for new mothers. Prior to that time, most women were expected to breastfeed their infants, as the alternatives were less than optimal. Now adequate substitute feedings are available that biochemically provide what scientists have identified as minimal nutritional support for the growth of a newborn infant. Given this contribution by medical science, each woman is faced with the decision about how she will feed her infant. The most important part of this decision is that the mother be well informed about the options and alternatives. She must select the choice that will work best for her. We are living in a bottle-feeding culture. Women may lack personal support for breastfeeding at home, and often do not have within their own personal family structure someone who is knowledgeable and experienced about breastfeeding. This does not mean that a woman cannot succeed at breastfeeding. It means that her health care support team will need to be more involved.

Major changes in the number of women breastfeeding their infants and the duration of breastfeeding will not take place until women grow up knowing about breastfeeding. Thus, making feeding one's young common knowledge in the school system will be part of that transition. In any event, a woman interested in breastfeeding her infant should seek out a health care professional who supports this option and a pediatrician who is knowledgeable about and supportive of it.

What are the issues a mother should consider? The benefits of breastfeeding as compared to bottle feeding with artificial formula, for both the infant and the mother, are the prime determinants.

WHY BREASTFEED?

The most compelling reason to consider breastfeeding one's infant is the fact that human milk is meant for the human infant. It has "species specificity." This means that of the 4,000 mammalian species known to science, each one produces a milk that is carefully designed and engineered to fulfill the needs of the offspring of that species. There are large differences in the composition of various mammalian milks, but each species provides the nutrients most important for the optimal brain growth, body growth, bone growth, and general development of the offspring. If one analyzes the special properties of human milk, one sees that they meet the special needs of the human infant who is born the most immature of all mammals (with the exception of the marsupials—e.g., the platypus and kangaroo). The human infant is very immature and is dependent on its caregiver for its needs. The human brain will double in size in the first year of life, and the neurological system will develop rapidly during the same time. The nutrient demands for brain and neurological growth are very specific in the human infant. Only human milk contains the special nutrients that are ideal for this growth. Recent studies in premature infants in Europe and in full-term infants in the United States confirm the fact that infants who are exclusively breastfed accelerate in their intellectual and motor development.

Nutritional Benefits

Other nutrients in human milk are especially adapted for digestion and absorption by an immature newborn. The protein is very different from that in other mammalian milks. It is rapidly digested and absorbed, so that the stomach is empty in a breastfed baby in 90 minutes to 2 hours, whereas it takes 3–4 hours to digest and absorb infant formula and 6 hours to digest cow's milk. Human milk contains dozens of active enzymes that facilitate the digestion and absorption of the nutrients, especially calcium, phosphorus, and the microminerals (e.g., iron, zinc, and copper). Enzymes are also known to affect the immature intestinal tract of the human infant, stimulating maturation so that nutrients are more readily absorbed. Much of the information about this has been accumulated by studying premature infants, who tolerate artificial formulas less well because their intestinal tracts are immature, and who benefit greatly from these active enzymes. There is a long litany of special enzymes with various functions, including infection protection and nutrient digestion and absorption. None has been developed synthetically.

Infection Protection

Apart from the fact that human milk is the ideal food for the human infant, human milk provides protection against infection. This protection for the newborn infant is very important in all species. It is well known in the field of animal husbandry that a newborn cannot be taken from its mother unless minimal amounts of early milk and its antibodies are provided, if the offspring is to survive against infection. For the human infant in developed countries, the benefits of being breastfed as protection against infection have been somewhat masked by the liberal use of antibiotics in artificially fed infants. In developing countries, where health care is less advanced and antibiotics are scarce or unavailable, being breastfed is a matter of life and death: Half the babies who are not breastfed will die from infections in the first year of life. In developed countries, which have better sanitation, better health care, and an abundance of antibiotics, the difference is not as blatantly obvious. Careful studies, however, have shown that there are few cases of otitis media, upper and lower respiratory infections, intestinal tract infections, and even urinary tract infections in infants who are exclusively breastfed. From a biochemical standpoint, several constituents of human milk protect against infection. These include antibodies, globulins, compounds that suppress the growth of pathogens and enhance the growth of normal bacteria, and living cells that destroy bacteria and viruses in the intestinal tract as they do in the rest of the body. In addition to providing protection against ordinary infections, breastfeeding is notable for furnishing protection against respiratory syncytial virus, which causes devastating pulmonary disease in young infants, and rota virus, which causes significant infection of the intestinal tract in artificially fed infants.

Immunological Protection

In the last decade, numerous studies have identified additional protective qualities of human milk, which have been attributed to its immunological constituents. Numerous studies have found that infants who are exclusively breastfed for at least 4 months have a reduced incidence of childhood-onset diabetes, especially among infants born to families with a strong family history of diabetes. Similar studies have demonstrated protective qualities against Crohn's disease and celiac disease. Epidemiological studies following large numbers of children in the United States have shown a clear association between exclusive breastfeeding for at least 4 months and a decreased incidence in childhood of specific malignancies, including lymphoma and acute lymphocytic leukemia. The association with the early onset of allergic symptoms such as eczema, rhinitis, and asthma also reveals that exclusive breastfeeding and other environmental protective procedures delay the onset of serious allergic disease, especially in children born into families with a high incidence of allergic phenomena.

Psychological Benefits

The one reason to breastfeed that withstood the competition when physicians were embracing the scientific, measurable constituents of artificial formula was that major psychological benefits are associated with the special relationship between the breastfeeding mother and her infant. The psychological bond between mother and infant is strong; it cannot be duplicated. The close physical contact, as well as the psychological impact of knowing that a mother is able to nourish her newborn baby completely with her own milk, is crucial. Evaluations of infants who were exclusively breastfed for 4–6 months have shown that at the age of 3, they are more self-assured, have greater self-esteem, and are more outgoing than comparable infants who were artificially fed. Breastfed infants have also been observed to progress along the developmental scales more rapidly than artificially fed infants.

Benefits for the Mother

The benefits of breastfeeding are not limited to benefits for the infant; there are many advantages for the mother as well. One of the first areas of interest has been the relationship of breastfeeding to breast cancer. Many years of following large groups of women have demonstrated that women who breastfeed their infants have a lower incidence of breast cancer than women who do not breastfeed their infants, and the difference is even greater between breastfeeding women and women who bear no children at all. A similar correlation has now been made with ovarian cancer, demonstrating the apparent protective qualities of breastfeeding for the mother. The explanation for this difference has been tentatively proposed to be related to the hormonal milieu of pregnancy and lactation, compared to the normal menstrual cycle over the years.

A point of great interest for women is the potential for developing osteoporosis. Logic might suggest that women who nurse their infants, particularly for many months, might easily be subject to greater leaching of calcium from the bone, setting themselves up for osteoporosis. Quite the contrary is true: Pregnancy and lactation change the body's ability to absorb and metabolize calcium. As a result, long-term studies have shown that although women who breastfeed their infants have decreased bone density at the end of lactation they actually have a lower incidence of long term osteoporosis.

Maintaining one's physiological weight and avoiding obesity are concerns of many young women. For many women, the experience of pregnancy involves the storing of additional weight beyond that required for the weight of the fetus and the gravid uterus. Many women have trouble losing that extra weight when they finally deliver their infants. Women who breastfeed tend to return to their prepregnancy weight more rapidly, with the final weight loss occurring when their babies are weaned. The postweaning weight of lactating women tends to be equal to the prepregnancy weight in a greater number of individuals. This suggests that lactation provides some degree of protection against obesity, which is one of the leading U.S. health problems today. It requires at least 500 calories a day to produce adequate milk for a newborn infant. Depending on the infant's intake, a mother may actually produce 1,000 calories of milk per day. The breasts are extremely efficient organs and do not require many additional calories for the "work of making milk." The body naturally stores extra weight during pregnancy, in anticipation of nourishing the infant once it is born.

The ovulation suppression effect of full lactation is yet another advantage of breastfeeding, since it decreases the probability of early return of ovulation and risk of early postpartum pregnancy. The practical application of this phenomenon is discussed by Labbok in her chapter on the lactational amenorrhea method of birth spacing.

Contraindications to Breastfeeding

The contraindications to breastfeeding are rare. There are, however, a few uncommon metabolic disorders of infancy that require very specialized feedings deficient in certain amino acids or galactose; in such cases, provision of human milk would not be appropriate. In the developed world, the risk of transmission of HIV (AIDS) via the breast milk, although slight, is an absolute contraindication to breastfeeding if the mother is HIV-positive. In developing countries, where survival itself depends on being breastfed, the risk of AIDS is the lesser of two evils.

The main reason for not breastfeeding is a lack of desire to do so on the part of the mother. It is a personal decision, and a mother should have every opportunity to consider her options. For many years some health care providers have hesitated to discuss infant-feeding options with their patients, for fear of making the mothers feel guilty if they did not choose to breastfeed. Careful studies of this question show that women who are provided the opportunity to make well-informed decisions are comfortable with the decisions they make for themselves and do not feel guilty.

PREPARING TO FEED THE NEWBORN

Once it has been established that pregnancy is in progress, a woman needs to begin to think about how she will manage her newborn infant. A baby changes the mother's life, and she will need to make many adaptations. If she decides to breastfeed, the mother should take comfort in the fact that Mother Nature is already preparing the breasts for this event. From the very early stages of pregnancy, the breasts begin to respond to the hormonal milieu of pregnancy and the establishment of the placenta. The hormones that develop the fetus and stimulate placental function also stimulate the breasts to grow and develop into a well-designed milk-producing system. Lactation is the physiological completion of the reproductive cycle, and the breasts are prepared to nourish the young after delivery any time after 16 weeks' gestation.

Full lactation is possible once the placenta has been delivered. The hormones produced by the placenta that have blocked the breasts from full milk production are gone. The breasts respond by filling with milk over the next few days. Full milk production depends on adequate stimulus of the breasts by the infant or a breast pump. Infants are born equipped to nurse at the breast. They have the appropriate reflexes (the rooting reflex and the suck-and-swallow reflex), and they know what to do. Women are not born knowing how to breastfeed; it is a learned skill.

In Western culture, where women now often do not grow up in large families where babies are being breastfed, women have to learn about this on their own. Reading books during pregnancy helps, but being in contact with women who have nursed their infants provides not only information but encouragement and support for a new mother. There are a number of mother-to-mother programs around the world. The best-known of these is La Leche League International. It has a network of mothers who are League leaders in almost every country of the world. They provide classes prenatally, to inform a woman about the process and to provide her with an opportunity to see a baby at the breast. A woman should talk with her obstetrical care provider and ask any questions that may arise about size and shape of the breast; changes during pregnancy; and the size, shape, and contour of the nipples. Even if a woman comes to the delivery with no preparation, her breasts are ready, her baby is ready, and the delivery and postpartum staff are ready to assist.

BREASTFEEDING AND SEXUALITY

Breastfeeding is physiologically and psychologically related to the reproductive cycle and to sexuality. The hormones that control the menstrual cycle are active in pregnancy and in lactation. The preparation of the breast for lactation during pregnancy, with the proliferation of the ductal system and the multiplication of the milk-producing lacteal cells, is an example of the effect of estrogens and progesterones. The two key hormones responsible for the production of milk in the lacteal cells and the ejection of milk from the duct system are prolactin and oxytocin, respectively. These hormones are also noted to act during lovemaking and sex in both the male and female. Although nursing an infant is not an erotic activity, on rare occasions in some women, it may cause a mild sensation of stimulation. On the other hand, a woman can experience normal sexual relations while lactating. In some studies, it has been noted that breastfeeding women are more ready to resume sexual relations after childbirth than are bottle-feeding women.

In the act of lovemaking, handling the breasts during lactation is acceptable. Some couples are distressed by the occasional dripping of milk. This can be minimized by feeding the infant or pumping the breasts beforehand. Some partners express concern about the mother's providing her breasts for the nourishment of the child instead of preserving them for the exclusive role in lovemaking. Although lactation is not incompatible with a good sexual relationship, some individuals (both male and female) have been unduly influenced by the public display of breasts and the sexual connotations the breasts are assigned, making it difficult for them to think rationally about breastfeeding. These individuals may be helped by counseling. Often this is only a symptom of a larger problem involving a woman's sexuality, rights, and behaviors.

FURTHER READING

Huggins, K. (1993). *The nursing mother's companion* (rev. ed.). Boston: Harvard Common Press. The author helps women through the decision making regarding infant feeding, and then explains how to breastfeed and what to do when small problems arise.

La Leche League International. (1997). *The womanly art of breastfeeding* (6th ed.). Shaumburg, IL: Author.
La Leche League International is a worldwide network of nursing mothers who help other mothers to breastfeed successfully. This is their guide to this womanly art.

Shevlov, S. P. (Ed.). (1993). *Caring for your baby and young child.* New York: Bantam Books.
The chapter on breastfeeding provides a discussion of the key reasons to consider breastfeeding and the basic information helpful in initiating the process. The text itself is a complete guide to child care for the first 5 years, written by pediatric experts.

82

The Lactational Amenorrhea Method

Miriam H. Labbok

WHAT IS THE LACTATIONAL AMENORRHEA METHOD?

Breastfeeding and lactation are inborn functions of the human body. The many roles of breastfeeding in the survival of the species have long been ignored. The benefits are taken for granted if breastfeeding occurs; the lack of these benefits goes unnoticed, and they are assumed to be nonessential, if breastfeeding is forsaken. Breastfeeding is now recognized as a public health intervention that has a major impact on many maternal and child health concerns. (For a fuller discussion of the advantages of breastfeeding, see Lawrence's chapter in this volume.)

Although it is by no means a new idea, the fertility-suppressing benefit of breastfeeding has received special attention in the last few decades. Although the "old wives' tale" that breastfeeding will delay pregnancy has frequently been dismissed, a small group of researchers has pursued the better understanding of breastfeeding-related infertility, some with the goal of providing women with a better understanding of their own bodies' potential. One of the results of this interest has been the development of an interim, introductory postpartum method of family planning now known as the "lactational amenorrhea method" (LAM). This method of family planning is now in use in more than 30 countries, and has been included in the family-planning and maternal and child health policies of several countries.

LAM is presented to a new mother as an algorithm (see Figure 82.1). It includes the three criteria for defining the period of lowest pregnancy risk, and then advises immediate commencement of another method that complements the effects of breastfeeding thereafter. The mother is asked, or asks herself, whether her menses have resumed, whether she is no longer fully or nearly fully breastfeeding (see Figure 82.2), and whether the infant is 6 months of age or older. If any of these three criteria is true, she is advised to begin the next method. If she is interested in and qualifies for LAM, she is advised to ask herself the same three questions in an ongoing manner, and to return to the clinic immediately if she has any questions as to whether or not the method still applies.

Ask the mother, or advise her to ask herself,
these three questions:

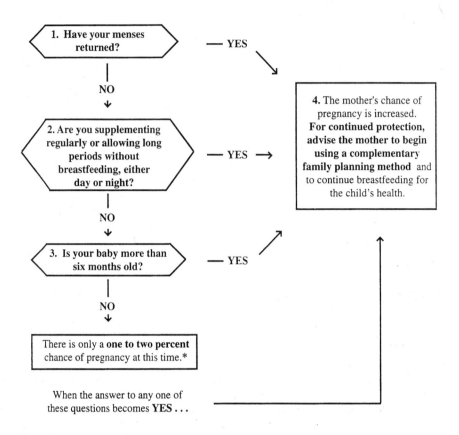

*However, the mother may choose to use a complementary family planning method *at any time.*

FIGURE 82.1. Algorithm for LAM; this is presented to a new mother who is considering the method. From Labbok, Cooney, and Coly (1994). Copyright 1994 by the Institute for Reproductive Health, Georgetown University. Reprinted by permission.

LAM serves as a vital adjunct and adds a special new perspective to family-planning programs and services. Not only does it provide a method free of drugs and devices, and therefore free of ongoing cost, it also encourages optimal breastfeeding behaviors, providing synergistic support for primary health of the mother and child.

Breastfeeding and LAM are complementary. Women who breastfeed their infants have, on average, longer intervals between births. This spacing alone is known to be independently associated with improved maternal and child survival. Furthermore, the occurrence of the next pregnancy is one of the major reasons women choose to stop or limit breastfeeding. Therefore, although breastfeeding enhances child spacing, the timely initiation of complementary family planning is necessary to ensure the recommended minimal child spacing of 3 years, which supports maternal recovery and allows for sustained breastfeeding.

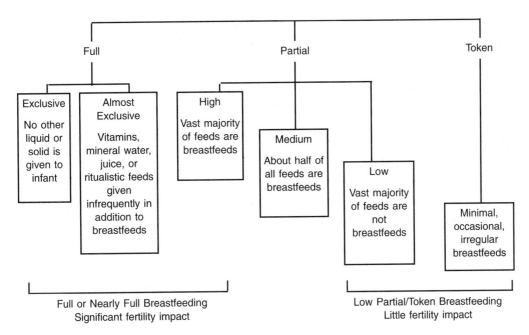

FIGURE 82.2. Definitions of "full," "parital," and "token" breastfeeding patterns. Intervals for full or nearly full breastfeeding should not exceed 4 hours during the day, 6 hours at night, and supplementation should not exceed 5–15% of all feeding episodes, preferably fewer. While the high–partial pattern is adequate for fertility suppression, women should be counseled that any supplementation or disruption of the breastfeeding pattern can increase the risk of fertility return.

THE HISTORY OF THE UNDERSTANDING
OF BREASTFEEDING AND FERTILITY

Women have long been aware that breastfeeding is associated with increased child spacing. First, Aristotle, then medical writers of the Renaissance, noted that women who suckled were less likely to become pregnant. When the phenomenon was forgotten in the age of infant-feeding substitutes, it became an "old wives' tale"; indeed, it has been actively refuted in our modern society, where proof and efficacy are scientific musts. However, today there is a melding of women's beliefs and science. Demographers have shown us the population-level impact of breastfeeding on fertility; medical and biological research has identified the biological basis of lactational infertility; and in the last 15 years, public health researchers and clinicians have discovered how we might optimize the fertility-suppressive effects of breastfeeding.

The World Fertility Surveys, among other surveys of the 1970s and 1980s, identified the association between breastfeeding and child spacing. In countries or regions with breastfeeding norms, the average birth interval (after family-planning use was controlled for) was longer than where breastfeeding norms had deteriorated. Furthermore, where breastfeeding was more intensive, with full breastfeeding patterns, this effect was augmented. Lactational infertility was shown to be associated with only a 2–15% chance of pregnancy, whereas nonlactating women experienced a 40–60% chance. Although these figures are not directly comparable, the effect is real and profound.

The biological basis of lactational infertility and its control have been studied more carefully only in the last 30 years. Data published in the early 1970s showed that women who breastfed were less likely to ovulate. When breastfeeding was more intensive, a triple phenomenon was found: delayed return of menses, less likelihood of normal ovulation in general, and less likelihood of normal ovulation prior to the first menstrual-like bleed. In the early 1980s, we proposed that contraception is not necessary until one of three criteria occurs: return of menses, less than full breastfeeding, or the infant's reaching 6 months of age (the time when supplement is suggested and when the infant's stomach is able to hold sufficient quantities that breastfeedings become more infrequent).

In the 1970s and 1980s, two major approaches were studied to assess whether this biological phenomenon could be exploited as a viable method for child spacing. Tyson proposed the use of thyroid-stimulating hormone to accentuate the ovulation suppression, whereas McNeilly, Howie, and Glasier explored behavioral factors associated with fertility suppression. Gray and colleagues followed a large cohort prospectively, tracking behaviors and hormones, and Perez and others began clinical testing of an algorithm. Additional researchers including Gross, Shaaban, and Parenteau-Carreau, worked with Kennedy on a multicenter trial, while Diaz and others looked at the issue as part of several postpartum contraception studies. In 1988, this work and the research of several centers around the world was shared at a meeting at Bellagio, Italy, and the scientists agreed that the three criteria noted above would be sufficient to serve as a method. This agreement became known as the Bellagio consensus; the consensus and the research supporting it are presented in a 1989 article by Kennedy and colleagues. A few months later, this approach was presented to a group of family-planning service providers at a meeting at Georgetown University, and the LAM was born.

DOES THE METHOD WORK, AND IS IT ACCEPTABLE?

The first major study of LAM actually began in 1987, based on the guidelines we proposed in the early 1980s, but it was rapidly adjusted following the birth of LAM. This controlled prospective clinical trial of the LAM was begun in Santiago, Chile. LAM users achieved 99.6% efficacy (6-month life table), confirming effectiveness comparable to that of most modern methods of contraception. Since that time many more studies have followed, each finding similar results.

LAM has been found acceptable worldwide in maternities, free-standing family-planning clinics, mother-to-mother counseling, and maternal and child health care facilities. Studies in the United States have found that women appreciate the period of time when they do not have to worry about pills or diaphragms, and men appreciate the ease and efficacy. Mothers and fathers alike note that LAM improves their understanding of the physiological importance of breastfeeding, and they are proud of the positive health benefits to their children.

Since this method is behavior-based, there is no organization in the United States with the mandate to review its safety. For this reason and others, the World Health Organization, Family Health International, and my own organization (the Institute for Reproductive Health, Department of Obstetrics and Gynecology, Georgetown University) assembled an internationally recognized panel sponsored by the Rockefeller Foundation to meet in Bellagio, Italy, in December 1995, to consider the safety and efficacy of the method. The conclusion of this expert panel was that the method is safe, efficacious, and ready for widespread introduction into family planning and health systems worldwide.

CONCLUSIONS

Today, the LAM parameters have been studied, considered, and accepted by organizations as diverse as the World Health Organization and UNICEF, and LAM is in use in nearly 40 countries. In addition to being a reliable method of contraception, LAM encourages the actions and behaviors that result in improved chances for optimal infant health and development, as well as optimal maternal health and survival. We cannot afford to continue to ignore the multiple benefits of breastfeeding, and LAM is one health care approach that creates a health synergy reinforcing both healthy child spacing and healthy breastfeeding at low monetary cost.

FURTHER READING

Cooney, K. A., Koniz-Booher, P., & Coly, S. (1997). *Taking the first steps: A decade of experience.* Washington, DC: Institute for Reproductive Health, Georgetown University.
This book reviews the many studies and trials of LAM as well as presenting major conclusions and field experiences.

Cooney, K., Labbok, M., & Coly, S. (Eds.). (1994). Breastfeeding as a woman's issue: A dialogue on health, family planning, work, and feminism. *International Journal of Gynecology and Obstetrics, 47,* 1–74.
Proceedings of a meeting and workshop on the subject of breastfeeding.

Hight-Laukaran, V., Labbok, M., Peterson, A., Fletcher, V., von Hertzen, H., & Van Look, P. (1997). Multicenter Study of the Lactational Amenorrhea Method (LAM): II. Acceptability, utility, and policy implications. *Contraception, 55,* 337–346.
This article contains the most up-to-date findings on LAM.

Kennedy, K., Rivera, R., & McNeilly, A. (1989). Consensus statement on the use of breastfeeding as a family planning method. *Contraception, 39,* 477–496.
This article served as the scientific base for the later codification of LAM at Georgetown.

Kennedy, K., Labbok, M., & Van Look, P. (1996). Consensus statement: Lactational Amenorrhea Method for family planning. *International Journal of Gynecology and Obstetrics, 54,* 55–57.
The 1995 consensus statement.

Labbok, M. (1983). Breastfeeding and contraception. *New England Journal of Medicine, 308,* 51.
The first version of a breastfeeding-based method to be presented in referred journal literature; it served as a basis for the structure of LAM.

Labbok, M., Cooney, K., & Coly, S. (1994). *Guidelines: Breastfeeding, family planning, and the lactational amenorrhea method (LAM).* Washington, DC: Institute for Reproductive Health. Georgetown University.
This booklet is derived from the Georgetown meeting of 1989. It includes an explanation of the development of LAM; clinical guidance for its use; descriptions of patterns of breastfeeding; and first-, second-, and third-choice family planning options for use during breastfeeding.

Labbok, M., Hight-Laukaran, V., Peterson, A., Fletcher, V., von Hertzen, H., & Van Look, P. (1997). Multicenter Study of the Lactational Amenorrhea Method (LAM): I. Efficacy, duration, and implications for clinical application. *Contraception, 55,* 327–336.
This article contains the most up-to-date findings on LAM.

83

Contraception

Susan A. Ballagh

An estimated 60 million women in the United States are at risk for unintended pregnancy each year. Of the 6 million pregnancies per year, 41% are unintended; half of these are attributable to the 10% of sexually active women who choose not to practice contraception. The other half of unintended pregnancies result from contraceptive method failures. Therefore, better use of existing methods and selection of more effective methods among women using contraception could have a dramatic impact on unwanted pregnancy.

The most effective method of contraception is abstinence, with only one recorded failure in literature. This and castration are the most effective methods available. Few are interested in such extreme measures, however. This chapter discusses other methods of contraception currently available in the United States (with the exception of the lactational amenorrhea method, which is discussed by Labbok in her chapter).

PERMANENT AND REVERSIBLE STERILIZATION METHODS

One third of sexually active couples rely on permanent sterilization to prevent pregnancy. These methods are not intended to be reversed (despite some success with surgical reversal). Male sterilization or vasectomy is used by 10% of couples. It is a 20-minute office procedure that interrupts the sperm exit tract from the testicle. The procedure is accomplished with a local anesthetic and becomes effective 3–6 months later, when all of the developing sperm have been flushed from the tract. Female sterilization or tubal ligation is used by one-fourth of couples, and is performed by interrupting or removing a portion of the fallopian tube. When this is done immediately following childbirth, a small incision is made in the navel, and a portion of the tube is removed from the incision. In other situations, the tube is interrupted by means of laparoscopy. When the procedure is uncomplicated, it can be done under local anesthesia, but many women opt for general anesthesia to avoid pain and to allow for successful completion in the event of unforeseen complicating factors. The complications of female sterilization are greater because a more involved surgical intervention is required. It is important to remember that either method fails about 1 time in 100 during the first year. Women experiencing pregnancy more than 1 year after tubal sterilization are more likely to have a tubal pregnancy.

Three reversible methods provide efficacy equal to that of permanent sterilization. One, the T-shaped intrauterine device (IUD) called the ParaGard, is inserted into the uterus in the office and provides protection for 10 years. The method works by killing sperm, thus preventing fertilization. Women in mutually monogamous relationships, with a low risk of acquiring sexually transmitted diseases (STDs), are good candidates for this method. It is a particularly good alternative for married women who have completed their families. This method is underutilized. Only 1% of U.S. women use this very effective method, compared to 12–25% of women in Canada and Europe. Unlike the Dalkon Shield, which had serious design flaws and is no longer marketed in the United States, the ParaGard is safe and has been thoroughly reviewed by the Food and Drug Administration (FDA). Women with multiple sexual partners, or women with very heavy menstrual cramping or flow, may be better off using a different method.

The other two methods with fewer than 1 pregnancy per 100 couples per year provide continuous release of an analogue of the female hormone, called progesterone, which is present in the second half of the menstrual cycle. Women with many symptoms during the week before their menses may experience similar sensations with these contraceptives. Both of the methods are associated with irregular bleeding, which is less than the normal blood loss but may be spread out over 20 or more days per month. One method, called Depo-Provera, is a shot given every 3 months. It is the most effective method and is very private. Irregular bleeding is reduced with continued use; 90% of women have no menses by the end of 2 years. It is associated with increased appetite and weight gain. The method should be discontinued at least 6 months before trying to conceive, as persistent hormones may delay pregnancy. The other method, Norplant, involves the insertion of six capsules beneath the skin of the upper arm and is done during an office visit. These capsules release levonorgestrel continuously for 5 years. Initial bleeding with this method may be irregular but infrequent. At least 1 year of frequent erratic bleeding is common, but with time this bleeding becomes more regular. There is no delay in the return of fertility after the capsules are removed. Women with previous tubal pregnancies, or those who easily develop ovarian cysts, may have difficulty with this method. Women with medical problems that prevent use of estrogen hormones can use Norplant or Depo-Provera successfully, as they have little effect on blood clotting.

ESTROGEN-CONTAINING ORAL CONTRACEPTIVES AND THE PROGESTERONE-RELEASING INTRAUTERINE DEVICE

The next tier of contraceptive effectiveness involves oral contraceptives and the progesterone-releasing IUD called Progestasert. Of 100 couples using these methods for 1 year, 2, or 3 will experience an unwanted pregnancy. The oral contraceptive is packaged with 21 hormone pills containing an estrogen (called ethinyl estradiol or mestranol) and a progestin (either norethindrone or its acetate, ethynodiol diacetate, levonorgestrel, norgestrel, desogestrel, or norgestimate). Some pill packages also contain inactive pills (which may contain iron or lactose) to be taken for 7 days between hormone cycles. There are many health benefits for women who use these combination oral contraceptives, including reduced ovarian and endometrial cancer; fewer benign breast or ovarian cysts; less anemia, less pelvic inflammatory disease, which can cause infertility; and fewer tubal (ectopic) pregnancies. There are nearly three dozen combinations of dose and medication types; most women can find a combination that is right for them. Some combinations can be used to treat acne, increased hair growth, endometriosis, or painful menses. Women who smoke and are over 35 years old are not good candidates for this method. If they cannot quit smoking, they should consider progestin-only methods or barriers. Women who have had a stroke or a heart attack because of blood clotting, or who have had blood clots in their legs, should not take these pills.

The progesterone-releasing IUD called the Progestasert is placed into the uterus through the cervix in the office. It releases progesterone continuously, making the uterine lining inhospitable for 1 year. It is recommended for women in mutually monogamous relationships, who are at low risk for STDs. Unlike the copper IUD, it does not increase bleeding or cramps. It is not effective in reducing tubal pregnancy, so women with prior ectopic pregnancies are better off choosing a method that prevents ovulation or fertilization. Women with prior difficulty with other IUDs have switched to this method successfully.

TRADITIONAL (MALE) CONDOMS AND PROGESTIN-ONLY CONTRACEPTIVES

Traditional latex condoms protect against STDs and prevent pregnancy. Since most contraceptive methods do not provide protection against STDs, condoms are often used in combination with other methods to prevent diseases while simultaneously improving protection against pregnancy. Dubbed a "male method," condoms can be supplied by the woman partner, since she is much more likely to suffer the consequences of STDs. Use of lubrication improves the protection of condoms by reducing tearing and leakage. When condoms are used in conjunction with vaginal spermicide, the unintended pregnancy rate per 100 couples is 5 per year. When they are used alone, the unintended pregnancy rate rises to 12 per year with typical use. The condom is applied to the erect penis and may interfere with normal sexual function for some couples. In addition, the rates given here are estimates and vary greatly with the consistency of practice. A condom can only work if it is used! For couples with latex allergy, polyurethane male condoms are available. While not yet confirmed, the new products are likely to have similar efficacy to the latex male condom.

Progestin-only birth control pills have efficacy similar to that of condoms when used alone. Each package contains 28 equivalent pills, and progesterone-type hormone is taken continuously with this method. Two types of pills are available: norethindrone or its acetate, ethynodiol diacetate, and norgestrel. They are most frequently used in breast-feeding women, since they do not reduce milk production. They can also be used in conjunction with other methods, such as condoms or vaginal spermicide, to provide greater efficacy. Irregular bleeding is common in women who are not breastfeeding. Absence of menses is more common in breastfeeding women using this method.

FEMALE BARRIER METHODS, FERTILITY AWARENESS, AND WITHDRAWAL

The next tier of contraceptive efficacy includes female barrier methods for women who have never delivered, fertility awareness, and withdrawal. These methods result in a 20% rate of unintended pregnancies per year.

The diaphragm and the cervical cap are rubber devices that are inserted into the vagina with spermicide to prevent entry of sperm into the cervix. The diaphragm, which must be fitted by a medical practitioner, can be placed up to 6 hours before intercourse without repeated application of spermicide. It is worn at least 6 hours following intercourse. To avoid infection, it should be worn a maximum of 24 hours. The diaphragm must be fitted correctly and is available by prescription only. Extra spermicide should be added in the vagina for subsequent ejaculations. The spermicide can be purchased without a prescription. Some women have difficulty with urinary tract infections with the diaphragm and prefer the cervical cap. The cap also requires fitting, and 6–10% of women cannot be fitted with this method. It is more difficult to learn to insert and remove initially, but women who have used both methods report the cap to be more comfortable. It can be worn up to 48 hours without needing additional spermicide. Petroleum products (such as Vaseline), heat, or sun exposure can damage either the diaphragm or the cervical cap. Both of these methods reduce the incidence of STDs, and both methods are much more effective in women who have not delivered a baby. The unintended pregnancy rate increases to 35 per 100 couples per year for women who have carried a pregnancy beyond 20 weeks.

The Reality female condom is a thin polyurethane sheath with two flexible polyurethane rings. One ring at the "bottom" of the bag is placed in the upper vagina, and the other ring forms a barrier outside. It is not used with spermicide and should not be used with the traditional (male) condom. Each condom can be inserted up to 8 hours before sex, but is intended for one-time use only. The female condom was designed to prevent the spread of STDs, but its lower success rate in preventing pregnancy compared to the male condom suggests that it may also provide less STD protection. The Today vaginal contraceptive sponge, which contained spermicide, is no longer manufactured because of changes in FDA requirements that were too costly to implement. Other forms of spermicide can be used in the vagina and have similar efficacy.

Fertility awareness, also called the "rhythm method" or "natural family planning," is estimated to have an unintended pregnancy rate of 20 per 100 couples per year overall. The rate varies dramatically, depending on the technique used, the number of days per cycle that abstinence is observed, and the regularity of the woman's menstruation. Calendar, basal body temperature, cervical mucus, and ovulatory symptoms may all be used to increase effectiveness.

Successful users of the withdrawal method also experience unintended pregnancy 20% of the time. Too often discounted, withdrawal is a male method that is used in many cultures. Couples using this method do not have sexual difficulties, provided that both partners can reach climax satisfactorily. The combination of these two methods offers a very low-cost alternative for some couples that does not require medical assistance.

FURTHER READING

Hatcher, R. A., Trussel, J., Stewart, F., Stewart, G. K., Kowal, D., Guest, F., Cates, W., & Policar, M. S. (1994). *Contraceptive technology* (16th rev. ed). New York: Irvington.

84

Abortion

Nancy E. Adler
Lauren B. Smith

*T*herapeutic abortion is one of the most commonly performed surgical procedures; over 1 million abortions are performed each year in the United States. Unlike other medical procedures, abortion involves a range of issues regarding the individual woman, her partner and family, the health care provider, and society. In addition to biomedical issues, abortion involves religious, moral, psychological, legal, and social considerations. The procedure has been subject to different legal constraints; since the U.S. Supreme Court decision in *Roe v. Wade* in 1973, abortion has been legal in all states. Current efforts to restrict access to abortion, particularly for adolescents, have focused in part on the psychological and medical risks of the procedure. In this chapter, we also review research on the consequences of abortion.

In any examination of the effects of abortion, findings must be placed in the appropriate context. Abortion occurs only in the context of an unwanted pregnancy. Thus, one cannot isolate the effect of abortion alone. Psychological reactions following abortion are not simply responses to the procedure, but to the entire experience of having had an unwanted pregnancy. The medical risks of abortion must be compared to those of childbirth, and the psychosocial risks must be compared to those experienced by women who carry an unwanted pregnancy to term. Under current conditions, where women who wish to terminate a pregnancy can do so, appropriate comparisons of women who *must* carry to term do not exist. However, through we cannot directly test the impact of termination per se, we can make inferences from the studies of women who have undergone abortion.

PROCEDURES AND MEDICAL RISKS

Vacuum aspiration is the most common procedure for abortions performed at 13 weeks of gestation or less. This procedure removes the contents of the uterus, can be done with local anesthesia, and is generally completed in about 15 minutes. Although some physicians perform vacuum aspiration in the second trimester, most second-trimester procedures are done by means of saline administration, which causes a miscarriage; women experience severe cramps similar to labor, although not as intense. The vast majority of abortions (almost 90%) are performed in the first trimester.

Induced abortion is a medical procedure, and it involves health risks. Potential complications of abortion include infection, hemorrhage, cervical injury, and uterine perforation. The death rate for abortion has been declining in the United States since abortion became legally available. In 1972, there were 4.1 deaths per 100,000 procedures, which dropped to 0.4 deaths per 100,000 procedures by 1987. Before 1977, causes of death most frequently involved infection and hemorrhage, but since 1983, complications with anesthesia have been the leading cause of death. In contrast, the death rate resulting from childbirth is 9 deaths per 100,000 cases, and 22% of pregnant women have predelivery complications that require hospitalization. Current data support the assertion that abortion involves far fewer maternal health risks than childbirth.

Recently, medical abortion through the use of mifepristone (RU-486) became an alternative. This involves administration of two pills a few days apart. The procedure has few medical side effects, but causes cramping and bleeding. It is, however, not always effective in inducing an abortion. About 4% of women who are given RU-486 subsequently have to undergo a surgical procedure in order to complete the abortion. RU-486 has been used by many women in other countries, but because of political restrictions it is currently available in the United States only to women participating in clinical trials.

DECISION MAKING

Many women reach the decision to have an abortion without significant difficulty. The vast majority are certain about their decision, and few women change their minds; indeed, most women have decided upon a course of action prior to seeking a pregnancy test. Many factors affect the decision to have an abortion. Since many women who have abortions already have children or plan to have them later in life, the decision to abort is strongly related to situational variables. Although most of the attention on psychological distress has focused on the postabortion period, longitudinal studies that have followed women from prior to the abortion until afterward find that the period of greatest distress is prior to the procedure. This distress may result from conflicts over decision making, from adverse reactions to having an unwanted pregnancy, or from anticipation of the procedure. Following abortion, indicators of distress begin to decline and continue to decline over time.

PSYCHOLOGICAL SEQUELAE

The psychological sequelae of abortion have received substantial attention. Clinical case studies predominated in the early research on psychological responses to abortion, and the focus was often on psychopathological responses. More empirical studies, based on more representative samples and using better measurement, have not revealed a high incidence of pathological responses. The predominant emotions reported after abortion are positive ones, most frequently happiness and relief. More recent studies have begun to include scales to capture the mixture of feelings that women may experience following abortion, in contrast to earlier research, which examined only negative emotions.

An alternative model to the psychopathological approach to postabortion responses is that of normal stress and coping. Stress results not simply from having an abortion, but from the entire experience of having an unwanted pregnancy that is terminated by abortion. Evidence from carefully controlled studies strongly support the theory that abortion is a relatively short-term stressor for the majority of women who undergo the procedure. Moreover, for some women it can be an empowering experience that increases positive feelings. Other women, however, do experience negative emotions following abortion, and it is important to determine the factors that are correlated with negative sequelae in these women who do not fare as well. Some of the key factors are described below.

Among the strongest predictors of poor psychological outcome are a woman's prior psychological functioning and psychiatric history. Prior mental health predicts responses to many kinds of stressors, including responses to spontaneous abortion. Although poor prior mental health would seem to be an obvious predictor of poor response to abortion, it has rarely been evaluated. A woman's prediction of how well she will cope with her decision is also related to her psychological response to abortion; coping expectancy is associated with the difficulty of the decision and the extent to which her partner and family support her decision to have an abortion.

Women who are terminating a pregnancy that was initially unwanted and unintended are less likely to show negative responses following abortion than those who are terminating for medical indications. The most adverse responses have been shown by women and their partners who have terminated a pregnancy following prenatal genetic testing that revealed a problem with the developing fetus. The sense of loss is likely to be much greater for those women (and their partners) than for those who are terminating an unintended and unwanted pregnancy. In addition, since genetic screening during pregnancy generally occurs in the second trimester, women who terminate because of genetic indications must undergo a second-trimester procedure.

As described earlier, the procedures for second-trimester abortions are more complicated and are experienced as being more stressful. Recent developments in prenatal diagnostic testing (e.g., chorionic villus sampling) provide information earlier in pregnancy and may reduce some of the problems for couples whose decision to terminate is based on adverse results. Prenatal genetic tests currently provide information on a range of diseases, including both childhood- and adult-onset diseases. Future testing may also include some cancers and behavioral traits. These developments will dramatically increase the complexity of the decision concerning whether to abort an affected fetus. Additional research on the psychological impact of these decisions will be a valuable extension of the current literature on abortion.

Finally, the context in which a woman makes her decision will influence her responses following abortion. Support from others, particularly from a woman's partner, is an important contributor to postabortion adjustment. Women who are pressured into terminating a pregnancy that they themselves wish to continue, and those whose partners oppose their decision to terminate, are both at greater risk for more adverse responses. Women who have strong religious beliefs or who are members of a religious community that opposes abortion may also have more difficulty following termination.

ADOLESCENTS

Several states have passed legislation mandating parental consent for abortion out of concern that adolescents lack sufficient cognitive abilities to make an informed choice and that they are at increased risk for adverse effects. There is considerable debate about whether adolescent women are competent to make a decision regarding abortion. It has been argued that adolescents do not have the necessary decision-making skills, including the capabilities to evaluate future consequences and to reason abstractly; however, studies empirically assessing adolescents' decision making have not borne this out. Although laboratory studies provide evidence that adolescents' reasoning differs from that of adults, naturalistic investigations of abortion decision making have not confirmed these findings, and it appears that adolescents' reasoning about abortion is similar to that of adults. Most adolescents consult with their parents regarding their decision. Even without mandated notification, the vast majority of adolescents voluntarily consult a parent or adult before obtaining an abortion (in one study, the rate of consultation was 95%). Adolescents who are younger and who are the most uncertain about abortion are the most likely to solicit parental guidance.

It is not clear whether, in fact, adolescents are at greater risk of negative responses following abortion than older women are. Several studies have found that age is negatively correlated with risk of negative responses: The younger the patient, the greater the likelihood of negative responses. However, most of these studies have included women across the entire childbearing age span, and there have not been separate analyses of adolescents in these studies. The few studies that focused specifically on adolescents have shown few adverse effects of abortion. One comparison of functioning over time among pregnant adolescents who had an abortion, pregnant adolescents who carried to term, and adolescents who had a negative pregnancy test found that, if anything, the abortion patients showed more favorable psychological responses 1 and 2 years later than the adolescents in the other two groups.

CONCLUSIONS

In the United States, political controversy over the legal status of abortion has complicated research on the psychological issues associated with the procedure. Assertions about the medical and psychological risks associated with abortion have been used to justify restrictions on the procedure, particularly for adolescents. Examination of the scientific literature, however, shows little evidence of severe negative responses when abortion is legal, is performed in the appropriate medical setting, and is freely chosen. Nevertheless, having to terminate a pregnancy, whether initially wanted or unwanted, can be a stressful experience. We need to continue our efforts to identify the factors that may contribute to more adverse responses, and to provide support and interventions for women who may be at greater risk. At the same time, we need to continue our research on determinants of unwanted pregnancy, in order to reduce the need for abortion.

FURTHER READING

Adler, N. E., David, H. P., Major, B. N., Roth, S. H., Russo, N. F., & Wyatt, G. E. (1990). Psychological responses after abortion. *Science, 248*, 41–44.
Report of an expert panel on the psychological responses of women to abortion.

Ambuel, B., & Rappaport, J. (1992). Developmental trends in adolescents' psychological and legal competence to consent to abortion. *Law and Human Behavior, 16*, 129–154.
A comprehensive study of pregnancy decision making and competence in different age groups of adolescents.

Cohan, C. L., Dunkel-Schetter, C., & Lydon, J. (1993). Pregnancy decision-making: Predictors of early stress and adjustment. *Psychology of Women Quarterly, 17*, 223–239.
Study demonstrating that women decide early in pregnancy regarding termination, that the timing of the decision is minimally related to later adjustment, and that negative responses resolve quickly following the procedure.

Koonin, L. M., Smith, J. C., & Ramick, M. (1995). Abortion surveillance—United States, 1991. *Morbidity and Mortality Weekly Reports, 44*, 23–53.
Provides the most recent statistics on abortion in the United States.

Lewis, C. C. (1987). Minors' competence to consent to abortion. *American Psychologist, 42*, 84–88.
Excellent discussion of issues surrounding adolescents' competence to make an informed decision regarding abortion.

Major, B., & Cozzarelli, C. (1992). Psychosocial predictors of adjustment to abortion. *Journal of Social Issues, 48*, 121–142.
Thorough review of the psychological and social factors that may influence responses following abortion.

Russo, N. F., Horn, J. D., & Schwartz, R. (1992). U.S. abortion in context: Selected characteristics and motivations of women seeking abortions. *Journal of Social Issues, 48*, 183–202.
Presents data on reasons why women in the United States choose to have an abortion.

Zabin, L., Hirsch, M. B., & Emerson, M. R. (1989). When urban adolescents choose abortion: Effects on education, psychological status and subsequent pregnancy. *Family Planning Perspectives, 21*, 248–255.
Two-year follow-up of adolescents who had an abortion, carried to term, or had a negative pregnancy test.

85

Reproductive Technologies

Linda C. Giudice

*I*nfertility affects approximately 15% of the U.S. population, and infertility resulting from a variety of causes can be cured by relatively simple therapies. However, infertility that is refractory to these treatments is approached by invoking the assisted reproductive technologies (ARTs). Since the birth of Louise Brown, the first "test tube" baby, in Great Britain in 1978, the ARTs leading up to her conception have advanced to the point of making most types of infertility curable in First World countries today. The wonders of these technologies are awe-inspiring. However, most couples, health care providers, and the general public are not well prepared for the emotional, ethical, financial, and legal consequences of ARTs. This chapter summarizes technical, emotional, and ethical aspects of ARTs.

WHAT IS A TYPICAL INFERTILITY WORKUP, AND WHAT ARE TYPICAL INFERTILITY THERAPIES?

About 40% of infertility can be attributed to a problem in the female partner ("female factor"), about 30% to a problem in the male partner ("male factor"), about 20% to problems in both partners ("combined factor"), and about 10% to neither partner ("unexplained" infertility). A typical infertility workup is shown in Table 85.1. This involves, for the male partner, evaluating the sperm by computer-assisted semen analysis; this is often accompanied by a mycoplasma culture of the seminal plasma. To evaluate compatibility between the woman's cervical mucus and the partner's sperm, a postcoital test is usually performed anywhere between 3 and 24 hours after coitus, around the middle of the woman's menstrual cycle. The workup for the female partner is more extensive and includes evaluating ovulation (by basal body temperature charting and endometrial biopsy); the anatomy of the uterine cavity and the fallopian tubes, as well as fallopian tube patency (by a hysterosalpingogram, a "dye" test); scar tissue (adhesions) or endometriosis in the pelvis (by laparoscopy); and endocrine and immune disorders that may contribute to poor implantation or inability to sustain a pregnancy (e.g., thyroid

TABLE 85.1. Typical Infertility Evaluation

Male partner	Both partners	Female partner
Semen analysis	Postcoital test	Basal body temperature chart
Mycoplasma		Endometrial biopsy
		Hysterosalpingogram
		Laparoscopy/hysteroscopy
		Hormonal evaluation
		Immune evaluation

disorders, pituitary gland dysfunctions, autoantibodies). Often laparoscopy is combined with hysteroscopy, a method of looking inside the uterine cavity with a fiber-optic lens. If poor ovulatory function is found then medications are administered to enhance ovulation. If the fallopian tubes are blocked, surgery may be performed. If there is a male factor, then ovulation enhancement (taking "fertility drugs" to increase the number of eggs [oocytes] matured and released) combined with intrauterine insemination is recommended. The latter is also recommended if no cause is found. If after several treatment cycles there is still no pregnancy, then the usual route is to proceed to ARTs.

ARE THERE MEASURES TO PREVENT INFERTILITY?

There are very few known causes of infertility that can truly be prevented. An exception is the avoidance of sexually transmitted diseases, which is critical for both women and men. The bulk of evidence indicates positive correlations between sexually transmitted diseases, such as gonorrhea and chlamydia, and scarred fallopian tubes and intrapelvic adhesions. Other healthy behaviors also have their advantages, although correlations between such behaviors and fertility are poorly understood. Avoidance of caffeine, alcohol, and cigarette smoking; minimizing stress; eating a well-balanced diet; and getting regular exercise have all been recommended for women (and men) attempting pregnancy. Doing all the "right things" will not necessarily improve fertility (although it cannot hurt), and it does contribute to one's state of well-being overall. In instances of known causes of infertility that have been treated, it is likely that there may still be elements of subfertility in one or both partners that remain unidentified, because the current state of our knowledge is incomplete with regard to the intricacies of the process of reproduction.

WHO NEEDS ASSISTED REPRODUCTIVE
TECHNOLOGIES, AND WHAT ARE THEY?

If (1) no pregnancy has occurred in patients who have undergone several cycles of ovulation enhancement and intrauterine insemination for unexplained or male factor infertility; (2) there is a severe male factor (very low count and motility, and a high percentage of abnormal sperm); or (3) the female partner has surgically incorrectable, scarred fallopian tubes, the next step is usually to proceed to ARTs. The age of the female partner is one of the critical determinants of success in ARTs, with fertility declining markedly after the age of 39 years.

The ARTs are a group of technologies that enhance fertility without natural intercourse. There are several groups, but the following are currently the most common:

classical *in vitro* fertilization and embryo transfer (IVF-ET), gamete intrafallopian transfer (GIFT), intracytoplasmic sperm injection (ICSI), assisted hatching (AH), and combinations thereof. IVF-ET and GIFT both involve (see Figure 85.1) administering a medication to inhibit a woman's ability to ovulate spontaneously on her own (a gonadotropin-releasing hormone agonist, or GnRHa), and then starting her on injectable gonadotropins (a combination of follicle-stimulating hormone and luteinizing hormone) to stimulate the ovaries to develop follicles that contain maturing oocytes. Monitoring of a cycle is usually done by means of serial ultrasound (US) and serum estradiol (E2) levels, to keep track of the sizes and numbers of follicles (by US) and the amount of estrogen (E2) produced by the follicles. Circulating E2 can reach levels that are 10-fold higher than in a natural, unstimulated cycle. When the follicles are of a certain size and the E2 level has reached a certain value, then human chorionic gonadotropin (hCG) is given intramuscularly, which begins the final process of oocyte maturation. Ovulation will occur within 36–48 hours of the hCG dose. For IVF-ET, the oocytes are retrieved 35 hours later (before spontaneous ovulation triggered by the hCG dose) with US guidance, transvaginally. When all of the oocytes are retrieved, then they are inseminated with sperm (the partner's or, in some instances, a donor's; see below). Fertilization, if it occurs, will occur *in vitro* in a petri dish, and the resulting embryos will be transferred into the woman's uterus 2 or 3 days after the oocyte retrieval. If there is a severe male factor, then ICSI is performed—a procedure in which a single sperm is injected directly into an egg. After cleavage and development *in vitro*, the resulting embryos are transferred to the woman's

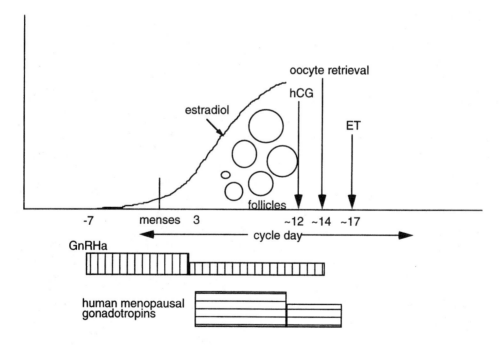

FIGURE 85.1. Schematic representation of a typical ART cycle. GnRHa is administered about 1 week before the expected menses. On day 3 of the subsequent cycle, the dose of the GnRHa is reduced, and human menopausal gonadotropins are begun. Estradiol is measured in the circulation, and follicle numbers and sizes are determined by ultrasound. Since different women respond differently to gonadotropins, approximate days for hCG, oocyte retrieval, and embryo transfer (ET) are illustrated.

uterus, as in classical IVF- ET. Pregnancy rates are typically about 25% for IVF-ET when four to six embryos have been transferred. The pregnancy rate increases with increasing numbers of embryos transferred, but so does the multiple-gestation rate (twins, triplets, and higher-order multiples). "Extra" embryos can be cryopreserved (frozen) indefinitely. With GIFT, as soon as the oocytes are retrieved, then they are placed in the fallopian tube along with sperm. The resulting conception occurs *in vivo*. If one wants to limit the number of oocytes replaced (to minimize the multiple-gestation risk), oocytes cannot currently be frozen and thawed successfully, and so insemination of the remaining oocytes is necessary with cryopreservation of any resulting embryos. GIFT has the advantage of *in vivo* conception (important to some couples) and a higher pregnancy rate (about 40%, compared to IVF-ET). It has the disadvantage of providing no information regarding fertilization (if a pregnancy has not occurred), and of requiring at least one normal fallopian tube. AH is a procedure in which the coat around the egg (the zona pellucida) is gently breached, to assist the blastocyst in hatching before it can implant in the uterus. It is not currently conducted for all procedures, although it is gaining in popularity.

SOME ETHICAL DILEMMAS IN ASSISTED REPRODUCTIVE TECHNOLOGIES

A number of issues immediately arise with regard to ARTs. How many embryos should be transferred in IVF-ET? How many oocytes should be transferred in GIFT? What should be done with the remainder? Should donor sperm be used? Are donor eggs a "better way to go"? If too many embryos have implanted, should "selective reduction" (a euphemism for abortion) be conducted? Are cryopreserved embryos the property or offspring of the genetic parents? What happens in the event of the death of one or both parents, or in the event of a divorce? What about surrogacy? ARTs have now provided couples with a variety of unconventional options to pursue having a family. For example, a woman without ovaries (but with a uterus) can now carry a conceptus (the union of a donated oocyte with her partner's sperm). A woman without a uterus can have her own genetic child (the union of her oocyte and her partner's sperm), carried by a gestational surrogate. If the male partner has no sperm (azoospermia), donor sperm can be used in the procedures described above. The laws regarding the use of donor sperm are well delineated in most states, whereas those regarding donor oocytes and donor embryos are not. The laws surrounding adoption are clear; however, most states discourage surrogacy because of the tremendous ethical, moral, and legal problems inherent in this form of reproduction. An ART child may have up to five potential "parents": the genetic mother, the gestating mother, the rearing mother, the genetic father, and the rearing father. Society is not ready for the ethical, legal, and moral dilemmas posed by such combinations. They are rare, but they do occur, and the societal infrastructure is not prepared to handle them.

EMOTIONS AND ASSISTED REPRODUCTIVE TECHNOLOGIES

Infertility can change the basic framework of an individual's existence and a couple's goals and aspirations. In addition to the realization that accompanies a "diagnosis," coping mechanisms are often compromised by the altered hormonal state that a woman may experience during infertility therapy. Loneliness, isolation, frustration, lack of control, hopelessness, anxiety, and sorrow may accompany the experience of infertility, as well as therapies aimed at correcting it. Being informed about "what's wrong," ways to solve it, and the chances of success are all very important in dealing not only with the emotional aspects of infertility, but with disappointments associated with failed therapies. Although scientific advances have abounded in understanding reproductive physiology, most attention over the years has been focused on the physical aspects of infertility, while the emotional ones have often gone ignored and untreated. The few studies conducted to date on the effects of stress and fertility have had conflicting results. There are currently national organizations in the United States that are dedicated to providing critical information, so that couples can make informed decisions during their infertility evaluation and treatment. As an example, a nonprofit agency, Resolve, Inc., serves as a counseling, referral, and support system for infertile couples; it also offers education and assistance to associated professionals.

CONCLUSIONS

The ARTs are pushing the boundaries of science, ethics, law, and genetics. Eventually they will serve as one avenue not only for widespread preimplantation genetic diagnosis (i.e., diagnosing a genetic disorder in the embryo), but also for gene therapy in the germ line (oocytes, sperm, and early embryos). Practitioners have the moral responsibility to see that human gametes and embryos are treated with the respect that distinguishes them from yet another group of cells. And all citizens have the responsibility to make sure that the ARTs for genetic diagnosis and therapy are judiciously used for the common good of individuals, and not to promote eugenics—the extreme outcome of such technology.

FURTHER READING

American Society for Reproductive Medicine. (1995). *Infertility: An overview.* Birmingham, AL: Author.
A comprehensive patient information booklet about infertility in general, including evaluation and therapies.

American Society for Reproductive Medicine. (1995). *IVF and GIFT: A guide to assisted reproductive technologies.* Birmingham, AL: Author.
A comprehensive patient information booklet about IVF and GIFT.

Serono Symposia, USA. *Infertility: The emotional roller coaster.* (1994, October). Norwell, MA: Author.
A patient information pamphlet produced by Serono Symposia, USA.

Society for the Advanced Reproductive Technologies (1994). Report 1994. *Fertility and Sterility, 63,* 237–248.
A report on the cumulative pregnancy rates in the United States and Canada in participating centers via IVF and GIFT.

Speroff, L., Glass, R. H., & Kase, N. G. (1994). Assisted reproduction. In L. Speroff, R. H. Glass, & N. G. Kase (Ed.), *Clinical gynecologic endocrinology and infertility* (pp. 931–946). Baltimore: Williams & Wilkins.
A comprehensive summary of assisted reproduction.

86

Menopause

Katherine A. O'Hanlan

PHYSIOLOGY OF HORMONES

During the reproductive years, estrogen is produced in varying amounts on a continuous basis by the cells surrounding the egg follicles in the ovary. Estrogen tells the cells in the uterine lining to grow. Once ovulation has occurred (usually about postmenstrual day 14), progesterone is secreted by the follicle for about 2 weeks; this causes the uterine lining cells to stop growing and to mature, ready for a potential pregnancy. If no pregnancy occurs, the lining of the uterus is shed as a menstrual period. Testosterone is also secreted by the ovaries in small amounts and may be important in maintaining libido in some women. Physiologically, menopause begins when the ovaries run out of eggs and the hormone-secreting follicles that surround them.

In addition to its role in the reproductive angle, estrogen supports the lining of the upper vagina and maintains a lush wall to allow secretion of lubrication during sexual excitement. It is responsible to some degree for libido in women, along with testosterone. It also supports the posterior wall of the bladder and helps maintain strength and continence, preventing bladder infections. Estrogen promotes bone maintenance by inhibiting osteoclastic calcium absorption. Furthermore, it induces favorable changes in the cholesterol profile by increasing high-density lipoprotein (HDL) and decreasing low-density lipoproteins (LDL). Estrogen causes direct arteriodilation and may reduce the incidence of coronary vascular disease in young women in a variety of other ways. Importantly, it is also trophic to breast ductal cells, while progesterone stimulates the glandular cells in the breast to proliferate. Estrogen is also implicated in the higher rates among susceptible women of gallstone formation, possibly by raising the saturation of bile cholesterols.

MENOPAUSE DEFINED

Menopause is clinically defined as the time after menses have ceased for at least 12 months. Many women will have multiple symptoms at the start of menopause, but a few have none at all. Symptoms can include typical hot flashes and palpitations; possibly alterations in mood, such as irritability and depression (which may be more closely related to sleep loss from hot flashes); and, usually later in the menopause, atrophic conditions such as vaginal dryness, painful sexual intercourse, and urinary incontinence, urgency, or infections. These symptoms usually abate after 1–5 years; however, some women have hot flashes all their lives after menopause. For some women these symptoms are not bothersome, but for other women they can be distracting to intolerable, requiring treatment for as long as they are present. Fortunately, there are multiple hormonal and nonhormonal modalities available to help menopausal women maintain a normal, functional, comfortable life.

DISEASE PREVENTION

Ideally, a woman's focus on health should be a continual one, heightened by information at each visit to the clinician, and augmented by self-education. Premenopausal diet and lifestyle habits have a significant impact on the health of menopausal women. With education about a cardiac-wise diet, quality exercise, and a healthy lifestyle, most women can avoid heart disease, stroke, and osteoporosis—the major diseases that have historically afflicted menopausal women. Estrogens have been variably shown to improve laboratory risk factors for heart disease, and to reduce bone absorption (The Writing Group for the PEPI Trial, 1995). Although hormones can play an important role in the maintenance of health, they should be treated as a medical intervention with risks and benefits, continued only for as long as they are necessary and effective, and not employed as "preventive" or as replacements for a healthy lifestyle and diet. Women of every age should be counseled that the evidence is strong that exercise—defined as 30-minute segments, three to four times weekly, of exertion resulting in a 1.5- to 2.0-fold increase in resting heart rate—reduces the risk of coronary vascular disease and osteoporosis. Cessation of smoking reduces risk for both vaso-occlusive diseases and osteoporosis. Although one alcoholic beverage daily may be beneficial in preventing cardiac disease, more than one beverage daily reduces bone density. Monitoring the blood pressure and cholesterol, and having a diet low in animal fat, reduce the risk of heart disease and stroke. Moderation of protein intake is associated with lower rates of osteoporosis. High calcium intake, both from the diet and from supplements, also reduces the risk of osteoporosis; total intake from both sources should be at least 1,000 mg of elemental calcium for women with either endogenous or exogenous estrogen, and 1,500 mg for women who do not have or take estrogens. Hormone therapy should be employed in women who have persistently elevated risk for or presence of these diseases despite counseling and sustained efforts at risk reduction.

INDICATIONS FOR ESTROGEN THERAPY

Figure 86.1 is a flowchart for use in deciding when short- or long-term estrogen therapy is indicated. The chart's recommendations are discussed in greater detail in this section.

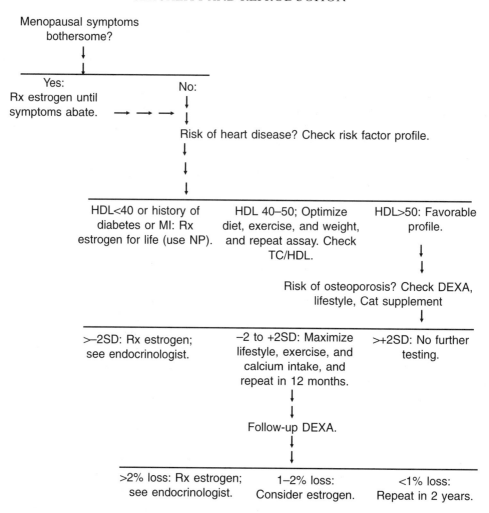

FIGURE 86.1. A flowchart for use in deciding when short- or long-term estrogen therapy is indicated. MI, myocardial infarctions; NP, natural progesterone; TC, total cholesterol; HDL, high-density lipoprotein; DEXA, dual-energy X-ray absorptiometry; 2SD, 2 standard deviations.

Symptom Amelioration

Bothersome systemic symptoms amenable to hormone therapy should be treated with the lowest effective dose. Estrogen in conjugated or esterified forms (0.625 mg) or as estradiol (1.0-mg tablets or a 0.05-mg continuous-release patch) will abate nearly all symptoms in most menopausal women. The estrogen can be taken daily, without stopping at the end of the month, as has been the tradition. It is not controversial that younger women entering the menopause before age 50 or so—either naturally or as a result of surgical extirpation of the ovaries—should receive hormone replacement until age 50, when they should then be evaluated for further need of hormone therapy. These younger women will often need higher doses of estrogens (0.9–1.25 mg of conjugated or esterified estrogens, 2.0 mg of estradiol, or 0.1 mg by patch). Usually women who are symptomatic but still having periods need very little supplemental estrogen to ameliorate their hot flashes, and can be given half the menopausal dose (0.3 mg of conjugated or esterified estrogen, or 0.5 mg of estradiol), which usually will not interfere with their cycles. When their cycles stop or become irregular, a progestogen can then be added.

On a yearly basis after age 50, each woman receiving hormones solely because of her symptoms should discontinue her regimen briefly to see whether her symptoms resume or persist. If her symptoms have abated, she should be evaluated for indications for long-term hormone therapy, such as the presence of, or unalterable risk factors for, osteoporosis or coronary vascular disease. In the absence of these indications, hormones should be stopped.

Cardiac Health

Women over 35 should know their serum cholesterol level and actively seek to optimize it. When menopause ensues, or when a woman in menopause has no symptoms requiring estrogens, the cholesterol profile is evaluated as an indication for initiating long-term postmenopausal hormonal therapy. Prospective studies have shown that estrogen can reduce the LDL, can raise the HDL and lower the fibrinogen for most women (The Writing Group for the PEPI Trial, 1995), and can reduce repeat myocardial infarction rates among the women who have already had one heart attack. These women should also be supported with consultation by a specialist in cardiac disease prevention, and should be encouraged to follow the recommendations for cardiac disease risk reduction. Lifelong estrogen may offer benefit to women whose HDL is under 40, whose LDL is over 150, or who have already had a heart attack. It must be recognized that estrogen may work to prevent cardiac disease in many ways other than improvement of the lipid profile, but until prospective trials show benefit to women with favorable profiles, only women with unfavorable profiles and previous myocardial infarction should receive estrogens for heart health (Grady et al., 1992).

Bone Density Maintenance

If the cholesterol profile is favorable, then the third indication for estrogen therapy should be investigated: bone loss. A dual-energy X-ray absorptiometry (DEXA) is the most reliable and reproducible method of assessing bone density. The DEXA is associated with less radiation exposure than a mammogram, and is useful in following bone density changes of even 2% with unparalleled accuracy. The spine and hip assessments are reported as direct bone density in grams per centimeter squared, and are also computed as standard deviations from the mean of women at that patient's age. These results are plotted on a chart showing the mean from ages 20 to 85, and the ranges (2 standard deviations) are easily understood.

Estrogen therapy is indicated for women with established osteoporosis because it inhibits bone resorption by osteoclasts. Women whose measurements are within 2 standard deviations of the mean (above or below) should be advised to maximize known effective osteoporosis prevention measures and to have a repeat measurement in 1–2 years. Women whose measurements are more than 1 standard deviation below the mean are up to three times more likely to develop fractures later, unless they begin to maintain the density they have through lifestyle change and calcium supplementation. Bone density loss of more than 2% in 1 year in women who are below the mean is an indication for lifelong estrogen therapy. If less than 2% is lost, then a second assessment in 1 year is indicated, as well as continued maintenance of a healthy diet and exercising lifestyle. It must be recognized that most of the bone density loss in the menopause occurs in the first 5 years after estrogen levels drop, with continued loss at a much slower rate thereafter, which emphasizes the need for lifelong weight-bearing exercise and calcium.

Women initially presenting for care well into their menopause should also have a bone density assessment as a screen. If their density is found to be low, further loss can be prevented, and appropriate consultation can be provided. All women who are 2 standard deviations below the norm, or who lose more than 2% of their density in 1 year, should be evaluated by a bone mineral endocrinologist for initiation not only of estrogen but possibly of one of the bisphosphonate drugs, which act to further retard bone loss.

Urinary Symptoms, and Vulvar and Vaginal Dryness

For women with favorable lipid profiles and bone densities, whose only symptoms are localized to the bladder and vagina (e.g., frequent urinary tract infections, mild incontinence or interstitial cystitis, and/or atrophic vaginitis or painful intercourse), the practitioner should consider administering a low-dose local regimen of estrogen cream, such as 1.0-gram conjugated estrogen cream. Multiple studies have shown that even after prolonged use, such low doses of estrogen are not associated with systemic elevations of serum estrogens or reflective of systemic estrogenic activity (van Haaften, Donker, Haspels, & Thijssen, 1989). The endometrium is not stimulated with this dose, which is one-fourth of the equivalent oral dose. This regimen is safe and useful even when systemic estrogens are contraindicated, such as for women with a history of breast cancer. Most women will need to use the cream nightly for at least 30 days, and then taper to the minimal frequency necessary to maintain the benefit.

RISKS AND SAFETY ISSUES

Increased Risk of Breast Cancer

The breast cancer risk of menopausal hormone replacement therapy appears minimal with short-term use of 1–5 years. After this duration, the risk of breast cancer is multiplied by a factor of 1.3–1.7. If the lifetime average risk of breast cancer among U.S. women is calculated as 11%, then women on prolonged use of hormones in the menopause will have lifetime rates of 15–20%. Menopausal estrogens also result in a higher concentration of saturated cholesterols in the bile, which favors stone formation, multiplying the risk for cholelithiasis by a factor of 2.0, and raising the lifetime risk from 2–4% to 4–8%. For these reasons, it is recommended that women take menopausal hormone regimens only for as long as they need them, and receive appropriate follow-up testing once the hormones are discontinued.

Previous Breast and Endometrial Cancers

A history of breast or endometrial cancer is seen by most as a contraindication to administration of systemic estrogens. Although most cases of breast cancer occur well into the menopause, many women are diagnosed in their 30s and 40s. The chemotherapy they often require results in ovarian failure and sudden severe menopausal symptoms. These women are subsequently at high risk for premature bone loss and heart disease; however, they usually seek treatment for relief of their hot flashes, dyspareunia, and insomnia. There are no prospective studies documenting that systemic estrogens actually cause breast cancer recurrence, and there are a few studies documenting the safety of administering replacement hormones to women with breast cancer. Breast cancer in pregnancy or followed by pregnancy, with its high levels of estrogens, does not have a worse survival probability than those cases not associated with pregnancy. Concerns about estrogen receptors in the remaining normal breast tissue, as well as potential "nests" of persistent or metastatic breast cancer, have brought about the widespread refusal to prescribe any estrogen regimen to breast cancer patients. Some oncologists are currently prescribing oral estrogen to select breast cancer patients who have early-stage disease and severe symptoms. Their unpublished accounts suggest no adverse effects; however, in the absence of controlled trials, few doctors are willing to risk being perceived to have stimulated an early recurrence or new occurrence of this cancer.

Although most women developing endometrial cancer are in the menopause, some women in the perimenopause develop endometrial cancer and notice significant changes after removal of the ovaries. Endometrial cancer is more highly curable than breast cancer, and patients can be categorized as having low, medium, or high risk for recurrent disease. Few gynecological oncologists would hesitate to prescribe estrogens to symptomatic low-risk women. The American College of Obstetricians and Gynecologists has endorsed the concept of providing estrogens for some women who have had endometrial cancer, because the well-being afforded by relief of menopausal symptoms in certain cases outweighs the theoretical risk of stimulating tumor growth.

Alternatives to Estrogens

Many partially effective regimens for abating the various symptoms are available and safe. Use of tamoxifen will often abate hot flashes and may already be indicated therapeutically for some younger patients. Patients who are not on a protocol may benefit from medroxyprogesterone acetate (MPA; 5–10 mg daily). A low-dose clonidine patch or oral tablets may be employed, with the limiting side effect of hypotension. Some patients report that vitamin E (alpha-tocopherol; 1,000–2,000 I.U.) ameliorates their flashes. Bellergal has been shown to reduce frequency of hot flashes as well. Troublesome insomnia can be treated with any of the fast-acting, rapidly metabolized benzodiazepines. Depression is a reasonable temporary response to developing breast cancer, but prolonged depression may be a result of insomnia and may require psychological counseling and possibly pharmacological therapy. Physicians must keep a patient, open mind to experimenting with some or all of these regimens, and should be open to their exceptional patients' bringing in ideas and regimens of their own. Natural and herbal remedies, including acupuncture, may be investigated by the patient and found to provide relief as well.

PROGESTOGENS

All women who have a uterus and require estrogen therapy should be given a cyclic or continuous progestogen, to prevent the expected overgrowth to hyperplasia and possibly cancer that occurs in one-third of cases when progestogens are omitted. Obese women have a higher level of endogenous estrogens and a 25–40% lifetime risk of endometrial cancer. Thus they also require systemic cyclic progestogen-stimulated "medical curettage" of the uterine lining, even if they are not using systemic estrogens.

Most women have no side effects from the cyclic or continuous progestogens, but some will describe psychological symptoms ranging from flattening of the affect to frank depression. These require experimenting with alternate oral progestogens, use of a progesterone-impregnated intrauterine device, or even cessation of all progestogens with yearly biopsy.

Whereas estrogen-only regimens improve the HDL by 11%, addition of micronized natural progesterone (NP) to estrogen results in an HDL rise of 8%, and addition of MPA results in an HDL rise of only 3%. Thus women with an abnormal lipid profile or a history of coronary vascular disease who have a uterus should use NP.

Cyclic Regimens

Cyclic regimens are the easiest to employ in the beginning of menopause, as they are associated with the lowest rates of unscheduled bleeding. The only detriment to this regimen is that most women will have a period at just the time of life when they thought they could become exempt from such issues. Use of 5–10 mg/day of MPA or 200 mg/day of NP for a minimum of 12 days per month, or 10 mg/day of MPA or 200–400 mg/day of NP for 14 days every 2–3 months, is sufficient to prevent hyperplasia in most women. Obese women may require 20 mg/day of MPA or 300–400 mg/day of NP if they wish to cycle every 2–3 months. A withdrawal bleed usually occurs just before or soon after completion of the progestogen cycle, but this is most often scant and gradually decreases to spotting with prolonged use. It is reasonable to stretch out the interval for women on monthly cycles who have only spotting or who do not have any withdrawal bleed, to permit them to cycle every 2–3 months. Should bleeding or spotting occur during the prolonged interval, then the interval should be shortened to prevent spotting. A biopsy or sonogram of the endometrium should be performed in the women who have unscheduled spotting if they have not had one in the preceding year.

Continuous Regimens

Most women with a uterus will prefer a continuous regimen, because it is usually associated with no bleeding on any scheduled basis. Nearly half of all women, however, will develop the most common side effect of this regimen—unscheduled bleeding, which may require more biopsies and visits to the doctor than the cyclic regimen. Use of 2.5 mg/day of MPA or 100 mg/day of NP will result in regression of the uterine lining to such an extent that spotting occurs and temporary or permanent use of the cyclic regimen may be required.

FURTHER READING

Colditz, G. A., Hankinson, S. E., Hunter, D. J., Willett, W. C., Mansom, J. E., Stampfer, M. J., Hennekens, C., Rosner, B., & Speizer, F. E. (1995). The use of estrogens and progestins and the risk of breast cancer in postmenopausal women. *New England Journal of Medicine, 332*(24).

This is prospective information about how the risk of breast cancer increases with increasing duration of use of estrogens and progestins: 1.3 times for 5 years, and 1.7 times for more than 10 years.

Ettinger, B., Selby, J., Citron, J. T., Vangessel, A., Ettinger, V. M., & Hendrickson, M. R. (1994). Cyclic hormone replacement therapy using quarterly progestin. *Obstetrics and Gynecology, 83*(5, Pt. 1), 693–700.

This study showed that progestins can be given only every 3 months with safe low rates of hyperplasia, but that the duration must be 14 days and the dose at least 10 mg/day.

Grady, D., Rubin, S. M., Petitti, D. B., Fox, C. S., Black, D., Ettinger, B., Ernster, V. L., & Cummings, S. R. (1992). Hormone therapy to prevent disease and prolong life in post-menopausal women. *Annals of Internal Medicine, 117*(12), 1016–1037.

This is a meta-analysis of risk of breast cancer, showing that combining all the good studies of breast cancer risk from hormone therapy does appear to indicate an increase in breast cancer rates.

Raz, R., & Stamm, W. E. (1993). A controlled trial of intravaginal estriol in postmenopausal women with recurrent urinary tract infections. *New England Journal of Medicine, 329*(11), 753–756.

See next entry.

van Haaften, M., Donker, G. H., Haspels, A. A., & Thijssen, J. H. (1989). Oestrogen concentrations in plasma, endometrium, myometrium and vagina of postmenopausal women, and effects of vaginal oestriol (E3) and oestradiol (E2) applications. *Journal of Steroid Biochemistry, 33*(4A), 647–653.

In these two studies, vaginal estrogens were shown to be safe and associated with virtually no absorption if given in low doses as vaginal creams.

The Writing Group for the PEPI Trial. (1995). Effects of estrogen or estrogen/progestin regimens on heart disease risk factors in postmenopausal women: The Postmenopausal Estrogen/Progestin Interventions (PEPI) Trial. *Journal of the American Medical Association, 273*(3), 199–208.

This is the first prospective long-term study of effects of various hormone regimens on the cholesterol profile, coagulation parameters, bone density, and many other health factors.

87

Sexuality and Aging

Antonette M. Zeiss

Sexuality in older women is rarely presented in the mass media, literature, art, or folklore. An occasional film, such as *Cocoon,* presents older people in sexual situations, but in such cases renewed sexuality is often presented as an aspect of renewed youth and health. Male film stars are more often presented as sexually appealing despite age, such as Sean Connery's appearance on the cover of *People* magazine as "the sexiest man alive" when in his 60s; female counterparts are rare. The more available female stereotype is the aging star from *Sunset Boulevard,* refusing to admit that she has lost attractiveness and sexual appeal. The covert message is that older women do not have legitimate sexual interests and should not be sexually active.

One purpose of this chapter is to examine these stereotypes about older women's roles, sexual interest, and sexual activity, in comparison to research on normal age-related changes in sexual function and behavior. A second purpose is to suggest useful approaches to clinical interventions for older women who do report age-related sexual concerns or dysfunction.

HORMONAL AND PHYSICAL CHANGES IN WOMEN WITH AGING

Aging is a gradual and highly individual process. None of the effects described below can be associated with a specific age. For example, some women may enter menopause at age 40, and others at 55 or even older. The processes described below are intended as guidelines for what a clinician should attend to in working with older people, not a fixed set of norms.

Menopause reflects a marked shift in hormones, initially seen as reduced production of estrogen. (For more details on the role of estrogen, and on estrogen therapy, see O'Hanlan's chapter on menopause in this volume.) Pituitary hormones (follicle-stimulating hormone [FSH] and luteinizing hormone [LH]) initially increase, in an unsuccessful attempt to stimulate the ovaries to produce more estrogen and to continue ovulation. Eventually, pituitary hormones decline, and postmenopausal women produce very low levels of estrogen, progesterone, FSH, and LH.

Before menopause, the ovaries also produce testosterone; they stop producing this hormone after menopause, although some is still produced by the adrenal gland. Research suggests that testosterone influences sexual desire in women (as well as men); the reduction of testosterone caused by menopause is significant and may influence older women's desire.

Reduced estrogen results in thinning of the tissues lining the vagina, reduced vaginal lubrication, and slower lubrication in response to sexual stimulation. These changes can result in pain with intercourse or other vaginal penetration; this is a problem for about one in three sexually active women over 65. Taking more time for foreplay can compensate for slower sexual response. Artificial lubricants, such as Astroglide or Replens, or hormone replacement therapy can also address the problems caused by reduced estrogen.

Vaginal penetration is also more difficult in older women because the vaginal lips (labia) no longer fully elevate during sexual arousal to create a funnel-like entrance to the vagina, as they do in younger women. In addition, the cervix may descend into the vagina, and cervical bumping during intercourse can be painful. For most aging women, clitoral response is unchanged, and clitoral stimulation continues as an important prelude to orgasm.

Older women may experience some changes with orgasm. Orgasm may involve weaker and fewer vaginal contractions and shorter duration of general body involvement in the orgasmic experience. Older women retain multiorgasmic ability. However, after completing the orgasmic phase, older women return to the prearoused state more rapidly than younger women.

"USE IT OR LOSE IT"

"Use it or lose it" has been a common injunction for older adults, but it is a potentially misleading one. Women over 60 who continue sexual activity with a partner are likely to experience vaginal lubrication almost as rapidly as younger women. In addition, the vaginas of postmenopausal women who have intercourse three times a month or more are less likely to become shorter and narrower with age. Women without a partner who masturbate regularly may also experience fewer physical changes in the vagina and more rapid vaginal lubrication. It is not necessarily true, however, that inactive women have permanently "lost" responsiveness. Older women who renew sexual activity after a period of abstinence can usually regain sexual functioning, but recovery may be a slow process.

OVERALL IMPACT OF AGE-RELATED CHANGES

Although these age-related changes in hormonal status and sexual response are meaningful, they do not, in themselves, cause a woman's sex life to end. Older women may need to plan for more time in a sexual encounter, to be sensitive to changes in their own bodies and their partners', and to use aids such as lubricants or vibrators to increase stimulation. They may want to emphasize sexual activities other than intercourse, such as oral stimulation, which can increase genital lubrication or can be an end in itself (e.g., for women who have pain during intercourse because the cervix gets bumped). Older women need to be able to talk about these changes, to be flexible in their thinking about the timing and nature of sexual contacts, and to be creative in working out activities that fit their own pattern of age-related changes.

BEHAVIORAL CHANGES WITH AGING

It is easy to say what healthy older women might do to maintain sexual satisfaction, but it is not always easy to do these things. Many women, at all ages, are uncomfortable talking candidly about sex, and few have been encouraged to think creatively and flexibly about sexuality. This may be even more true for the current cohort of older women, who were raised in a less sexually open time. It would not be surprising, then, if the typical sexual behavior of older women showed more change than one would expect solely from the physical changes described above.

The best longitudinal research on aging women studied only married women and their husbands in long-lasting relationships over a 10-year span, starting when couples were in their 60s and 70s. This sample excludes the situations of many older women (e.g., those who are single or whose partners are women). However, the study does shed light on the interplay between biological changes and cultural expectations in aging adults. The most common pattern for couples in this study was to maintain a steady level of sexual activity, at whatever the initial level had been. The second most common pattern was for couples to maintain sexual activity until a point of fairly sudden, dramatic decline or cessation of sexual activity for both the husband and the wife. These sudden declines in sexual activity generally occurred because of health changes in the man. For example, if a husband died, his wife usually ceased all sexual activity. When a husband developed medical problems that interfered with erections, he and his wife often ceased all sexual activity. However, reversing the genders did not have the same result. When a wife died, her husband often remained sexually active, either in masturbation or with a new partner. When a wife developed medical problems that made sexual activity more difficult, she and her husband usually remained sexually active nonetheless.

This second pattern suggests that both genders believe that men must have erections for heterosexual couples to have satisfactory sexual lives. When health problems affect erection, many couples do not communicate, plan, or change their behavior; instead, they give up on sex. Although medical problems, especially in men, clearly play a major role in sexual functioning in older couples, the changes in behavior are also the result of a psychosocial construction of sexuality that emphasizes the passive, receptive role of women and the centrality of intercourse in sexuality.

THE ETIOLOGY OF SEXUAL CONCERNS
AND PROBLEMS IN OLDER WOMEN

These behavioral patterns suggest that psychological problems can affect the sexuality of older women. These are probably rooted in the negative cultural stereotypes discussed, but can also be considered from the point of view of the particular woman expressing sexual concern. Commonly reported concerns include relationship issues, intrapersonal issues (e.g., difficulties accepting aging), psychopathologies, grief, and adjustment to illness or loss of a partner. None of these problems are exclusive to older women, but the prevalence of many of these factors increases with age.

A full clinical syndrome of depression is not more common in older women than in younger women (it may even be less common), but reports of some depressive symptoms are elevated. Loss of sexual desire is a common component of depression and can combine with hormonal changes and reduced comfort to result in reports of sexual uninterest or even aversion. Changes in roles, through changes in health status, widowhood, adapting to retirement, or the assumption of a patient or caregiver role, can also have a negative impact on sexual feelings and activity in older women. The transition from an equal partnership to one of caregiver and patient may disrupt sexual functioning in the relationship. The death of a partner may require the survivor to use skills for establishing a new relationship that have been long dormant. Establishment of a new romantic or sexual relationship also may require frank discussion of sexual interests, habits, and needs with potential new partners—a difficult task for anyone.

Women experience various physical changes with aging, such as wrinkling skin, graying and sometimes loss of hair, sagging breasts, and loss of muscle tone. Psychological reactions to these changes may be dramatic, especially when women have been heavily invested in their personal appearance. Illnesses such as heart disease or lung disease, which have increased incidence with age, can lead to loss of stamina; breast cancer may necessitate a mastectomy. With the cultural definition of sexuality as being for the young and healthy, it is not surprising that an older woman, especially one who is medically compromised, may find it difficult to overcome physical changes and to maintain an identity as a sexually active and attractive person.

In addition to psychological factors, medical problems can affect sexual expression in older women. Unfortunately, most research on the impact of disease and medications has been done with older men; only recently have researchers been encouraged to study older women. Thus, the information currently available is scanty and inconclusive. Many physical systems are involved in sexuality; thus, a huge array of illnesses and treatments can disrupt sexuality. Cardiovascular diseases (including hypertension, coronary artery disease arrhythmias, and heart failure) may affect sexual functioning in women, as they are known to do in men. For example, the processes during sexual stimulation that result in the increased blood flow responsible for penile erection are paralleled by processes responsible for vaginal lubrication. Diseases impeding blood flow, such as atherosclerosis, thus can affect vaginal lubrication (just as they affect erection).

Diabetes is notorious for its link to erectile dysfunction, and diabetes in women may be associated with sexual problems also. Some research suggests that diabetes may be associated with desire disorders, reduced vaginal lubrication, and painful intercourse in older women. However, these are common problems for older women, and the additional contribution of diabetes (if any) is not clearly understood. The incidence of these problems in older diabetic women actually may be no greater than in the general population.

Many health problems that occur more frequently in the older population do not directly affect sexual organs or functioning, but they have an indirect effect. One that is particularly common, especially for women, is arthritis. Arthritis, with its stiffness and joint pain, interferes with sexual activity itself, as well as with pleasure and satisfaction. Use of the "missionary" position can be especially painful for women with arthritis in their hips, but it is the most common position for sexual intercourse. Alternate positions can ease the strain of painful joints. For example, the "spoon" position allows both partners to lie on their sides, the woman in front of the man, so he can enter her vagina from behind and she need not support his weight.

Although all of these psychological and medical factors can have important effects as single factors, it is difficult to overemphasize the cumulative effect of multiple simultaneous causes for sexual dysfunction in older women. It is common to see a postmenopausal woman who is widowed, with a long history of smoking and arthritis, who does not lose adequate lubrication and sexual desire until she develops an additional problem (e.g., depression). The physical basis of sexual responses is vulnerable, in that it is dependent on many systems, but it is also resilient. It often takes multiple problems to overcome that innate resilience.

PSYCHOLOGICAL TREATMENT: APPLYING THE PLISSIT MODEL WITH OLDER WOMEN

The PLISSIT model is a four-level conceptual framework that guides the therapist from simple to more complex interventions. PLISSIT is an acronym for four progressive levels of sex therapy: "permission," "limited information," "specific suggestions," and "intensive therapy." If problems are not resolved with a simple intervention, the therapist adds more complex interventions as needed. With older women, interventions at the first three levels can be especially helpful.

In the first level, the therapist gives permission for sexual activities and fantasies, reassuring patients that these are normal. For instance, an older woman may need permission to masturbate as an alternative to sex with a partner who is uninterested or ill. Women in the current group of older adults have not heard accepting messages about their own sexuality very often; if such messages are given well, the therapist can provide much-needed support for older women's right to sexual expression.

In the next level, limited information, a clinician provides psychoeducational information. Older women rarely know much about normal, age-related changes in sexual functioning, let alone changes caused by illness or medications, and they may misinterpret these changes. For example, an older woman whose husband obtains decreased erections because of diabetes may fear that he does not find her sexually desirable because of changes in her appearance. Discussion of the physical basis of his problem can be helpful to his wife, as well as to the diabetic older man.

The third step of the model, specific suggestions, involves simple problem-solving interventions. For example, an older man and woman who used to have sex after romantic evenings out will need to change their pattern if they can no longer drive after dark. An older woman who always considered the man's erection to be the signal to begin sexual activity will need suggestions on changes in the initiation and orchestration of sex, since the older man will probably need direct penile stimulation to obtain an erection. If a postmenopausal woman experiences painful intercourse, she and her partner can use vaginal estrogen cream in a sensual way as part of foreplay, rather than having her apply it by herself before sex.

Intensive therapy, the fourth level of intervention, is used when brief therapy is ineffective or when specific suggestions are not carried out. With any age group, a specific program drawing on empirically tested sex therapy and couple therapy procedures is developed. It is important that the treatment incorporate information on age-related changes in functioning, but the therapeutic techniques (e.g., sensate focus exercises) are similar to those used with younger adults.

Often, older women will need intensive therapy if they are unable to discuss sexual concerns and wishes. In many older couples, both partners believe that only men discuss or initiate sex, and that men should always be ready for sex. Although these beliefs may not have presented problems when a couple was younger, they can prevent flexible adaptations to age-related changes. Therapy can provide the opportunity to develop a new pattern, in which both partners can talk intimately about the physical aspect of their relationship and express interest in sex (or lack of interest if timing is wrong).

THE IMPACT OF DEMENTIA ON SEXUALITY IN OLDER WOMEN

The prevalence of dementia, as a result of several factors, increases directly with age; only recently has its influence on sexuality been examined. Dementia has serious sexual implications for both patient and caregiver, and the impact may differ according to the gender of the demented partner.

Men with Alzheimer's disease are more likely to have problems with erections than men of similar age without Alzheimer's, but the disease does not seem to affect men's sexual interest directly. Consequently, an older woman who is a caregiving spouse may need to work out strategies for dealing with sexual overtures from a husband who cannot successfully initiate intercourse and who is unlikely to be able to orchestrate a complex sexual interaction. A female caregiver may also lose interest in sex because of the lack of satisfaction for her in these sexual interactions, the loss of intimacy with a demented partner, or the exhaustion and emotional distress created by the overall burden of caring for a demented spouse.

Women with Alzheimer's disease do not seem to lose sexual interest or responsiveness, although, like men, they will be less able to orchestrate a fulfilling sexual encounter. Male caregivers have been reported to feel hesitant about having sex with demented wives who are unable to indicate clear consent or refusal. This may be a remnant of double-standard thinking: The central principle seems to be adherence to the assumption that generally men are interested in sex and women are not. Given this assumption, only women who directly and cogently describe sexual interest are appropriate as sexual partners; this is something a woman with dementia cannot do.

It is often assumed that dementia will result in inappropriate sexual behavior, such as masturbating in public or initiating sex promiscuously. Research shows that this is very unlikely. Demented women (and men) demonstrate little public sexual behavior of any kind, either appropriate or inappropriate. For the occasional patient who does demonstrate this problem, the caregiver can be trained to handle the behavior calmly and to provide privacy or distraction.

If a caregiver decides to discontinue sexual activity with a demented partner, the caregiver can be encouraged to satisfy his or her own sexual desires through self-stimulation. If a demented partner initiates sexual activity, the caregiver can distract the patient or focus him or her on other physical contact, such as massage, hugging, cuddling, and kissing. Both the patient's and the caregiver's need for touch can also be met through these activities.

FURTHER READING

Arthritis Foundation. (1990). *Living and loving: Information about sex.* Atlanta: Author.
An excellent pamphlet providing information on the impact of arthritis on sexuality, and suggesting positions for successful intercourse and alternatives to intercourse.

Davies, H. D., Zeiss, A., & Tinklenberg, J. R. (1992). 'Til death do us part: Intimacy and sexuality in the marriages of Alzheimer's patients. *Journal of Psychosocial Nursing, 30,* 5–10.
Provides an overview of research on dementia and sexuality, and suggestions for therapeutic interventions with patients and their spouse caregivers.

George, L. K., & Weiler, S. J. (1981). Sexuality in middle and late life. *Archives of General Psychiatry, 38,* 919–923.
Longitudinal study of sexual activity in older married couples.

Kaiser, F. E. (1994). Sexuality. In P. D. O'Donnell (Ed.), *Geriatric urology* (pp. 493–502). Boston: Little, Brown.
Provides an overview of medical conditions affecting sexual functioning.

Morrissette, D., Zeiss, R. A., & Zeiss, A. M. (1996). Assessment and management of sexual problems. In J. Sheikh (Ed.), *The management of psychiatric problems in the elderly.* San Francisco: Jossey-Bass.
Provides a thorough overview of issues in sexuality and aging for both men and women. Provides more detailed information on etiology of sexual problems, assessment, and intervention with older adults.

Schover, L. R. (1986). Sexual problems. In L. Teri & P. M. Lewinsohn (Eds.), *Geropsychological assessment and treatment: Selected topics* (pp. 145–187). New York: Springer-Verlag.
Provides an overview of psychological factors affecting sexuality in the elderly.

Sherwin, B. B. (1991). The psychoendocrinology of aging and female sexuality. In J. Bancroft, C. M. Davis, & H. J. Ruppel (Eds.), *Annual review of sex research* (pp. 181–198). Lake Mills, IA: Society for the Scientific Study of Sex.
Provides a scholarly review of the role of sexual hormones (including testosterone) in sexual functioning, and describes menopausal changes, their consequences, and criteria for determining appropriate hormone therapy.

Section VII

PHYSIOLOGICAL DISORDERS WITH BEHAVIORAL AND PSYCHOSOCIAL COMPONENTS

88

Section Editors' Overview

Beth E. Meyerowitz
Gerdi Weidner

*I*n this section, experts on psychological and medical aspects of chronic physiological diseases, disorders, and dysfunctions provide up-to-date overviews of research findings targeted to health care providers and concerned women. Since illness cannot be understood separately from normal functioning, we also include chapters on some basic physiological systems, particularly those such as the endocrine and immune systems, which play key roles in the mechanisms underlying many physiological disorders in women. In the chapters on specific diseases and disorders, special attention is paid to medical, behavioral, and psychosocial issues of relevance to women. In some cases there are multiple chapters that offer different perspectives on topics of particular importance or complexity, and/or on areas in which sufficient medical and psychological research is available to allow for extended discussion. (For the sake of simplicity, the chapters in this section are arranged in alphabetical order by title.)

The information contained in this section is vital for health care providers working with women and for women themselves. Virtually every woman who lives a normal lifespan can expect to suffer from the adverse effects of a chronic illness or disorder. Most adult women report at least one chronic health problem. The problems increase with aging, so that by age 55 more than 80% of women experience at least one chronic health problem, and over half have multiple chronic problems.

It is a well-known paradox that mortality rates are higher for men, whereas morbidity rates are higher for women. Recent data from the National Institutes of Health (NIH) indicate that for every cause of mortality, annual death rates are higher for men than for women.[1] In contrast to the mortality data, for nearly two-thirds of both the acute and the chronic causes of morbidity (which do not include cancer and mental illness in NIH's data base), women have higher rates than men. For men, most of the reported morbidity is related to injury and impairment, whereas for women the morbidity is more likely to result from illnesses and disorders.[2] Since many of the most common causes of morbidity progress with aging, the longer lifespans of women increase gender differences (see the chapter by Wisocki).

These differences in morbidity are clear from the chapters in this section. In addition to illnesses that essentially occur only in women (such as gynecological cancers and breast cancer; see the chapters by Andersen, by Rowland, and by Ganz), many other chronic illnesses are substantially more common in women than in men. Autoimmune disorders occur far more frequently in women, as described for rheumatoid arthritis in Zautra's, Roth's, and Wisocki's chapters; for multiple sclerosis in Foley's chapter, and for lupus in Newell and Coeshott's chapter. Whitehead lists several gastrointestinal disorders that are more prevalent among women than among men (including irritable bowel syndrome, gallstones, constipation, and general gastrointestinal symptoms) and notes that these disorders may be related to slower colonic transit time and inhibited gallbladder motility in women, as well as to the gastrointestinal side effects of medications taken for other disorders (see also Roth's discussion of medication for rheumatoid arthritis). Other diseases and disorders with higher prevalence rates among women include Alzheimer's disease (see Haley's and Siegler's chapters), migraine headaches (see Blanchard's chapter), osteoporosis (see Wisocki's chapter), and Raynaud's disease (see Freedman's chapter). Even illnesses that are not more prevalent in women may have female-specific forms, such as gestational diabetes (see the chapters by Ruggiero and by Wylie Rosett) and menstrual epileptic seizures (see the chapter by Newsome).

In most cases, these illnesses are associated with significant pain, disability, and disruption in quality of life, but do not necessarily lead to shortened lifespan. Women live longer than men and are likely to live many years with medical and psychosocial problems related to chronic illnesses or disorders, as documented in the chapters in this section. In some cases, in fact, the very mechanisms that protect women against mortality may be responsible for increased morbidity. Both Claman and Laudenslager raise this intriguing possibility in their discussions of female superiority in antibody production and the possible association of high antibody levels with the much higher rates of autoimmune diseases in women. Moreover, as Haley and Siegler point out in the chapters on Alzheimer's disease, many women will be caregivers for aging parents or spouses and can expect to deal with chronic illness in their loved ones.

---

[1]Although mortality rates are substantially higher for blacks than for whites in the United States, the sex difference in mortality rates holds within race. Rates for black women are lower than for black men (with the exception of diabetes mellitus). However, black women have higher death rates than white men for several causes of mortality. NIH does not provide separate data for other racial or ethnic groups.

[2]The morbidity rates for acute and chronic conditions that the NIH reports are age-adjusted, and therefore do not result from the longer lifespans of women and the associated greater morbidity in old age. Without this adjustment, the comparative rates of morbidity would be even higher.

RESEARCH PROGRESS

Fortunately, medical and psychological researchers have made substantial progress over recent years in understanding, preventing, and treating some of the most common causes of morbidity and mortality among women. The chapters in this section highlight these advances and point to two positive trends that have been particularly helpful in advancing understanding.

First, there has been an increasing awareness of the importance of acknowledging sex differences and of doing research with specific relevance to women. For many years, medical research focused on the study of men, except in the case of a few illnesses that occur only in women. Even when women were included in research, they were often outnumbered by men; female-specific issues such as cyclical endocrine functioning were overlooked; and sex differences were rarely explored.

Many chapters in this section make it clear that it is a grave mistake to assume that research findings with men will generalize to women. For example, the discussions of coronary heart disease in the chapters by Jenkins, Stoney, and Sholinsky demonstrate how many aspects of disease process and treatment can differ between genders. Although heart disease is the leading cause of death for both men and women, women get the disease approximately 10 years later than men on average; current treatments are less effective for women; and survival rates after the first myocardial infarction are worse. Even the basic physiological processes involving stress reactivity, the presenting symptoms of the disease, and the impact of comorbidities differ between men and women. Other examples of gender differences described in this section include mechanisms regulating finger blood flow in Raynaud's disease (see Freedman's chapter), symptom presentation and survival in HIV (see Richardson's chapter), and the etiology and treatment of pain (see Bodnar's chapter). These examples confirm that even when disease is not clearly a function of sex hormones, there may be important differences in basic physiological functioning, disease etiology, prognosis, symptom presentation, treatment effectiveness, and treatment side effects between the genders.

A second recent research trend that has yielded important insights has been the recognition that physiological functioning and disorders cannot be fully understood if mind and body are dichotomized and if the social contexts of women's lives are ignored. Nearly every chapter in this section demonstrates this point. The authors provide numerous examples of the complex interactions in which psychosocial and behavioral variables can be viewed as both causes and outcomes of chronic illness. Only complex biopsychosocial models will yield a comprehensive understanding of these complicated phenomena. The importance of such models is demonstrated in the chapter by Andersen, in which she provides an excellent example of the value of a biobehavioral model in breast cancer.

Comprehensive models will need to integrate consideration of gender-specific medical issues, as indicated by the examples discussed above. Similar to this need to consider gender differences in medical research is the fact that psychosocial research in behavioral medicine cannot necessarily be generalized from one gender to the other. Chapters in this section suggest, for example, that the impact of social support, psychosocial stressors, and behaviors such as smoking on health may be moderated by gender (see Stoney's, Laudenslager's, and Hermanoff's chapters for examples). The impact of illness on psychological well-being and role functioning also appears to differ in some cases on the basis of gender.

VARIABLES TO INCLUDE IN COMPLEX
MODELS OF WOMEN'S HEALTH

Clearly, it is essential to continue research that considers women's health issues within the context of a multidimensional, nonlinear model. Such a research agenda will not be easy, however. If anything is clear from the chapters in this section, it is that the relationships among physiological, psychological, behavioral, social, and cultural variables are far from simple and straightforward. It is no longer possible to conceptualize the etiology for the onset and progression of chronic disease as either psychological/behavioral or physiological; in almost every case it will be both.

The chapters in this section give important leads as to five categories of variables that should be included in comprehensive models: underlying physiological functioning; disease and treatment characteristics; health care behaviors; psychosocial variables and quality of life; and contextual issues. The relationships of variables both within and among these categories are typically multidirectional, often with mediators and moderators that further complicate the picture. Moreover, in addition to the sex differences discussed earlier, other individual differences such as race/ethnicity and socioeconomic status need to be considered within each category (see the chapters on arthritis, asthma, cardiovascular disorders, diabetes, and hypertension for examples of the importance of these variables in predicting disease onset, prognosis, and treatment efficacy).

Physiological Functioning

Many chapters in this section point to the centrality of endocrine and immune functioning in determining disease etiology, prognosis, and symptom exacerbation in women. The functioning of the immune and endocrine systems is interdependent, with each system influencing the other. Both systems are also subject to the influences of stress and can mediate the important relationships between stress and illness that are highlighted in many chapters in this section. Disruptions in immune and endocrine functioning can, in turn, cause changes in stress levels. The basic mechanisms underlying these interrelationships are described in the chapters by Norris, by Claman, and by Laudenslager; many other chapters provide cogent examples of the complexity of this psychological–physiological interface.

Links with endocrine functioning require special attention in women, in light of the changes in hormone levels that take place over the lifespan with the menstrual cycle, pregnancy, and menopause. In addition, many women will experience hormonal changes caused by exogenous hormones taken as birth control pills, hormone replacement therapy, or prescribed medication (see, e.g., chapters by Rowland and by Ganz on cancer treatments). As the chapters in this section make clear, the relationships between hormone levels and disease onset or symptom exacerbation are not straightforward. Menopause is associated with increased risk for some conditions (see the chapters on arthritis and osteoporosis, coronary heart disease, and hypertension) and with decreased risk for others (see the chapters on gastrointestinal disorders, headache, and lupus). Hormonal fluctuations associated with the menstrual cycle and with pregnancy appear to influence the symptoms of several conditions (see e.g., the chapters on asthma, diabetes, headache, epileptic seizures, lupus, multiple sclerosis, and pain). Curiously, the changes in severity of symptoms are often not in a uniform direction. As both Schmaling and Hermanoff point out, for example, pregnancy is associated with symptom exacerbation for some women with asthma and with symptom improvement for others.

Disease and Treatment Characteristics

Much of the research reported in this section focuses on specific disease processes and treatments. It is obvious from reading these chapters that the unique components of each illness and treatment require continued disease-specific research. It is also clear that important commonalities allow researchers to study broader, underlying mechanisms across related illnesses. The chapters in this section make apparent both the similarities and the differences among autoimmune diseases, for example. In addition to considering underlying biological/medical mechanisms, these chapters suggest common themes that may allow researchers to develop taxonomies based on key elements of disease and treatment that have psychological import. For example, several authors point out the adverse impact on quality of life and stress level when illnesses and treatment side effects are uncontrollable and/or unpredictable. Other common themes that emerge across chapters include the extent to which illness is incurable or fatal, and the extent to which illness and treatment are disabling, painful, disfiguring, or stigmatizing. Many of these issues are considered in depth in other sections of this volume. As is true for each of the model's five categories, disease and treatment characteristics are likely to influence and be influenced by the other categories. For example, Stanton discusses how coping strategies may interact with site of cancer to predict quality of life.

Health Care Behaviors

Many chapters in this section document that disease etiology, progression, and symptom control are related to health care behaviors. Healthy lifestyles—including such behaviors as smoking cessation, weight control, exercise, and good nutrition—are related to almost every condition described in this section. Even when behavior does not appear to play a causal role in disease onset or progression, it may be helpful for symptom control. Chapters on illness prevention are included in Section III of this volume.

Adherence behaviors are of particular relevance to the illnesses discussed in this section. Both Ruggiero and Wylie Rosett, for example, describe the complicated adherence regimens that are required to maintain disease control and extend life for diabetics, and Wassertheil-Smoller provides specific suggestions for enhancing compliance with hypertension treatment. Adherence can be especially difficult with treatments that have iatrogenic effects, which compromise quality of life and sometimes health. For example, as Rowland and Ganz point out, cancer treatments can cause nausea, vomiting, hair loss, weight gain, pain, sexual dysfunction, disfigurement, menopausal symptoms, and a variety of other distressing and disruptive side effects. However, refusal to accept treatment can seriously compromise patients' chances for disease control. Andersen provides a detailed description of how behavior, quality of life, immune functioning, and disease control are interrelated in the case of breast cancer.

Psychosocial Variables and Quality of Life

The chapters in Section II of this volume offer detailed discussions of psychosocial variables that can affect and be affected by health. This section provides examples of these relationships for chronic illnesses. Stress emerges in many chapters as both a cause and an effect of disease onset and progression, symptom exacerbation, and quality of life. The impact of stress varies on the basis of the nature of the stressor and the woman's approach to coping with it. As examples, Bodnar discusses the differences between chronic and acute stressors in analgesia production, and Laudenslager describes how personality interacts with gender in predicting coping strategies in stressful situations. Other psychosocial characteristics with empirically demonstrated importance include personality, social support, active coping, attitudes, and beliefs.

Contextual Issues

There is a growing awareness that comprehensive biopsychosocial models require consideration of the contexts in which women live their lives. Several chapters in this section, for example, point to the importance of family and social networks. Access to supportive relationships—with family members, friends, and health care providers—can be pivotal in adjusting to illness. However, as Zautra points out in his discussion of social support for arthritis patients, the types of social support that are available and the ways in which that support interacts with a patient's needs are more important than simple quantity of support. A woman's life stage, work situation, and role responsibilities also provide contexts that bear on illness and quality of life. Laudenslager provides a compelling picture of the complexity of the relationships between multiple roles and health outcomes in women, for example. Occupational health hazards are also mentioned by several authors (see, e.g., Stoney's and Hermanoff's chapters). In addition, under-standing the impact of any illness or treatment requires placing it within the context of comorbid conditions that it may cause or exacerbate.

Two other contextual issues have traditionally received somewhat less attention in behavioral medicine research: cultural contexts and health care contexts. The United States is a multicultural society, with increasing ethnic and cultural diversity. Almost all of the research in behavioral medicine, however, has focused on the majority culture. When race or ethnicity is considered, it is typically in terms of disease epidemiology. Moreover, research is often limited to comparisons of blacks and whites, without consideration of other rapidly growing ethnic groups. Yet attitudes toward illness and provision of health care, culturally valued coping responses, and perceptions of optimal quality of life may vary across cultures. Research has indicated, for example, that ethnicity can be a primary predictor of patients' attitudes toward autonomy and decision-making preferences. Section IX of this volume considers ethnicity in greater detail.

Obviously, the nature and quality of the provision of health care can influence health outcomes and quality of life. Other sections of this volume offer information on health care policies and approaches that promote women's health. The data provided in this section suggest that women do not always receive optimal care. In some cases, different patterns of symptom presentation lead physicians to overlook serious illness in women (see the examples given by Richardson of HIV infection, by Foley of multiple sclerosis, and by Stoney of coronary heart disease) or to misdiagnose it (see, e.g., the diagnosis of chronic obstructive pulmonary disease as asthma, described by Hermanoff). Misdiag-nosis, as well as lack of access to care, can lead to failures to provide women with adequate care (see, e.g., Richardson's discussion of treatment for women with HIV). It is especially likely—as Stoney, Foley, and Bodnar point out—that symptoms of illness will be attributed to emotional problems in women. Finally, Siegler, Roth, Jenkins, and Richardson underscore the importance of considering the broader social–economic–political context in which health care is administered.

INTERVENTIONS BASED ON MULTIDIMENSIONAL MODELS

One advantage of viewing illness within a complex causal model is that such models allow for psychosocial, behavioral, medical, and public health interventions at several levels. Interventions have been developed to influence physical and psychological well-being in each of the five components of the comprehensive model suggested above. For example, the chapters in this section provide examples of successful nonmedical interventions that help to improve immune functioning, to increase longevity, to decrease treatment side effects, to control pain, to decrease unhealthy behaviors, to teach effective coping skills, to enhance quality of life, and to improve medical care. Effective approaches described here include psychoeducational interventions, social support groups, family therapy, cognitive-behavioral therapies, hypnosis, biofeedback, and progressive muscle relaxation. As Stanton points out in regard to cancer, further research is needed to identify which components of these treatments are most effective for which women.

Behavioral and psychological treatments have further advantages, in that they may be less likely than medical treatments to have negative side effects. They also emphasize teaching skills that a woman can maintain and generalize to other areas of her life. However, several authors caution that psychotherapeutic interventions developed to treat psychological disorders may need to be adapted to be optimally effective for women with chronic physical illnesses. Foley, for example, offers recommendations for altering psychological interventions to meet the needs of people with multiple sclerosis. The examples provided in this section also demonstrate that effective treatment planning requires selecting and adapting interventions targeted to specific disease mechanisms. For example, Freedman documents that temperature feedback is successful in raising finger temperature for women with Raynaud's disease, whereas frontalis electromyographic feedback and autogenic training do not lead to temperature elevations. Similarly, Blanchard indicates that the effectiveness of interventions for treating headaches may depend on the type of headache.

Interventions are also available for family members or people at high risk of developing illness. As several authors in this section explain, a woman's chronic illness can increase stress and disrupt quality of life for her entire family. Illnesses with established genetic bases may be especially upsetting for family members who must deal with the awareness of their own susceptibility, as well as their loved one's illness. Medical genetics is a rapidly growing area of research that is having great success in identifying the genetic markers for specific disease susceptibilities (see, e.g., the chapters on cancer, coronary heart disease, lupus, multiple sclerosis, and Syndrome X). Behavioral medicine researchers and practitioners must be prepared to meet the psychological and ethical challenges that genetic testing will bring. Rowland provides a detailed discussion of these challenges as they relate to women with genetic susceptibility to breast cancer.

CONCLUSION

This section includes essential information for women and their health care providers. The authors describe the physiological, behavioral, and psychosocial aspects of the chronic medical conditions that are most common among women. They offer clear evidence of the importance of considering women's health as a distinct area of inquiry not limited to reproduction and direct endocrine functioning. They also highlight the need to continue the study of behavioral medicine in women. Recent advances document the impossibility of drawing a clear distinction between physiological/medical disorders and behavioral/psychological disorders. Future advances will require a multidisciplinary approach to research and patient care.

The chapters in this section raise as many questions as they answer. We suggest that these questions can best be addressed by considering women's health within a complex, multidirectional, biopsychosocial model. There is still much to learn about how physiological, medical, behavioral, psychosocial, and contextual components interrelate. The research described in this section documents that each of these components can have a bidirectional causal relationship with the others. Much further research will be necessary to understand fully the causal, mediational, moderating, and interactional mechanisms involved in these relationships. Clearly, individual studies will be limited in the questions and processes that they can examine. However, as a collaborative and multidisciplinary field, behavioral medicine holds great promise for answering these questions and for improving the health and well-being of women.

FURTHER READING

Aponte, J. F., Rivers, R. Y., & Wohl, J. (Eds.). (1995). *Psychological interventions and cultural diversity.* Needham Heights, MA: Allyn & Bacon.
This edited volume provides an overview of basic issues relevant to treating culturally diverse patient populations. Although the focus is on interventions for mental health problems, much of the research that is reviewed is applicable to physiological conditions, as well. For example, the book includes chapters on topics such as acculturation, symptom expression, ethnic minority physical health, and clinical issues with ethnic minority women.

Blumenthal, S. J., Matthews, K., & Weiss, S. M. (Eds.). (1994). *New research frontiers in behavioral medicine: Proceedings of the national conference* (Publication No. 94-3772). Washington DC: National Institutes of Health.
This publication includes sections on disease processes, biobehavioral risk factors, treatment interventions, and disease prevention/health promotion across the lifespan. Each section contains an overview and a series of task group reports that summarize current knowledge and suggest promising areas for future research.

Hall, N. R. S., Altman, F., & Blumenthal, S. J. (Eds.). (1996). *Mind–body interactions and disease and psychoneuroimmunological aspects of health and disease.* Orlando, FL: Health Dateline.
This book contains the proceedings of an NIMH conference on psychological and behavioral influences on health and disease. There is a series of brief chapters, each of which is followed by a discussion by the conference participants. The emphasis is on the multifactorial nature of disease.

Stanton, A. L., & Gallant, S. J. (Eds.). (1995). *The psychology of women's health: Progress and challenges in research and application.* Washington, DC: American Psychological Association.

This volume includes chapters on the chronic diseases that account for much of the morbidity and mortality among women. The editors provide an introduction to these topics and suggest challenges for future research.

89

Alzheimer's Disease: A General View

William E. Haley

*A*lzheimer's disease (AD) and related disorders are rarely considered to constitute an important topic in behavioral medicine. These neurological disorders are in fact a major public health problem, affecting up to 4 million U.S. residents and leading to progressive disability and tremendous economic costs associated with their care. In addition, AD commonly takes a heavy toll on family members, who commonly experience severe psychological stress and high rates of depression as they provide care for their relatives in the community. AD takes its greatest toll on women, who not only are at higher risk than men of suffering from AD, but also most commonly take on the role of family caregivers for impaired relatives.

DEFINITION AND DESCRIPTION

"Dementia" is the term used to describe a syndrome of cognitive impairment characterized by a generalized deterioration of intellectual functioning. Patients with dementia experience declines not only in memory, but also in other higher cognitive functions; for example, they exhibit aphasia, constructional apraxia, and alterations in judgment, reasoning, and personality. AD is the most common cause of dementia, followed by vascular or multi-infarct dementia, although dementia can be caused by such diverse processes as Parkinson's disease, AIDS, head trauma, and alcohol dependence. Conceptually, dementia must be distinguished from "amnestic disorder" (e.g., Korsakoff's disease), in which the patient experiences deterioration in memory but not in other cognitive functions, and "delirium," in which cognitive impairment is associated with an acute and often reversible reaction to trauma, medications, or an acute illness.

AD typically has a gradual and insidious onset. In its early stages, patients commonly exhibit such symptoms as forgetfulness, difficulty in remembering names, and mild anxiety and depression; these are often mistakenly attributed to aging, retirement, or psychosocial stresses. As AD slowly progresses, patients develop characteristic impairments in cognitive functioning, self-care skills, and personality and behavior. As memory progressively worsens, patients become disoriented, get lost in unfamiliar settings, and ask the same questions repeatedly. In later stages, memory impairment is so severe that patients may not recognize their homes, their family members, or their own reflections in the mirror. Other higher cognitive functions progressively deteriorate as well. Thus, the patients will show increasingly poor judgment; their language becomes impoverished and repetitive; and concreteness in thinking predominates.

These cognitive impairments lead to characteristic self-care deficits. Patients show reduced abilities in higher-level functions that they were previously capable of performing well, including balancing a checkbook, shopping, preparing meals, housekeeping, and making household repairs. As dementia progresses, patients become unable to dress, bathe, or feed themselves without assistance; urinary and fecal incontinence occurs as well. In end-stage dementia, the patients may become incapable of ambulation, unable to chew or swallow food, and at risk for developing bed sores and opportunistic infections.

Personality and behavioral changes are other common consequences of the cognitive deterioration seen in AD. Patients may develop depression, anxiety, or delusions that people are stealing things from them. Agitation, excessive dependency (e.g., shadowing a caregiver), and resistance to taking baths or medications are also common. A patient may become unsafe without supervision (e.g., leaving the stove on, wandering from the home). Low frustration tolerance and egocentricity are common. In later stages, family members often comment that the patient, though still physically alive, does not seem to be the same person they have known and loved for years. Most patients deny that they have significant cognitive impairment, further complicating their care.

On autopsy, the brains of AD patients show characteristic changes, including atrophy, with particular loss of cholinergic neurons. Neuropathological examination reveals neuritic plaques and neurofibrillary tangles concentrated in the hippocampus and temporoparietal regions. Autopsy studies demonstrate a significant relationship among severity of dementia, number of plaques, and synaptic loss.

EPIDEMIOLOGY AND ECONOMIC IMPACT

As noted above, epidemiological studies suggest that up to 4 million people in the United States have AD or a related dementia. Prevalence is closely associated with age; whereas only 3% of individuals ages 65–74 have AD, about 47% of individuals over age 85 have the disorder. Because of the increasing aging of the U.S. population (individuals over age 85 are the fastest-growing segment of the population), projections suggest that over 14 million U.S. residents will have AD by the year 2050.

Despite extensive research, the causes of AD are presently poorly understood. Women experience higher rates of AD not only because of their greater life expectancy, but even after age is controlled for. Documented risk factors besides age and gender include family history of AD, presence of certain genetic markers, and lower educational and occupational attainment, although the mechanisms through which these factors communicate risk are unclear.

Because AD patients typically need care over a 5- to 10-year period of progressive decline, the costs to society are high. Economic studies suggest that AD and related disorders cost about $40 billion per year from all causes (including nursing home care), and this cost is rapidly increasing.

DIAGNOSIS AND ASSESSMENT

The diagnosis of AD requires cognitive assessment to document changes in cognitive functions; history taking to confirm the characteristic progression of dementia; functional assessment to demonstrate impairment in daily activities; psychological/psychiatric assessment to rule out depression and other mental disorders that can mimic dementia symptoms; and medical assessment to rule out other possible causes of cognitive impairment. Because the only positive confirmation of AD comes through autopsy examination of central nervous system tissue, diagnosis of AD results from a process of exclusion. In specialized AD centers, diagnostic accuracy of over 90% (confirmed through postmortem examination) is attained through judicious use of neuropsychological testing (particularly vital in assessing early AD) and careful consideration of the numerous complex problems of later life that can produce cognitive impairment, including medications, previously undetected illnesses, malnutrition or dehydration, and traumatic injuries caused by falls or other mishaps. Many primary care physicians are poorly prepared to diagnose AD; many patients receive inappropriate diagnoses such as senility, or hardening of the arteries, or have their problems dismissed as "old age."

Neuropsychological assessment is fundamental to the care of AD patients. Such assessment is not only vitally important in distinguishing between early AD and normal age-related changes in memory, but provides a means of monitoring disease progression. Neuropsychological testing also provides critical information in evaluating the effectiveness of treatments for AD, and feedback to caregivers concerning patients' specific cognitive strengths and weaknesses.

CAREGIVING ISSUES

Contrary to the stereotype that families readily abandon their relatives to nursing homes, the majority of patients with AD are cared for in the community by family members. For men with AD, their wives are the most common caregivers; because most women over age 75 are widows, their daughters most commonly assume the caregiving role.

Caregiving in AD is highly stressful, because families must provide increasing levels of assistance with daily care activities to relatives who are often difficult, demanding, and unappreciative of the effort because of their dementia. A patient's behavioral and personality changes are particularly upsetting to a caregiver, because these problems can occur unpredictably, deprive the caregiver of sleep, and threaten the patient's safety. The caregiver must also manage such demanding problems as incontinence in a close family member who was once an active and vital loved one.

Caregiving often leads to other secondary stressors, including financial strain, complications on the job for caregivers who are employed, family conflict, and social isolation. Caregivers have been repeatedly shown to have high rates of depression and may have health problems associated with chronic stress, although there is a great deal of individual variability in coping with caregiving stress. Better adjustment to caregiving is commonly found to be associated with greater social support and activity, more benign appraisals of stress, and problem-focused coping. African-Americans show fewer negative effects of caregiving than European-Americans do, perhaps because of cultural factors that support and normalize the caregiving role.

Although most care of AD patients occurs in the community, patients with dementia constitute about 50% of nursing home residents. Patients with dementia can present severe challenges for professional caregivers as well, who must often manage incontinence, disruptive behaviors, and other disabilities in an environment that is short of resources. Family caregivers experience ongoing strain with institutional care and often show chronic stress-related problems after the death of the patients.

INTERVENTIONS FOR PATIENTS AND FAMILIES

Experimental drug therapies have focused on efforts to improve cholinergic functioning in the brain of the AD patient. Two drugs, tacrine and donepezil hydrochloride, have been approved for the treatment of mild to moderate AD by the U.S. Food and Drug Administration. Tacrine has been shown to produce significant improvements in neuropsychological functioning. However, its use is controversial because many patients experience significant side effects; the clinical significance of these changes is uncertain; and treatment does not prevent the eventual deterioration of the patients. Donepezil hydrochloride has also been shown to lead to significant improvements compared to a placebo, but little is currently known about its practical or long-term impact on AD. Thus the treatment of AD is generally aimed at managing the behavioral and functional losses that occur as the disease progresses, controlling comorbid problems, and helping caregivers to care successfully for the patients while avoiding depression and social isolation themselves. Although psychotropic medications are most commonly used to manage behavioral problems, behavior management approaches that teach caregivers appropriate patient care strategies are effective and preferable where possible. Behavioral approaches have also been used successfully in institutional settings, not only to control patients' disruptive behavior, but also to reduce incontinence and excess disability.

A number of psychosocial programs, including individual and family therapy, support groups, and respite care, have been developed to assist family caregivers. These caregiver interventions have been shown to reduce caregiver depression and burden significantly, and some studies indicate that psychosocial intervention can significantly delay nursing home placement of patients. Ideally, the care for patients with AD and their family caregivers should be provided by an interdisciplinary team, including physicians, psychologists, nurses, social workers, and others who can address the wide range of problems in AD. Such teams are generally available only in specialized AD or geriatric clinics. In other settings, collaboration among health care providers will be essential in assuring appropriate care for patients and families.

FURTHER READING

Aneshensel, C. S., Pearlin, L. I., Mullan, J. T., Zarit, S. H., & Whitlatch, C. J. (1995). *Profiles in caregiving: The unexpected career.* San Diego: Academic Press.
Reviews family caregiving research and reports results of a unique longitudinal study following caregivers through the institutionalization and death of AD patients.

Graves, A. B., & Kukull, W. A. (1994). The epidemiology of dementia. In J. C. Morris (Ed.), *Handbook of dementing illnesses* (pp. 23–69). New York: Marcel Dekker.
Reviews the epidemiology of AD as well as future projections for the disorder.

Haley, W. E., Clair, J. M., & Saulsberry, K. (1982). Family caregiver satisfaction with medical care of their demented relatives. *The Gerontologist, 32,* 219–226.
Reviews problems that families encounter in gaining an accurate diagnosis of AD and appropriate referrals for information, particularly in primary care settings.

Haley, W. E., Roth, D. L., Coleton, M. I., Ford, G. R., West, C. A. C., Collins, R. P., & Isobe, T. L. (1996). Appraisal, coping, and social support as mediators of well-being in black and white Alzheimer's family caregivers. *Journal of Consulting and Clinical Psychology, 64,* 121–129.
Reviews evidence on predictors of successful adjustment to AD caregiving, and reports findings of a study showing mechanisms producing relatively better adjustment among African-American caregivers.

Knight, B. G., Lutzky, S. M., & Macofsky-Urban, F. (1993). A meta-analytic review of interventions for caregiver distress: Recommendations for further research. *The Gerontologist, 33,* 240–248.
Meta-analysis showing that psychosocial interventions lead to demonstrable benefits for caregivers.

LaRue, A. (1992). *Aging and neuropsychological assessment.* New York: Plenum Press.
Reviews the role of neuropsychological testing in diagnosing AD and monitoring its progression.

Mace, N. L., & Rabins, P. V. (1991). *The 36-hour day* (rev. ed.). New York: Warner Books.
A book written as a family guide to AD, but full of practical tips for the management of AD that will also prove helpful for health care professionals.

Mayeux, R., & Schofield, P. W. (1994). Alzheimer's disease. In W. R. Hazzard, E. L. Bierman, J. P. Blass, W. H. Ettinger, & J. B. Halter (Eds.), *Principles of geriatric medicine and gerontology* (3rd ed., pp. 1035–1050). New York: McGraw-Hill.
An excellent overview of the scientific and clinical literature on AD, emphasizing biomedical issues.

90

Alzheimer's Disease: Impact on Women

Ilene C. Siegler

Gender inequality in survival during the period of old age is quite staggering. To put this in perspective, at ages 65–69 there are 127 women per 100 men; at age 85 and older the ratio moves to 220 women per 100 men. Consequently, there are many issues and concerns pertaining to the health care of women in old age. Old age is a status primarily filled by women; functional health is a major link between physical and psychological disorders; and gender predicts marital status, living arrangements, and economic status in later life. Thus, increased survival with decreased resources makes aging particularly challenging for many women. The social–economic–political context, which is often ignored in behavioral medicine research, may need to be considered more often in research dealing with aging women. For older women with Alzheimer's disease (AD), there are two additional concerns: (1) their own risk as patients with AD; and (2) their risk of becoming caregivers for others with AD, and the associated risks that caregiving poses for health and quality of life.

There are also gender differences in functional health and physical disability, as noted by Guralnik and Simonsick in their review of the evidence. The prevalence of disability increases sharply by age. Persons aged 85 and older are in the most difficult circumstances, with these differences magnified by gender for the very old. From ages 65 to 74, 90% of men versus 89% of women live independently, with 1% of each gender in nursing homes. By age 85 and older, 54% of the men and 38% of women live independently at home; 31% of men and 37% of women live at home with help; and 15% of men and 25% of women live in nursing homes.

The difficulties inherent in a diagnosis that is only definite upon autopsy make good data on AD hard to collect. Survey data are generally variable in diagnostic specificity and may represent a cognitive impairment of unknown etiology. Jorm,

Korten, and Henderson provided the classic review on the prevalence of dementia. After reviewing the literature from 1945 to 1985, they concluded that AD is more common in women than in men, whereas multi-infarct dementia is more common in men. Breteler and colleagues provided an excellent review of epidemiology of AD, with particular attention to international studies. Limiting their reports of prevalence from European studies that used diagnostic criteria accepted at that time (DSM-III; DSM-III-R, NINCDS-ADRA) they presented prevalence rates by ages. At ages 60–69, 70–79, and 80–89, the respective rates were 0.4%, 3.6%, and 11.2% for women and 0.3%, 2.5%, and 10.0% for men. Thus, a slight increase for women at each decade was reported. Gender differences were minimal in incidence. Overall, gender plays a relatively small role compared to age as a risk factor.

Other risk factors studied in case–control studies include the family history of dementia, family history of Parkinson's disease, family history of Down's syndrome, head trauma, hypothyroidism, depression, and smoking (protective). The associations with depression and smoking may have gender implications. Heyman and colleagues present some of the very best current data available. They suggest the possibility of two types of survivor confounds. Not only do more women survive until the onset of AD, but, once affected, they survive longer with AD. Also, it is interesting that in those with AD, race and low socioeconomic status do not further increase mortality rates.

Henderson and colleagues found that postmenopausal estrogen replacement therapy may be associated with a decreased risk of AD, and that estrogen replacement may improve cognitive performance with this illness. If these findings can be confirmed, they will be extremely important. Data collection in the ongoing Women's Health Study, as well as from a new clinical trial being conducted by the Alzheimer's Disease Cooperative Study Group, should help provide some answers. Two studies completed while this book was in production have confirmed that estrogen use is protective for AD (Paganini-Hill & Henderson, 1996; Kawas et al., 1997).

When we look at caregivers for older persons, the burden falls on women: 23% of care for older persons is provided by wives, 13% by husbands, 29% by daughters, 8% by sons, 20% by other women, and 7% by other men. However, when we look at studies of caregiving, such as that by Light, Niederehe, and Lebowitz, the design is to use spouse caregivers and matched controls; gender is not a major variable in the analyses. Therefore, the conclusions are indirect. There is little reason to assume that the processes that increase stress and potential for cardiovascular disease, immune breakdown, and depression affect aging men differently from aging women. In a 1992 meta-analysis of gender differences in caregiving, Miller and Cafasso reported that they found 99 studies conducted on caregiver issues between 1980 and 1990. Of these, only 14 had sufficient data to be used in the meta-analysis they performed. Results indicated that over the studies that included the variables of interest, there were no differences in the level of impairment of the patients cared for by men and women caregivers, in caregiver involvement, or in the types of tasks carried out. There was a significant finding that women caregivers were more likely to report a higher burden.

As the "baby boom" generation enters old age (the 1946 cohort will be 65 in 2011) in better shape, what will the future hold for it? Along with better education and health promotion activities comes a youth culture with extremely high expectations for its own old age. Because more and more people are products of blended families with fewer siblings and few children, we can only predict that family patterns will change, and that the inequalities seen now can be expected to increase in the future.

FURTHER READING

Breteler, M. M. B., Claus, J. J., van Duijn, C. M., Launer, L. J., & Hofman, A. (1992). Epidemiology of Alzheimer's Disease. *Epidemiologic Reviews, 14,* 59–82.
Classic international review.

Guralnik, J. M., & Simonsick, E. M. (1993). Physical disability in older Americans. *Journal of Gerontology, 48,* 3–10.
Good description of gender differences.

Henderson, V. W., Paganini-Hill, A., Emanuel, C. K., Dunn, M. E., & Buckwalter, J. G. (1994). Estrogen replacement therapy in older women: Comparisons between Alzheimer's disease cases and nondemented control subjects. *Archives of Neurology, 51,* 896–900.
Speculative hypothesis.

Heyman, A., Peterson, B., Fillenbaum, G., & Pieper, C. (1996). The Consortium to Establish a Registry for Alzheimer's Disease (CERAD): XIV. Demographic and clinical predictors of survival in patients with Alzheimer's disease. *Neurology, 46,* 565–660.
Best current data.

Jorm, A. F., Korten, A. E., & Henderson, A. S. (1987). The prevalence of dementia: A quantitative integration of the literature. *Acta Psychiatrica Scandinavica, 76,* 465–479.
Classic review.

Kane, R. L., Ouslander, J. G., & Abrass, I. B. (1994). *Essentials of clinical geriatrics* (3rd ed.). New York: McGraw Hill.
Textbook.

Kawas, C., Resnick, S., Morrison, A., Brookmeyer, R., Corrada, M., Zonderman, A., Bacal, C., Donnell Lingle, D., & Metter, E. (1997). A prospective study of estrogen replacement therapy and the risk of developing Alzheimer's Disease: The Baltimore Longitudinal Study of Aging. *Neurology, 48,* 1517–1521.
Provides support for the protective effect of estrogen.

Light, E., Niederehe, G., & Lebowitz, B. D. (Eds.). (1994). *Stress effects in family caregivers of Alzheimer's patients.* New York: Springer.
Comprehensive set of chapters on caregiving.

Miller, B., & Cafasso, L. (1992). Gender differences in caregiving: Fact or artifact? *The Gerontologist, 23,* 498–507.
A review of gender differences in caregiving.

Paganini-Hill, A., & Henderson, V. W. (1996). Estrogen replacement therapy and the risk of Alzheimer's Disease. *Archives of Internal Medicine, 156,* 2213–2217.
Supports role of estrogen.

Stanford, E. P., & Du Bois, B. C. (1992). Gender and ethnicity patterns. In J. E. Birren, R. B. Sloane, & G. D. Cohen (Eds.), *Handbook of mental health and aging* (pp. 99–117). San Diego: Academic Press.
Useful statistics from a useful volume.

91

Arthritis: Behavioral and Psychosocial Aspects

Alex J. Zautra

Of the over 100 forms of arthritis, two types predominate: rheumatoid arthritis (RA) and osteoarthritis (OA). RA is a systemic autoimmune disease that affects approximately 3% of older adult women. The disease is characterized by unpredictable episodes of painful swelling and tenderness in multiple joints, and by progressive destruction in those joints. Its onset is typically between the ages of 30 and 45; women are three times more likely to contract RA than men. OA is a more common disease. It affects over 50% of those over the age of 70, and is more evenly distributed across the genders, with men just as likely to have OA as women. OA is known as a "wear-and-tear" disease, caused by the breakdown of cartilage between the bones. Often only one joint is involved, with progressive deterioration in function and increased pain over time as the space in the joint capsule narrows, leading to bone-to-bone contact. Like RA, OA is highly painful and disabling in its most severe forms.

Together, these two diseases pose the primary threat to quality of life among older adult women. Not only are these forms of arthritis the chief cause of disability among adults, but there is also no known means of preventing these diseases, and no treatments have been proven to arrest the disease course. According to the Centers for Disease Control and Prevention, nearly 40 million U.S. residents have some form of arthritis. As the average age of the population increases, the prevalence of these diseases also is also growing; a 57% increase in the number of people with arthritis is expected by the year 2020.

BEHAVIORAL AND PSYCHOSOCIAL IMPACTS OF ARTHRITIS

Pain and activity limitation are the twin perils of arthritis, and to this list may be added sleep disturbance and fatigue, which often accompany the disease. There are also many side effects of medications used to control the inflammatory processes of arthritis, including severe gastric distress, ulceration, and liver damage from the use of nonsteroidal anti-inflammatory drugs, and bone loss and muscle atrophy from long-term use of steroid medications. In addition, there are the social consequences of joint disfigurement, especially in the hands and wrists of women with RA. Arthritis is a silent disease. When there is no visible impairment of limbs, even those close to a patient are often unaware of the extent of pain and limitation, and may question the patient's claims of disability. These difficulties are present not only among those with RA or OA; other forms of arthritis, such as systemic lupus erythematosus (SLE) and fibromyalgia, can also lead to severe joint pain, fatigue, and disability. (For a fuller discussion of SLE, see Newell and Coeshott's chapter in this volume.)

In light of these symptoms, it is not surprising that many women with arthritis suffer from psychological distress. An appropriate term for these psychological reactions may be the one coined by Jerome Frank, "demoralization"—that is feelings of helplessness and hopelessness, a loss of self-esteem, a sense of loss, and anxiety over the future. Three related problems in living are most responsible for this demoralization: pain, activity limitation, and the strain from troubled interpersonal relationships (which often worsen for those with a chronic illness).

Underlying these difficulties is a fundamental psychological threat—a threat to autonomy. Physical restrictions force a change in future goals; plans and dreams for a vigorous life are disrupted; and the frequent, if not constant, struggle with chronic pain begins to consume daily life. Many older adult women see caregiving as a central aspect of their identity. Limitations on their activity often restrict their ability to fulfill their role of caring for other family members, principally their husbands, who often have disabling illnesses as well.

Apart from its impact on mental health, arthritis can profoundly affect quality of life. Clearly, pain and activity limitation increase the negative affect usually associated with psychological states of depression and anxiety. The disease also reduces opportunities for engagement in everyday life experiences that promote positive affect, a separate component of a person's psychological well-being. Frequently, these deficiencies in quality of life will go unnoticed by practitioners adhering to a medical model for assessing and treating arthritis-related symptoms. Behavioral interventions designed to assist these women ought to include not only ways of coping with pain, but methods of enhancing a sense of well-being through attention to needs for active engagement in life concerns.

ADAPTIVE AND MALADAPTIVE COPING STRATEGIES

Current research on psychological adjustment to arthritis focuses on the identification of forms of coping that help patients adapt to the negative impacts of the disease, as well as maladaptive forms of coping associated with poor adjustment. The key ingredient in all adaptive forms of coping is an increase in patient's beliefs that they can effectively control the most distressing aspects of the disease. In treatment of chronic arthritis pain, patients are typically offered training in a variety of active coping strategies, including progressive deep muscle relaxation, activity pacing, visualization and imagery training, meditation and deep breathing, physical exercise, and methods of cognitive distraction. Any one or a combination of these techniques may prove successful in providing a patient with a greater sense of mastery over the pain that accompanies the disease. In addition to professional services, self-help manuals are available, and the local chapters of the

Arthritis Foundation run self-help groups that provide instruction to those with arthritis on how to cope with the illness. These self-help groups are effective in increasing self-efficacy among arthritis patients.

Maladaptive forms of coping include passive withdrawal, catastrophizing, and wishful thinking. Cognitive models of depression are applied here to understanding and treating problems of adjustment to the chronic pain and limitations of arthritis. Indeed, there is strong empirical evidence that these forms of coping are most common among those arthritis patients with the greatest distress. Therapies that have been directed toward reducing these cognitions have generally been successful in the short run in reducing pain, psychological distress, and "psychological" disability among those with OA and RA.

Active acceptance of the disease is generally associated with better psychological adjustment, but passive resignation, or giving up, is not. Denial is common among women who first learn they have RA; they often refuse to accept the illness in part because they fear the loss of control implied by passive resignation. Such women are often helped by learning to distinguish passive from active acceptance of their condition. Education about the disease's course, and instruction on what patients can do to help themselves early in the disease process, are also useful.

THE ROLE OF INTERPERSONAL
RELATIONSHIPS IN COPING

One of the most frequent responses to arthritis pain and activity limitation is to seek social support. Whether this coping strategy is adaptive or maladaptive depends both on the type of support sought and on the nature of response from significant others. For a marital couple, there are two related issues: the quality of the marital relationship independent of the disease, and the way in which the partners respond to each other when coping with the challenges presented by the disease. Strains caused by marital problems are exacerbated by pain and activity limitation. In such a relationship, fatigue, pain, and depression are often misinterpreted as a form of malingering or a willful disregard of the other spouse's needs. Patients with highly critical spouses report using more maladaptive coping strategies; those who perceive their spouses to be more supportive use more active and adaptive methods. My colleagues and I have found that patients' beliefs in the efficacy of their coping efforts are also adversely affected by troubled interpersonal relationships.

Even a couple with a good relationship may be challenged by the disease-related changes imposed. Neither the patient nor the spouse/partner may know how best to help each other cope with the pain and physical limitations. A spouse/partner must learn how best to provide caregiving responses that assist the arthritis patient in her coping efforts. One approach that my colleagues and I have taken is not only to identify the extent of support (and the presence of negative social interactions), but also to examine the supportive message itself. Table 91.1 shows one typology we have found useful in classifying the caregiving responses of spouses of RA patients: (1) self-reliance encouragement; and (2) other-reliance encouragement. A spouses/partner may unwittingly increase a patient's pain and dependency through attempts to take command of the patient's illness. Encouragement of self-reliance is usually associated with better psychological adjustment and a greater sense of self-efficacy in the patient.

TABLE 91.1. Assessing Partners' Styles of Encouragement

Self-reliance encouragement

1. Told her she could make her own decisions.
2. Suggested that she should work on her problems in her own way.
3. Told her that she can pretty much determine what will happen in her life.
4. Asked her to "stand on her own two feet," emotionally.
5. Encouraged her to be more self-reliant.

Other-reliance encouragement

1. Suggested that she be more reliant on others.
2. Encouraged her to feel that others know what's best for her.
3. Suggested that she let others take more responsibility for solving her problems.
4. Suggested that others may be more capable of handling her problems than she is.

We have found some exceptions to this general principle in our study of RA couples. Older women with an external locus of control are sometimes helped by other-reliance encouragement from their spouses, perhaps because that type of support matches their expectations for the type of help they believe they need. Furthermore, during those times that the disease is most painful, encouragement of self-reliance may not be beneficial. The key point is that the spouse/partner needs to be flexible in providing supportive help, and needs to understand that the ill partner's needs may change over the course of the illness and during peak flare-ups of the disease.

ARTHRITIS AND STRESS

There is mounting evidence in arthritis research that chronic stress can worsen the disease itself. There are a number of potential mechanisms for such effects. First, it appears that some forms of chronic stress can increase pain sensitivity among arthritis patients, and are also likely to reduce efforts to cope effectively with the disease. For RA patients, the research evidence suggests that the inflammatory processes themselves are affected by stress via hormonal responses in the hypothalamic–pituitary–adrenal axis. We have found evidence to suggest that RA patients are more reactive to interpersonal stressors physiologically as well as psychologically. Normally, cortisol elevations following stressful encounters serve to lower immune activity. In patients with RA, however, stress reactivity may be accompanied by a blunted cortisol response, which may lead to a failure to down-regulate immune cell proliferation provoked by immune-stimulating hormones such as prolactin. Increased inflammation and eventual joint damage may result. These last pieces of the puzzle are not yet in place, but they provide increasingly strong support for the role of psychosocial factors both in disease progression and in the patient's quality of life.

FURTHER READING

Bandura, A. (1992). Self-efficacy mechanism in psychobiologic functioning. In R. Schwarzer (Ed.), *Self-efficacy: Thought control of action* (pp. 355–393). Washington DC: Hemisphere.

This chapter examines the research evidence from a number of studies on the importance of perceptions of self-efficacy for the preservation of health and well-being.

Chrousos, G. P. (1995). The hypothalamic–pituitary–adrenal axis and immune-mediated inflammation. *New England Journal of Medicine, 332,* 1351–1362.
This author presents a comprehensive review of current knowledge on the influence of hypothalamic, pituitary, and adrenal hormones on immune system functioning.

Frank, J. D. (1961). *Persuasion and healing.* Baltimore, MD: Johns Hopkins University Press.
This classic book describes the factors that all therapies have in common and how they assist in the restoration of morale.

Keefe, F. J., Caldwell, D. S., Williams, D. A., Gil, K., Mitchell, D., Robertson, C., Martinez, S., Nunley, J., Beckman, J., Crisson, J., & Helms, M. (1990). Pain coping skills training in the management of osteoarthritic knee pain: A comparative study. *Behavior Therapy, 21,* 49–62.
This paper examines the success of a cognitive-behavioral program in pain management for patients with OA of the knee, in comparison to a control population.

Lorig, K., & Fries, J. F. (1996). *The arthritis helpbook* (4th ed.). Reading, MA: Addison-Wesley.
This self-help manual provides an introduction to arthritis-related illnesses, and ways in which patients can help themselves manage the disease successfully.

Manne, S., & Zautra, A. J. (1989). The effects of spouse critical remarks on psychological adjustment to rheumatoid arthritis. *Journal of Personality and Social Psychology, 56,* 608–617.
This empirical study examines the role of the spouse in the coping efforts of the patient with RA.

Yelin, E. (1992). Arthritis: The cumulative impact of a common chronic condition. *Arthritis and Rheumatism, 35,* 489–497.
This paper provides an overview of the broad social impact of arthritis on family and community life.

Zautra, A. J., Burelson, M., Matt, K., Roth, S., & Burrows, L. (1994). Interpersonal stress and disease activity in rheumatoid arthritis. *Health Psychology, 13,* 139–148.
This study tests the proposition that flare-ups of RA are related to interpersonal stressors as mediated by immune-stimulating hormones.

Zautra, A. J., Reich, J. W., & Newsom, J. T. (1995). Autonomy and sense of control among older adults: An examination of their effects on mental health. In L. Bond, S. Culter, & A. Grams (Eds.), *Promoting successful and productive aging* (pp. 153–170). Thousand Oaks, CA: Sage.
This chapter reviews concepts of control as they relate to older adults who are coping with a loss of autonomy caused by disabling medical conditions.

92

Arthritis: Medical Aspects

Sanford H. Roth

*T*he term "arthritis" refers to a group of diseases characterized by joint inflammation. The most common form of crippling arthritis is rheumatoid arthritis, with at least a 3:1 female-to-male ratio. Osteoarthritis represents the most common form of arthritis in general and is associated with an equal gender distribution in the population. Typically more women than men seek treatment, according to our national data bank, the American Rheumatism Association Medical Information System (ARAMIS). Infectious forms of arthritis were formerly on the wane; however, with more common immunosuppression and glucocorticosteroid use in arthritis, and further immunocompromise by aging, diabetes, or poor nutrition, secondary infectious forms of arthritis and sexually transmitted forms of antibiotic-resistant arthritis are increasingly seen. Nevertheless, there is a dissociation between rheumatoid arthritis, which is immune-T-cell-expressive, and AIDS, which is immune-T-cell-compromised. Thus, there are virtually no cases of comorbid rheumatoid arthritis and AIDS.

Rheumatoid arthritis is used here as the prototype for arthritis models and management, since it represents the inflammatory rheumatic spectrum of the most devastating of systemic diseases. It tends to occur in three phases of the female host population: at menarche, during the early childbearing years, and postmenopausally. The hormonal associations with these events have been studied, and the basis for this point prevalence remains unknown but important.

The economically disadvantaged minority female suffers the consequences of rheumatoid arthritis disproportionately. A major epidemiological study at Vanderbilt University has documented that level of education, rather than socioeconomic factors, has the strongest impact on prognosis. The less educated appear to have more severe rheumatoid arthritis and arthritis-related compromising outcomes.

DRUG THERAPY FOR RHEUMATOID ARTHRITIS

Pharmacotherapy of rheumatoid arthritis has changed drastically in the past decade. Aggressive immunomodulation (most often with methotrexate and antimetabolite therapy such as azathioprine) is started at the earliest stage, before erosive, destructive disease progresses. Corticosteroids are still commonly used to bridge more active stages of the arthritis until the slower-acting disease-modifying agents become effective. Nonsteroidal anti-inflammatory drugs (NSAIDs) are ubiquitously used because of both their symptomatic analgesic and useful anti-inflammatory properties. The therapeutic toxicity consequences of all these drugs in women are especially expressed in relation to age.

Corticosteroids are poorly tolerated in postmenopausal women, with osteopenia and potential for compression fractures, as well as adverse hormonal metabolic consequences. However, corticosteroids may be tolerated and useful in lower doses in younger women and males. NSAIDs are associated with the most common severe events reported for all forms of medication—NSAID gastropathies. In particular, the ulcer problems (usually affecting the stomach) are more dangerous in elderly females than in any other subset of the population, according to both retrospective and prospective studies. These complications result in considerable morbidity, are highly expensive, and may account for up to 10,000 iatrogenic deaths annually. They have resulted in a new industry: developing potentially gastrosparing NSAIDs and gastroprotective medication. The focus of this industry is predominantly the female health consumer.

Immunomodulating drug therapy has brought about some recent changes in outcome expectations. For the first time, reports of long-term successful depression of disease activity are entering the literature. Disease-suppressive pharmacotherapy at the earliest stage, before mobilization of immune-expressive momentum, appears to be critical to these improved outcomes.

THE NEED FOR A TEAM APPROACH

Despite the recent advances in drug therapy, it is increasingly documented that pharmacotherapeutics are only part of the challenge of managing problems related to rheumatoid arthritis. Psychosocial factors, as discussed by Zautra and Wisocki in their chapters, appear critical to both disease exacerbation and progression. Psychoendocrine immunopathy correlation indicates that behavioral intervention with social structuring is key to the long-term successful management of patients with this incurable chronic disorder.

Physical and occupational rehabilitation efforts should be continual and should be integrated into a team program, along with obvious nutritional and orthopedic programs. However, such highly structured and essentially lifelong programs are significantly threatened by the new directions of managed care in medicine. The enormous pressures for short-term, cost-effective outcomes too often mitigate against quality-of-life issues, with long-term consequences that can only be measured over the years and even decades.

CONCLUSIONS

A team approach combining behavioral, psychosocial, and educational support with pharmacological, rehabilitative, and at times orthopedic intervention is the recommended approach to treatment of rheumatoid arthritis. Reinforcement and continuing review of goals and alternative measures are necessary to help patients adjust to such a chronic and variable disease. Again, however, the short-term goals of managed care, in the absence of monitoring and a more comprehensive health care program, can result in long-term severely compromised outcomes with larger public health consequences. This is a particular concern in this era of single mothers, working mothers, and disparities in availability of affordable health care. Only a well-educated public health sector can respond to this challenge in an already frayed fabric of health care support. Pharmacotherapeutic advances, with the discovery of biological agents that affect the cellular receptors responsible for abnormal disease-related immune expression, may be the wave of the near future. But the health care consumer must have access to a committed health care provider to maintain quality of life and wellness.

FURTHER READING

Roth, S. H. (1995). Role of the rheumatologist in 1995: Leadership [Editorial]. *Journal of Rheumatology, 22*(1).
Defines the management programs for the various arthritis and rheumatic disorders so common in women.

Roth, S. H. (1996). NSAID gastropathy: A new understanding. *Archives of Internal Medicine, 156,* 96.
This is an overview of the most devastating and dangerous consequences of long-term NSAID use, particularly in elderly women, offering a basis for prophylaxis and alternative therapies.

Zautra, A. J., Burleson, M. H., Matt, K. S., Roth, S. H., & Burrows, L. (1994). Interpersonal stress, depression, and disease activity in rheumatoid and osteoarthritis patients. *Health Psychology, 13,* 139–148.
This is the first documented study that corroborates the relationship between stress/coping mechanisms and serological endocrine and immune responses correlated with actual clinical arthritis changes in disease activity.

93

Arthritis and Osteoporosis

Patricia A. Wisocki

Health status often defines the quality of a person's older years. If an older adult is in good health, worries are fewer, levels of functioning are higher, and life satisfaction is greater. Unfortunately, more than two-thirds of people over age 65 have at least one chronic medical condition, and more than 50% have at least two chronic illnesses. Adults over 65 have the highest overall rate of illness, disability, and restrictions on their activities when all population groups are considered. Older adults also use health care services more often and incur more health-related expenses than any other age group.

As a woman ages, she experiences diminished efficiency on both physiological and behavioral levels. These changes occur gradually, however, and vary among individuals. Tissues, body systems, and cells age differently both among and within people, perhaps because of genetic mandates, the health practices of a lifetime, or both.

Decline usually occurs in the nervous system, resulting in decreased reaction time, performance speed, and flexibility. The cardiac, pulmonary, sensory, and immunological systems also diminish in efficiency. Immune responsivity decreases on both the humoral and cellular levels, correlating with increased incidence of infection, malignancy, and autoimmune diseases. The performance of complex, coordinated activities becomes more difficult as one ages.

The three leading causes of death for adults over the age of 65, regardless of sex, are cardiovascular disease, cancer, and stroke. The most common chronic health problems for older adults are hypertensive disease, arthritis, and osteoporosis, each of which is related to such lifestyle variables as diet, cigarette smoking, excess weight, and lack of exercise. Of particular concern for older adult women are the two diseases of arthritis and osteoporosis, because they occur more often among women than among men of a similar age, and because they often result in extreme disability and lead to home confinement or nursing home care.

ARTHRITIS

"Arthritis" refers to a collection of nearly 100 inflammatory and noninflammatory joint diseases that are chronic, degenerative, and debilitating. The most common forms of inflammatory joint diseases include rheumatoid arthritis, ankylosing spondylitis, and systemic lupus erythematosus. These disorders begin with the precipitating symptom of joint inflammation, principally in the synovial membrane, which then damages the joint capsule, supporting ligaments, cartilage, and subchrondal bone. This tissue damage places mechanical stress on the joint structures, making them extremely vulnerable to over-stretching; if the stress is severe and prolonged, joint destruction and residual deformity may occur, accompanied by pain and protective muscle spasm. Systemic inflammation can affect connective tissue throughout the body, and a small percentage of patients may also experience damage in the eyes, nerves, heart, blood vessels, and lungs. In osteoarthritis, the most common arthritic condition, joint damage is caused by degeneration rather than by inflammation, although secondary inflammation may be present. Osteoarthritis is characterized by stiffness, muscle weakness/atrophy, deformity caused by degeneration of the cartilage, and pain upon weight bearing. When secondary inflammation is present, pain and muscle spasm may coexist. Taken together, the various forms of arthritis afflict about 38 million U.S. residents, a substantial portion of whom are older adult women. They are the primary causes of disability in older adults, affecting 60–90% of people over the age of 60. (For further discussions of osteoarthritis and, in particular, rheumatoid arthritis, see Zautra's and Roth's chapters; for more details on systemic lupus erythematosus, see Newell and Coeshott's chapter.)

Endocrine, nutritional, and metabolic factors and a variety of occupational, psychosocial, and geographic factors have some influence over the course of arthritis, although they do not contribute to its cause. Researchers have hypothesized that the pathology of the disease may have its basis in the autoimmune mechanisms, the genetic predisposition, or the impact of direct trauma or neoplastic lesions.

Treatment for arthritis includes exercise to strengthen supporting muscles, weight loss if necessary, stress reduction, anti-inflammatory drugs, and bed rest. A number of behavioral techniques may be used to reach these goals, such as relaxation or biofeedback to reduce muscle tension; programs for pain management, weight control, and stress management; and reinforcement programs to enhance compliance with exercise and medication schedules. There is a substantial amount of literature documenting the value of these procedures for a variety of health-related problems, but few studies have included older adults in their treatment protocols.

Four studies have been published describing the application of behavioral or cognitive-behavioral procedures to the treatment of arthritis for older adults. In three of the studies, a cognitive-behavioral treatment package was compared with either a symptom-monitoring condition or an educational program in which arthritis sufferers learned about various aspects of the disease and its treatment. In the first two studies, by Appelbaum and colleagues and by Keefe and colleagues, behavioral treatment was superior to both of these conditions in subjective measures of pain perception, control of pain sensations, and use of coping techniques. Appelbaum and colleagues also reported that patients were more functionally active and demonstrated moderate improvement in range of motion, but Keefe and his colleagues did not find improvement in physical ability or pain behavior in any group. Calfas and colleagues did not find that a cognitive-behavioral treatment program was any better than an educational program for pain relief; patients improved in both conditions. The fourth study, by Radojevic and colleagues, involved a comparison of the benefits of enlisting family support in a behavioral pain management program versus no family support for patients with rheumatoid arthritis. Family support did not add significantly to the benefits of the treatment program.

An educational program developed by Lorig and her colleagues has been used throughout the country as a helpful adjunct to other treatment methods. The course is taught by two trainers for six weekly 2-hour sessions, with a primary theme of achieving a sense of control over the disease. Patients taking the course are given a wide range of information about arthritis and its management, including the importance of exercise, relaxation, and nutrition, and they have opportunities to practice new and previous learned techniques during each session. A group of participants was evaluated at 4, 8, and 20 months after the course was completed. Compared with a control group, the participants significantly increased their knowledge and self-management behavior while significantly decreasing their pain.

Exercise, particularly walking, is a highly recommended intervention for elderly arthritis sufferers. Exercise training produces gains in physical capacity and decreases in pain and disability. Despite these findings, however, physicians do not routinely recommend exercise to their older arthritic patients, according to interviews with a large sample of older adults. Dexter found that only a small percentage of the adults interviewed exercised in a therapeutically beneficial way, even when they were advised to exercise; this indicates a need for proper training in exercise methods.

OSTEOPOROSIS

Osteoporosis is a disease which affects between 25 and 30 million people in the United States. It is characterized by low bone mass and deterioration of bone tissue, which lead to enhanced skeletal fragility, increased risk of fractures, and sometimes death. It is almost exclusively a problem for older adults and occurs four times more often in women than in men, probably because of estrogen withdrawal. Nutritional impoverishment of calcium and phosphorus in early life may also be associated with later-life development of this disorder.

Treatment for this disorder mainly consists of a calcium-rich diet, Vitamin D supplements, and estrogen supplements to reduce further bone resorption. There are no studies describing the use of psychological procedures to enhance compliance with dietary requirements for osteoporotic women, but evidence from other areas in which nutrition was improved through behavioral technology supports its value in this case. Because older adults typically consume fewer calories than nutritionists recommend, nutrient intake must remain at normal levels or even increase if patients are to maintain good health.

Exercise is also a critical factor in treatment, as it is in arthritis. Studies consistently indicate that women participating in strength training programs demonstrate maintenance or positive gains in bone density, whereas patients in control groups experience corresponding decreases.

FURTHER READING

Appelbaum, K., Blanchard, E., Hickling, E., & Alfonso, M. (1988). Cognitive behavioral treatment of a veteran population with moderate to severe rheumatoid arthritis. *Behavior Therapy, 19,* 489–502.
Behavioral treatment was more effective in reducing arthritis pain than was symptom monitoring, but the effects were not maintained at an 18-month follow-up.

Calfas, K., Kaplan, R., & Ingram, R. (1992). One year evaluation of cognitive-behavioral intervention in osteoarthritis. *Arthritis Care and Research, 5,* 202–209.

Although arthritic patients given a cognitive-behavioral intervention initially showed more improvement on various measures of psychological and physical functioning than patients given an educational program did, no differences were noted between the groups at the end of a year.

Dexter, P. (1992). Joint exercises in elderly persons with symptomatic osteoarthritis of the hip or knee: Performance patterns, medical support patterns, and the relationship between exercising and medical care. *Arthritis Care and Research, 5,* 36–41.

Although exercise is regarded as a standard treatment for osteoarthritis, and most arthritic patients have seen physicians, few physicians advise patients to exercise.

Ettinger, W., & Afable, R. (1994). Physical disability from knee osteoarthritis: The role of exercise as an intervention. *Medicine and Science in Sports and Exercise, 26,* 1435–1440.

Exercise training corrects deficits in physical capacity of older adult patients experiencing osteoarthritis of the knee.

Keefe, F., Caldwell, D., Williams, D., Gil, K., Mitchell, D., Robertson, C., Martinez, S., Nunley, J., Beckman, J., Crisson, J., & Helms, M. (1990). Pain coping skills training in the management of osteoarthritic knee pain: A comparative study. *Behavior Therapy, 21,* 49–62.

Training in pain coping skills, compared to education about arthritis or standard care, lowered levels of pain and psychological disability, but did not improve physical disability on pain behaviors.

Lorig, K., Laurin, J., & Holman, H. (1984). Arthritis self-management: A study of the effectiveness of patient education for the elderly. *The Gerontologist, 24,* 455–457.

A self-management program involving training in relaxation, problem-solving, exercise, and education was effective for reducing the pain of elderly arthritis sufferers.

Nelson, M., Fiatarone, M., Morganti, C., Trice, I., Greenberg, R., & Evans, W. (1994). Effects of high intensity strength training on multiple risk factors for osteoporotic fractures: A randomized controlled trial. *Journal of the American Medical Association, 272,* 1909–1914.

Strength training for postmenopausal women preserved total body bone mineral content, along with muscle mass, muscle strength, and dynamic balance.

Radojevic, V., Nicassio, P., & Weisman, M. (1992). Behavioral intervention with and without family support for rheumatoid arthritis. *Behavior Therapy, 23,* 13–30.

Family support did not add significantly to the treatment benefits of behavioral interventions for pain behavior associated with rheumatoid arthritis.

94

Asthma

Karen B. Schmaling

Breathing is a basic human function, essential for life, and under voluntary control; yet asthma and other respiratory disorders have been afforded little attention by behavioral scientists.

EPIDEMIOLOGY, PHYSIOLOGY, AND MEDICAL TREATMENT OF ASTHMA

Asthma is a significant public health problem that affects 4–5% of the U.S. population. The number of deaths resulting from asthma has been increasing in the last 15 years, especially among the poor, those living in urban areas, and African-Americans. Reliable gender differences in mortality have not been found. The reasons for increased mortality are unclear, but they may be associated with changes in environmental factors (e.g., pollution), overuse of asthma medications with potentially fatal side effects, undertreatment or delayed treatment seeking by patients, limited availability of health care for patients in lower socioeconomic strata, or a combination of these factors. Paradoxically, this increase in asthma deaths has occurred in an era of development of new and improved asthma treatments.

Asthma is a multifactorial illness characterized by reversible obstruction or narrowing of the airways through edema and inflammation, hyperresponsiveness, increased mucus secretion, and changes in smooth muscle tone. Asthma symptoms may be triggered by a variety of factors, including extrinsic agents (e.g., allergens, irritants, and exercise) and intrinsic factors (e.g., strong emotions or behavior associated with strong emotions, such as laughing or crying).

Stimulation of the sympathetic division of the autonomic nervous system is associated with bronchodilation; conversely, increased parasympathetic activity and activation of the vagus nerve are associated with bronchoconstriction. Asthma has been characterized as a state of parasympathetic dominance. Thus, most inhaled asthma drugs act as beta-adrenoceptor stimulants and may be referred to as "sympathomimetic"; that is, they mimic the effects of stimulation of the sympathetic nervous system and result in bronchodilation.

Asthma symptoms may include coughing, wheezing, shortness of breath, and sensations of tightness in or pressure on the chest. Asthma "attacks" may be characterized by an acute onset of symptoms, but because symptoms can occur insidiously, "attack" may be a misnomer for some patients' experience of their asthma. Treatment involves medications that control acute attacks, as well as medications that are used for long-term maintenance and prophylaxis of acute episodes of symptoms. Patients with mild asthma may use an inhaled bronchodilator on an as-needed basis only; patients with severe asthma may require regular use of bronchodilators and anti-inflammatory preparations, such as inhaled or oral corticosteroids. The latter medications taken orally may be associated with the development of a variety of unpleasant side effects, including weight gain, mood lability, and delirium.

Parameters of normal lung function are well established. The peak flow meter is a self-monitoring device that can be very useful for patients. Clinically significant deviations from a patient's normal range of maximal expiratory flow (e.g., a decrement of 15–20%) signal the need to change behavior, such as taking extra medication or calling one's physician.

COMPLIANCE WITH MEDICAL TREATMENT

Effective asthma control requires a lifelong commitment to its treatment. Patients may be asked to comply with a number of emotionally challenging recommendations, such as giving away cherished pets to whom they are allergic, isolating themselves from valued people or activities in settings where smoke or other irritants are present, and taking medications that may result in a variety of unwanted side effects. Taking medication is an omnipresent reminder of having asthma. Patients whose asthma is well controlled may have fewer reminders to use their medications, which in turn may put them at risk for an exacerbation.

HOW DO PSYCHOLOGICAL FACTORS AFFECT ASTHMA, AND VICE VERSA?

Asthma is a physical illness, and its primary treatment should be medical. However, because psychological factors can influence the expression of asthma disease-related activity, psychological treatments are often effective adjuncts to medical treatment. Emotional problems may "switch on" asthma in a vulnerable individual—that is, an individual with a combination of factors possibly including genetic predisposition, a history of respiratory infections, and exposure to allergens or irritants in the environment. In the context of an individual with an established asthma diagnosis, strong emotions may be the triggering antecedent for an exacerbation of asthma symptoms; strong emotions can represent a state of parasympathetic dominance, as does asthma.

Having asthma is stressful. A variety of emotional reactions may be the consequences of having asthma or being intimate with someone who is living with asthma. Systematic examinations of the prevalence of psychiatric diagnoses among asthmatics have revealed that as many as one-third of patients meet criteria for a major psychiatric disorder.

Anxiety disorders, especially panic disorder and generalized anxiety disorder, are particularly prominent and occur among asthmatics at much higher rates than in the general population. The similarity in the symptomatic presentations of asthma and panic attacks may make differential diagnosis and treatment a challenge for patients and caregivers alike.

Studies have found modest associations between daily variation in mood and peak flow. However, it appears that the mood–bronchoconstriction relationship may differ by person (i.e., mood is a trigger for bronchoconstriction in only some individuals) and by mood (i.e., among mood-responsive asthmatics, anger may be the salient trigger for some, sadness for others). Similarly, some asthmatics are responsive to suggestion; responses to suggestions for bronchoconstriction are somewhat stronger than responses to suggestions for bronchodilation.

PSYCHOLOGICAL TREATMENTS FOR ASTHMA

As noted above, psychological treatments can have a useful adjunctive role to sound medical treatment. Psychoeducational asthma programs have repeatedly been shown to increase knowledge about asthma, compliance, and self-monitoring. However, this research has been criticized for employing overly short posttreatment follow-up intervals, having high dropout rates that threaten the validity of the results, and needing enhancement by better integration of state-of-the-art behavioral techniques. These programs enhance asthmatics' ability to manage their illness by teaching them facts about asthma and asthma medications; self-monitoring skills for the early recognition of an asthma exacerbation through the use of a peak flow meter and other strategies; and relaxation and coping skills, including diaphragmatic breathing to prevent hyperventilation.

Progressive muscle relaxation has been found to produce bronchodilation, though not of a clinically significant magnitude. There is some evidence that both generalized progressive muscle relaxation and facial or trapezius muscle electromyographic biofeedback are especially helpful for dilation of the upper airways. However, increased asthma symptoms have been reported during relaxation—a seemingly paradoxical response. A similar phenomenon, relaxation-associated panic attacks, has been observed. Since carbon dioxide pressure increases during relaxation and sleep (nocturnal asthma attacks are common), a common pathway of sensitivity to hypercapnia may trigger panic and asthma.

The limited research on family therapy for asthmatic children has found that improved family interaction has resulted in better asthma management. The mechanism underlying these effects is not clear. More functional family interaction may result directly in more effective use of asthma monitoring and treatment; may reduce family stress; or may help the family cope with stress more effectively, thereby reducing asthma triggers and decreasing bronchoconstriction indirectly.

In summary, the behavioral clinician must know the objective parameters that characterize the severity of a patient's asthma and medication needs, and engage in a process of collaborative discovery to elucidate irritants and triggers of asthma attacks. It is also important to assess the following areas: psychiatric diagnosis, mood reactivity, quality of social supports and reactions of significant others to asthma, compliance, coping skills repertoire, and cognitive variables related to asthma (e.g., use of denial vs. catastrophizing).

SPECIAL CONCERNS FOR WOMEN WITH ASTHMA

Women with asthma face unique challenges during pregnancy and as parents. Pregnancy usually changes the severity of women's asthma, although not in a uniform direction. Pregnancy is associated with an apparent worsening of asthma symptoms for some women and an apparent improvement for others.

Some degree of genetic predisposition is probably necessary for the development of asthma. Yet not all genetically at-risk individuals develop asthma, nor do similarly at-risk individuals develop asthma of similar severity. Prospective research of children genetically predisposed to asthma has found that children whose parents had difficulty coping and parenting were more likely to develop asthma in the first 2 years of life than were children whose parents had adequate parenting and coping skills. Furthermore, mothers of preadolescents with asthma were found to make more critical remarks while interacting with their children than mothers whose children did not have asthma.

As primary child caregivers, women shape and are shaped by their children's behavior. The issue of cause and effect is an important one that cannot be adequately addressed on the basis of the research to date. Intuitively, it would be good clinical practice to help adult asthmatics learn to cope optimally with their asthma and to enhance general life coping skills, in order to pass on these skills to their children and perhaps to decrease the stress that may trigger the development of asthma in some cases. Emotional stressors for a primary caregiver probably affect a child; conversely, having a child who is ill is stressful for a caregiver.

FURTHER READING

Busse, W. W., Kiecolt-Glaser, J. K., Coe, C., Martin, R. J., Weiss, S. T., & Parker, S. R. (1995). Stress and asthma. *American Journal of Respiratory and Critical Care Medicine, 151,* 249–252.
Recent outline of needed research in the area of stress and asthma.

Isenberg, S. A., Lehrer, P. M., & Hochron, S. (1992). The effects of suggestion and emotional arousal on pulmonary function in asthma: A review and a hypothesis regarding vagal mediation. *Psychosomatic Medicine, 54,* 192–216.
Comprehensive review of research on the effects of suggestion and emotions on asthma.

Lehrer, P. M., Sargunaraj, D., & Hochron, S. (1992). Psychological approaches to the treatment of asthma. *Journal of Consulting and Clinical Psychology, 60,* 639–643.
Review of psychological treatments for asthma.

Mrazek, D. A., & Klinnert, M. (1991). Asthma: Psychoneuroimmunological considerations. In R. Ader, D. L. Felten, & N. Cohen (Eds.), *Psychoneuroimmunology* (2nd ed., pp. 1013–1035). San Diego: Academic Press.
Review of the various mechanisms for bronchoconstriction and interactions between psychological and physiological factors in asthma.

95

Breast Cancer: Biobehavioral Aspects

Barbara L. Andersen

*F*or decades the understanding of the psychological processes and outcomes of breast cancer was largely clinical, consisting of detailed case studies of women coping with mastectomy. The message from these reports was that the psychological trajectory was guarded at best. However, within the last 15 years, controlled research on the behavioral and psychological aspects of cancer has described the specific difficulties that women may face, has tested psychological interventions to enhance coping, and has proposed models of the interaction of psychological/behavioral factors and disease outcome. The importance of the third approach—using biobehavioral models to understand the cancer experience—has been underscored by data suggesting that psychological interventions may affect disease outcomes.

FACTS AND FIGURES ABOUT THE DISEASE

For women, cancer is a leading cause of death; it ranks either first or second across age groups, with the top killers of women being breast, colon/rectum, lung, and uterine (gynecological) cancers. These four types of cancers account for approximately 70% of all cancers in women. Breast cancer alone accounts for 32%. Incidence rates are higher for white than for black females, but survival rates are consistently lower for black women. There has been an increased incidence of breast cancer, about 2% a year, since 1980. The overall stability of the death rates in breast cancer over the last 30 years, and the apparent increases in incidence, have been two important factors underscoring arguments that significant resources should be placed into prevention. The empirical basis for some of the proposed strategies comes from prior data on risk factors for breast cancer. For example, sociodemographic data indicate that factors such as increased age, white race, Jewish ethnicity, and higher socioeconomic status place a woman at higher risk. Other risk factors—such as family history (e.g., women who are daughters or siblings of women with breast cancer), never having been pregnant or having a first child after the age of 30, and early age at menarche or late age at menopause—implicate genetic or hormonal (estrogen) factors.

Available data suggest that it may take from 3 to 30 years for breast cancer to develop. This lengthy interval suggests that there may be opportunities to interrupt the natural history of the disease. At least three major prevention trials are under-way to test this possibility. The first trial, which is part of the Women's Health Initiative, will test the hypothesis that a diet that is very low in fat and high in fruits and vegetables (fiber) will lower breast cancer incidence in postmenopausal women. This trial is 10 years long, because it intervenes at the earliest possible stage in the natural history of breast cancer.

The second trial will only take 5 years to complete, because it intervenes much later in the natural history of the disease. Healthy women who are at higher risk for breast cancer—for example, older women (>60 years old) and younger women whose risk is higher for other reasons, such as history of benign disease or family history—will be randomly assigned to placebo or tamoxifen treatment. The notion that tamoxifen, an antiestrogen compound (see description below), might be useful in prevention is based on the observation that primary breast cancer patients treated with tamoxifen appear to have a lower risk of developing a new cancer in the opposite breast. The third prevention effort is a mammography screening trial. The goal of this effect is to detect cancers at the earliest of stages, when treatments are more effective and the disease is not disseminated (e.g., 5-year survival rates are approximately 90% for Stage I, 66% for Stage II, and 44% for Stage III disease).

The majority of breast cancers are now detected on mammography. When detected manually, a cancer may appear as a painless, mobile lump (usually in the upper outer quadrant). Other symptoms include swelling, skin irritation, scaliness, pain, and nipple discharge. Breast cancer spreads by local infiltration, moving directly into surrounding breast tissue and eventually involving the overlying skin or the underlying muscle. As many as 40% of patients have regional disease, usually involving the axillary lymph nodes, at original diagnosis and treatment. The presence and extent of nodal disease at diagnosis are the most important prognostic factors for survival.

In the last 30 years, there have been dramatic changes in the recommended therapies for breast cancer. Before the 1970s, radical mastectomy was used and consisted of removal of the entire breast as well as the underlying muscles, leaving a significant chest wall defect. However, clinical trials indicated that less radical surgery (e.g., modified radical mastectomy or lumpectomy with or without radiotherapy) can significantly reduce unpleasant side effects (e.g., problems with arm mobility and body image) without compromising mortality. Studies generally find no psychological benefit per se for lumpectomy, yet do find more positive sexual outcomes for women receiving this procedure. For example, lumpectomy patients report less alteration in body image, greater comfort with nudity and discussing sexuality with their partners, few changes in intercourse frequency, and a lower incidence of sexual dysfunction.

Women with regional disease usually receive chemotherapy and/or hormonal therapy following surgery, with or without radiotherapy. A significant factor that influences adjuvant therapy choice is the estrogen receptor status (positive vs. negative) of a woman's tumor. Women with receptor-positive tumors are typically offered tamoxifen hormonal therapy, which blocks estrogen uptake at the receptor level. The functional result of receiving this antiestrogen treatment is that women undergo a menopause-like experience.

Thus, women may experience hot flashes, mood lability, and the gynecological symptoms of estrogen deficiency (in which the vaginal mucosa can thin and become dry).

Some women undergo a premature menopause as a result of chemotherapy, and others are postmenopausal at the time of diagnosis. Many of these women would like to receive hormonal replacement therapy to control menopausal symptoms, yet the concern of the medical community is that such therapy might be a promoter of their disease. In fact, the data are not clear on the role of exogenous hormones in breast cancer incidence, whereas the picture is clearer for the role of endogenous estrogen in risk (hence the tamoxifen prevention trial discussed above). Until the picture is clarified, the majority of breast cancer patients will not be offered estrogen replacement therapy.

THE BIOBEHAVIORAL MODEL

Psychological/behavioral research documents that the psychosocial burdens of cancer may be notable in number, severity, and scope. Finding strategies to reduce stress and prevent deteriorations in quality of life (QoL) is now a research objective, particularly for breast cancer. The importance of such an initiative is underscored by three contextual factors. First, breast cancer mortality rates have remained essentially stable for the past 30 years (and have even shown a 6% *increase* in mortality), despite the fact that hundreds of breast cancer treatment clinical trials have been conducted. It is imperative that innovative treatments be developed to improve survival rates. Second, research has demonstrated that psychological interventions result in significant improvements in QoL, and the findings are particularly impressive for breast cancer patients. Third, both qualitative and quantitative summaries of the psychoneuroimmunology (PNI) literature conclude that psychological distress and stressors (i.e., negative life events, both acute and chronic) are reliably associated with changes—that is, down-regulation—in immunity.

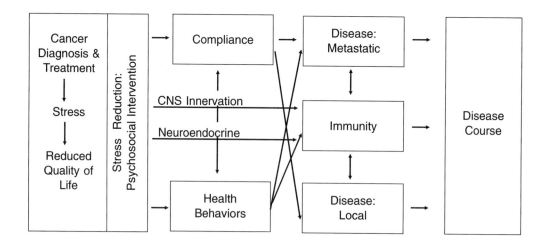

FIGURE 95.1. A biobehavioral model of the psychological (stress and quality of life), behavioral (compliance and health behaviors), and biological pathways from cancer stressors to disease course. CNS, central nervous system.

Figure 95.1 provides a conceptual model of the psychological, behavioral, and biological factors and mechanisms by which health outcomes and cancer progression might be influenced. The majority of the paths in the diagram move in one causal direction.

The Cancer Stressor and Lowered Quality of Life

Data from many studies document severe, *acute* stress at diagnosis. However, it is also clear that lengthy cancer treatments and disruptions in major life areas occur, producing *chronic stress*. Emotional distress, in combination with the other life disruptions, can result in a stable, lower QoL. Permanent sequelae of cancer treatments, such as sexual problems and/or sterility, can have an impact on intimate relationships and social support. Unemployment, underemployment, job discrimination, and difficulty in obtaining health insurance can also be problems for a substantial minority. Thus, many chronic stressors may occur for survivors.

Health Behaviors and Compliance

The biobehavioral model suggests that the cancer stressor and reduced QoL may have important health behavior sequelae—specifically, an increase in negative behaviors and/or a decrease in positive behaviors. There are many manifestations of negative health behaviors. Individuals who are depressed and/or anxious are more likely to self-medicate with alcohol and other drugs, and alcohol misuse can potentiate distress. Distressed individuals often have appetite disturbances or dietary changes, which are manifested by eating less often or eating meals of lower nutritional value. Although there appear to be individual differences in this phenomenon, women may be more vulnerable, and women who have undergone changes in their eating habits (e.g., restrictions because of cancer treatments) may have heightened vulnerability. On the other hand, there is a tendency for some women to gain weight; this is most often the complaint of breast cancer patients receiving adjuvant chemotherapy. Distressed individuals may report sleep disturbances, such as early-morning awakening, sleep-onset insomnia, and middle-of-the-night insomnia. Cigarette smoking and caffeine use, which often increase during periods of stress, can intensify the physiological effects of psychosocial stress (e.g., by increasing catecholamine release). Conversely, individuals who are stressed may not begin positive health behaviors or may abandon previous positive health behaviors such as regular physical activity. Data suggest a positive relationship between physical activity or fitness and psychological health. Positive mood effects as well as increased functional capacity have been found for women with breast cancer receiving chemotherapy who were also participating in a program of aerobic interval training.

The model suggests that health behaviors may in turn affect immunity (see the arrow from "Health Behaviors" to "Immunity" in Figure 95.1). Immunity has been found to covary with objective measures of sleep, alcohol intake, smoking, and drug use. Also, problematic health behaviors interact to produce detrimental immune consequences. For example, substance use problems (e.g., alcoholism) have direct effects, as well as indirect effects via alterations in nutrition. Conversely, there is growing evidence that physical activity may have positive consequences for both the immune and endocrine systems, even among individuals with chronic diseases.

The model also suggests that health behaviors may be directly related to disease progression (see the arrow from "Health Behaviors" to "Disease: Metastatic" in Figure 95.1). Among all the health behaviors noted above, the strongest case can be made for the importance of nutrition and diet in breast cancer. Findings from various disciplines link nutrition/dietary factors and risk for breast cancer (e.g., epidemiological data; animal models of high-fat diet and tumor growth; studies of obesity and the increase of breast cancer incidence). More germane to human behavioral studies are the data suggesting that increased fat intake, obesity at diagnosis, and weight gain may be related to recurrence and survival. Alternatively, some researchers suggest that fiber, rather than fat, is the critical dietary factor, because fiber is postulated to modify serum estrogen levels by increasing fecal excretion of estrogens. Finally, related data link weight gain after breast cancer to an increased risk of recurrence. Taken together, these data suggest that behavioral factors relevant to nutrition, fat–fiber balance, and energy expenditure (vis-à-vis weight gain) may be relevant to disease progression.

The second behavioral factor noted in the model is treatment (non)compliance, as the available data suggest that psychological factors may be important. Compliance problems cross a wide range of diseases, therapies, and individual patient characteristics. With cancer treatments, some patients become discouraged and drop out. A general implication of such behaviors is the invalidation of clinical trials, with an eventual adverse effect on overall patient survival. Noncompliance may influence, a range of treatments and regimen characteristics in a range of ways, as the data suggest that there are different correlates for different compliance behaviors. The model suggests that poor compliance can affect local and/or metastatic control of the disease; which route is affected depends on the treatment regimen, as well as the characteristics of an individual's noncompliance.

The model also specifies that the processes governing compliance and health behaviors may interact or may be synergistic. Specifically, women who are compliant may expect better health outcomes; moreover, they not only may comply with individual recommendations (diet, exercise, sleep, etc.), but may adopt other behaviors indicative of "good health" or may engage in higher levels/rates of healthy behaviors. Despite their importance, health behavior and compliance variables have been understudied in psychological intervention studies, including those with immune-related outcomes.

Biological Pathways

Stress sets in motion important biological effects involving the autonomic, endocrine, and immune systems. Stress may be routed to the immune system by the central nervous system via activation of the sympathetic nervous system or through neuroendocrine–immune pathways (i.e., the release of hormones; see Figure 95.1). In the latter case, a variety of hormones released during stressors have been implicated in immune modulation (e.g., catecholamines, cortisol, prolactin, and growth hormone). Without any stress pathway (effect) to immunity, there is evidence for the importance of the immune responses in host resistance against cancer progression, and hence the arrows in Figure 95.1 go in both directions from "Immunity" to "Disease: Local" and "Disease: Metastatic."

Experts in the immunology and cancer areas cite the following important findings with regard to the specific importance of natural killer (NK) cell activity: (1) Patients with a variety of solid malignancies and large tumor burdens have diminished NK cell activity in the blood; (2) low NK cell activity in cancer patients is significantly associated with the development of distant metastases; and (3) in patients treated for metastatic disease, the survival time without metastasis correlates with NK cell activity. These effects have also emerged specifically for women with breast cancer. NK cells have been shown to play an important role in the surveillance of tumor development and the occurrence of metastases. Also, the level of NK activity has been correlated with prognostic factors, including tumor burden and estrogen receptor status. Moreover, cancers that are etiologically linked to hormonal stimuli, such as breast cancer, may be more responsive to stress effects.

Mediation of the Immune Response

Summaries of the PNI literature conclude that psychological distress and stressors (i.e., negative life events, both acute and chronic) are reliably associated with immune system down-regulation in noncancer populations. Time-limited (acute) stressors can produce immunological changes in relatively healthy individuals, and chronic stressors are associated with down-regulation rather than adaptation, with some of the largest NK cell effects found for lengthy stressors and/or stressors that have interpersonal components. Many of the qualities of chronic stressors—such as continued emotional distress, disrupted life tasks (e.g., employment), and disrupted social relationships—occur with the decrements in QoL found in studies of cancer patients.

Studies with breast cancer patients provide data linking QoL aspects and immunity. Data from Andersen and colleagues are in line with data from healthy individuals; that is, stress predicts lower NK cell lysis and T-cell function.

Stress, Quality of Life, and Health Consequences: Direct Effects and Indirect Effects via Immune Mediation

Data on the health (illness) consequences of stress or data linking the two via immunity, are accumulating. One example comes from Cohen and colleagues, who found that in healthy volunteers who were inoculated with either a cold virus or a placebo, rates of both respiratory infection and clinical colds increased in a dose–response manner with increases in psychological stress across five different strains of cold viruses. Data from cancer samples reveal that conceptually consistent variables (e.g., negative mood) are correlated with disease endpoints (e.g., nodal status), but experimental data are needed. The biobehavioral model is presented as one strategy to examine this important question.

FURTHER READING

American Cancer Society. (1994). American Cancer Society Conference on Behavioral and Psychosocial Cancer Research [Whole issue]. *Cancer, 74*(Suppl.).
Progress report and statement of future directions for psychological/behavioral research by the American Cancer Society.

Andersen, B. L. (1992). Psychological interventions for cancer patients to enhance the quality of life. *Journal of Consulting and Clinical Psychology, 60,* 552–568.
A comprehensive review of the intervention components and treatment outcomes of psychological interventions for cancer patients.

Andersen, B. L., Farrar, W. B., Golden-Kreutz, D., Kutz, L. A., MacCallum, R., Courtney, M. E., & Glaser, R. (in press). Stress and immune responses following surgical treatment for regional breast cancer. *Journal of the National Cancer Institute.*
A study that demonstrates a significant negative correlation between higher levels of psychological distress and lower NK cell and T-cell responses.

Andersen, B. L., Kiecolt-Glaser, J. K., & Glaser, R. (1994). A biobehavioral model of cancer stress and disease course. *American Psychologist, 49,* 389–404.
Theoretical model considering the psychological (stress and QoL) and behavioral factors (compliance and health behaviors) and immune mechanisms that may influence disease progression.

Cohen, S., Tyrrell, D. A., & Smith, A. P. (1991). Psychological stress in humans and susceptibility to the common cold. *New England Journal of Medicine, 325,* 606–612.
Empirical demonstration of the dose–response relationship between stress and viral infection and cold symptoms.

Fawzy, F. I., Cousins, N., Fawzy, N., Kemeny, M. E., Elashoff, R., & Morton, D. (1990). A structured psychiatric intervention for cancer patients: I. Changes over time in methods of coping and affective disturbance. *Archives of General Psychiatry, 47,* 720–725.
Data from a randomized intervention design (psychoeducational group intervention vs. assessment only) for melanoma patients and the significant findings on the psychological and coping outcomes.

Fawzy, F. I., Kemeny, M. E., Fawzy, N., Elashoff, R., Morton, D., Cousins, N., & Fahey, J. L. (1990). A structured psychiatric intervention for cancer patients: II. Changes over time in immunological measures. *Archives of General Psychiatry, 47,* 729–735.
Data from a randomized design (psychoeducational group intervention vs. assessment only) for melanoma patients, and the significant findings at follow-up on immune parameters.

Institute of Medicine. (1993). *Strategies for managing the breast cancer research program: A report to the U.S. Army Medical Research and Development Command.* Washington, DC: National Academy Press.
Special report that provided guidelines for the special federal research initiative in breast cancer.

Kiecolt-Glaser, J. K., & Glaser, R. (1992). Psychoneuroimmunology: Can psychological interventions modulate immunity? *Journal of Consulting and Clinical Psychology, 60,* 569–575.
A comprehensive review of data on changes in immunity following psychological interventions.

Spiegel, D., Bloom H. C., Kraemer, J. R., & Gottheil, E. (1989). Effect of psychosocial treatment on survival of patients with metastatic breast cancer. *The Lancet,* 888–901.
Long-term follow-up of a randomized study (group support vs. assessment only) for women with metastatic breast cancer, which reported a longer survival interval for the intervention participants.

96

Breast Cancer: Psychosocial Aspects

Julia H. Rowland

With one in every eight women in the United States expected to develop breast cancer in her lifetime, this disease has become a national health concern. Indeed, probably no other type of malignant disease has been more thoroughly researched with respect to its psychosocial impact. This is attributable only in part to breast cancer's prevalence and the attendant threat it poses to an organ intimately associated with self-esteem, sexuality, and femininity. The fact that studies of breast cancer serve as a paradigm for understanding a wide range of social, emotional, and behavioral issues associated with life-threatening illness and care is equally important. All the major treatment modalities (surgery, radiotherapy, chemotherapy, hormonal therapy) are used in treating and controlling the disease. The broad age range at time of diagnosis means that patients and their families cover the developmental spectrum. Finally, increasing numbers of women are living longer with the disease cured or controlled.

In the past decade, the two most important changes in the breast cancer area have been the growing emphasis on choices in treatment, and the broadening array of psychosocial interventions available to women and those caring for them. Research has begun to show that psychological and social variables may influence not only risk for developing and detecting breast cancer, but also adaptation to and survival from this illness. A number of factors go into a woman's adaptation to breast cancer (see Table 96.1). These are covered in more general detail in Chapters 97 and 98 of this volume. In this chapter, research addressing specific aspects of women's responses to the diagnosis, treatment, and outcome of breast cancer will be reviewed.

DIAGNOSIS

Increasing numbers of women with breast cancer are diagnosed at an early stage, where the chance for cure is 70% or better. The broader availability of mammography, and

TABLE 96.1. Factors Contributing to the Psychological Responses of Women to Breast Cancer

Current sociocultural context, treatment options, and decision making

- Changes in surgical management from a uniform approach
  Breast-conserving management; more acknowledged uncertainty
- Social attitudes
  Public figures disclose having had breast cancer
  Autobiographic accounts of and "how to" guides for treatment of breast cancer in popular press
- Ethical imperative for patient participation in treatment issues; legal imperative for knowledge of treatment options
- Variations in care by ethnicity, location, age
- Public awareness of treatment and research controversies; advocacy for more funding and lay oversight

Psychological and psychosocial factors

- Type and degree of disruption in life cycle tasks caused by breast cancer (e.g., marital, childbearing)
- Psychological stability and ability to cope with stress
- Prior psychiatric history
- Availability of psychological and social support (partner, family, friends)

Medical factors

- Stage of cancer at diagnosis
- Treatment(s) received: mastectomy/lumpectomy and radiation, adjuvant chemotherapy, hormonal therapy, bone marrow transplant
- Availability of rehabilitation
  Psychological (partner, support groups)
  Physical (reconstruction)
- Psychological support provided by physicians and staff

Note. From Rowland and Massie (1977). Copyright 1997 by Raven Press. Reprinted by permission.

behavioral and educational programs to enhance the use of routine mammographic screening, have significantly improved detection. Also, the last decade has seen a dramatic rise in the use of breast-sparing approaches to surgical management or local control of disease. At the same time, the use of adjunctive treatment (e.g., radiotherapy, chemotherapy, and hormonal therapy) has become more widespread. These latter changes have occurred in part as a function of the growing attention to quality-of-life issues in women's care; more critically, they reflect the greater appreciation of breast cancer as a systemic (vs. local) disease. These trends, coupled with concerns about providing adequate informed consent and greater emphasis on patients' involvement in their care, have led to new— and for some women overwhelming—stresses centering around the decision-making process.

Although most women wish to have complete and accurate information about their illness and treatment, many may not wish to make the final decision about which course to pursue. Physicians' recommendations continue to play a critical role in choice of treatment. Various models for informing women about their illness and determining what role they wish to play in their care are currently being studied. It is clear that no single strategy works for all women. Furthermore, because important material may be missed or processed in different ways, most information needs to be conveyed in a variety of formats (e.g., written material, audiotape/videotape, direct contact). Importantly, research suggests that women who are given a choice in treatment options exhibit better psychological adjustment to their illness than those who are provided with no choice. Furthermore, inclusion of the spouse/partner in the decision-making dialogue appears helpful to the woman's and the couple's subsequent functioning.

TREATMENT

Surgery: Lumpectomy versus Mastectomy

Today, most women with early-stage disease have a choice between modified radical mastectomy and lumpectomy (or breast conservation) with radiation as primary treatments for breast cancer. Although women undergoing lumpectomy report feeling less self-conscious, having a better body image, and experiencing somewhat better sexual functioning than those undergoing mastectomy, posttreatment data from over two dozen studies have found few differences between the two groups with respect to other parameters of psychosocial or emotional functioning. Given the expected dramatic emotional benefit that saving the breast was expected to provide women, some have argued that the differences seen between the two groups are less than might have been predicted. Others have noted that women in the lumpectomy group may fare worse in the short term, as they must undergo 6 weeks of additional radiation therapy as part of their primary care.

The National Cancer Institute has stated that breast conservation should be recommended whenever possible. It is not clear, however, how often such a recommendation is made. Epidemiological information suggests that conservation rates are higher in those states in which the law mandates that information be provided to women about their options. These data also suggest that conservation may be offered less often to older women and may be performed in the absence of additional radiation treatment. Given that few differences in quality of life can be attributed to the different surgical approaches to management, greater attention to women's personal preferences is warranted. Women selecting lumpectomy over mastectomy tend to be younger, more concerned about insult to body image, more dependent on their breasts for self-esteem, and more convinced that they would have difficulty adjusting to loss of the breast. In contrast, women choosing mastectomy are often older, more fearful of leaving cancer cells behind, more fearful of exposure to additional radiation, and in some cases less willing to commit to the time demanded for the added weeks of radiation treatment. Although accurate figures are hard to come by, it is estimated that half of women offered a choice will select conservation; of those undergoing mastectomy, an estimated 20% will go on to have breast reconstruction.

Surgery: Postmastectomy Breast Reconstruction

Like conservation, reconstructive surgery is an option that may decrease the adverse physical and emotional consequences of breast cancer surgery. Research suggests that women who seek postmastectomy breast reconstruction, though younger, are no different in terms of psychosocial functioning than those not pursuing this option. With respect to outcome, reconstructed patients, similar to those selecting breast conservation, report better body image, sense of femininity, and sexual functioning than their mastectomy-alone peers. In terms of timing of reconstructive surgery, it appears that the sooner the better. The few studies that compare a lumpectomy group with a mastectomy-plus-reconstruction group report few differences between the two, with slight advantages in sexual and body image areas going to the conservation group. However, women who pursue reconstruction to please others or to resolve long-standing difficulties are at significant risk for dissatisfaction with outcome.

Recent concern about and litigation associated with the potential health risks posed by use of silicone implants has created alarm and worry for many breast cancer survivors with these devices in place. Substitution of saline implants and development of alternative methods of reconstruction (e.g., tissue flaps) have offered newer, safer options for restoration of the breast. However, because use of autologous tissue flaps is still relatively new, there is as yet little information on women's long-term satisfaction and delayed physical problems associated with this more extensive surgery. (For a fuller discussion of breast implants, see the chapter by Pruzinsky in this volume.)

Radiotherapy

Most women undergoing breast conservation will also receive several weeks of adjuvant radiation therapy for local control of their disease. Radiation treatment is often associated with symptoms of fatigue, breast tenderness, swelling, and skin changes. Most of these symptoms resolve once treatment is completed; however, about 15% of patients can expect to experience long-term cosmetic changes that may be mildly to markedly disfiguring (e.g., permanent tattooing, changes in skin coloring, hardening of the breast tissue). A significant proportion of women may experience depression and anxiety across the course of treatment. Furthermore, the need for daily treatments over several weeks can pose considerable disruption to a woman's daily routine. Careful education of women about what to expect, evaluation of their responses over time, and provision of additional support as necessary can reduce the levels of both anxiety and mood disturbance seen in association with radiation.

Chemotherapy

Anticipation of chemotherapy can be difficult. Women's fears of the side effects arise from common knowledge of the distressing effects of chemotherapy. Since many women with early breast cancer now receive some form of adjuvant therapy, the association of these treatments with "more serious disease" has diminished. Despite having fears, few women refuse treatment, and most comply with their regimen.

Many of the common side effects of adjuvant chemotherapy, once feared and dreaded by patients, are now well controlled with pharmacological and behavioral interventions. Nausea and vomiting are generally well controlled with the use of antiemetic drugs. The use of simple behavioral interventions (e.g., hypnosis, visualization, distraction, and relaxation exercises) provides a means of regaining a sense of self-control over symptoms while also reducing anxiety.

Three additional troublesome side effects of adjuvant therapy that have psychological consequences are hair loss, weight gain, and problems with sleep and concentration. Although hair loss may be anticipated, its impact can be devastating for many women.

In my colleagues' and my research, many women noted that hair loss was as distressing as hearing the diagnosis. In addition to being disfiguring, alopecia may be the first visible indicator of disease. Early discussion of this potential side effect, purchase of a wig or head coverings, and participation in programs such as the American Cancer Society's *Look Good . . . Feel Better* can reduce distress related to hair loss.

The cause of weight gain remains unclear. At least one study has shown that weight may be negatively associated with mortality. This potential risk, and the added insult to self-esteem posed by significant weight gain, suggest that more attention should be paid to this problem. Difficulties with concentration and memory are also reported by many women undergoing chemotherapy. Not well researched or clearly documented, these symptoms may be associated with the stress of illness, antiemetic drugs, sleep disorders, the chemotherapy itself, and/or (for younger women) hormonal changes secondary to chemotherapy-induced menopause.

A final troublesome effect of chemotherapy in younger women is premature menopause. Threatened or actual loss of fertility and acute onset of menopausal symptoms can be very distressing in the group of women affected. Unlike those associated with natural menopause, the hot flashes, night sweats, vaginal dryness, and vaginal atrophy caused by chemically induced menopause appear to produce more severe discomfort. The latter symptoms may lead to emotional distress and dyspareunia. Although instruction in the use of vaginal lubricants is helpful, thinning of the vaginal mucosa may still result in irritation on intercourse. A further effect of chemotherapy is loss of libido, probably associated with a reduction in circulating androgens. For many women, loss of desire is a difficult symptom to treat. Although longitudinal data are lacking, it can be expected that early loss of ovarian function also increases the risk in these young patients of later morbidity associated with osteoporosis and cardiovascular disease. Use of estrogen replacement in this population of women remains controversial because of concerns about inducing recurrent or second (e.g., endometrial) malignancies. Although potentially useful for addressing libido problems, administration of androgen supplements poses problems of its own and has been little researched in this population. With growing numbers of younger women now being treated for breast cancer, greater research attention needs to be given to addressing these special problem areas.

Most women experience acute symptoms related to their treatment at some point in time. Many women report coping with treatment by "staying busy," "getting information about the treatment," and "keeping a positive, hopeful outlook." It is clear that others cope with the short-term adverse psychological effects by focusing on delayed benefits (e.g., reassurance that they have done everything possible to eradicate their disease) or applying adaptive denial (e.g., ignoring the negative and focusing on the positive aspects of illness). Some researchers suggest that women who exhibit a "fighting spirit" or an active coping stance adjust better and survive longer than those who manifest a helpless or hopeless attitude. Critical to adaptation is an ability to be flexible and to draw upon available resources both within and outside the medical system.

The extent to which emotional or physical symptoms may persist after treatment ends is unclear. Although overall quality of life is expected to improve following treatment, a half to a third of women may experience long-term effects, particularly with respect to sexual dysfunction and fatigue. Few studies have followed women longitudinally beyond 12 months, and only recently has research been instituted to delineate more clearly the prevalence and etiology of functional difficulties in these latter two problem areas.

Psychological preparation for chemotherapy is essential and should incorporate patient education, nursing input, and an outline by the physician of the disease- and treatment-related expectations. Assessing social support and supplementing this as needed are other important parts of the preparatory process. It is equally important to anticipate and plan for emotional reactions to ending treatment, when (as with completion of radiotherapy) fears of recurrence peak. Although patients are relieved to be finished with intensive care, concern about potential regrowth of the cancer without treatment, as well as anticipation of the loss of close monitoring and frequent visits with the doctor and staff, may create ambivalence toward ending treatment. Reassurance about the commonness of this paradoxical effect, as well as of continued staff availability and plans for follow-up care, can reduce distress. Fears of disease recurrence remain high in many women and can reach distressing levels before follow-up visits and scans and while waiting for test results. Anxiety generally returns to usual levels with news of normal findings.

Hormonal Therapy

Long used in the care of women with advanced breast cancer, hormonal therapy—more specifically, the antiestrogen drug tamoxifen (Nolvadex)—is being increasingly used in the context of early disease to prevent cancer in the remaining breast. Appreciation of its psychosocial impact is only just beginning to be addressed, largely because of the interest generated by tamoxifen's use as a chemopreventive (or breast cancer prevention) agent for healthy women at high risk for breast cancer. Intensification of menopausal symptoms (such as hot flashes, sweats, and vaginal discharge) can be a side effect limiting its use. It has also been suggested that the drug may induce depression in a small set of women. Concern about increased risk for uterine cancer has led to the recommendation that any women taking this medication have careful gynecological monitoring. Other agents, such as megestrol acetate, progestins, aminoglutethimide, luteinizing hormone-releasing hormone analogues, and estrogens, may be associated with weight and appearance alterations and need to be administered in the context of counseling about these expected effects.

Bone Marrow Transplant

Bone marrow transplant (BMT) is playing a growing role in the treatment of locally advanced breast cancer. Developed as a curative therapy for patients with hematological cancers and autoimmune disorders, BMT is used in the breast cancer setting as a "rescue" procedure to permit the administration of higher, potentially fatal doses of anticancer drugs. Although much has been written about the psychological stages in patients' adaptation to BMT, this has focused largely on hematologic patient samples, receiving allogeneic (or donor) transplants. Long-term follow-up of patients undergoing BMT suggests that although most patients do well, 12–20% may continue to experience distress and might benefit from psychological or psychiatric intervention. At least one study reports that despite the additional strain and longer hospitalization associated with BMT, no difference could be seen in psychological or social functioning between BMT survivors and those treated with conventional chemotherapy alone.

Breast cancer patients undergoing BMT today represent the new vanguard of survivors. Less is known about their experience and how it may resemble or differ from that of patients treated with allogeneic (vs. autologous—using the patient's own marrow or stem cell products) transplants, or in an earlier period without benefit of growth factor support, effective antiemetics, and shorter hospitalization. Consequently, anticipatory anxiety in this group tends to be high. As with other intensive therapies, the toll on quality of life is often very high; the equation must be balanced by hope for the results and the desire to live. Ensuring that optimal support is provided across the course of transplant and into follow-up is critical. Although psychiatric problems may or may not alter survival, they can have a dramatic impact on quality of survival and should be rapidly diagnosed and treated.

ADVANCED DISEASE

Women who present with advanced disease, or whose cancer progresses, require more intensive psychosocial and supportive intervention. Care in these patients is generally aimed at comfort and control of symptoms. Contrary to the approach in early-stage disease, where short-term costs in quality of life are accepted to achieve long-term gain in disease-free survival, quality-of-life issues become paramount in any decision to pursue experimental or even palliative treatment. Among the psychiatric symptoms of most concern, anxiety and depression are the most frequent and the most disabling. Depression may reach significant proportions. Although suicide is unusual, suicidal ideation is common. A management approach that combines psychological support with psycho-pharmacological use of antidepressants is often helpful.

INTERVENTIONS

Although most women with breast cancer adjust well to their illness, specific risk factors may put a woman at risk for problems in adapting and warrant immediate attention. These include a past history of psychiatric problems, young age, pain, delirium, lack of social support, multiple life stresses, and/or a hopeless/helpless outlook. Because of the demands of illness, the majority of women benefit from support across the course of care. Psychosocial interventions are both broadly advocated and widely available in breast cancer care settings. These vary greatly by type (e.g., individual vs. group), orientation (e.g., behavioral vs. cognitive vs. supportive vs. . . .), duration (time-limited vs. open-ended), and target populations served (early-stage vs. advanced, under 40 vs. older, partnered vs. single, European-American vs. African-American, or mixed). Nevertheless, the fundamental purpose of all the interventions developed has been the same: to provide each woman with the skills or resources necessary to cope with her illness and to improve the quality of her life.

Taken as a whole, researchers have found that those women who received an intervention designed to improve knowledge or coping or to reduce distress did better than those who did not (the control group often being "standard care"). Specifically, provision of or random assignment to some form of individual or group intervention can result in less anxiety and depression, increased sense of control, improved body image, greater satisfaction with care, better sexual functioning, and improved medication adherence. Importantly, no studies to date in which women received additional help have shown that these women have done worse than their "standard care" peers.

Surveys show that most cancer treatment centers in the United States provide counseling services to their patients and families. This reflects not only patients' demand for supportive care, but growing recognition that addressing psychosocial issues may improve outcomes for patients. In their landmark study, Spiegel and colleagues at Stanford University found that women with metastatic breast cancer randomly assigned to participate in a year of weekly supportive group therapy (which included instruction in self-hypnosis for pain) survived an average of 18 months longer than did nonintervention controls. In attempting to explain their surprising findings, Spiegel et al. emphasized the multiple support functions such groups may serve.

The results of this study have been very encouraging. However, a number of questions still remain regarding the efficacy of interventions in breast cancer. In particular, these questions concern when to conduct such interventions and for whom. Studies that help identify women who are at risk for problems in adjusting and who might be singled out for more support, as well as those who might be better served by individual rather than group interventions, would be beneficial. Furthermore, greater attention is needed to identify those aspects of interventions that are most helpful and the mechanisms by which they may operate.

IMPACT ON THE FAMILY

There is a positive relationship between social support and health or illness outcome. This is well illustrated in the context of breast cancer, where adequate social support has been found to be integral not only to positive adjustment, but also to length of survival. For most breast cancer patients, primary support comes from the family. At the same time, however, new stresses have taxed this resource. Greater demands on family decision making, the lengthened course of treatment with more aggressive therapies, and the shift of care into the outpatient setting have all served to place renewed focus on the family in the management of care.

Despite their recognized importance, the impact on partners and families of the diagnosis of breast cancer in a loved one has been the subject of few studies. What research exists suggests that family members often constitute second-order patients, exhibiting levels of distress comparable to that seen in cancer patients themselves. Patients' and their husbands'/partners' levels of adjustment may be significantly related, such that if one partner is experiencing difficulties adjusting, the other is more likely to be having problems as well. Factors that may promote adaptation include the husband's/partner's involvement in the decision-making process, hospital visitation, early viewing of scars, and early resumption of sexual activity. Couples at risk for problems in coping include those with a history of marital problems, concurrent competing stresses (e.g., work, family, finances), or difficulty communicating, and those in which the partners are younger or in a new relationship. Patients and their partners identify emotional support, information, attitude, and religion as factors helpful in coping.

The traumatic effect on children, both sons and daughters, is great when mothers develop breast cancer. Behavioral disorders, conflicts with parents, and regressive and acting-out behaviors have been seen to increase during a mother's illness. The mother–child relationship may deteriorate; this is a particular problem in those situations in which the mother has a poor prognosis, extensive surgery, poor psychological adjustment, or (to a lesser degree) difficulty adjusting to chemotherapy or radiotherapy. Mothers' relationships with daughters may be more stressed than those with their sons. This may be attributable in part to the observations that mothers rely more often on daughters than on sons during illness, and that adolescent daughters in particular may be vulnerable to disruption in their lives. In turn, daughters are found to be more likely than sons to show signs of fearfulness, withdrawal, and hostility, which probably reflect both the greater demands placed on them and their greater fears of developing the disease. Problems may carry into adulthood in some cases; daughters of breast cancer patients have been reported to experience decrements in the frequency of and satisfaction with sexual activity, when compared to nonaffected peers.

The monitoring of all children, especially when a mother's breast cancer is advanced, is important. The opportunity for parents to discuss how and what to tell their children about the mother's illness early in the course of care is also important and should include advice on tailoring these conversations to meet appropriate developmental needs of their offspring. Health care professionals need to encourage women to identify the key providers in their support network and to involve them in appropriate aspects of care. They also need to recognize that these individuals may or may not be spouses or even family members, depending on a woman's particular situation.

HIGH-RISK FAMILY MEMBERS AND THE IMPACT OF GENETIC TESTING

For immediate female relatives, breast cancer in a sister, mother, or daughter is known to mean heightened risk for all, particularly if the disease has occurred before menopause. This group of "at-risk" women (at times referred to as "the worried well") has become the focus of growing attention as a function of concern about the impact of risk status on physical and emotional well-being and health practices, as well as about the proper identification and support of individuals and families who might benefit from genetic testing and counseling.

Several studies have indicated that as many as a quarter to a third of female first-degree relatives of breast cancer survivors exhibit clinically elevated levels of psychological distress that warrant further counseling. Many such relatives report intrusive thoughts about breast cancer, impairment in daily functioning because of breast cancer worries, and sleep disturbance—symptom patterns similar to those observed in populations exposed to a traumatic stressor. Such patterns of distress warrant special attention as excessive psychological distress can interfere not only with family functioning, but also with adherence to subsequent cancer screenings. At-risk women tend to overestimate their actual chances of developing breast cancer. If worry becomes excessive, a woman may be at risk for poor adherence to recommended guidelines for mammographic screening, breast self-exams, and comprehensive breast exams. Research has already indicated that women with high levels of breast cancer concerns are significantly less likely to improve their comprehension of personal risk when offered counseling. This is consistent with various studies showing that stress and anxiety can interfere with comprehension of complex information and lead to ill-considered decisions.

Health care providers can play an important role in educating high-risk women about breast cancer risk factors and motivating adherence to recommended surveillance. The impact of a simple recommendation can be enhanced by emphasizing the benefits of continued breast screening, such as the potential for detection of early-stage cancers, which can result in more treatment options and a better rate of cure. Communications that heighten perceived vulnerability to breast cancer must be balanced by such reassuring messages. Providers can also address known barriers to mammographic screening adherence, including fear of radiation, embarrassment, and anxiety about positive results. High-risk women should be instructed in breast self-exam to increase their confidence in lump detection and reduce anxiety about self-examination.

Identification of breast cancer susceptibility genes (i.e., *BRCA1* and *BRCA2*) have raised hopes for early recognition of women at familial risk of breast cancer. Mass media coverage and clinical experience already suggest that public demand for genetic testing for breast cancer risk is likely to be high. Although enhanced risk comprehension may motivate better screening adherence, research suggests that cancer risk notification may have psychological costs, even for women not found to be gene carriers. Culturally appropriate methods to facilitate decision making about testing are needed, as is more research on the consequences of notification. In some cases, prophylactic surgery (bilateral mastectomy) may provide important psychological benefits (e.g., reduction in chronic worry and in dependence on breast cancer screening), especially for women who are found to have an altered breast cancer susceptibility gene. However, the psychological impact of such surgery has not been determined. This is especially important, given that the efficacy of this procedure has not been carefully documented. The rapid growth of knowledge about genetic risk and testing means that health care providers and researchers alike must work toward a fuller understanding of the behavioral and psychosocial factors that contribute to optimal use of these technologies, with minimal adverse cost to women's ultimate quality or length of life.

CONCLUSION

Research on the psychosocial aspects of breast cancer indicates that a range of psychosocial and behavioral factors mediate a woman's response to and recovery from this disease. While most women adapt well, few obtain optimal outcomes in the absence of good multidisciplinary care and adequate social support. The growing numbers of women treated for and surviving breast cancer, greater complexity of care, and increasing demand for patient, family, and societal involvement in this process have placed considerable demands on the medical community to identify and address psychosocial issues across the course of care. Importantly, extension of this research into the area of social and cultural differences in response and outcomes is also needed. While much is known about the psychosocial impact of breast cancer, this information derives largely from work with white, middle-class women, the majority of whom were treated in academic medical settings. In this context, clinicians and researchers in behavioral medicine have an important role to play.

FURTHER READING

National Cancer Institute (NCI). (1994). *Breast cancer in younger women.* (National Cancer Institute Monograph No. 16). Bethesda, MD: U.S. Department of Health and Human Services.
Volume of the proceedings of an NCI-sponsored conference on state-of-the-art knowledge regarding the epidemiology, treatment research, and clinical care of younger women diagnosed with breast cancer.

Fawzy, F. I., Fawzy, N. W., Arndt, L. A., & Pasnau, R. O. (1995). Critical review of psychosocial interventions in cancer care. *Archives of General Psychiatry, 52,* 100–113.
Thoughtful review of the available information on the most common types of psychosocial interventions being used today, and their efficacy.

Glanz, K., & Lerman, C. (1992). Psychosocial impact of breast cancer: A critical review. *Annals of Behavioral Medicine, 14,* 204–212.
Focused review of the literature that emphasizes the roles that time since diagnosis, type of treatment, and a woman's individual characteristics play in moderating the impact of breast cancer on her psychological health.

Kiebert, G. M., de Haes, J. C. J. M., & van de Velde, C. J. H. (1991). The impact of breast conserving treatment and mastectomy on the quality-of-life of early-stage breast cancer patients: A review. *Journal of Clinical Oncology, 9,* 1059–1070.
Comprehensive review of controlled studies showing that compared with mastectomy, breast conservation is more or less equivalent to more extensive surgery with respect to women's overall quality of life, and can lead to improved body image and sexual functioning in women treated.

Lerman, C., & Schwartz, M. (1993). Adherence and psychological adjustment among women at high risk for breast cancer. *Breast Cancer Research and Treatment, 28,* 145–155.
A review of the adverse impact a family history of breast cancer can have on women's psychological health and their adherence to breast cancer screening practices, and a discussion of interventions to improve functioning in both.

Rowland, J. H., Dioso, J., Holland, J. C., Chaglassian, T., & Kinne, D. (1995). Breast reconstruction after mastectomy: Who seeks it, who refuses? *Plastic and Reconstructive Surgery, 95,* 812–822.
Well-controlled study demonstrating that women who opt for breast reconstruction after mastectomy are, with few exceptions, similar to women who do not pursue reconstruction.

Rowland, J. H., & Massie, M. J. (1996). Psychological reactions to breast cancer diagnosis, treatment and survival. In J. R. Harris, M. E. Lippman, M. Morrow, & S. Hellman (Eds.), *Diseases of the Breasts.* Philadelphia: Lippincott-Raven.
Comprehensive review of the literature on the psychological aspects of breast cancer across the course of care.

Schover, L. R. (1991). The impact of breast cancer on sexuality, body image, and intimate relationships. *CA-A Cancer Journal for Clinicians, 41,* 112–120.
Thoughtful overview of the research on women's sexual and intimate functioning following breast cancer that highlights a general lack of information in this area and the need for clinicians to ask about and treat sexual problems when they arise.

Spiegel, D., Bloom, J. R., Kraemer, H. C., & Gottheil, E. (1989). Effect of psychosocial treatment on survival of patients with metastatic breast cancer. *Lancet, ii,* 888–891.
Presentation of important follow-up data from an earlier randomized study, suggesting that a psychosocial intervention (supportive–expressive group therapy) may improve not only quality of life, but possibly even length of survival in women with metastatic breast cancer.

Simonoff, L. A. (1989). Cancer patient and physician communication: Progress and continuing problems. *Annals of Behavioral Medicine, 11,* 108–112.
Excellent review of the importance of and current barriers to effective communication in the medical setting with practical guidelines for addressing these barriers.

97

Cancer: Behavioral and Psychosocial Aspects

Annette L. Stanton

*A*lthough a diagnosis of cancer presents profound challenges to women's intra- and interpersonal functioning, most women remain resilient in the face of diagnosis and treatment. The psychological status of women diagnosed with cancer is likely to be indistinguishable from that of physically healthy women by 12–24 months after diagnosis, given that treatment is complete and the cancer controlled. However, some women experience severe life disruption at particular points, often manifested in symptoms of depression, anxiety, or posttraumatic stress disorder (PTSD). For example, Andersen found elevation in depressed mood in women with gynecological cancer at the point of diagnosis and at recurrence, as compared with women with recent benign gynecological diagnoses and healthy women; Cordova and colleagues estimated that 5–10% of women would meet diagnostic criteria for PTSD associated with breast cancer.

Given the apparent diversity in women's reactions to a cancer diagnosis, it is important to specify factors that facilitate and hinder behavioral and psychosocial adjustment, in order to target for intervention those who may be most at risk for adverse outcomes. What we know and do not know about these factors is summarized in this chapter. Research on the effectiveness of psychological interventions to enhance adjustment and quality of life is also reviewed. Two caveats are important in interpreting this literature. First, the great majority of studies focus on women with cancer of the breast, as opposed to other sites. Second, participants in studies of behavioral and psychosocial issues in cancer are in the main white women of relatively high education and affluence.

CORRELATES OF BEHAVIORAL AND PSYCHOSOCIAL ADJUSTMENT TO CANCER

Demographic and Disease-Related Characteristics

Perhaps the most consistent demographic characteristic associated with adjustment to cancer is age; younger women report greater distress, at least in the face of a breast cancer diagnosis. Some evidence also suggests that less affluent women experience greater life disruption. However, these two factors have been related to distress in general community samples as well, suggesting that these associations may not be unique to those with cancer. Psychosocial adjustment also varies as a function of disease- and treatment-related characteristics, including extent of disease, treatment regimen toxicity, and side effects, and point in the chronology of cancer diagnosis. These data are summarized well by Rowland in her chapter on psychosocial aspects of breast cancer.

Premorbid Psychological Characteristics

A history of psychological disorder, particularly depression, is related to poorer adjustment to cancer. Personality characteristics also predict adjustment. For example, Carver and colleagues found that optimism (defined as a dispositional expectancy for favorable outcomes) at the point of breast cancer diagnosis predicted lower distress over the following year. In general, personality attributes that promote productive engagement with the stressor may confer benefit.

Coping Strategies

Women use diverse strategies to cope with the demands of having cancer. Among these, perhaps the strongest predictor of psychological distress is avoidant coping. Women who attempt to disengage from their experience of cancer, either cognitively or behaviorally, are likely to evidence poorer psychological adjustment. For example, Stanton and Snider found that women who reported greater distress prior to breast biopsy were younger, less optimistic, and more threatened by the possibility of a cancer diagnosis, and that they engaged in more cognitive avoidance coping. Avoidant coping prior to biopsy also predicted more distress after cancer was diagnosed and after completion of surgery, even when initial distress was controlled statistically. The association between avoidant coping and distress has emerged in both cross-sectional and longitudinal studies, with coping assessed at the point of diagnosis or at some other point in the cancer trajectory, and with follow-up assessment as long as 1 year. Indeed, of 14 published studies reviewed for this chapter that assessed the relation of avoidant coping and distress in cancer patients, 12 yielded significant associations. Of importance is the recent finding of Epping-Jordan and colleagues in a sample of patients (80% women) with various cancers that greater use of avoidant coping shortly after diagnosis predicted cancer progression 1 year later.

In contrast, coping strategies aimed at active engagement with one's experience of cancer are related to more positive adjustment. Strategies such as active acceptance of the reality of the cancer diagnosis, positive appraisal of one's experience of cancer, information seeking, and seeking of social support may protect women from adverse psychological effects.

Interpersonal Resources

Receipt of social support is an important predictor of adjustment. Helgeson and Cohen reviewed the literature on social support and adjustment to cancer, many studies for which were conducted with breast cancer patients. The review revealed that perceptions of greater emotional support by significant others were associated consistently with positive psychological adjustment to cancer. Perceived informational and instrumental support evidenced less consistent associations with adjustment, although fewer studies tested these relations.

Inadequate communication with and support by health professionals may also confer psychological risk. For example, Lerman and colleagues found that 84% of a sample of breast cancer patients reported problems communicating with the health care team. Most frequent were difficulty understanding physicians, problems expressing feelings to the medical team, desire for more control, and difficulty asking questions of physicians. Communication problems were associated with greater distress at a 3-month follow-up.

Although their results were not uniform, several studies have demonstrated an association between the presence of social support and more positive medical outcomes. For example, Maunsell and colleagues reported that self-reported use of confidants by breast cancer patients in the 3 months after surgery, particularly when the confidant included a physician or nurse, was associated with greater likelihood of survival 7 years later.

Remaining Questions and Future Directions

Although the research to date provides a portrait of which women might be most at risk for significant life disruption following cancer diagnosis, many questions remain. Whether findings to date apply to diverse groups requires exploration. As noted above, the knowledge base to this point primarily pertains to white women of relatively high education and socioeconomic status who are coping with early-stage breast cancer. Further examination of the impact of cultural and economic factors on quality of life and health is required. Such study is rendered more important, given findings that women without private health insurance are less likely to be screened for breast cancer, more likely to present with advanced disease, and are less likely to survive than privately insured women, as well as the finding that breast cancer survival rates are lower for African-American than for European-American women.

Further delineation of contributors to adjustment for women experiencing various cancer diagnoses and treatments is also needed. Coping tasks and predictors of adjustment may be different for women with ovarian cancer (70% of whom present with advanced disease), for example. More generally, active, problem-focused coping strategies may prove most effective at the point of diagnosis of early-stage cancer, whereas unremitting attempts by a woman with cancer or her loved ones to seek information and new treatments may impede quality of life when the woman faces terminal disease. That different predictors may be important for different quality-of-life outcomes also deserves study. For example, some evidence indicates that negative indicators of quality of life (e.g., depression, anxiety) may be influenced by different factors than more positive indicators (e.g., vigor, joy). It should also be noted that many women report that the experience of cancer provides the opportunity for enhancing their lives, whereby intimate relationships are enriched and priorities strengthened. Resources that promote the ability to garner psychosocial benefits in the face of adversity deserve study. In addition, Meyerowitz and Hart observed that women are most frequently studied when quality-of-life outcomes include emotional status and social relationships, whereas men are more likely to be participants when the outcomes examined are somatic discomfort and functional ability. In general, fine-grained longitudinal analyses of contributors to specific domains of life quality in diverse groups of women with various cancers are needed.

Whether there are gender-specific predictors of adjustment to cancer remains virtually untested. The preponderance of research on adjustment to cancer has been conducted with women participants. In mixed-gender samples, testing for gender-related effects is often not reported, or testing is only for mean differences rather than for differential relations of predictors with adjustment for women and men. In one of the few tests of these relations, Fife and colleagues found that perceived support from family members was a significant correlate of adjustment for women with various cancers, whereas perceived support from health professionals was a correlate for men. Studies of adjustment to cancers of similar prevalence and prognosis in women and men would reveal whether any important gender-specific relations emerge, and mechanisms for these effects could then be explored.

PSYCHOLOGICAL INTERVENTIONS FOR CANCER PATIENTS

Research Findings

Interventions designed to enhance the adjustment of those with cancer are diverse; they include information provision about the disease and treatment, techniques to ameliorate specific cancer-related symptoms (e.g., treatment of anticipatory nausea during chemotherapy), and more general approaches to foster emotional support and adaptive coping. Interventions demonstrated to improve both quality of life and physical health outcomes have generated particular interest in the scientific and lay communities. Spiegel and colleagues reported that women with metastatic breast cancer who were randomly assigned to weekly, year-long supportive–expressive group therapy had significantly less mood disturbance than controls. Those whose group therapy included hypnosis reported half the pain of those in the control group. A 10-year follow-up revealed that women in the intervention group lived on average twice as long (36.6 vs. 18.9 months from study entry to death) as women in the control group. More recent research by Fawzy and colleagues has also documented the survival benefit of psychological interventions. Their 6-week structured intervention involves health education, stress management, and coping skills training conducted in a supportive group format. The approach was developed with malignant melanoma patients and is being extended to breast cancer patients. Findings for melanoma patients (54% women) revealed greater use of active coping, greater reduction in psychological distress (e.g., depressed affect, fatigue), enhanced immune parameters, and greater rate of survival (after 6 years) for intervention than for control participants. Although immune function was not significantly related to survival, higher baseline distress and an increase in active behavioral coping were related to better survival.

Reviews of the literature on psychological interventions demonstrate their positive effects on quality of life. Meyer and Mark conducted a meta-analysis of 45 published, randomized, controlled studies of these interventions, in which the majority of participants were women. Beneficial effects of the interventions were demonstrated with regard to emotional (e.g., mood state, self-esteem) and functional (e.g., return to work, role performance) adjustment, as well as disease- and treatment-related symptoms (e.g., pain, chemotherapy-related nausea). No significant effect emerged on medical status (e.g., leukocyte activity), and several different treatment approaches (e.g., cognitive-behavioral treatment, educational methods, organized social support) were found to be equally effective, although statistical power to detect these effects was low.

Reviewing many of the same studies, Andersen noted that individual and group therapeutic interventions have yielded equivalent outcomes, and that structured interventions appear more effective than those with no structured content. She suggested that components of effective interventions include (1) an emotionally supportive context; (2) provision of information about cancer and its treatment; (3) instruction in active behavioral and cognitive coping strategies; and (4) relaxation training.

Remaining Questions and Future Directions

Reviews of the literature clearly indicate that psychological interventions can be effective for enhancing quality of life, and perhaps improving survival, for women with cancer. Again, a number of questions remain. The first concerns the particular patients to whom such an intervention should be targeted. Although most women with cancer adjust successfully without formal psychological aid and report satisfaction with the support they receive, Massie and colleagues estimated that at least one-quarter of cancer patients need more structured intervention, and many well-functioning women actively seek formal support. Information regarding psychological resources can be offered to all who receive a cancer diagnosis, and preventive interventions might be targeted toward women who display the risk factors previously discussed (e.g., young women with low social support).

A second question involves what intervention components are most effective. With the exception of treatments targeted to specific cancer-related symptoms (e.g., treatment for anticipatory nausea), most psychological interventions have included multiple components, and maximally effective ingredients need to be identified. Mechanisms for beneficial effects also require examination. For example, the survival advantage demonstrated in some intervention studies may be a consequence of increased medical regimen adherence and patient advocacy, enhanced health behaviors, immune or endocrine changes, or some other factor.

Whether matching particular treatments with women who have specific characteristics produces the best outcomes is an important question. For example, it is clear that women who cope through avoidance are at risk for greater distress. Would an emotionally evocative therapy such as Spiegel et al.'s be especially effective to counter avoidant coping, or would avoidant copers be more at risk for dropout or adverse outcomes in such expressive therapies? Would treatment targeted primarily toward enhancing social support confer benefit for those who already possess rich support resources? Furthermore, group formats may be a successful and cost-effective mode of intervention delivery for most women. However, not all women will elect to join a group, and the conditions under which other formats are more beneficial warrant study. Careful selection of participants with specific attributes for entry into interventions designed to address their most central psychosocial needs represents a next step in intervention research. In addition, testing the generalizability of effective interventions to diverse groups of women is necessary.

CONCLUSIONS

Implicit assumptions regarding the concerns of women were present in the early literature on adjustment to cancer. Fortunately, research has been conducted to test these assumptions. For example, some writers assumed that breast loss would be the most significant (and often devastating) concern of women with breast cancer. Research has shown that threat to life and fears about the future are greater concerns, and that most women are psychologically resilient after breast loss. Also, substantial research has been devoted to examining the presumed psychosocial benefits of breast-conserving surgical procedures over mastectomy, and findings have revealed more circumscribed advantages than originally assumed. As Rowland notes in her chapter, although breast conservation (e.g., lumpectomy) confers some benefit in the realms of body satisfaction and sexual functioning, it has not been shown to yield broader positive psychosocial effects as compared with mastectomy. Women have been the most frequent participants in psychological oncology research; thus, our accurate understanding of risk and protective factors for women's adjustment and of effective psychological interventions to enhance quality of life is burgeoning. The next generation of research requires sophisticated methodologies (e.g., longitudinal and experimental designs) to explore theory-driven conceptualizations of adjustment to cancer and associated psychological interventions for women.

FURTHER READING

Andersen, B. L. (1992). Psychological interventions for cancer patients to enhance quality of life. *Journal of Consulting and Clinical Psychology, 60, 552–568.*
Review of research on psychological interventions for cancer patients.

Andersen, B. L., Anderson, B., & deProsse, C. (1989). Controlled prospective longitudinal study of women with cancer: II. Psychological outcomes. *Journal of Consulting and Clinical Psychology, 57, 692–697.*
Exemplary study of adjustment in women with gynecological cancer.

Carver, C. S., Pozo, C., Harris, S. D., Noriega, V., Scheier, M. F., Robinson, D. S., Ketcham, A. S., Moffat, F. L., & Clark, K. C. (1993). How coping mediates the effect of optimism on distress: A study of women with early stage breast cancer. *Journal of Personality and Social Psychology, 65, 375–390.*
Longitudinal study illustrating the relations among optimism, coping strategies, and distress in breast cancer patients.

Cordova, M. J., Andrykowski, M. A., Kenady, D. E., McGrath, P. C., Sloan, D. A., & Redd, W. H. (1995). Frequency and correlates of posttraumatic-stress-disorder-like symptoms after treatment for breast cancer. *Journal of Consulting and Clinical Psychology, 63, 981–986.*
Study estimating the prevalence of symptoms of PTSD in women with breast cancer.

Epping-Jordan, J. E., Compas, B. E., & Howell, D. C. (1994). Predictors of cancer progression in young adult men and women: Avoidance, intrusive thoughts, and psychological symptoms. *Health Psychology, 13, 539–547.*
Study in which avoidant coping predicted cancer progression one year later.

Fawzy, F. I., Fawzy, N. W., Hyun, C. S. Elashoff, R., Guthrie, D., Fahey, J. L., & Morton, D. L. (1993). Malignant melanoma: Effects of an early structured psychiatric intervention, coping, and affective state on recurrence and survival 6 years later. *Archives of General Psychiatry, 50, 681–689.*
Controlled experimental study of psychological intervention for melanoma patients.

Fawzy, F. I., & Fawzy, N. W. (1994). A structured psychoeducational intervention for cancer patients. *General Hospital Psychiatry, 16, 149–192.*
Treatment manual for effective psychological intervention, with application to breast cancer.

Fife, B. L., Kennedy, V. N., & Robinson, L. (1994). Gender and adjustment to cancer: Clinical implications. *Journal of Psychosocial Oncology, 12*(1/2), 1–21.
Study examining gender differences in adjustment to cancer.

Helgeson, V. S., & Cohen, S. (1996). Social support and adjustment to cancer: Reconciling descriptive, correlational, and intervention research. *Health Psychology, 15*, 135–148.
Review of literature on social support and cancer.

Lerman, C., Daly, M., Walsh, W. P., Resch, N., Seay, J., Barsevick, A., Birenbaum, L., Heggan, T., & Martin, G. (1993). Communication between patients with breast cancer and health care providers. *Cancer, 72*, 2612–2620.
Study illustrating the importance of communication between breast cancer patients and health care providers for patients' adjustment.

Massie, M. J., Holland, J. C., & Straker, N. (1990). Psychotherapeutic interventions. In J. C. Holland & J. H. Rowland (Eds.), *Handbook of psychooncology* (pp. 455–469). New York: Oxford University Press.
Description and review of psychotherapeutic interventions for cancer patients.

Maunsell, E., Brisson, J., & Deschenes, L. (1995). Social support and survival among women with breast cancer. *Cancer, 76*, 631–637.
Representative study of the link between social support and enhanced survival in breast cancer patients.

Meyer, T. J., & Mark, M. M. (1995). Effects of psychosocial interventions with adult cancer patients: A meta-analysis of randomized experiments. *Health Psychology, 14*, 101–108.
Meta-analysis of 45 controlled psychological intervention studies with cancer patients.

Meyerowitz, B. E., & Hart, S. (1995). Women and cancer: Have assumptions about women limited our research agenda? In A. L. Stanton & S. J. Gallant (Eds.), *The psychology of women's health: Progress and challenges in research and application* (pp. 51–84). Washington, DC: American Psychological Association.
Chapter exploring implicit assumptions in research on women and cancer.

Spiegel, D., Bloom, J. R., Kraemer, H. C., & Gottheil, E. (1989). Effect of psychosocial treatment on survival of patients with metastatic breast cancer. *Lancet, ii*, 888–891.
Study demonstrating survival advantage in women with metastatic breast cancer randomly assigned to supportive–expressive psychological intervention.

Stanton, A. L., & Snider, P. R. (1993). Coping with a breast cancer diagnosis: A prospective study. *Health Psychology, 12*, 16–23.
Longitudinal study demonstrating relations of coping strategies and adjustment in breast cancer patients.

98

Cancer: Medical Aspects

Patricia A. Ganz

EPIDEMIOLOGICAL FACTORS

Cancer will affect one in three individuals and is second only to heart disease as the leading cause of mortality in the United States. The absolute number of new cancer cases will increase as the population ages, as cancer is primarily a disease of the elderly. This is a particularly important issue for women, since their life expectancy exceeds that of men, and they are at increasing risk of certain cancers as they age (e.g., breast and colorectal cancer). For example, at age 35 years, the incidence of breast cancer is about 50 women per 100,000 in the population; this climbs to over 300 per 100,000 after age 60 years. Although cancer is more than 100 different diseases (based on the tissue site of origin), the age-specific pattern of incidence will vary among cancer sites, more than 50% of all cancers occur in people over age 60 years.

What does age have to do with the development of cancer? Although some rare forms of childhood cancer may be genetic or relate to *in utero* exposures or risks, the majority of cancers occur because of long-term and gradual changes in normal tissues, which then lead to transformations in cells and thus to cancer. Therefore, it takes many years for an individual to be sufficiently exposed to one or more carcinogens for a cancer to develop. Throughout a woman's lifetime, her tissues are constantly being exposed to carcinogenic agents (e.g., sunlight, radiation, tobacco products). Most tissues are capable of repairing the damage to cells, but over time these mechanisms do not work as well, and some abnormal cells will be allowed to continue growing. In addition, the body's natural immunity tends to wane with age, and there is a decline in the ability of naturally occurring immune cells to identify and suppress abnormal cells that are cancerous. Thus, a number of factors conspire to make cancer a disease that is more frequent in later life.

What role does inheritance play in the development of cancer? We know that cancer tends to run in some families, whereas it is infrequent in others. When cancer occurs in a family, it may have what is called a "genetic basis"; that is, an actual genetic abnormality is passed in the DNA of the germline tissue (eggs and sperm) to the offspring, who then have the abnormality in all cells of their bodies. Usually, in genetic forms of the disease, the same type of cancer (e.g., colorectal or breast) occurs in multiple generations (e.g., grandparents, parents, aunts, uncles, children, and cousins) and tends to occur at an early age (e.g., as early as 20 years). In contrast, cancer has a "familial risk" in some individuals; that is, several members of a family may have cancer of differing types, but occurring at the usual older age of onset. In these situations, family members may share some common lifestyle habits or exposures, rather than a specific genetic abnormality in the inherited DNA. For example, several family members may develop lung, bladder, and pancreatic cancer. These are all smoking-related cancers and may be present in a family because the members are smokers or have a gene that makes them more susceptible to the carcinogens in cigarette smoke. Although many people commonly believe that cancer only occurs in individuals with a family history of cancer, this is incorrect; most newly diagnosed patients with cancer do not have a notable family history. Everyone is at risk. Those with a family history may be at somewhat increased risk, depending on whether their family pattern of inheritance appears genetic or familial.

What types of exposures lead to an increased risk of cancer? Almost half of all cancers are related to exposure to tobacco products (in all forms, including cigarettes, cigars, and chewing tobacco). The carcinogenic effects of tobacco have been known for over 30 years, yet consumption has only begun to drop in recent years. Unfortunately, this is an area where women's equality has resulted in a substantial increase in all tobacco-related cancers—particularly lung cancer, the leading cause of cancer death in women. Women have generally been protected from a variety of other occupational exposures to cancer-causing agents. Known carcinogens such as asbestos, aniline dyes, nickel, uranium, and the like have increased the risks of cancer in men, largely by virtue of their occupational history. Another type of cancer risk is from infections—in particular, certain types of viruses. For example, cervical cancer is related to certain strains of the papillomavirus, a sexually transmitted disease that women often acquire from exposure to multiple sexual partners at an early age. Other viruses associated with the development of cancer include hepatitis B virus, Epstein–Barr virus, and certain viruses that infect T lymphocytes. These viruses are not gender-specific in their pattern of infection.

Female hormones (estrogen and progesterone), which are produced in a woman's own body from puberty to menopause, are factors in the development of certain cancers that occur primarily in women (e.g., breast cancer, endometrial cancer). Hormone exposure can also come from exogenous sources, such as contraceptive hormones and noncontraceptive estrogens and progestins given at various times during a woman's life. Although endogenous and exogenous female hormones are growth factors for both normal and cancerous tissues in general, some agents, such as diethylstilbestrol, may act as carcinogens. Currently, there is considerable interest in the estrogen-like effects of environmental pesticides, which may have effects on tissues that are normally responsive to estrogens.

Other lifestyle factors also influence the risk of cancer in women. Sun exposure, especially sunburns at an early age, can increase the risk of skin cancers and the lethal form of skin cancer called melanoma. Use of sunscreen and avoidance of sunburns are important preventive strategies. Oral contraceptives have generally been found to be cancer-protective, especially with regard to the risk of ovarian cancer; however, some earlier formulations may have contained synthetic hormones that have been associated with a risk of uterine and breast cancer. The age at first childbirth can also influence the risk of breast cancer. The older a woman is at the time of her first full-term pregnancy, the greater her relative risk of breast cancer. Thus, the increase in late pregnancies (e.g., first pregnancy over age 30 years) may be contributing to the small but increasing rates of breast cancer during the past 30 years. Finally, the sexual revolution and contraceptives have increased the risk of sexually transmitted diseases. Some of these infections can increase the risk of cervical and anogenital cancers in women.

WHAT IS CANCER?

Cancer is a state characterized by the disorderly growth of cells within a tissue. In general, the earliest pathological transformation of a tissue from normal is represented by "hyperplastic changes," an exuberant overgrowth of normal-appearing cells. Eventually, some of the cells will develop atypical features (e.g., they look more abnormal and begin to develop some features of cancer cells). Further along this continuum of tissue transformation are "dysplastic change" (highly abnormal-looking cells) and a state called "in situ cancer." In this latter situation, there is a localized growth of malignant cells that does not invade the adjacent tissues. *In situ* cancers are low-grade malignancies because they rarely "metastasize" (spread to distant parts of the body). When the malignant cells frankly invade the adjacent tissue, this is a true cancer. Under these circumstances, the prognosis is directly related to the size or dimensions of the primary tumor and the extent to which it has spread to local lymph nodes or distant organs.

The entire process described in the preceding paragraph takes decades to occur under most circumstances. Cancer is a multistep process that requires a series of critical insults to the DNA of a cell. It may take 20–30 years for a known carcinogen to cause sufficient damage to a tissue to force the cells through the phases of hyperplasia, atypia, dysplasia, and *in situ* cancer. Finally, when the first cancer cell develops, it may take another 8–10 years of repeated doublings of the cells before the tumor reaches a size that is detectable with screening (e.g., by mammography), and additional years may ensue before any symptoms occur from dissemination of the cancer to vital organs.

For example, from the evaluation of serial cytological examinations from the cervix (Papanicolau or Pap smears), we know that the first abnormalities preceding an *in situ* cancer are hyperplasia, atypia, and dysplasia. Not all dysplastic changes will progress to cancer, but some will. Careful monitoring of individuals with dysplastic Pap smears allows the early detection of the first malignant cells and the complete cure of *in situ* cancers with local therapy by surgical removal of the involved tissue. However, if a woman neglects to have routine Pap smear screening, or does not return for follow-up examinations when a Pap smear abnormality is found, she puts herself at risk for allowing these abnormal cells to continue to grow and ultimately lead to an invasive cancer that is locally advanced (many centimeters in size), with a high risk for dissemination to other parts of the body. Under these circumstances, more extensive surgery, radiation, and chemotherapy may be required. Even when they are used appropriately, cure is not assured for patients with advanced disease.

Many years ago, medical practitioners used to think of a cancer diagnosis as an emergency and would often take patients for surgery within days of diagnosis. For instance, no less than 20 years ago, women would have a breast biopsy under general anesthesia and then immediately have a mastectomy without waking up in between. These women would give consent for mastectomy in anticipation of the results of the frozen section biopsy evaluation. Practitioners now know that there is no urgent need to remove a cancer immediately, as many years have preceded the time of diagnosis, during which time the risk of dissemination was present. Although a treatment plan should be defined promptly for a patient (i.e., within several weeks), cancer is rarely viewed as a medical emergency. Now a woman with a suspicious abnormality in the breast usually undergoes a two-step procedure, which first requires a biopsy to determine whether the abnormality is cancer. If it is, she can then see several consultants to discuss her treatment options. She and her partner or family can then have time to adjust to the shock of the diagnosis and can participate in the treatment planning—all of which have important psychological implications.

In general, some form of "staging" is performed for most cancers. This means that the physician will clinically determine the extent of the cancer (locally and in distant parts of the body) prior to making a treatment recommendation. The treatments and prognosis are directly related to how extensive the cancer is. Treatment options and prognosis are best when the cancer is small and localized. Depending on the type of cancer, staging may require a minimum of tests, or it may require extensive tests as well as surgical staging (e.g., ovarian cancer). Anyone who is interested in learning more about specific cancers and their staging and prognosis may want to consult one of the general texts listed at the end of this chapter. In addition, the National Cancer Institute's Cancer Information Service (1-800-4-CANCER) can provide technical information about the current staging and treatment of particular types of cancer.

TREATMENT ADVANCES

In the past two decades, there have been tremendous changes in the management of cancer. Previously most patients with cancer received either surgery or radiotherapy as the primary treatment. Chemotherapy was reserved for palliation of patients with advanced cancer. With the success of chemotherapy in the treatment of childhood leukemia in the late 1960s, chemotherapy treatment was expanded to the treatment of various cancers in adults. Systematic clinical trials identified promising chemotherapy drugs and combinations of drugs, often with cure of widespread disease becoming a reality (as in the case of Hodgkin's disease in the 1970s). Finally, research expanded to the testing of multiple modalities (surgery, chemotherapy, radiation, immunotherapy) in the treatment of cancer, with the ultimate goal of higher rates of cure. This has occurred for several diseases; however, the cost of this advance is more complex and prolonged treatment. This approach has also increased the widespread application of organ-sparing treatments (e.g., for larynx cancer, breast cancer, rectal cancer, and bladder cancer), which may offer better quality of life to some patients.

In addition to these traditional approaches to cancer treatment, a new and exciting area of research and treatment is in the area of chemoprevention. As the medical profession becomes increasingly able to identify early events in the development of a cancer (e.g., hyperplasia, atypia, dysplasia), new agents are being evaluated and tested for their ability to interfere with the further transformation of these tissues to frank malignancy. The Breast Cancer Prevention Trial, which is evaluating the efficacy of the drug tamoxifen as a chemopreventive agent for breast cancer, is an example of one of several large trials currently underway. In this study, 13,000 women at high risk for breast cancer (based on tissue changes and strong family history) are randomly assigned to receive either a placebo or tamoxifen for a 5-year period of time. This trial began in 1992, and by the end of this century we should know whether this agent is effective in reducing the incidence and death rate from breast cancer in this high-risk population of women.

COMMON CANCERS IN WOMEN

Breast Cancer

Breast cancer is the most common malignancy in women, with about 180,200 cases in 1997. Through intensive use of screening with clinical breast examination and mammography, the number of women being diagnosed with very small tumors in the breast (less than 2 centimeters in size) has been increasing. An analysis of all the mammographic screening trials conducted throughout the world has shown a consistent 25–30% decrease in mortality from breast cancer because of screening (mammography every 1–2 years on a regular basis). The mortality benefit from screening in women less than 50 years of age is uncertain, and guidelines on this issue are conflicting (see the chapters by Mayer and Kaplan in Section III of this volume). For women with a family history of breast cancer, screening should be started at an earlier age; most experts would agree on a baseline between the ages of 35 and 39 years, with additional screening at 1- to 2-year intervals between the ages of 40 and 49 years. A mammogram is not a substitute for a biopsy, and any lump in the breast should be biopsied even if a mammogram is negative!

Studies performed during the past 10–15 years have demonstrated that there is no difference in survival between breast-conserving treatment (removal of the breast tumor and lymph node dissection, followed by radiation to the breast) and total mastectomy (removal of the entire breast and lymph nodes). Women should be offered a choice of treatments, as long as breast-conserving surgery is technically feasible and is likely to lead to a good cosmetic result. Alternatively, a woman who either chooses or requires a total mastectomy can be offered immediate surgical reconstruction of the breast. In either case, research has shown that offering women a choice is critical to psychological acceptance and recovery after breast cancer. Whichever treatment a woman chooses should be her decision, to the extent possible. Quality-of-life outcome studies have shown few differences between these two procedures.

After surgical treatment, most women are seen in consultation by a medical oncologist to determine whether any additional treatment is necessary. Depending on the size of the tumor, its microscopic and biological characteristics, and whether it has disseminated (especially to the adjacent lymph nodes), a decision will be made about subsequent treatment (adjuvant therapy). If the tumor is an *in situ* cancer or is very small, no further therapy may be required. Some women may require adjuvant therapy with the antiestrogen tamoxifen; others may require chemotherapy treatments; and some may be given both. For women who are at very high risk of cancer recurrence, experimental treatments with very high doses of chemotherapy are under evaluation (also known as autologous bone marrow transplant therapy or peripheral stem cell transplant therapy). Overall, a woman with a diagnosis of breast cancer can anticipate some form of additional therapy after surgery, and the intensity of the therapy will relate to her risk of recurrence. With the advances that have been made in breast cancer treatments during the past two decades, we have begun to see a decrease in deaths from breast cancer. Overall, 75% of early-stage breast cancer patients can expect to be alive 5 years after diagnosis. Some women with very early disease can anticipate nearly normal life expectancy.

In spite of these encouraging statistics, some women will have a recurrence of their breast cancer several years after diagnosis, and a small number (about 10–15%) will have metastatic disease at the time of diagnosis. Although cure occurs seldom in this situation, many women will have prolonged survival with the use of hormone therapies and chemotherapy. For many women with metastatic breast cancer, the disease is slowly progressive and leads to minimal disruption in daily life. An unfortunate few may have rapidly fatal disease that is unresponsive to intensive treatments.

Colorectal Cancer

Cancers of the large bowel and rectum are the next most common cancers in women. They are most common after the age of 50 years, but occasionally occur in younger women, especially those with a family history of colon cancer or polyps. These latter individuals can benefit from early screening with colonoscopy. In addition, a number of chemoprevention studies are underway in high-risk groups. In general, colorectal cancer is detected because of a change in bowel habits, blood in the stool, or anemia that may gradually result from chronic low-grade blood loss. These symptoms of cancer will prompt an evaluation to detect the source of bleeding or the cause of the change in bowel habits.

Similar to other cancer sites in the body, cancers of the colon and rectum usually arise from hyperplastic changes in the lining of the bowel wall, which gradually transform into a cancer over many years. The earliest visible precursor to a bowel cancer is a polyp, a small growth that is usually on a stalk. Screening examinations of the large bowel with a flexible fiber-optic scope can detect these polyps and remove them, leading to a reduction in colon cancers in some studies. Although larger trials are underway to evaluate the exact mortality benefit from this type of screening, most scientific groups suggest a screening examination of the lower segment of the rectum and large bowel every 5 years after the age of 50 years.

When a cancer of the colon or rectum is diagnosed, surgery is usually the initial treatment. The local tumor and draining lymph nodes are removed and examined under the microscope. As in the case of breast cancer, the extent of disease and microscopic findings will determine whether additional treatment is warranted. Often radiation is given in association with a rectal cancer. Adjuvant chemotherapy is also given with either colon or rectal cancer. For cancers in the lowest portion of the rectum, the surgical procedure may require a colostomy (in which the rectum is completely removed and an opening is created on the abdominal wall for fecal excretion). Often the rectum can be conserved (similar to breast conservation treatment) by using a combination of limited surgery, chemotherapy, and radiation.

A fair number of patients (40–50%) will have evidence of metastatic disease at the time of diagnosis. For these individuals, treatment with chemotherapy is primarily palliative. Unlike the situation with breast cancer, there are relatively limited options for treatment of colorectal cancer, and new experimental approaches are needed.

Lung Cancer

The increased adoption of cigarette smoking by women during the latter half of the 20th century has accelerated the rate at which lung cancer occurs in women. It is now the leading cause of cancer death in women, having surpassed breast cancer several years ago. In absolute numbers, the incidence of lung cancer in women is lower than that of either breast or colorectal cancer, but the survival rate from this cancer is exceedingly poor, thus accounting for its status as the most lethal cancer in women. (This is the case in men too, but for men it is also the most common cancer.) The major reason for these ominous statistics is that there are no useful techniques for early detection of lung cancer, and most individuals are diagnosed only when symptoms occur. At that point the cancer has been present for many years and is usually widely disseminated. If it is localized (only about 10–15% of cases), surgery can offer a chance of cure. Chemotherapy and radiation are both used in the treatment of lung cancer. They offer some minimal prolongation of life and may be useful in the palliation of symptoms. Overall, the best way to address this cancer is through prevention of the risk behavior—smoking—that etiologically accounts for the overwhelming number of cases of lung cancer. Behavioral and pharamacological approaches (nicotine replacement) have been evaluated and are useful in encouraging smoking cessation.

Gynecological Malignancies

Cancers of the cervix, uterus, ovaries, and vulva are unique to women. Although numerically not as frequent as the previously described cancers, they are important sites for cancer in women. Cancer at each of these sites has a unique epidemiology, etiology, and age distribution. From the perspective of the behavioral scientist, these cancer sites are important because of the effects of treatment on the reproductive and sexual functioning of women. Cervical cancer, although completely preventable through screening and early treatment, still accounts for a substantial number of deaths, particularly in socioeconomically disadvantaged groups. Behavioral interventions to increase adherence to screening and follow-up of abnormalities are critical. Uterine, ovarian, and vulvar cancers are also more amenable to treatment when diagnosed early. Unfortunately, they occur in older women who often do not regularly obtain gynecological evaluation. As with other cancers described earlier, the more limited the disease, the less complex the treatment. Surgery, radiation, and chemotherapy are used to treat all three of these cancers when the disease is advanced.

Lymphomas

The two major types of primary lymph gland tumors are called Hodgkin's disease and non-Hodgkin's lymphoma. These are important cancers to know about, since they are highly responsive to chemotherapy and radiation therapy treatments and are often cured with these treatments. Again, as in the other cancers, the stage or extent of disease and the microscopic evaluation of the tumor are critical in determining the type of treatment and estimating prognosis. Lymphomas have a bimodal incidence pattern, with the first peak in late adolescence and the 20s, and the second in adults over age 60 years. The treatment regimens are often complex and toxic but have high rates of cure. Patients who have been treated for lymphoma are among the growing numbers of cancer survivors.

MEDICAL ISSUES IN CANCER SURVIVORS

Late Effects of Treatment

The overall survival rate for cancer is in excess of 50%, and for some of the selected cancer sites discussed earlier, 75–90% survival can be expected. These treatment gains have not been achieved without cost. The complex, multimodal therapies described earlier are effective in curing the cancer, but they often do not spare normal tissues. Late effects of treatment on normal tissues can be subclinical or clinical, and may cause minor symptoms or be disabling. Often they will require additional medical treatments that are bothersome for the cancer survivor. Examples include injury to the heart (radiation pericarditis, congestive heart failure, premature heart attacks), lung fibrosis, kidney failure, and neurological syndromes. With the growing number of cancer survivors (6–7 million and increasing), many physicians are beginning to describe these sequelae and are modifying the initial therapy as a result.

Sexual Dysfunction

Sexual problems may result directly from the cancer treatment (e.g., treatment of gynecological cancer) or may be secondary to the psychological and endocrine effects of the treatment. Often, with chemotherapy and radiation treatments, there is a loss of libido and decrease in sexual activity. Furthermore, many women become menopausal prematurely as a result of chemotherapy or oophorectomy, and this may lead to drastic changes in vaginal lubrication and libido. For patients with breast cancer, estrogen replacement therapy is relatively contraindicated, so that nonestrogen alternatives for symptoms must be considered. Other cancer survivors may be candidates for hormone replacement therapy (e.g., patients with lymphoma). For patients who undergo extensive gynecological surgery, anatomical changes in the vagina secondary to surgery or radiation may pose important difficulties for sexual rehabilitation. Overall, the area of sexual health after cancer is largely overlooked by medical professionals, and is an area that needs further attention from behavioral scientists and cancer clinicians.

Second Cancers

Finally, another risk that cancer survivors face is the occurrence of second malignancies. These may be secondary effects of radiation treatment (e.g., patients who were treated for Hodgkin's disease are at increased risk for breast cancer a decade later) or of some forms of chemotherapy. Although the benefits of the original treatment in relationship to cure outweigh the long-term risk of a second cancer, a second bout with cancer can be very traumatic for a patient and her family.

CONCLUSIONS

Cancer is such a common disease that most behavioral scientists have frequent experience with cancer among their patients, their patients' family members, or their own circle of friends. The medical outlook for women with cancer has improved substantially in the past few decades, and future cancer control strategies (e.g., identification of high-risk groups, chemopreventive agents, better screening tests) will almost certainly have an impact on reducing the burden of cancer. Nevertheless, as the population ages, cancer will soon become the leading cause of death, and therefore it will continue to affect women of all ages and their families. This brief introduction to the medical aspects of cancer should provide a framework for understanding current and future strategies aimed at the treatment and control of this disease.

FURTHER READING

American Cancer Society. (1997). *Cancer Facts and Figures—1997,* p. 4.
Most recent cancer statistics.

DeVita, V. T., Hellman, S., & Rosenberg, S. A. (Eds.). (1997). *Cancer: Principles and practice of oncology* (5th ed.). Philadelphia: Lippincott-Raven.
Standard encyclopedic reference text on cancer and its treatment.

Harris, J. R., Lippman, M. R., Morrow, M., & Hellman, S. (Eds.). (1996). *Diseases of the breast.* Philadelphia: Lippincott-Raven.
Comprehensive text of breast diseases, benign and malignant, including treatment with surgery, radiation, and chemotherapy, as well as rehabilitation and psychosocial support.

Haskell, C. M. (Ed.). (1995). *Cancer treatment.* Philadelphia: W. B. Saunders.
Excellent standard text describing cancer diagnosis and treatment.

National Alliance of Breast Cancer Organizations. (1997). Hard won consensus on screening younger women. *NABCO News, 11*(2), 1–6.
This is not a reference but a news article describing the mammography screening controversy.

Schottenfeld, P., & Fraumeni, J. F. (1996). *Cancer epidemiology and prevention.* New York: Oxford University Press.
Comprehensive text describing epidemiological aspects of cancer and potential means of cancer prevention.

99

Cardiovascular Disorders

C. David Jenkins

Cardiovascular diseases have constituted the leading cause of death in most industrialized countries since at least the year 1900. They have been subjected to intensive study, and much has been learned not only about their causes and cures, but also about how they can be prevented. Although the pathological changes that mark the major cardiovascular diseases are measured in terms of biological processes and tissue changes, psychosocial and behavioral forces are the primary contributing causes.

Research into cardiovascular diseases over the past 50 years has been primarily conducted with men. Men have greater mortality from cardiovascular diseases early in life than do women. Nevertheless, cardiovascular diseases rank second only to cancers as a cause of death in women in the United States prior to age 65 years and take the first position thereafter. Only recently have the U.S. National Institutes of Health mandated a research policy of gender equality. Consequently, only limited numbers of long-term studies are currently available for cardiovascular disorders in women.

HYPERTENSION

Hypertension is diagnosed by repeated measures of elevated blood pressure (BP). Sustained over years, hypertension causes damage to heart muscle, brain, kidneys, and other organs. It is a risk factor for stroke (cerebrovascular accident) and heart attack (coronary heart disease [CHD] and myocardial infarction). High BP is about equally frequent in women as in men among European-Americans; however, it is about twice as frequent in African-Americans, especially in women, as in European-Americans. Blood pressure goes up with age. High BP has no accompanying symptoms, except in rare instances of acute BP crises.

Contrary to the implication of its name, hypertension is not a high level of nervous tension, in terms either of its causes or its manifestations. Population screening studies show that people with hypertension are no more anxious or tense than their normotensive neighbors. Some people, however, show an increase in anxiety and physical complaints after being told that their BP is high. Work absences also increase.

Although there is hereditary contribution to some cases of hypertension, there are many things a person can do to help maintain BP as close to normal as possible. These include maintaining a normal weight, exercising regularly, and avoiding or minimizing alcohol consumption. There is considerable debate about the role of salt intake in raising blood pressure. Epidemiological studies show that populations of people having high salt intake tend to have higher average BPs and more pronounced rise in BPs with aging compared to groups having low salt intake. At the individual level, however, it appears that fewer than half the persons in most groups are salt-sensitive, and only these persons receive a BP reduction from dietary restriction of sodium. Most people consume far more salt with their foods than is nutritionally needed, and so salt reduction would certainly do no harm. This is useful information for a family in which one member requires reduced salt. The whole family can eat the same food, and the craving for salt typically declines after about one month.

Stress raises blood pressure over the short term, but there is only limited evidence that it might create sustained hypertension. Data are particularly lacking for the psychosocial antecedents of sustained hypertension in women. The combination of hostile outlook and a frustrating situation has been shown to raise BP temporarily in women more sharply than the presence of either condition alone. Other research shows that it is the expression of anger, in angry talk or gestures, that raises BP, not just experiencing anger as thoughts or feelings. Monitoring BP while women were speaking showed that they could lower their BPs simply by speaking more slowly and softly.

The question, then, is whether to try to keep calm and maintain lower current BP with some risk of continuing resentment over time, or to gain the immediate relief of discharging anger, with its brief rise in BP. If many brief surges in BP over time tend to reset stable BP levels higher—an argument often offered, but not well proven yet—then the prudent individual would seek either to reduce hostile outlook or to minimize exposure to anger-provoking situations.

Stress also raises BP. Laboratory studies show that having to do mental math causes bigger rises in BP in nurses than does moderate physical exertion. The combination of constant mental challenge and the disastrous cost of errors appears to be responsible for the high incidence of hypertension among air traffic controllers.

The psychobiological role of anger and hostility is real even in biologically determined hypertension. In one study, women and men with mild to moderate hypertension received less treatment benefit from diuretic drugs if they were hostile, suspicious, and resentful. Levels of anxiety and depression had no effect on treatment results.

Antihypertensive drugs have increased in number, effectiveness, and freedom from side effects over the last 30 years. In addition to drugs, five health-promoting behaviors have been shown by research in many parts of the world to help reduce BP. These are weight reduction in the overweight; regular aerobic exercise (such as walking, biking, swimming, or active sports); reduction of alcohol intake; reduction of sodium intake; and the regular practice of relaxation, such as progressive relaxation, "the relaxation response," or certain breathing exercises. Doing relaxation sessions daily has been shown not only to lower mild BP elevation in many people, but also to reduce the medication dosage needed in moderate hypertensives. Hypertension is an illness that needs to be managed by a physician, and people should not introduce their own lifestyle changes without first getting the approval of their doctor.

For a more detailed discussion of hypertension, see the chapter by Wassertheil-Smoller in this volume.

CORONARY HEART DISEASE

Called "coronary artery disease," "ischemic heart disease," or "heart attack" almost interchangeably, coronary heart disease (CHD), develops from atherosclerotic deposits of hardened fat and calcium inside arteries in the heart. When these deposits block the arterial openings sufficiently to reduce blood flow or set up a narrowing that can easily be blocked by a tiny blood clot, the symptoms of angina pectoris, myocardial infarction, or coronary thrombosis occur. Rates of CHD increase with age. Men have three to five times the incidence rate of women prior to age 50; the rate of CHD in women accelerates after menopause, but never catches up with the male rate.

CHD is a lifestyle disease. Mortality rates for CHD differ sharply across countries, being four to five times as high for men (ages 45–64) in the United States and Finland as for men in Japan. For women across the same countries, the ratio is about 2.5:1. Within all 26 countries reported by the World Health Organization, women have only from one-half to one-third the mortality of men of the same age and nationality. There have also been great changes in mortality rates the last 25 years, with U.S., Swiss, and Japanese rates declining by more than 30% for both men and women. In contrast, Eastern European and developing countries have experienced equally dramatic increases in CHD mortality over the same years. The consensus of cardiovascular researchers is that the major declines in CHD mortality have followed declines in the lifestyle risk factors: cigarette smoking, elevated serum lipids, uncontrolled high BP, obesity, and sedentary lifestyle. Over recent decades cigarette smoking has become distinctly unfashionable, as well as prohibited in many public places. The fitness craze has recruited men and women of all ages. Low-fat prepared foods are more widely available, and fatty meats and dairy products are being used more sparingly. Hypertension and serum cholesterol screening programs are finding and helping people before their atherosclerosis progresses.

Despite this great progress, there is still too much CHD occurring too early in the lives of both women and men. Perhaps 25–30% of CHD cases occur in the absence of high levels of any of the above-described risk factors. Some psychosocial indicators identify additional cases. It has not yet been demonstrated that changing these psychosocial indicators will necessarily reduce CHD rates, but they are worth knowing about.

Low socioeconomic status (SES), especially little education, is a strong risk factor for hypertension, stroke, and CHD for both women and men. The higher CHD rates among persons with less than a high school education are partly explained by their higher rates of CHD risk factors, such as cigarette smoking, obesity, high BP, high blood lipids, and sedentary lifestyle. Thus women and men who did not have the opportunity to complete high school can offset the SES risk factor by prudent lifestyle. In addition, low-SES persons often have a smaller social network and less social support, both of which are risk factors for CHD (apparently more so in men than in women). People who live alone, have no close friendships, and belong to no groups are at higher risk of overall mortality, especially mortality due to cardiovascular diseases.

Studies of large groups (such as college students) who have taken psychological tests show, after many years of follow-up, that persons who give more hostile, cynical responses are more likely to develop CHD and die prematurely. This risk has been confirmed in a study of women undergoing clinical heart examinations (thallium scans). Those with greater expressed hostility had worse atherosclerosis.

Population research has sometimes found that the Type A behavior pattern—a response style marked by competitive striving, constant hurry, impatience, irritability, and hostility—is associated with future CHD in both men and women. Other risk factors include suppressed (rather than expressed) hostility, tension, chronic conflict, depression, and sleep problems. The strength of these factors differs across subpopulations. Experts are debating both whether they have causal significance and what mechanisms might be involved.

The common element in most of these psychosocial risk factors is sustained struggle, including struggle against other people, life circumstances, and time limitations, and struggles involving emotions. Lower SES and lack of social support reduce a person's resources for coping with such struggles. This explanation connects nicely with the known biology of stress and its cardiovascular effects. Struggle activates the endocrine and central nervous systems, which in turn raise blood pressure, irritate the artery linings, increase oxygen demand, and increase the potential for blood platelet aggregation and clotting. The hygienic measures called for to protect oneself against excessive struggles include changing one's social environment, changing one's expectations (demands) on oneself and others, and learning new physical and mental coping strategies. A comprehensive stress management book has much to offer.

For a fuller discussion of CHD, see Stoney's chapter of this volume.

RECOVERY FROM HEART ATTACK OR HEART SURGERY

Psychosocial and behavioral factors not only govern the risk of getting a disease; they also help determine whether recovery after an illness or major surgery will be rapid, slow, or indeed whether a patient fails to survive. In the U.S. population as a whole, women are more likely to die from their first heart attack than men; women also have higher mortality after coronary artery bypass surgery.

A prospective community-based study in New Haven, Connecticut, measured many health and social variables in healthy older people. The study found that, among those who later had a myocardial infarction, the persons who had lacked previous emotional support were three times as likely to die as those with adequate support, even after controlling for severity of the infarction and the presence of other illnesses and risk factors. Other population studies show that people with small or absent social networks have only slightly higher incidences of CHD and stroke, but significantly higher mortality. This suggests that social networks play a stronger role in supporting recovery than they do in preventing disease.

A prospective study of 536 men and women undergoing coronary artery bypass or cardiac valve surgery found many psychosocial predictors of postoperative recovery, above and beyond the medical/surgical predictors. Women tended to recover less well than men, but this difference was eliminated when other factors were taken into account. The best relief of cardiac symptoms came to patients who had higher preoperative levels of social support, social participation, activities and hobbies, self-esteem, and sense of well-being, and lower levels of anxiety, depression, sleep problems, fatigue, and fewer life change stresses. Some of these same variables also predict recovery after surgery and illnesses of other organ systems, and hence may participate in a general "force for health."

FURTHER READING

Adler, N., & Matthews, K. (1994). Health psychology: Why do some people get sick and some stay well? *Annual Review of Psychology, 45,* 229–259.
A thoughtful summary of research on what protects health, with a special emphasis on women.

Anastos, K., Charney, P., Charon, R. A., et al. (1991). Hypertension in women: What is really known? *Annals of Internal Medicine, 115,* 287–293.
A critical effort to separate knowledge from guesswork about hypertension in women from mixed population data.

Jenkins, C. D., Stanton, B. A., & Jono, R. T. (1994). Quantifying and predicting recovery after heart surgery. *Psychosomatic Medicine, 56,* 203–212.
Quantitative research identifying the biopsychosocial contributors to more complete recovery in men and women.

Kaplan, N. M., & Stamler, J. (Eds.). (1983). *Prevention of coronary heart disease: Practical management of the risk factors.* Philadelphia: W. B. Saunders. (See especially Chapter 8.)
A preventive cardiology textbook written in lay terms. This gives an excellent summary of all the risk factors, how they operate, and how to control them.

Siegman, A. W. (1993). Cardiovascular consequences of expressing, experiencing and repressing anger. *Journal of Behavioral Medicine, 16,* 539–569.
A review of experimental studies linking emotions with cardiovascular responses.

100

Coronary Heart Disease

Catherine M. Stoney

*H*eart disease is the leading cause of death among women, and the clinical manifestations of the disease are most prevalent among postmenopausal women over the age of 60 years. The progression of coronary heart disease (CHD) is delayed roughly 10 years in women relative to men. One unfortunate consequence of this advantage is that most research and resources have been focused on CHD in men rather than women. This pattern has been remedied somewhat recently with the initiation of the Women's Health Initiative, sponsored by the National Institutes of Health, and other new research programs. As researchers learn more about the physiological and anatomical aspects of CHD in women, important psychosocial issues relating specifically to women are also becoming apparent.

For both men and women, CHD is a progressive, lifelong, chronic disorder; this makes the identification of the links between psychological factors and the initiation and progression of the disease difficult. Nonetheless, several behavioral and psychosocial antecedents and consequences of heart disease in women can be identified. What follows is a brief discussion of some of these psychosocial aspects of CHD, particularly as they relate to the disease in women.

ANTECEDENTS

Health Behaviors

Among health behaviors, cigarette smoking is arguably the most important, because it is the leading cause of preventable CHD. Although the overall smoking rate in the United States is declining, smoking prevalence among women is declining at a slower rate than among men. Women are smoking in greater numbers, and women smokers are smoking more than ever before. Women may also have lower cessation rates and higher relapse rates than men. Distressingly, smoking initiation among young girls is increasing at an alarming rate; the public health impact is underscored by the fact that the 1-year smoking cessation rates in the general public are under 1%. Women and girls are increasingly being targeted by the advertising campaigns of the tobacco industry, but clinical treatments for smoking cessation are failing to target women smokers similarly. Several factors that are specific to women smokers include concern about weight gain associated with smoking cessation; smoking for affect regulation; comorbidity of psychiatric disorders; and the interaction of reproductive hormones, menstrual cycle phase, pregnancy, and the postpartum period with smoking patterns. Of these, it has been argued that the most important issue for women smokers is the concern about weight gain.

Many smoking relapse prevention programs with weight control components have been unsuccessful, perhaps because of the emphasis these programs place on simultaneously extinguishing two health-damaging behaviors. One unique set of treatment programs for smoking cessation has been developed specifically for women smokers. The programs focus on women's concerns about weight gain by combining a smoking cessation program with an exercise adherence program. Not only does the exercise portion of the program help to counteract the weight gain typically associated with metabolic changes during smoking cessation; exercise is also a positive health behavior that diminishes appetite, increases fitness, and provides a healthy alternative for stress reduction. (Maheu's chapter in Section III of this volume describes worksite programs that combine smoking cessation and exercise components.) Although the true efficacy of these multicomponent programs is still unclear, such treatments that are designed with a particular focus on women may help to isolate and target methods for improving health behaviors in women.

Work Stress and Role Stress

Over 65% of women in the United States work outside the home for pay, and this number is steadily increasing. Because child care and the bulk of household responsibilities typically fall to women, employed women work over 3,900 hours per year in their paid and unpaid jobs combined, or approximately 500 hours more than the number of hours that employed men work. This difference translates into about 2.5 more hours of work per day for women than for men. These relative differences are maintained throughout the lifespan and are even more substantial for unemployed men and women. In part because of the dual roles assumed by employed women, and in part because of the stress typically associated with employment in general, there was an overall expectation that the incidence of CHD would rise with increasing numbers of women in the work force. Quite the contrary has occurred. Although the number of women in the work force has increased by over 60% over the last 25 years, the incidence of CHD has diminished (particularly for women) in this same time period. Overall, employed women with or without children do not have an increase in risk of CHD, although several factors moderate the relationship between work and CHD. For example, the Framingham Heart Study data showed that employed women of lower socioeconomic status (SES) and with more than three children had an increase in CHD, whereas higher-SES working women with the same number of children did not. In addition to SES and number of children, satisfaction with one's work also affects the CHD mortality rate for women, as does the emotional response to working outside the home. For example, women who report working by choice have a lower incidence of hypertension than those who report working reluctantly. Similarly, perceived control at work is a more important predictor of CHD risk than is the fact of employment. Increased rates of hospitalization for myocardial infarction have been noted among women with monotonous, irregular, demanding, and low-control positions (high job strain). Thus, a positive work environment outside the home generally has a positive impact on risk of CHD, but for employed women with poor job satisfaction, low decision latitude, and high stress, CHD risk is greater than for nonemployed women. As more and more women are given the choice to work in employed positions with high levels of control, the positive impact of employment on women's CHD risk may become even greater.

Reactivity

Women's psychophysiological responses to both short- and long-term stress have been investigated with respect to the cardiovascular, neuroendocrine, metabolic, and immunological response systems. Only a few studies have controlled or assessed menstrual cycle phase, menopausal stage, and reproductive hormone levels when monitoring physiological stress responses. Nonetheless, relatively consistent findings emerge from this literature. During acute stress, women generally report levels of experienced stress similar to those of men, but have smaller-magnitude blood pressure, vasoconstriction, neuroendocrine, and lipid responses to those stressors. Gender also moderates the underlying processes of blood pressure control during stress. When cardiac impedance measures are evaluated during stress, sex differences in cardiac output, peripheral resistance, stroke volume, and myocardial contractility have all been noted.

Two factors that have been tested as potential moderators of women's stress responses are reproductive hormones and ethnicity. Regarding hormonal influences, the physiological responses of women are not greatly modified by small fluctuations in reproductive hormones (such as those occurring during the menstrual cycle), but do appear to be sensitive to larger-magnitude fluctuations in hormonal levels (such as those occurring during menopause and exogenous hormone use). Postmenopausal women experience larger physiological stress responses than do premenopausal women. Although the findings are inconclusive, preliminary data suggest that premenopausal women taking oral contraceptives and postmenopausal women taking hormone replacement therapy may have somewhat altered patterns of physiological reactivity to stress, relative to women who are not taking exogenous hormones.

Regarding ethnic influences, black women show greater vasoconstriction and attenuated heart rate responses to stress than do white women, although these ethnic influences depend in large measure on the particular stressors evaluated. Interestingly, this same pattern of ethnic differences may also be apparent for adolescents and children, and may thus reflect neural regulatory differences in beta-receptor activity and/or sensitivity.

The significance of these findings is best illustrated by innovative animal studies showing that large cardiovascular responses to stress in macaque monkeys are associated with greater atherosclerotic lesions. To the extent that physiological reactivity is important in the initiation and progression of CHD, further examination of reactivity among women is warranted.

Social Support and Social Relationships

After many decades of research, it is now clear that there is a significant relationship between social relationships and health. Risk of death from CHD and other causes is demonstrably higher among those with either poor or inadequate social support networks. The effects are approximately equal to the relationship between smoking and health and are consistently weaker for women than for men. Marriage has been shown in many studies to be associated with longevity in general and cardioprotection in particular. Most investigations have demonstrated that the effect is more prominent for men than for women; that is, men derive more health benefits from marriage than do women. Because marriage is one of the few known determinants of social support, the female disadvantage probably mirrors the weaker effects of social support on health found among women. However, men and women appear to benefit equally (from a health perspective) from social ties with friends and relatives. The relationship is maintained for the elderly and for those with serious illness. These findings parallel animal and human investigations demonstrating that physical contact reduces both cardiovascular reactivity to stress, as well as atherosclerotic plaque formation (in rabbits fed a high-fat diet).

The mechanisms responsible for the effects of social support on cardiovascular health are likely to include environmental, social, psychological, economic, and selection processes. Whether social support operates to attenuate the negative consequences of stress by reducing psychophysiological reactivity, or whether it acts more globally during both high- and low-stress periods, is controversial; this should be further examined in longitudinal studies of both men and women. Most importantly, the mechanisms for gender differences in the protective effects of social support must be examined further. Although they may simply be reflecting methodological issues (measurement of social support quality and quantity), they may also be reflecting a real difference, which may help to elucidate the ways women develop CHD.

Social Control

Kaplan, Manuck, and colleagues demonstrated the impact of social control and dominance on atherosclerosis in cynomolgus macaque monkeys. They showed that among dominant male macaques, unstable (stressful) social environments led to more severe atherosclerosis than did stable environments. Interestingly, this relationship was not apparent among the nondominant males, and the pattern was reversed among the females. That is, the *subordinate* female macaques were more vulnerable to the negative cardiovascular effects of social instability. This relationship between gender and social control may also be relevant to men and women. In general, attempts to influence or control strangers are associated with increased blood pressure in both men and women. Among married couples, however, efforts to control or influence one's spouse vary with gender. As examination of the physiological effects of social interaction on women and men showed that husbands who attempted to exert control over their wives had increases in angry, hostile displays and in blood pressure; when wives attempted to influence their husbands, no increases in blood pressure or anger were apparent. Under conditions where husbands and wives were asked to discuss issues related to marital conflict situations, but were not asked to deliberately exert control, women did have elevated blood pressure responses. These findings suggest that social control specifically may be a particularly salient variable in blood pressure reactivity, and suggest possible links between social influence and CHD.

CONSEQUENCES

Several investigations on the psychological adjustment to CHD are available, but virtually all are restricted to male cardiac patients, and frequently women are included only in the role of the patients' (presumably) healthy spouses. Thus, the unique psychosocial adjustments that women with diagnosed CHD make often must be inferred from other information available on how women cope with chronic disease.

Coping with Chronic Disease

The effects of chronic illness, particularly CHD, commonly include lifestyle change, marital adjustment, and physical and psychological coping. Very few data are available on psychosocial consequences or coping patterns among women with CHD. Although several investigations have examined women's coping responses to stress in general, very few have specifically examined the stress of CHD diagnosis. One limited study of 50 CHD men and women and their spouses found that women with CHD did not alter health-related lifestyle behaviors, and appeared to cope somewhat differently with a diagnosis of CHD (by engaging in more planned problem solving and being more accepting of responsibility) than did their male counterparts.

Interfacing with the Health Care System

Several recent investigations have demonstrated unique issues that women with CHD face when interacting with the health care system. Men are more frequently diagnosed with CHD than are women, even when only documented CHD patients are examined, and even when the diagnoses are made by a cardiologist. Once women are correctly diagnosed, there are gender differences in how men and women CHD patients are treated. In a recent study, for example, only 4% of women with abnormal thallium scans were referred for cardiac catheterization or surgery, while 40% of men were referred. The problem of gender differences in misdiagnosis and treatment stems from several sources and has multiple psychosocial consequences. First, because the symptoms of cardiac ischemia can be similar to symptoms of nonspecific anxiety, many women with CHD are misdiagnosed as anxious or as having other psychiatric disorders. Second, many women themselves do not recognize symptoms of angina or ischemia as being cardiac in nature. In fact, symptoms for these diseases may be manifested differently in women than they are in men, and the typical episodes of severe chest pain typically associated with signs of CHD may not be valid for women. The prevalence of angiographically documented coronary artery disease (CAD) in women referred for chest pain is typically less than 50%, while for men this percentage typically exceeds 95%. The extent to which this is a function of referral practices, differential symptomatology, or differential disease progression is not known. Third, the anatomy of CAD may play an important role in the prediction of CAD severity. At the same ages, single-vessel disease is more common in women than men, whereas triple-vessel disease is more typical in men than women. Some evidence indicates that the locations of the lesions also differ between men and women, and the extent of collateralization of the stenosed coronary arteries is better in men than in women. Thus, the progression of CAD among men occurs at earlier ages.

Once women are correctly diagnosed, other psychological issues that are unique to women also surface. The prognosis for a woman diagnosed with CHD is worse than for a man, because of the later development of CHD in women, the delay in diagnosis of the disease, and the poorer efficacy of both surgical and pharmacological treatments in women. The extent to which the later development *and* delayed diagnosis of CHD in women are responsible for the poorer response to treatment is unknown. However, it is clear that a cycle exists, in which delayed treatment (for fear of a negative outcome) leads to a sicker and older patient. The psychological consequences to the patient and her family are variable and may depend on the social support available from the medical community.

FURTHER READING

Frankenhaeuser, M., Lundberg, U., & Chesney, M. (Eds.). (1991). *Women, work, and health: Stress and opportunities*. New York: Plenum Press.
This text provides an epidemiological overview of how work affects women's health.

Goldman, N., Korenman, S., & Weinstein, R. (1995). Marital status and health among the elderly. *Social Science and Medicine, 40*(2), 1717–1730.
This article empirically illustrates gender differences in the relationships between marital status and health.

House, J. S., Landis, K., & Umberson, D. (1988). Social relationships and health. *Science, 241,* 540–545.
This is a landmark article reviewing how social support relates to health in men and women.

Kaplan, J. R., Adams, M. R., Clarkson, T. B., Manuck, S. B., Shively, C. A., & Williams, J. K. (1996). Psychosocial factors, sex differences, and atherosclerosis: Lessons from animal models. *Psychosomatic Medicine, 58,* 598–611.
This review of the animal literature suggests strong links between social support, gender, and the development of heart disease.

Kyriakidis, M., Petropoulakis, P., Androulakis, A., Antonopoulos, A., Apostolopoulos, T., Barbetseas, J., Vyssoulis, G., & Toutouzas, P. (1995). Sex differences in the anatomy of coronary artery disease. *Journal of Clinical Epidemiology, 48*(6), 723–730.
Although a small study, this important research illustrates significant sex differences in the anatomical progression of CAD.

Marcus, B. H., Emmons, K. M., Simkin, L. R., Albrecht, A. E., Stoney, C. M., & Abrams, D. B. (1994). Women and smoking cessation: Current status and future directions. *Medicine, Exercise, Nutrition, and Health, 3,* 17–31.
This is a review of clinical and epidemiological aspects of smoking cessation in women.

Ory, M. G., & Warner, H. R. (Eds.). (1990). *Gender, health, and longevity.* New York: Springer.
This text broadly addresses the finding that women report more illness and spend more health care dollars relative to men, yet have a higher life expectancy.

Shumaker, S. A., & Czajkowski, S. M. (Eds.). (1994). *Social support and cardiovascular disease.* New York: Plenum Press.
This book examines the research demonstrating that health is positively affected by social support, and negatively affected by a lack of supportive interactions.

Stoney, C. M. (1992). The role of reproductive hormones in cardiovascular and neuorendocrine function during behavioral stress. In A. S. J. R. Turner & K. C. Light (Eds.), *Individual differences in cardiovascular response to stress* (pp. 147–163). New York: Plenum Press.
Both exogenous and endogenous reproductive hormones are considered possible influences on physiological adjustments to stress.

Stoney, C. M., Davis, M. C., & Matthews, K. A. (1987). Sex differences in physiological responses to stress and in coronary heart disease: A causal link? *Psychophysiology, 24,* 127–131.
This editorial includes a meta-analysis of sex differences in cardiovascular reactivity, and an overview of the potential implications for these sex differences.

101

Diabetes:
Biopsychosocial Aspects

Laurie Ruggiero

Diabetes mellitus is a serious chronic illness that affects millions of people in the United States. Furthermore, estimates suggest that there is one undiagnosed case for each one currently diagnosed with diabetes. Although Type I diabetes is equally common in men and women, the incidence of Type II is greater in women, especially in age groups over 65. In general, ethnic minority populations are more likely to develop diabetes mellitus and more likely to develop diabetes-related complications. For example, in 1990, age-adjusted prevalence of known diabetes was almost twice as high in African-Americans as in non-Hispanic white individuals, and more than twice as high in Mexican-Americans and Puerto Ricans. For women in particular, black females have the highest prevalence rates, surpassing other groups at all ages. In women over 65 years old, diabetes is twice as prevalent in black women as in white women. Black women also have the highest rates of mortality for diabetes as the underlying cause of death, while white women have the lowest.

Given the high prevalence rates of diabetes mellitus in the general population; the elevated risk of diabetes and its complications in certain subgroups of women; and the fact that one variant of diabetes, gestational diabetes, is strictly a women's disorder, it is important to understand the specific biopsychosocial impact of this condition on women. Although diabetes has a number of biopsychosocial aspects, such as depression and adherence, the specific focus of this chapter is on three primary topics that both uniquely affect women and have received empirical investigation: weight control, diabetes in pregnancy, and sexual functioning. Other topics that are also very important to women with diabetes, but have not yet received much empirical investigation, are highlighted in the "Future Directions" section of this chapter.

A LANDMARK STUDY IN DIABETES MANAGEMENT

Before I describe the biopsychosocial aspects of diabetes for women, it is important to put this discussion in the current context of the field of diabetes management. Diabetes management is undergoing revolutionary changes resulting from the findings of a major study. This study, called the Diabetes Control and Complications Trial (DCCT), compared conventional diabetes management with an intensive management approach. The intensive approach included multiple daily insulin injections, frequent blood glucose self-testing, and following a special dietary and exercise plan. The results of this study indicated that maintaining blood glucose levels in a "normal" range was associated with fewer long-term complications of diabetes, and that the intensive management approach best achieved this goal. Therefore, it is clear that intensive management is the ideal approach to managing diabetes. Although this study was conducted on individuals with insulin-dependent diabetes mellitus (IDDM or Type I), these results may generalize to those with non-insulin-dependent diabetes mellitus (NIDDM or Type II) as well. Interpretation of previous research and planning for future research on the biopsychosocial factors associated with diabetes should be done with the findings of the DCCT in mind.

WEIGHT CONTROL AND DIABETES IN WOMEN

Dietary adherence and weight control are key aspects of the management of diabetes. For individuals with IDDM, close adherence to a healthy diet that is consumed on a consistent schedule is critical to the day-to-day management of blood glucose levels. For individuals with NIDDM, weight control, along with adherence to a specific dietary plan, is critical in the management of diabetes. Individuals with NIDDM constitute the great majority of all individuals with diabetes, and the majority of them are obese. Therefore, weight management is considered the cornerstone of diabetes management for obese individuals with diabetes and poses a particular challenge for individuals and professionals alike.

Weight Loss and Type II Diabetes

Weight loss intervention research with persons with NIDDM has indicated that weight loss is associated with important health benefits. For example, weight loss has resulted in improved glycemic control, increased insulin sensitivity, and decreased risk of coronary heart disease. Since, again, Type II diabetes accounts for the largest proportion of individuals with diabetes, and weight loss is the treatment of choice for the majority of this group, this topic has received ongoing empirical investigation.

It has been recommended that the ideal weight management program for obese persons with NIDDM be provided by a multidisciplinary team, including at least a physician, a dietitian, a health psychologist, an exercise physiologist, and a diabetes educator. The core components of such a program include: individualized dietary recommendations and nutrition education; increased physical activity, including both structured exercise and lifestyle activity; cognitive-behavioral strategies to achieve attitude and behavior change; medical monitoring to track metabolic changes and identify any need for medication adjustments; social support to facilitate and reinforce positive changes; and continued long-term follow-up and intervention to facilitate maintenance of the weight loss.

The research on weight loss in diabetes parallels that in the general population indicating that behavioral weight management programs (including both dietary and exercise recommendations) lead to modest weight loss, and that no single intervention approach is best for all obese persons. Furthermore, long-term maintenance of the lost weight is the greatest challenge across all populations of obese individuals. It is therefore recommended that a "best-fit" approach be used to match the most appropriate intervention components to the special needs of a particular individual, and that this matching approach be used for both weight loss and maintenance. In this light, a small number of studies have examined gender differences in weight loss, and the results of these studies may help begin to identify the best weight management approach for obese women with diabetes.

Although few studies have been conducted on weight loss in people with diabetes, it is notable that the majority of participants in studies of behavioral weight control programs for individuals with diabetes have been women. Therefore, it is likely that the results of the general research on weight loss in persons with diabetes reflect the impact specific to women. Social support has been identified as an important component of weight management programs for women with diabetes. Specifically, the results of one study indicated that women with diabetes do better when their spouses are included in the weight management program. Therefore, it is important to include social support as a component of treatment matching in attempts to maximize weight loss in women with diabetes. As in research on the general population, research on diabetes has demonstrated that exercise is important in weight loss and maintenance. Also paralleling the general body of literature, very-low-calorie diets have shown promise in individuals with diabetes.

More research is needed to continue identifying the best intervention components for women with diabetes, as well as the most important variables on which to base treatment-matching decisions. In particular, the specific dietary approaches (e.g., very low calorie diet, low fat diet), exercise approaches, and even pharmacological approaches should be further examined to help determine the best interventions for these women. Furthermore, biopsychosocial variables that may help predict outcome of behavioral weight loss programs, such as readiness for change, fat distribution (e.g., upper-body-type vs. lower-body-type obesity) and weight cycling, should be examined in women with diabetes to help establish realistic expectations for outcome. In addition, since little is known about the best weight maintenance approach for obese women with diabetes, research should be conducted on this important topic with this special population.

Eating Disorders and Diabetes

It is well known that weight control through maladaptive means, such as fasting and purging, is much more common in women than in men. Tight control of blood glucose in a narrow target range is the key to avoiding both short-term and long-term complications of diabetes. It is believed that two aspects of diabetes management may pose a special challenge for women with diabetes who are concerned about their weight. First, an important component of the management of diabetes involves following a specific eating plan on a regular schedule, and dietary restraint is likely to be a problem. Dietary restraint has been found to be associated with the development of eating disorders. Second, insulin use is another important component of the diabetes management program for many women. Research indicates that insulin use is associated with weight gain. For example, the DCCT found that people on an intensive insulin management program were more likely to gain weight and gained an average of 4.6 kg more than the conventional group after 5 years of treatment. Therefore, one of the costs of obtaining tight control to prevent or delay complications of diabetes is an increased risk of weight gain. This weight gain may pose an added challenge for women. Since these factors suggest that women with diabetes may be more vulnerable to developing eating disorders, researchers have focused their attention on this question.

To date, the primary focus of research in this area has been on examining the occurrence of eating disorders in individuals with diabetes. Research on the prevalence of eating disorders, such as anorexia nervosa and bulimia nervosa, in women with Type I diabetes have found that although the consequences of eating disorders are clearly more serious in this group, eating disorders do not necessarily occur more often than in the general population. Binge eating, however, has been found to be a common problem for obese individuals with NIDDM, especially for women. Furthermore, one unique maladaptive mechanism of weight management that is sometimes seen in individuals with diabetes is insulin manipulation. For example, women with diabetes may adjust their insulin dose to attempt to lose weight or to compensate for a specific binge episode. The consequences of this approach are very serious and require immediate intervention if identified.

Research should continue in this area, but with more of a focus on identifying the biopsychosocial risk factors for developing eating disorders, such as body image disturbance, in this group and the most effective ways to treat these disorders in women with diabetes. In addition, since one important negative consequence of intensive insulin management is weight gain, future research should focus on understanding the use of maladaptive weight management approaches (such as insulin manipulation, fasting, and purging) in women with diabetes.

DIABETES IN PREGNANCY

The presence of diabetes during pregnancy puts both the mother and fetus at increased risk of many medical complications. Common maternal complications include Cesarean section, hypertension, hydramnios, and diabetic ketoacidosis. The rates of perinatal mortality and neonatal complications, such as congenital malformations and macrosomia (i.e., being large for gestational age), are higher in this group. The rates of maternal and infant complications can be greatly reduced by maintaining tight glycemic control during pregnancy. Therefore, close adherence to the complex, daily diabetes self-care regimen and close medical monitoring are critical in the management of this disease state during pregnancy.

There are two subgroups of women with diabetes during pregnancy. One group includes women who have diabetes, either Type I or Type II, and become pregnant: the other group includes women who develop diabetes during pregnancy (i.e., gestational diabetes). For both groups of women with diabetes during pregnancy, adherence to a complex set of lifestyle behaviors is critical. For individuals with pregestational diabetes who become pregnant, more intensive management is generally needed to best manage blood glucose levels during pregnancy. Both groups are expected to follow a specific eating plan and to test their blood glucose levels frequently. Many also need to take diabetes medication, either insulin injections or oral agents. For both groups, the additional behavioral demands of diabetes pose a particular challenge during pregnancy.

Few studies have been conducted examining the biopsychosocial aspects of diabetes during pregnancy. Research has focused on identifying the levels of adherence in these groups, identifying the facilitators and barriers of adherence, and examining psychological adjustment in women with newly diagnosed gestational diabetes. For those who are newly diagnosed, the challenge is to learn the information needed to best manage the disorder, cope with the emotional challenges of this new diagnosis, and initiate and maintain the necessary daily regimen behaviors. One encouraging finding from this area is that little difference has been found in psychological adjustment between pregnant women with gestational diabetes and those without diabetes, suggesting that the former women quickly adapt to their new diagnosis.

Research examining the rates of self-reported self-management adherence in women with diabetes during pregnancy indicates high levels of adherence. Paralleling the data on general populations of individuals with diabetes, differences have been seen across regimen areas. Studies examining the impact of biopsychosocial factors including stress, diabetes knowledge, and social support on self-management adherence, found that these variables may be important influences on adherence for pregnant women with diabetes. This research further indicates that these biopsychosocial factors may have differential impacts on specific self-management regimen tasks. These findings can help guide the development of interventions to enhance diabetes self-management during pregnancy. More research is needed, however, to clarify the relationship of these and other biopsychosocial variables to self-management adherence in pregnant women with diabetes.

One area that is important and needs further empirical examination is family planning for individuals with diabetes. Some researchers have focused on the use of oral contraceptives in women with diabetes. Such research can help identify the impact of different contraceptive approaches on glycemic control and provide guidance in the safest choices. Regarding pregnancy planning, women may be better able to make the necessary changes in their daily regimen and to manage their blood glucose during pregnancy if they are knowledgable early in the childbearing process about the impact of pregnancy on diabetes. Since behavioral self-management is critical in controlling blood glucose levels to reduce complications during pregnancy, future research should focus on identifying factors associated with diabetes self-management and on developing appropriate interventions for enhancing self-management during pregnancy. Furthermore, following women with diabetes or at risk of developing diabetes longitudinally, from early in the childbearing process through at least 1 year after delivery, would be a valuable contribution to the literature in this area. Such a study would help clarify the naturalistic patterns of self-management adherence and the need for interventions at various points in the childbearing process.

SEXUAL FUNCTIONING IN WOMEN WITH DIABETES

The prevalence and correlates of sexual dysfunction in men with diabetes have been well studied. Research has identified a higher prevalence of sexual dysfunction in men with diabetes that in those without diabetes. As is true in many areas of health research, the research on sexual dysfunction in women with diabetes lags behind that of men. The research that has been conducted on women has not resulted in such clear findings as the research with men has produced. In general, it has been found that sexual dysfunction occurs in about 27% of women with diabetes. The findings specific to problems of sexual desire have not found differences between women with diabetes and a general population of women. The findings specific to sexual arousal suggest that women with diabetes may experience lower levels of arousal. However, since the results of subjective and physiological measures of arousal are often discordant, more research that uses physiological measures of arousal to examine this question is needed before confident conclusions may be established. To date, the research specific to orgasmic difficulties in women with diabetes has led to inconsistent findings.

Numerous factors could influence the sexual functioning in women with diabetes. These include the typical individual factors (e.g., mood disorders, misinformation) and interpersonal factors (e.g., communication problems), which may be further exacerbated by the chronic disease condition. Furthermore, the presence and process of the chronic disease may be associated with additional potential contributing factors. That is, diabetes may affect sexual functioning through at least two pathways—physiological and psychological. Diabetes may affect sexual functioning through such physiological mechanisms as changes in neurological (e.g., neuropathy) and vascular functioning, as well as through medication-related physiological changes. Psychological sequelae, for example, include mood changes (e.g., depression), relationship or role changes, and body image changes.

Research investigating the physiological correlates of sexual dysfunction in women with diabetes has consistently found no relationship with nephropathy, retinopathy, or macrovascular disease, but has found mixed results regarding neuropathy. Very few studies have examined psychosocial correlates of sexual dysfunction in women with diabetes. Although it is premature to draw conclusions from these data, the findings suggest that such areas as diabetes adjustment, marital adjustment, coping, and depression should be more fully investigated. Future research should focus on the impact of these variables on sexual functioning and should include a matched control group without diabetes.

Although this area of women's health has received more attention than many others for women with diabetes, there are still more questions than answers emerging from the literature to date. For example, type of diabetes has not been adequately investigated for its impact on sexual functioning. Given the differences in the onset and course of these two subtypes of diabetes, it is possible that they affect sexual functioning differently. For example, one consistent finding for women with Type II diabetes or NIDDM is that they experience decreased vaginal lubrication compared with other women. Therefore, future research should compare matched groups of women with NIDDM and IDDM. Furthermore, there is much room for improvement in the methodology used to examine these questions. Future research should (1) include both subjective and physiological measures of sexual functioning; (2) compare women with IDDM and NIDDM; (3) examine women with different degrees of diabetic complications, especially neuropathy, and duration of diabetes; and (4) include matched nondiabetic control group. In addition, two potential confounds have been totally ignored in the research to date. Menopause and obesity may influence sexual functioning through both physiological (e.g., hormonal) and psychological (e.g., mood, body image) mechanisms. Researchers should therefore also examine these important variables when studying sexual function in women with diabetes.

FUTURE DIRECTIONS

In addition to continuing to examine the topics addressed in this chapter, investigators need to examine several other important issues concerning the health of women with diabetes. In particular, the biopsychosocial aspects of diabetes may change through the lifespan of women. For example, since a woman's body contains different proportions of sex hormones than a man's body, and release of these hormones differs at varying points in a woman's life, this process is likely to have a differential impact on diabetes management across the genders. The impact of these hormonal changes on diabetes across the lifespan needs to be closely examined in women. Although few empirical data are available, anecdotal information suggests that women with diabetes mellitus may experience delayed menarche, early onset of menopause, increased incidence of menstrual irregularities, and greater incidence of infertility problems (see Hartman-Stein & Reuter, 1988, for an excellent overview of the developmental issues affecting women with diabetes). Since the U.S. population is aging and there is a high prevalence of diabetes in this older population, special attention should be focused on important physiological factors in women with diabetes as they age. Identifying the special needs of women with diabetes as they experience menopause would be one important area to study.

In addition to the biological processes that may have an impact on women with diabetes throughout the lifespan, several associated psychosocial factors should be examined empirically. For example, women with diabetes may have special needs in regard to body image and weight control; coping with illness; sexuality and use of contraceptives; and pregnancy planning and motherhood. For example, since women are generally the primary caregivers in families, any medical condition that affects a mother's health and health behavior generally affects the entire family as well. Research on the effects of maternal diabetes on the family is lacking, and this topic should be a focus of future research. Longitudinal research following a group of women with diabetes throughout their lives would greatly improve our knowledge and understanding of the special needs of women with diabetes throughout their lives.

It is also of special concern that there is a paucity of literature on cultural diversity issues among individuals with diabetes in general and among women in particular. As noted in the introduction to this chapter, diabetes is more prevalent and more problematic in certain cultural subgroups. Therefore, future research should focus on identifying the biopsychosocial influences on these groups and on developing appropriate interventions to address any special needs identified.

Finally, as a new standard of care, intensive management is being established in the medical management of diabetes; the energy of behavioral medicine researchers and practitioners should also be focused in this direction. Future research should focus on better understanding the biopsychosocial impact of intensive management. Such research will help guide the development of behavioral medicine interventions to assist individuals in adhering to their increasingly complex daily self-management regimen; it will also assist with special problems (e.g., weight gain) that may arise from this new management approach.

FURTHER READING

Diabetes Control and Complications Trial Research (DCCT) Group. (1993). The effect of intensive management on the development and progression of long-term complications in insulin-dependent diabetes mellitus. *New England Journal of Medicine, 329,* 977–986.
Landmark study showing that tight metabolic control achieved by intensive management results in reduced long-term complications of diabetes.

Hartman-Stein, P., & Reuter, J. M. (1988). Developmental issues in the treatment of diabetic women. *Psychology of Women Quarterly, 12,* 417–428.
Review of the developmental issues across the lifespan specific to females with diabetes.

Jensen, S. B. (1986). Sexual dysfunction in insulin-treated diabetics: A six-year follow-up study of 101 patients. *Archives of Sexual Behavior, 15*, 271–283.
A long-term follow-up study on sexual dysfunction in individuals with diabetes, with a focus on prevalence, patterns, and correlates of sexual dysfunction.

Marcus, M. D., Wing, R. R., Jawad, A., & Orchard, T. J. (1992). Eating disorders symptomatology in a registry-based sample of women with insulin dependent diabetes mellitus. *International Journal of Eating Disorders, 12*, 425–430.
Study showing that women with diabetes are not more likely to report eating disorders symptomatology, but that such symptomatology is associated with poorer diabetes control.

Mestman, J. H., & Schmidt-Scarosi, C. (1993). Diabetes mellitus and fertility control: Contraception management issues. *American Journal of Obstetrics and Gynecology, 168*, 2012–2020.
Review of issues of fertility and contraception in women with diabetes.

Ruggiero, L., & Clark, M. M. (Eds.). (1992). Obesity management in people with diabetes: An update [Special section]. *Diabetes Spectrum, 5*, 199–237.
Review and expert commentary on key articles in the area of obesity management in diabetes.

Ruggiero, L., Spirito, A., Bond, A., Coustan, D., & McGarvey, S. (1990). Impact of social support and stress on compliance in women with gestational diabetes. *Diabetes Care, 13*, 441–443.
Study showing that social support and stress are associated with compliance in women with gestational diabetes.

Spector, I. P., Leiblum, S. R., Carey, M. P., & Rosen, R. C. (1993). Diabetes and female sexual function: A critical review. *Annals of Behavioral Medicine, 15*, 257–264.
A review of the research on diabetes and female sexual functioning.

Spirito, A., Ruggiero, L., Duckworth, M., Low, K. G., Coustan, D. R., McGarvey, S. T., & Koury, M. R. (1993). The relationship of diabetes knowledge to regimen compliance and metabolic control during pregnancy. *Psychology and Health, 8*, 345–353.
Study showing that diabetes knowledge is associated with regimen compliance in pregnant women with preexisting diabetes.

Spirito, A., Williams, C., Ruggiero, L., Bond, A., McGarvey, S. T., & Coustan, D. (1989). Psychological impact of the diagnosis of gestational diabetes. *Obstetrics and Gynecology, 73*, 562–566.
Study showing that pregnant women newly diagnosed with gestational diabetes do not differ from nondiabetic pregnant women on psychological status.

Wing, R. R., Marcus, M. D., Epstein, L. H., & Jawad, A. (1991). A "family-based" approach to the treatment of obese Type II diabetic patients. *Journal of Consulting and Clinical Psychology, 59*, 156–162.
Controlled study showing that women do better in a weight control program when their spouses are also included.

Wing, R. R., Marcus, M. D., Epstein, L. H., Blair, E. H., & Burton, L. R. (1989). Binge eating in obese patients with Type II diabetes. *International Journal of Eating Disorders, 8*, 671–679.
Study showing that binge eating is common in individuals with Type II diabetes and is strongly associated with depressive symptomatology.

102

Diabetes: Medical Aspects

Judith Wylie-Rosett

Diabetes is a leading cause of premature mortality and excess morbidity among women. Advances in diabetes management can greatly reduce the long-term health risk posed by diabetes. This chapter reviews the prevalence rates for each type of diabetes and the diabetes-related health problems in women. Techniques for treatment and prevention of diabetic complications are presented. Information about the impact of stress on metabolic control and the behavioral therapy in diabetes management are discussed.

TYPES OF DIABETES AND PREVALENCE RATES

The American Diabetes Association estimates that in the United States 16 million people have diabetes, and that half of them are undiagnosed. Diabetes is a heterogeneous disorder of fuel metabolism characterized by glucose intolerance. Table 102.1 lists the diagnostic criteria for diabetes and impaired fasting glucose (IFG). Diabetes has been classified into several types based on the clinical manifestations.

Insulin-dependent diabetes mellitus (IDDM) or Type I, which is characterized by severe insulin deficiency and ketosis, accounts for approximately 10% of diabetes cases. Although the concordance for identical twins is only 25–50% for IDDM, a defect in chromosome 6 appears to cause autoimmune destruction of the beta cells in the pancreas.

Non-insulin-dependent diabetes mellitus (NIDDM) or Type II, which is characterized by a limited secretory insulin response to compensate for insulin resistance (usually related to obesity), accounts for 90% of cases. Glucose intolerance increases with age. Individuals of Hispanic, African, Asian, and Native American heritages are at greater risk for developing NIDDM. There is a 50–75% concordance among identical twins, and women are slightly more likely to develop NIDDM than men. However, the role of genetics in developing NIDDM is largely unknown.

TABLE 102.1. Diagnostic Criteria for Diabetes Mellitus

Diabetes in nonpregnant adults

A fasting plasma glucose level of $\geq$ 126 mg/dl on more than one occasion, or an unequivocal glucose level of 200 mg/dl and symptoms, would be considered diagnostic.

A fasting plasma glucose level $\geq$ 110 and < 126 mg/dl is considered impaired fasting glucose.

Gestational diabetes

All pregnant women who have not been identified as glucose-intolerant should be screened between 24 and 28 weeks of gestation, using a 50-gram glucose challenge. If the 1-hour postchallenge glucose level is $\geq$ 140 mg/dl, a glucose tolerance test is required.

The diagnosis can be made using a 100-gram glucose challenge, if two more plasma glucose levels meet or exceed the following: fasting, 105 mg/dl; 1-hour, 190 mg/dl; 2-hour, 165 mg/dl; 3-hour, 145 mg/dl.

Gestational diabetes is defined as diabetes that develops during pregnancy; it occurs in approximately 2–5% of all pregnancies. Between 20% and 50% of women who have gestational diabetes will subsequently develop NIDDM.

HEALTH COMPLICATIONS OF DIABETES IN WOMEN

Diabetes increases the risk of congenital anomalies, blindness, coronary disease, stroke, end-stage renal disease, and lower-extremity amputation. Data from the Framingham Study indicated that women with diabetes lose the premenopausal protective effect of gender with respect to cardiovascular disease and have rates of disease that are three- to fivefold greater than those of their age-matched counterparts. Although the rates of complications are greater among individuals with IDDM, the absolute number of complications associated with NIDDM is greater because of the much greater prevalence of NIDDM. Neuropathic and vascular complications of diabetes are established causes of impotence in men and may also cause sexual dysfunction in women.

Women with preconception diabetes have an increased risk of congenital anomalies in their infants, caused by the effects of elevated glucose on cell division. Having an elevated glucose level later in pregnancy is associated with an increased risk of a large-for-gestational-age infant, delivery complications, and infant respiratory distress during the neonatal period.

PREVENTION OF COMPLICATIONS

After years of debate, the results of the Diabetes Control and Complications Trial indicate that the risk of complications can be reduced by 40–75% through achieving blood glucose levels very close to the normal range. Clinical trials in diabetic eye disease indicate that early detection and treatment can reduce the risk of blindness by half. There is evidence that foot self-care and early professional intervention, when needed, can cut the risk of amputation in half as well. The individual with diabetes needs to be actively involved in self-management of blood glucose and foot hygiene, as well as having screening and early intervention for other complications (or for related risk factors) in order to reduce the risks of complications.

TREATMENT MODALITIES AND PROBLEMS

The standards of medical care and the educational goals for diabetes management focus on early detection and treatment of complications, as well as on achieving metabolic control to prevent them. The medical care standards listed in Table 102.2 address health professional and patient behaviors. For many patients, adjusting to the diagnosis of diabetes is difficult, and treatment priorities need to be negotiated. However, insulin therapy must be initiated and maintained in patients with IDDM to prevent ketoacidosis and coma, even when a "vacation" from the burden of more intense management may be indicated.

TABLE 102.2. Minimal Standards of Medical Care for Diabetes Management

Annual examination

Dental referral
Dilated fundoscopic eye examination
Comprehensive foot exam (pulse/vascular, neurological, and skin)
Blood tests
    Total cholesterol
    HDL cholesterol
    Triglycerides
    Glycogylated hemoglobin (4 times per year)
    Assessment of renal status (microalbuminuria)
    Influenza immunization

All visits

Blood pressure
Weight
Foot examination
Review of metabolic control and strategies to improve control

Education, evaluation, and intervention

Nutrition and exercise related to:
    Weight
    Metabolic control
    Risk factors for complications
    Smoking habits
Daily self-care
    Monitoring glucose control
    Modifying habits to improve glucose control
    Foot hygiene
IDDM
    Possible insulin adjustment related to habits/glucose levels
    Management of intercurrent illness

In IDDM, intensifying diabetes management to achieve near-normal glucose levels usually involves injecting insulin three or more times daily (or using a continuous-infusion insulin pump), self-monitoring capillary blood glucose four or more times each day, and achieving consistency in the timing and macronutrient composition of food intake. Adjustment are made in the timing and amount of insulin therapy when physical activity or food intake changes, or when blood glucose monitoring indicates that values are out of the target range. Having impaired hypoglycemia awareness is a barrier to achieving a near-normal blood glucose, but most individuals can improve their level of glycemic control even if near normal glucose levels are not realistic. Although the rates of eating disorders among adolescent females with diabetes are consistent with those among their peers, the techniques used may vary. Using poor blood glucose control to promote loss of calories via urinary excretion can result in ketoacidosis and increases the risk of long-term complications.

In NIDDM, lifestyle modification to achieve weight control is usually the primary focus of treatment. Oral hypoglycemic agents may be added to the treatment if glucose control is not achieved through dietary treatment alone. Insulin may be used in treatment as well. If weight loss is achieved, pharmacological therapy can often be discontinued or dosage decreased.

In gestational diabetes mellitus, achieving normal blood glucose reduces the risk of having a large-for-gestational-age infant and the associated perinatal complications. Six feedings a day are used to control postprandial glucose levels. If the fasting glucose level exceeds 105 mg/dl, or postprandial glucose levels exceed 120 mg/dl, insulin therapy is recommended.

STRESS AND GLUCOSE

The effects of stress on metabolic control of diabetes are mediated through the glucocorticoid hormones that counterregulate the action of insulin. This counterregulatory response to stress can be triggered by infection, the metabolic stress of pregnancy, or wound healing, as well as by emotional forms of stress. Such stresses often precede the development of overt diabetes, but diabetes occurs only if insulin deficiency (either relative or absolute) is present. How stress affects IDDM is much less clear. In clinical management of IDDM, the effects of stress on metabolic control are highly variable. In response to experimental stress conditions, glucose levels may increase, decrease, or be unchanged.

Many women report that their blood glucose levels vary by the phases of the menstrual cycle. The extent to which these changes are attributable to changes in eating behavior needs to be studied. Little is known about how the hormonal shifts during the menstrual cycle affect insulin resistance and requirements. Therefore, trial and error may be used to adjust medical nutritional therapy if this is considered to be a problem.

ROLE OF BEHAVIORAL THERAPY IN TREATING WOMEN WITH DIABETES

The treatment of diabetes is complex and can be overwhelming. Patient education needs to be tailored to the needs of the individual woman with diabetes. The treatment needs to focus on health and quality-of-life outcomes. A number of instruments have been developed to facilitate psychosocial assessment and behavioral management of diabetes. For example, the concept of avoiding foods such as sugar does not link behavioral changes to the overall treatment goals. Furthermore, the American Diabetes Association no longer recommends such restrictions; it focuses instead on individualized dietary changes based on the glucose, lipid, blood pressure, medical treatment, and other factors related to the risk of complications.

The transtheoretical model of behavioral change has been applied to diabetes. Some behaviors, such as exogenous insulin therapy, are essential to avoid a medical crisis in IDDM. Other behaviors can be approached more gradually, based on readiness to change behavior.

FURTHER READING

American Diabetes Association. (1994). Standards of medical care for patients with diabetes mellitus. *Diabetes Care, 17,* 616–623.
Consensus guidelines for managing diabetes are presented. These guidelines focus on initial and ongoing care issues.

American Diabetes Association. (1995). *Medical management of pregnancy complicated by diabetes.* Alexandria, VA: Author.
Overview and practical treatment issues for managing diabetes in pregnancy are addressed.

American Diabetes Association. (1995). *Diabetes education goals.* Alexandria, VA: Author.
Educational goals for managing various types of diabetes are presented.

Bradley, C. (Ed.). (1994). *Handbook of psychology and diabetes.* Chur, Switzerland: Harwood Academic.
An edited book that includes assessment instruments as well as an overview of psychological issues in diabetes management.

Diabetes Control and Complications Trial (DCCT) Research Group. (1993). The effects of intensive management on the development and progression of long-term complications in insulin-dependent diabetes mellitus. *New England Journal of Medicine, 329,* 977–986.
A review of results from the DCCT, which demonstrated that glycerine control could prevent or delay development of complications affecting a number of organ systems.

Ruggiero, L., & Prochaska, J. O. (1993). From research to practice: Readiness for change. *Diabetes Spectrum, 6,* 21–59.
Summaries of research papers addressing the transtheoretical model for behavioral change. Clinical commentaries discuss the applicability of this model to clinical diabetes management.

Surwit, R. S., & Schneider, M. S. (1993). Role of stress in the etiology and treatment of diabetes mellitus. *Psychosomatic Medicine, 55,* 380–393.
A comprehensive review of how stress affects metabolic control and affects the management of diabetes.

Tinker, L. F. (1994). Diabetes mellitus: A priority health care issue for women. *Journal of the American Dietetic Association, 94,* 976–985.
A comprehensive review of the nutritional issues for managing diabetes in women.

103

The Endocrine System and Endocrine Disorders

David O. Norris

An endocrine gland secretes one or more specific chemicals, called hormones, into the blood. Hormones travel through the blood to target cells or tissues located elsewhere in the body. Once they bind to protein receptors in or on the surface of a target cell, they elicit a particular response or action. Typically, hormones control and time the occurrence of processes essential to survival and reproduction. The main hormone-secreting structures include the pituitary, thyroid, adrenals, ovaries, parathyroids, and pancreas. Among these structures, the pituitary is responsible for secreting the largest proportion of hormones; the release of tropic hormones by the pituitary is controlled by the release of other hormones from the hypothalamus. The major pituitary tropic hormones in women are listed in Table 103.1, and the major hypothalamic hormones affecting pituitary hormone release are given in Table 103.2. In addition, many other organs secrete hormones but are often not suspected to be endocrine glands; these include the thymus, heart, liver, and kidneys.

Disorders of the endocrine system are among the most common medical problems faced by women. Diabetes mellitus, a disease resulting from impaired insulin secretion or function, is one of the leading causes of death in the United States (see the chapters by Ruggiero and Wylie-Rosett in this volume). Reproduction is regulated by the endocrine system and has its own impacts on health. Younger women suffer from a variety of reproductive disorders, including production of ovarian cysts, fibroid uterine growths, premenstrual syndrome (PMS), and amenorrhea. Fertility problems are among the most common of the endocrine disorders younger women face. Menopause is brought about by the failure of the aging ovary to produce sufficient estrogens to maintain normal reproductive structures and functions; this can exacerbate loss of minerals from the skeleton, making it brittle and subject to fracture. Thyroid imbalance can produce weight problems and unstable neural function. Excessive stress causes hyperactivity of the adrenal glands, which produces negative effects on reproduction as well as a depression of the immune

TABLE 103.1. Major Pituitary Tropic Hormones in Women

Pituitary tropic hormone	Actions
Gonadotropins	
Luteinizing hormone (LH)	Stimulates synthesis of androgens in ovary, which can be converted to estrogens; causes ovulation and formation of corpus luteum from cells of ruptured follicle.
Follicle-stimulating hormone (FSH)	Stimulates follicle growth, synthesis of inhibin, and conversion of androgens to estrogens in ovary.
Thyrotropin (thyroid-stimulating hormone; TSH)	Stimulates cells of thyroid gland to secrete thyroid hormones (T_3 and T_4).
Corticotropin (adrenocorticotropic hormone; ACTH)	Stimulates adrenal gland to secrete glucocorticoids such as cortisol.
Growth hormone (GH)	Stimulates growth of skeletal muscle, cartilage, bone; important metabolic hormone associated with storing dietary nutrients and mobilizing stored nutrients during starvation.
Prolactin (PRL)	Stimulates synthesis of milk in mammary glands.

Note. The more commonly used name appears first, and only the major abbreviation is given.

response system. These few examples illustrate why it is important to understand the basics of endocrine system function when interpreting causes, symptoms, and understanding the treatments employed for endocrine disorders.

THE REPRODUCTIVE AXIS

The ovaries contain structures called follicles. Each follicle contains a growing oocyte that will possibly become a mature ovum or egg cell. The walls of each follicle are

TABLE 103.2. Hypothalamic Hormones Affecting Pituitary Tropic Hormone Release

Hypothalmic releasing hormone	Actions
Gonadotropin-releasing hormone (GnRH)[a]	Stimulates release of FSH, LH.
Thyrotropin-releasing hormone (TRH)	Stimulates TSH release; also stimulates PRL release under certain conditions.
Corticotropin-releasing hormone (CRH)	Stimulates ACTH release.
Arginine vasopressin (AVP)	Increases sensitivity of pituitary ACTH cells to CRH.
Somatostatin (SS)[b]	Inhibits GH release; also inhibits TSH release.
Growth hormone-releasing hormone (GHRH)[c]	Stimulates GH release when SS is absent.
Dopamine (DA)	Inhibits PRL release.
Vasoactive intestinal peptide (VIP)	Stimulates PRL release during lactation.

[a] Also known as luteinizing hormone-releasing hormone (LHRH or LRH).
[b] Also known as growth hormone release-inhibiting hormone (GRIH or GHRIH).
[c] Also known as somatocrinin.

separable into two distinct regions. The outermost region is composed of layers of thecal cells, and the inner region consists of granulosa cells that immediately surround the oocyte. The ovary undergoes a cycle consisting of two phases. The follicular phase involves development of the follicles and is terminated by ovulation, which involves the rupture of the largest follicle and release of the egg. The ovulated egg then passes into the open end of the fallopian tube. Ovulation is followed by the luteal phase, which is dominated by the corpus luteum derived from the ruptured follicle.

The pituitary gland secretes two gonadotropic (gonad-stimulating) hormones that control ovarian functions: follicle-stimulating hormone (FSH) and luteinizing hormone (LH). Growth of the ovarian follicles is regulated by FSH, whereas both LH and FSH are necessary for estrogen synthesis (the major estrogen is estradiol). LH also stimulates progesterone and androgen synthesis in the ovary. The androgen is a precursor for estrogen synthesis and this step is regulated by FSH. In addition, LH is responsible for ovulation. Following ovulation, LH causes the granulosa cells and some thecal cells of the ruptured follicle to transform into the corpus luteum, which secretes primarily progesterone and some estrogen during the luteal phase.

Release of LH and FSH from the pituitary is regulated by a single hypothalamic hormone called gonadotropin-releasing hormone (GnRH; formerly called luteinizing hormone-releasing hormone, or LHRH) (see Figure 103.1). However, the pattern of LH and FSH secretion varies independently at times during the ovarian cycle because of differences in feedback mechanisms. For a time, estrogens secreted by the growing follicle have a positive feedback effect, causing release of more GnRH, which causes production of more estrogen. Once estrogens reach a critical level near the end of the follicular phase, a massive release of GnRH occurs. This in turn produces a surge of LH release, but only a minor increase in FSH release. The LH surge causes ovulation within about 24 hours. Under the influence of FSH, the ovary also has been releasing a hormone called inhibin, which makes the pituitary mechanism for FSH release relatively insensitive to GnRH. Hence, only a small peak in FSH occurs. During the luteal phase, the high levels of progesterone and estrogen produce negative feedback at the hypothalamus, and GnRH, LH, and FSH levels diminish.

During the follicular phase, estrogen stimulates cell proliferation and glandular formation in the lining (endometrium) of the uterus to prepare it for pregnancy. During the luteal phase, progesterone and estrogen are necessary to retain the condition of the endometrium and stimulate its secretory activities. The corpus luteum soon begins to degenerate so that in 3–10 days there is a drop in progesterone and estrogen, allowing the endometrium to break down. The outer portion of the endometrium, containing trapped blood, is sloughed off and becomes the menstrual discharge that characterizes the ovarian cycles of humans and some other primates. Once the hypothalamus is freed from inhibitory effects of estrogens and progesterone, initiation of LH and FSH secretion begins the cycle anew.

PREGNANCY

If the ovulated egg is fertilized while in the fallopian tube, the resulting zygote begins to divide and forms a simple, multicellular form called a blastocyst. The inner part of the blastocyst will become the embryo, and the outer portions form extraembryonic membranes that will aid development throughout pregnancy. One of these membranes, the

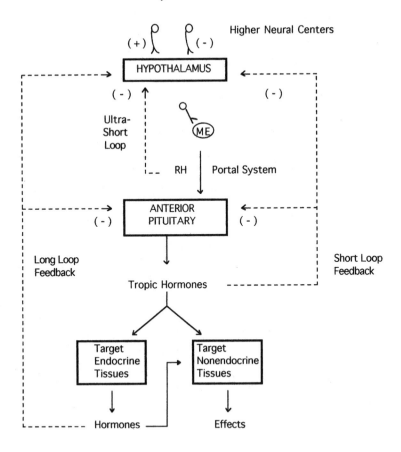

FIGURE 103.1. The hypothalamus–anterior pituitary system. Releasing hormones (RH) made in the hypothalamus are stored in the median eminance (ME) until they are released into the portal vessels that carry them to the anterior pituitary. Listings of these hormones are provided in Tables 103.1 and 103.2. In response, most tropic hormones are released into the blood, travel to specific endocrine glands, and cause release of other hormones into the blood. Two tropic hormones have nonendocrine gland targets. Feedback loops that can reduce secretion of tropic hormones are indicated by dashed lines for the final hormones like thyroid hormones and steroids (long loop), tropic hormones (short loop), and releasing hormones (ultrashort loop), that affect the pituitary and/or hypothalamus.

chorion, begins to secrete an LH-like gonadotropin that prevents degeneration of the corpus luteum and stimulates it to continue to produce progesterone and estrogen. This hormone is called human chorionic gonadotropin (hCG). Consequently, the endometrium will be maintained, allowing the blastocyst to erode its way into the vascularized endometrium. The chorion will contribute to formation of the placenta, a complex organ that assists development through physiological processes (e.g., supplying oxygen and nutrients while removing carbon dioxide and nitrogenous wastes) and through endocrine functions.

At about 2 months of pregnancy, the corpus luteum degenerates, even though the placenta is still making hCG. However, at about this time the adrenal gland of the embryo (now called a fetus) begins secretion of androgens that the placenta requires for conversion to estrogen. The placenta takes over production of progesterone on its own. If dependence upon the corpus luteum for maintaining the endometrium does not shift smoothly to dependence on the placenta, a miscarriage or spontaneous abortion occurs, primarily because of the drop in estrogen. Most miscarriages occur near the end of the first trimester (3 months) of pregnancy, and in most cases the cause is related to an abnormal fetus that cannot provide androgens for the placenta to convert to estrogen. This early dependence on a normal fetus for continuation of pregnancy seems to be nature's way of eliminating nonviable fetuses.

The placenta secretes a number of other hormones that are important in pregnancy, including a hormone called human chorionic somatomammotropin (hCS; formerly called human placental lactogen, or hPL). Progesterone and estrogen are primarily responsible for enlargement of the mammary glands during the later part of pregnancy, but hCS stimulates the machinery for making milk. Prior to birth, the placenta secretes another hormone called relaxin, which softens the pelvic ligaments and the cervix to facilitate passage of the fetus through the pelvis (birth canal) during birth (parturition).

The endocrine factors responsible for parturition are not understood fully. One of the best-known participants is oxytocin, a hypothalamic hormone that is stored in the posterior pituitary. The initiation of contraction by the uterine muscles during labor involves the release of this hormone. Synthetic forms of oxytocin are often used to induce labor. Oxytocin also can reduce postpartum bleeding by causing the uterus to contract after detachment of the placenta (the afterbirth). The fetus also participates in the birth process, but the details are not understood completely.

LACTATION

The synthesis and ejection of milk are controlled by the hypothalamus and pituitary. Suckling on the breast by the newborn (neonate) causes neural stimulation that travels from the nipple to the brain and quickly to the hypothalamus, resulting in release of oxytocin from the posterior pituitary. Oxytocin causes contraction of cells lining the mammary gland ducts, so that milk is ejected into the mouth of the neonate. Association of the neonate's hunger cries with suckling may even induce this milk ejection reflex in a conditioned mother.

Prolactin, a tropic hormone of the anterior pituitary, is released after a suckling bout through a similar neural reflex. Prolactin then stimulates milk synthesis during the interim between feedings. This reflex is not always ready to function at birth, and several suckling attempts may be required before prolactin release is sufficient to provide the amount of milk demanded by the neonate's metabolism.

There is evidence to show that suckling also can prevent GnRH release and prevent the recurrence of follicular development. Follicle growth is blocked during pregnancy through negative feedback by high levels of progesterone and estrogen. Although lactation prevents conception in some women, there are many cases of lactating women becoming pregnant; breast feeding in and of itself should not be considered a safe birth control method. (However, see Labbok's chapter on the lactational amenorrhea method of birth control in Section VI of this volume.)

In addition to providing nutrients and antibodies to the neonate, milk contains numerous hormones. Although the mammary glands are not considered to be endocrine glands, they concentrate hormones in milk and pass them to the neonate.

THE PANCREAS AND DIABETES MELLITUS

Insulin release is caused by an increase in blood sugar (glucose) following a meal. The complex regulation of metabolism by insulin and other hormones is too involved for this discussion, but the following account will serve as an introduction. There are two forms of diabetes mellitus that are characterized by high blood glucose levels and appearance of glucose in the urine. Normally, in the presence of adequate insulin, blood glucose is low enough that the kidney can prevent transfer of glucose to the urine.

The better-known but less common form of diabetes is called insulin-dependent diabetes mellitus (IDDM). IDDM most commonly is caused by the inability of the pancreas to secrete insulin, following destruction of the insulin-secreting cells by antibodies the patient has made against those cells. Formerly IDDM was called "juvenile-onset diabetes" because it was most commonly diagnosed among children. IDDM is incurable and ultimately shortens the lifespan of the patient, often leading to blindness and loss of limbs in later life. Treatment involves administration of insulin by injection or chronic-infusion pumps, as well as careful attention to diet. Currently, experimentation with implanted chambers containing insulin-secreting cells may provide means of restoring the ability to secrete insulin in a more natural way.

The more common form of diabetes in the United States occurs in the "over" group—those who are overweight and over 40. These patients exhibit insulin resistance; that is, insulin levels are normal or slightly greater than normal yet insulin is ineffective at controlling blood sugar. The failure of insulin to bring about its normal effects in these patients is not understood completely. Although this disease was formerly called "maturity-onset diabetes," it is now called non-insulin-dependent diabetes mellitus (NIDDM). Every 10% increase in body weight or decade of life doubles a person's probability of developing NIDDM. Loss of excessive weight and control of diet are necessary to bring the system back into balance. If the condition is severe, special drugs called "oral insulins" may be administered to increase the effectiveness of the insulin already being secreted. Although it is easier to bring the NIDDM patient back into balance than the IDDM patient, careful attention to diet and body weight regulation are important to prevent recurrence of the symptoms.

Insulin has several metabolic actions including effects on proteins and fats. One of its important roles is to promote storage of glucose in both liver and muscle tissue. Another is to prevent fat use and promote fat storage. In its absence, glucose is taken out of liver storage and added to the blood. Fat is broken down, and the products are used to synthesize more glucose, contributing further to the rise in blood sugar. In addition, conversion of fats to glucose results in release of byproducts called ketone bodies. These acidic molecules normally are excreted by the kidneys, but if they are produced in excess (as when insulin is absent or not working properly), they cause increased acidity of the blood and can induce coma.

Diabetics produce large volumes of urine because of the presence of glucose and ketone bodies in the urine, which makes it more difficult to conserve water. This causes dehydration and, if unchecked, can lead to reduced blood volume, heart failure, and death.

CALCIUM REGULATION AND OSTEOPOROSIS

Regulation of blood calcium is vital to nerve and muscle function, and many cellular processes are dependent on calcium. Three hormones regulate calcium metabolism. The parathyroid glands, mentioned earlier, secrete parathyroid hormone (PTH) in response to a decrease in blood calcium. PTH stimulates certain bone cells to dissolve or resorb the bone and calcium enters the blood. It also reduces calcium loss to the urine. A separate hormone called calcitonin (CT) is secreted by cells located in the thyroid gland, and it can stimulate calcium deposition in bone. The third hormone involved is a derivative of vitamin D (cholecalciferol) and is known as dihydroxycholecalciferol (DHC). Absorption of dietary calcium by the intestine is facilitated by DHC.

Pregnancy and lactation can place a major strain on bones and teeth unless dietary calcium and DHC are adequate to provide for absorption. PTH acts mainly on the kidneys to conserve calcium, and its usual effect on bone resorption is prevented by CT as long as the calcium demand is met and normal calcium levels are maintained through the diet. Otherwise, more PTH is released, and bone and teeth are resorbed. Hence, calcium supplements typically are encouraged by physicians for pregnant and lactating women, as well as for pre- and postmenopausal women (Table 103.3).

Menopause has several unique features and creates another challenge to the skeleton. As a woman grows older, her ability to absorb dietary calcium decreases. The lack of estrogen results in elevated secretion of PTH and increased loss of calcium through the urine. However, there is no reduction in blood calcium, but rather a transfer of bone calcium to the blood to replace that lost in the urine. Progressive loss of bone calcium leads to the condition of osteoporosis. Because blood levels of calcium remain normal, it is important for women to have a bone scan performed to determine bone density (a reflection of calcium content)—preferably before menopause, to provide baseline data for comparison of bone density later in life and to ascertain whether they are at risk.

The most effective therapy to prevent skeletal bone loss involves a combination of treatments. Prior to menopause, exercise and often calcium supplements are recommended to increase bone density. A vitamin D derivative often is included to ensure adequate absorption of the supplemental calcium. Exercise must be weight-bearing and place stress on bones, which favors deposition of bone matrix and calcium salts. Swimming, for example, is an excellent aerobic activity, but it does not stress the skeleton as walking or cycling does. The swimmer experiences an almost weightless environment; among athletes, swimmers have the lowest bone densities. Similarly, immobilization of a limb or confinement to bed favor bone loss. It is interesting that regular activity of elderly nursing home residents can produce a marked increase in bone density and reduce the risk of bone fractures.

Once menopause is reached, exercise, calcium supplements, and in some cases estrogen replacement is recommended. There are pluses and minuses to weigh before electing estrogen therapy. Women should consult one or more knowledgeable physicians.

TABLE 103.3. Recommendations for Calcium Intake, Based on Report of National Institutes of Health Panel, 1995

Age	mg Calcium/day (all sources)[a]
Infants up to 6 months	400
Infants 6 to 12 months	600
Children 1 to 10 years	800
11 to 24 years	1,200 to 1,500
Women 25 to 50 years	1,000
Postmenopausal women	1,000 to 1,500

[a]*Caution:* More than 2,000 mg/day could cause kidney stones.

Current practices of estrogen therapy prevent bone loss when administered in conjunction with calcium supplements and weight-bearing exercise. Increases in bone density have been reported even when estrogen replacement was not begun until the patients were over 70 years old. Furthermore, estrogens relieve many postmenopausal symptoms and markedly reduce the incidence of heart attack. However, there is increased risk of developing breast cancer with estrogen administration, and women with a familial history of breast cancer should be especially concerned (see Andersen's and Rowland's chapters in this volume). Some studies show that although there is a greater incidence of breast cancer in women receiving estrogen replacement, there is a higher cure rate, probably related to earlier detection through awareness of this possibility and regular examinations. In the final analysis, each woman must obtain expert advice, weigh the pros and cons, and determine her own comfort zone.

THE ADRENAL CORTEX AND STRESS

The stress response is a reaction to harmful or potentially harmful stimuli, either real or imagined. It is especially adaptive for responding to long-term or chronic stresses. During the stressful period, its purpose is to provide nutrients for heightened brain activity and to suppress other activities (e.g., reproduction) until the source of the stress has been eliminated.

Two hormones from the adrenal gland are important in the stress response. The first is epinephrine, which is produced in the central part of the gland (the adrenal medulla). Epinephrine is involved in emergency reactions (e.g., the flight-or-fight response to danger) and causes an elevation of blood sugar. It also prevents release of insulin, which normally would counteract any increase in blood sugar. The second hormone is cortisol, a steroid produced in the outer region of the gland called the adrenal cortex. Hence, cortisol and related molecules are called corticosteroids. Cortisol also elevates blood sugar in part by stimulating production of glucose from fats and by preventing uptake of glucose from the blood by other tissues such as muscle. Release of cortisol is controlled by corticotropin (ACTH) from the pituitary and corticotropin-releasing hormone (CRH) from the hypothalamus.

The adrenal cortex produces another corticosteroid called aldosterone, which is not directly controlled by the hypothalamus and pituitary. Aldosterone controls sodium and potassium balance, with the kidneys being its major targets. Hence, aldosterone is often termed a mineralocorticoid for its effect on mineral balance, whereas cortisol is called a glucocorticoid because of its effects on carbohydrate metabolism (especially glucose). The adrenal cortex is also the source of weak androgens, such as androstenedione and dehydroepiandrosterone (DHEA). Impaired secretion of these adrenal androgens has been linked to decreased sexual appetite, increased breast cancer, and aging, but their physiological roles are not yet clear. As a result of recent animal studies, health enthusiasts are advocating over-the-counter preparations of DHEA as an anti-aging or anti-cancer agent. However, the Endocrine Society, a prestigious organization of professional medical and research endocrinologists, cautions that although DHEA has been shown to be beneficial in rodent studies, human studies involving DHEA treatment have not shown consistent and confirmed beneficial actions. Furthermore, they caution that DHEA may have harmful effects, especially in women who may become masculinized.

The first phase of the stress response is the alarm phase, which involves secretion of both epinephrine and cortisol. If the stress persists, the resistance phase, which involves prolonged elevated secretion of cortisol but not of epinephrine, develops. Should the intensity and/or duration of the resistance phase deplete the body's capacity to provide cortisol and nutrients to produce glucose, the individual may enter the exhaustive phase, which can lead to death if the stressor is not removed or eliminated soon.

Chronically elevated cortisol is a well-known inhibitor of reproductive function by preventing GnRH release. It also can suppress the immune response system and lower resistance to disease. Because of their ability to reduce inflammation, synthetic glucocorticoids are used therapeutically for treating muscle injuries. Topical creams containing glucocorticoids are available for relief of minor skin irritations. Glucocorticoids often are prescribed for relieving the symptoms of rheumatoid arthritis, an autoimmune disorder resulting in inflammation of joints, making them stiff and painful (see Zautra's, Roth's, and Wisocki's chapters). Massive quantities of glucocorticoids are used to prevent rejection of transplanted organs by suppressing the entire immune response system.

Since glucocorticoids elevate blood sugar, their extended use can cause chronic stimulation of the endocrine pancreas and release of insulin. Prolonged glucocorticoid therapy often impairs the ability of the pancreas to maintain insulin secretion, and permanent IDDM can result. However, the therapeutic value of glucocorticoids for relief of arthritis or immune suppression associated with life-saving organ transplants probably outweighs the risk.

THE ADRENAL CORTEX AND CONGENITAL ADRENAL HYPERPLASIA

The inability of the fetal adrenal cortex to secrete glucocorticoids and mineralocorticoids in response to ACTH leads to excessive mitosis of cells and enlargement of the adrenal cortex (hyperplasia) and excessive production of adrenal androgens. This condition is known as congenital adrenal hyperplasia (CAH). In a female fetus, these androgens can induce development of external genitalia toward the male condition, resulting in ambiguous determination of sex at birth. Furthermore, if not treated with adrenal corticosteroids, both genetic male and female children whose adrenal cortex makes only or mostly androgens may soon die of mineral imbalance. Fortunately, the more severe cases of CAH lacking adrenal corticosteroids are relatively uncommon, but milder forms are very common and may go clinically undetected for years. Body shape and muscular development in girls may be influenced in the male direction. Another effect in these children is premature termination of normal growth.

THE THYROID GLAND: DEVELOPMENT AND METABOLISM

The hypothalamus secretes thyrotropin-releasing hormone (TRH), which stimulates the pituitary to release thyrotropin (TSH), which in turn activates secretion of thyroid hormones. The thyroid gland primarily secretes two thyroid hormones: the iodine-containing thyroxine (T_4) and a small amount of triiodothyronine (T_3). Thyroid hormones are carried in the blood bound to blood proteins with only a small percentage free in the blood to enter target cells. An important role of the liver is to remove one iodide from T₄ and convert it to the more active form, T_3, which binds more strongly to thyroid hormone receptors in target cells than does T_4. Common diagnostic tests for thyroid activity include measurement of total T_4, total T_3, free T_4, and/or free T_3. Uptake by the thyroid of radioactive iodide or technetium is also used as a measure of thyroid gland activity and can be used to identify hyperactive or underactive tumors. Large dosages of radioactive iodide also are used to destroy overactive thyroid tissue, such as that found in Graves' disease (see below). Thyroid disorders are more frequent in women than in men, in part because of enhancement of thyroid hormone levels by estrogens.

Thyroid hormones are essential for normal development and function of the nervous system. They also regulate growth in children and metabolic rate in adults. Hypothyroidism (underactive thyroid) at birth is relatively common (1 per 1,000 births), but can be corrected easily if detected early. If not corrected, it can lead to poor growth and severe mental retardation. Hypothyroidism is especially important in older adults, in whom these symptoms often are attributed simply to aging, and thyroid state is not assessed.

Hypothyroidism is most commonly caused by inadequate dietary iodine (iodine deficiency). This makes production of thyroid hormones impossible. Iodine deficiency is a serious problem in mountainous areas and other locations where iodine is low in the soil and hence in the local diet. The absence of sufficient thyroid hormones causes excessive production of TRH and TSH, which overstimulates the thyroid gland, causing it to enlarge and form a goiter. Sometimes hypothyroidism results from destruction of the thyroid by antibodies produced by the immune system against certain thyroid gland proteins. This general condition is called thyroiditis and has several clinical forms (e.g., Hashimoto's thyroiditis).

Hyperthyroidism is less common than hypothyroidism, and the symptoms are the opposite (Table 103.4). One form of hyperthyroidism is Graves' disease, in which the immune system makes an antibody that actually binds to the TSH receptor on the thyroid cell and activates it. Graves' disease is 20 times more common in women than in men and occurs with greater frequency in young women. Among older women, Graves' disease accounts for about half of the thyroid disorders involving hyperthyroidism. In other hyperthyroid cases, a thyroid tumor (usually benign) secretes excessive amounts of thyroid hormones even in the absence of TSH. Rarely, a TSH-secreting tumor can bring about hyperthyroidism. In this latter case, and sometimes with thyroid tumors, the thyroid gland may enlarge to form a goiter.

TABLE 103.4. Comparison of Some Hypothyroid Symptoms in Adults

Hypothyroid	Hyperthyroid
Sluggish, mentally and physically	Mentally quick, restless, hyperkinetic, irritable, anxious
Sensitive to cold	Sensitive to heat
Sleep excessively	Wakeful
Low metabolic rate	High metabolic rate
Poor appetite yet tendency toward obesity	Voracious appetite but tend to be thin
Muscular weakness	Muscular weakness with tremors
Constipation	Diarrhea

Note. Patients may not exhibit all of these symptoms.

Pregnancy typically induces a mild form of hyperthyroidism in the mother and often slight goiter formation. This often results in a rebound hypothyroidism after birth, but thyroid function usually returns to normal in about 6 weeks. Autoimmune-based hypothyroidism may develop after birth because of a rebound in immune system activity, following its repression during pregnancy.

SUMMARY

The major components of the endocrine system are the pituitary and the hypothalamus; the hypothalamus controls the release of tropic hormones from the pituitary. Some tropic hormones direct other endocrine glands—those involved with reproduction (ovaries), stress (adrenal cortex), development (thyroid), and metabolism (liver, thyroid, adrenal cortex). Other tropic hormones affect growth, metabolism, and reproduction directly. Additional endocrine glands independently control such things as calcium balance (parathyroids, thyroid), glucose metabolism (pancreas), and sodium balance (kidneys, adrenal cortex). Imbalances within the endocrine system can have profound effects on the health and well-being of women at different stages in their lives.

FURTHER READING

Goodman, H. M. (1994). *Basic medical endocrinology* (2nd ed.). New York: Raven Press.
A brief but thorough introduction of endocrine disorders. Written as a textbook for introductory medical students. Also available in economical paperback.

Griffin, J. E., & Ojeda, S. R. (Eds.). (1992). *Textbook of endocrine physiology* (2nd ed.). New York: Oxford University Press.
This is a generally readable, scholarly account of the basics on how endocrine systems work. It is available in paperback.

Jones, R. E. (1997). *Human reproductive biology* (2nd ed.). San Diego: Academic Press
An excellent, thorough, and highly readable discussion of all aspects of human reproduction, from AIDS to population control. This text assumes the reader to have a very minimal background.

Mendelsohn, G. (1988). *Diagnosis and pathology of endocrine diseases*. Philadelphia: J. B. Lippincott.
Although slightly dated, this is a thorough introduction to a wide variety of clinical disorders.

Norris, D. O. (1997). *Vertebrate endocrinology* (3rd ed.). San Diego: Academic Press
This is the latest edition of a textbook that covers general endocrinology in considerable detail and includes discussions of numerous human disorders.

104

Gastrointestinal Physiology

William E. Whitehead

ANATOMY

The gastrointestinal tract (see Figure 104.1) is divided by sphincter muscles into four distinct regions: the esophagus, stomach, small intestine, and colon. Each of these regions has a distinct physiological function, and is therefore characterized by distinct patterns of motility (contractions) and secretion.

Esophagus

The esophagus is a tube approximately 25 cm long, which is closed at the upper end by the upper esophageal sphincter, and at the lower end (where it joins the stomach) by the lower esophageal sphincter. This tube is normally collapsed, but can stretch to accommodate a bolus of at least 2.5 cm. However, the sphincters remain tightly closed until reflexively opened in response to a swallow. The esophagus is unique in that it consists of striated (skeletal-type) muscle in its upper third, smooth (visceral-type) muscle in its distal third, and a transition zone in the middle composed of a mixture of striated and smooth muscle.

The principal function of the esophagus is to transport food, water, and secretions to the stomach. This function is served by a pattern of motility in which a swallow, or any distention of the esophagus, triggers a ring of contraction that progresses toward the stomach. The swallow also triggers a simultaneous relaxation of the lower esophageal sphincter to allow the bolus of food to pass into the stomach, after which the sphincter closes. This peristaltic reflex is so efficient that healthy persons can swallow water while standing on their heads and have it delivered into their stomachs.

The most common symptom associated with the esophagus is heartburn, which is caused by the reflux of acid from the stomach into the esophagus, where it causes irritation. This may occur if the lower esophageal sphincter is lax and does not provide an effective barrier to reflux, or if the stomach bulges up through the diaphragm (hiatal hernia) and weakens the effectiveness of the lower esophageal sphincter. Dysphagia (food

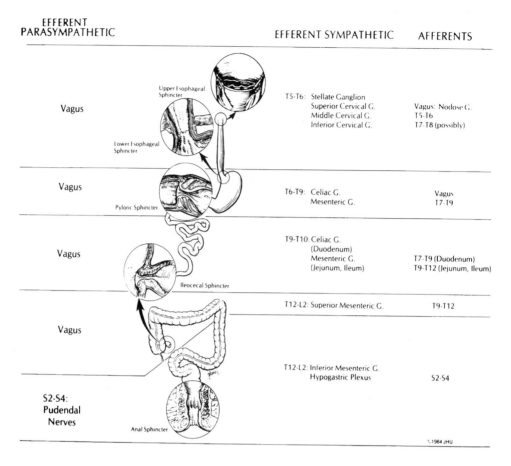

EFFERENT PARASYMPATHETIC   **EFFERENT SYMPATHETIC**   **AFFERENTS**

FIGURE 104.1. Schematic representation of the gastrointestinal tract, showing innervation. The gastrointestinal tract can be divided into four compartments—esophagus, stomach, small intestine, and colon—that are separated from each other by sphincters. These compartments serve different functions and have different innervations and different patterns of motility. From Whitehead and Schuster (1985). Copyright 1985 by Academic Press, Inc. Reprinted by permission.

becoming stuck in the esophagus) may result from disorganized or ineffective contractions in the body of the esophagus or from failure of the lower esophageal sphincter to relax (achalasia). Chest pain, which can be mistaken for ischemic heart disease, may also result from disorganized esophageal contractions or from acid reflux.

Stomach

The stomach is a stretchable bag 25–30 cm in length, which is bounded by the lower esophageal sphincter at the top and by the pyloric sphincter at the bottom. It has a capacity of approximately 1,000 ± 500 ml, with a wide variation depending on a person's usual eating habits. The primary physiological functions of the stomach are (1) storage of a meal, (2) mixing of ingested food with digestive enzymes, (3) breaking down of food particles to a diameter of less than 0.5 mm, and (4) controlled emptying of food into the small intestine. Because of this complex group of functions, the stomach has well-differentiated patterns of motility.

The top of the stomach (fundus) primarily serves to store food. The relaxation of the lower esophageal sphincter is accompanied by a receptive relaxation of the stomach, so that even if the stomach is very full, the new bolus of food can still pass from the esophagus into the stomach. In addition to this phasic (brief) relaxation that accompanies each swallow, there is a tonic relaxation of the stomach muscles as a meal accumulates in the stomach; this prevents intragastric pressure from increasing significantly until the maximum capacity is approached.

The lower portion of the stomach (antrum) has a pattern of motility that is optimal for mixing stomach contents, grinding down particle size, and emptying the contents of the stomach into the small intestine. This is accomplished by forceful rings of contraction, occurring at a frequency of 3 cycles per minute, which begin in the middle of the stomach and propel the contents toward the pyloric sphincter. The pylorus may be completely closed, or it may have a pinhole opening as the contraction approaches. If there is a small opening, this closes almost immediately, allowing only a small squirt of liquid contents to pass through. When the advancing contraction reaches the closed sphincter, the stomach contents are forced back against pressure. This creates a grinding motion, which reduces particle size and mixes the food with digestive enzymes.

The pyloric sphincter is the principal mechanism for regulating gastric emptying. During and immediately after a meal, it will only allow particles smaller than 0.5 mm in diameter to pass through. Large particles that cannot be broken down remain in the stomach and are emptied by a unique pattern of motility, the migrating motor complex, which only occurs between meals. The migrating motor complex consists (in the stomach) of (1) stronger contractions of the gastric antrum and (2) a wide-open pylorus. During meals, the pylorus also controls the rate of caloric emptying (2 calories per minute) through a reflex mechanism, with the result that meals are emptied more slowly if the caloric density is high.

The most common disorder of gastric motility is delayed gastric emptying, which causes symptoms of nausea and vomiting. Delayed gastric emptying can be caused by decreased contractions of the stomach, disordered regulation of the pyloric sphincter, or mechanical obstruction (in which indigestible food particles prevent the stomach from emptying). Abnormally rapid gastric emptying can also occur, leading to postprandial diarrhea (dumping syndrome). This typically only occurs following surgical alteration of the stomach.

Small Intestine

The small intestine is divided into three regions: the duodenum, which involves the first 30 cm of bowel; the jejunum, which involves the next 2–2.5 meters; and the ileum, which involves the distal 3 meters. The physiological function of these regions are similar (principally absorption of nutrients), and the patterns of motility are similar. The ileum terminates in the ileocecal junction, which acts like a sphincter to prevent reflux of contents from the colon into the ileum.

The motility of the small intestine following a meal consists of mixing waves, which are characterized by adjacent segments of bowel contracting more or less independently of each other. This pattern of motility propels food particles over only short distances (3–9 cm).

Between meals (when there is no significant amount of nutrient in the upper small intestine), the motility is dominated by the migrating motor complex. This regularly occurring cycle of motility is divided into three phases: Phase I, in which there are no contractions; Phase II, which is identical to the fed motility pattern; and Phase III, which consists of a burst of rhythmic contractions that migrate along the small intestine over long distances. Phase III, sometimes called the "housekeeper" phase, sweeps bacteria and undigested food particles from the small intestine into the colon. During Phase III, the small intestine contracts at its maximum frequency, which is 12 cycles per minute in the duodenum and decreases to 8–10 cycles per minute in the terminal ileum.

The motility disorders that affect the small intestine are divided into myogenic and neurogenic types and are referred to as pseudo-obstruction (because they cause symptoms of obstruction that are attributable to abnormal motility rather than to mechanical obstruction). Myogenic pseudo-obstruction is said to occur when there are decreased numbers or reduced amplitudes of contractions, but the contractions that do occur show normal organization into the three phases of the migrating motor complex. Neurogenic pseudo-obstruction is associated with disorganized, nonperistaltic motility and/or the failure of a meal to stimulate increased numbers of mixing waves. The symptoms of pseudo-obstruction include rapid abdominal distention, abdominal pain, and vomiting. Abnormally rapid transit through the small intestine is also theoretically possible, but it has not been identified as a motility disorder. Failure of the intestinal mechanism for absorbing water and electrolytes from the lumen of the small intestine may result in diarrhea.

Colon

The colon is 90–125 cm long and is bounded by the ileocecal sphincter and the anal sphincters. Its primary functions are the storage of fecal material and the reabsorption of water. More than 95% of the contractions in the colon are segmental (i.e., segments close to each other contract independently), with the result that there is little net progression of stool toward the rectum. However, high-amplitude propagated contractions sweep around the colon about six times per day, moving fecal material toward the rectum. These high-amplitude propagated contractions usually precede defecation or the desire to defecate.

The most common disorder of colonic function is constipation. This may result from decreased numbers of high-amplitude propagated contractions in the colon (colonic inertia) or from an inability to relax the pelvic floor muscles and anal sphincter when straining to defecate (pelvic floor dyssynergia). Diarrhea (frequent loose or watery stools) is also a common symptom, but it does not result from altered colonic motility so much as from increased volumes of fluid or undigested carbohydrate reaching the colon from the small intestine.

The rectum is a specialized segment of the colon that has two important characteristics: compliance and afferent innervation. As the rectum fills with fecal material, it relaxes to accommodate increased volumes with little increase in pressure, in a manner similar to the fundus of the stomach. This receptive relaxation continues until the mechanical limit is approached or until the person voluntarily initiates a rectal contraction by straining to defecate. Incontinence may result if rectal compliance is significantly reduced by inflammation or other causes. The sensory innervation of the rectum is also important to continence, because the perception of rectal distention is a critical cue to tell the person when to contract the external anal sphincter in order to avoid incontinence.

There are two types of anal sphincter muscles: the internal anal sphincter, which consists of smooth muscle that normally stays tightly closed; and the external anal sphincter, which consists of striated muscle that can be voluntarily contracted to prevent defecation. In addition, other striated muscles of the pelvic floor influence the ability to defecate and the ability to hold back stool. The most common disorders affecting the rectum and anus are fecal incontinence, which may be attributable to weak pelvic floor muscles; chronic rectal pain, which may result from chronically tense pelvic floor muscles; and pelvic floor dyssynergia-type constipation, which may result from the inability to relax the pelvic floor muscles during attempts to defecate.

NEURAL CONTROL

There are two levels of neural regulation of the gastrointestinal tract. The enteric nervous system is a complex network of neurons and interconnecting fibers in the walls of the gastrointestinal tract from esophagus to anus (see Figure 104.2). This neural network contains as many neurons as the spinal cord, and it is able to regulate the reflex activity of the gastrointestinal tract even when it is completely isolated from the central nervous system (CNS).

The vagus nerve provides most of the parasympathetic input to the gastrointestinal tract (see Figure 104.1); it innervates the gut down to the level of the distal colon. Sacral parasympathetic fibers innervate the rectum. Sympathetic fibers, which primarily inhibit the motility and secretion of the gastrointestinal tract, are also present. Two principles are important to understanding the role of the extrinsic nerves from the CNS. First, most

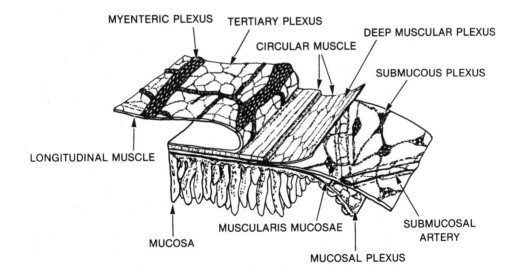

FIGURE 104.2. Section of small intestine showing the enteric nervous system. The outer (longitudinal) muscle layer is peeled back to reveal the myenteric nerve plexus (also called Auerbach's plexus). The submucosal plexus of nerves (also called Meissner's plexus) is seen to lie between the inner (circular) muscle layer and the mucosa. Adapted from Furness and Costa (1980). Copyright 1980 by Pergamon Press, Inc. Adapted by permission.

of the efferent fibers to the gut from both the parasympathetic and sympathetic nervous systems synapse on neurons in the enteric nervous system rather than on muscle cells, and they exert their influence through the enteric nervous system. Second, 80–90% of the vagal and sympathetic fibers to the gut are afferent fibers, which bring information back to the CNS about what is going on in the gut. In general, the vagus carries information on intraluminal pH, osmolarity, and other conditions in the gut, which are important to homeostatic regulation but which are not available to awareness. Sympathetic fibers carry information on intraluminal distention from stretch receptors in the muscle wall or surrounding mesentery, and this information is available to conscious awareness.

HUMORAL CONTROL

Three types of chemical signaling systems are recognized: neurocrine or synaptic transmission, in which chemicals released by axons affect receptors on dendrites or nerve bodies only within a synapse; paracrine transmission, in which chemicals released from axons can affect multiple neurons at a distance of a few millimeters; and endocrine transmission, in which chemicals released into the blood can affect cell bodies at a long distance from the site of release. All three types of chemical transmission occur in the gastrointestinal tract, and the same chemicals can serve all three functions.

GENDER DIFFERENCES IN GASTROINTESTINAL TRANSIT AND PHYSIOLOGY

Women have slower colonic transit than men, and they report more symptoms of constipation. The slowing of transit time may be related to decreased levels of bile acids in the colon, since bile acids stimulate colonic motility.

EFFECTS OF THE MENSTRUAL CYCLE AND PREGNANCY

Gastrointestinal symptoms of diarrhea, bloating, and abdominal pain are more common during menses. They are probably associated with the release of prostaglandins during menses since prostaglandins are known to be powerful stimulants to smooth muscle contractions, including contractions of the gastrointestinal tract, and they are released at a high concentration from the uterus during menses.

Progesterone, and possibly estrogen, inhibit the motility of the gallbladder and the sphincter of Oddi (which regulates gallbladder emptying); this effect may be responsible for the increased incidence of gallstones and of sphincter-of-Oddi dysfunction in women of childbearing age. One group of investigators reported that mouth-to-cecum transit time was delayed in the luteal phase of the menstrual cycle, but other investigators have not been able to replicate this. There is no convincing evidence that either gastrointestinal transit or gastrointestinal symptoms differ significantly between the luteal and the follicular phases of the menstrual cycle.

Another factor accounting for increased numbers of gastrointestinal symptoms in women may be indirectly related to the menstrual cycle. Nonsteroidal anti-inflammatory drugs are taken frequently by many women for the relief of menstrual cramps, and these produce gastrointestinal complications that are more common in women than in men.

Pregnancy is associated with nausea and vomiting during the first trimester and with gastroesophageal reflux and constipation later in gestation. Reflux is associated with decreased pressure in the lower esophageal sphincter, and constipation is associated with slowed transit through the small intestine and colon, both of which appear to be mediated by progesterone. The nausea of pregnancy is associated with abnormal myoelectric activity, but the mechanism by which reproductive hormones modify gastric myoelectric activity is not known.

FURTHER READING

Baron, T. H., Ramirez, B., & Richter, J. E. (1993). Gastrointestinal motility disorders during pregnancy. *Annals of Internal Medicine, 118,* 366–375.
Summary of the effects of pregnancy on gastrointestinal physiology and symptoms.

Furness, J. B., & Costa, M. (1980). Types of nerves in the enteric nervous system. *Neuroscience, 5,* 1–20.
Detailed analysis of the organization of the neural network in the walls of the gastrointestinal tract, and of the types of neurotransmitters involved.

Heitkemper, M. M., & Jarrett, M. (1992). Pattern of gastrointestinal and somatic symptoms across the menstrual cycle. *Gastroenterology, 102,* 505–513.
Study that used a daily symptom diary to investigate the effects of the menstrual cycle on gastrointestinal symptoms and physiology during two menstrual cycles in healthy women.

Henry, D., Dobson, A., & Turner, C. (1993). Variability in the risk of major gastrointestinal complications from nonaspirin nonsteroidal anti-inflammatory drugs. *Gastroenterology, 105,* 1078–1088.
Study showing that the number of upper gastrointestinal complications from ingestion of nonsteroidal anti-inflammatory drugs is nearly threefold greater in women than in men.

Koch, K. L., Stern, R. M., Vasey, M., Botti, J. J., Creasy, G. W., & Dwyer, A. (1990). Gastric dysrhythmias and nausea of pregnancy. *Digestive Diseases and Sciences, 35,* 961–968.
Electrogastrograms recorded from 26 pregnant women experiencing nausea showed abnormalities, whereas pregnant women with minimal or no nausea had normal electrogastrograms.

Lampe, J. W., Fredstrom, S. F., Slavin, J. L., & Potter, J. D. (1993). Sex differences in colonic function: A randomised trial. *Gut, 34,* 531–536.
Study comparing whole-gut transit time, stool volumes, and bile acid secretion in men and women on identical diets.

Smout, A. J. M., & Akkermans, L. M. A. (1992). *Normal and disturbed motility of the gastrointestinal tract.* Stroud, England: Wrightson Biomedical.
Comprehensive review of the anatomy and physiology of the gastrointestinal tract, written in nontechnical language and with helpful illustrations.

Whitehead, W. E., & Schuster, M. M. (1985). *Gastrointestinal disorders: Behavioral and physiological basis for treatment.* Orlando, FL: Academic Press.
Chapter 3 is a concise review of anatomy and physiology; the book also contains a detailed review of gastrointestinal disorders and their behavioral treatment.

105

Gastrointestinal Syndromes and Disorders

William E. Whitehead

IRRITABLE BOWEL SYNDROME

Definition and Diagnostic Criteria

Irritable bowel syndrome (IBS) is defined as follows: The patient experiences abdominal pain or discomfort that is relieved by defecation or that is associated with a change in the frequency or consistency of stools; and these symptoms are not explained by another recognized disease process, such as bacterial infection, lactase deficiency, or inflammatory bowel disease. Research diagnostic criteria additionally require that the patient report two or more of the following symptoms on at least one-fourth of occasions or days: (1) altered stool frequency (more than three stools per day or fewer than three per week); (2) altered stool form (lumpy, hard, loose, or watery stools); (3) altered stool passage (straining, urgency, or feeling of incomplete evacuation); (4) passage of mucus; and/or (5) bloating.

Epidemiology

IBS is more common in women (14.5%) than in men (7.7%) by a ratio of approximately 2:1 in the community and by a ratio of approximately 4:1 among medical clinic attenders with this diagnosis. The gender difference is so striking that some investigators have suggested that the symptom criteria used to diagnose the disorder are not valid or are less reliable in men than in women. However, this appears not to be the case. When factor analysis is used to identify clusters of symptoms that covary across large numbers, the symptoms defining IBS cluster together as strongly in men as in women. There are simply fewer men reporting these symptoms. Possible explanations for the greater prevalence of IBS symptoms among women are as follows:

1. *Physiological differences.* As I have noted in the preceding chapter, women have a slower whole-gut transit time than men, leading to a greater prevalence of constipation. In addition, prostaglandins released during menstruation may contribute to increased colon motility. The effects of reproductive hormones on the gastrointestinal tract are poorly understood, but they represent a possible source of increased IBS symptoms in women.

2. *Abuse.* Approximately 40–60% of women with IBS report a history of sexual or physical abuse. Although the reasons for this association are not fully understood, it is speculated that a history of pelvic trauma leads to conscious or unconscious distortion of the significance and intensity of visceral sensations.

3. *Cultural influences and childhood social learning.* If parents respond to their children's somatic complaints by giving them special privileges and gifts, these children tend to report more somatic complaints even after they become adults. This pattern of childhood social learning contributes to the presentation of functional bowel disorders. Parents may be more likely to respond in this fashion to young girls than to young boys, leading to a greater tendency for women to notice, to report, and to seek treatment for gastrointestinal symptoms related to IBS.

Treatment

Conservative treatment of IBS consists of education and reassurance, a high-fiber diet for constipation, and anticholinergics (e.g., dicyclomine, hyoscyamine) for pain and diarrhea. Antidepressants (either tricyclics or selective serotonin reuptake inhibitors) are rapidly becoming a routine part of the management of patients with abdominal pain, including those who are not clinically depressed, because antidepressants have been shown to be superior to placebo for the relief of visceral pain. Conservative treatments such as these described above are effective for approximately 70% of patients consulting for IBS when provided by a primary care physician.

When conservative treatment fails to provide sufficient benefit, psychological treatment may be tried. There are controlled trials supporting the efficacy of interpersonal psychotherapy, cognitive-behavioral therapy, progressive muscle relaxation training, and hypnosis. These psychological interventions are helpful in patients who have diarrhea-predominant symptoms and intermittent or variable abdominal pain; they are not beneficial for the symptom of constipation. Except for hypnosis, these psychological treatments are more effective in patients who can associate their symptoms with psychological stress and in patients with some degree of anxiety and depression. Hypnosis appears to work best in people who are younger than age 55 and who do not have significant psychopathology.

CONSTIPATION

Definitions

There is widespread confusion about what constipation means. Physicians have traditionally defined it as infrequent passage of hard stools, but patients usually refer to difficulty evacuating stool from the rectum or a feeling of incomplete evacuation. This confusion arises because there are three different types of constipation associated with different physiological mechanisms:

1. *Colonic inertia.* This refers to slow transit through the colon (i.e., to whole-gut transit times greater than 67 hours). Colonic inertia is associated with infrequent, hard stools and is believed to be attributable to decreased numbers of peristaltic contractions in the colon. It is more common in women than in men.

2. *Pelvic floor dyssynergia.* When a person is straining to defecate, the normal response includes a reflex inhibition of the striated pelvic floor muscles. However, some patients fail to relax these muscles when straining, or they paradoxically contract them. This creates a functional outlet obstruction and results in the accumulation of stool in the rectum and sigmoid colon. It is associated with symptoms of excessive straining or a feeling of incomplete evacuation. Pelvic floor dyssynergia is frequently associated with chronic rectal pain (levator ani syndrome), because the pelvic floor muscles may be tonically overly contracted.

3. *Constipation-predominant IBS.* Patients with IBS who report constipation as their predominant stool pattern typically have a stool frequency and consistency within the normal range. The most frequent symptoms reported are straining, feeling of incomplete evacuation, and constant urge to defecate (often resulting in frequent, unsuccessful attempts to defecate). The physiological mechanism is thought to be increased numbers of nonperistaltic contractions in the distal colon.

Epidemiology

Epidemiological studies have usually not tried to distinguish among subtypes of constipation and have allowed patients to use their own definitions. Self-defined constipation is reported by 20.8% of adult females and 8.0% of adult males. Self-defined constipation is more common in sedentary than in physically active individuals, more common in the elderly (possibly because they tend to be more sedentary), and more common in African-Americans than in European-Americans.

Role of Psychological Symptoms

In every published study in which psychological tests have been administered to patients with chronic constipation, abnormal test scores were found. Depression and anxiety were the most common findings, and the severity was typically mild to moderate. No specific pattern of psychological traits or symptoms has been identified for colonic inertia or constipation-predominant IBS. However, there is evidence to suggest that pelvic floor dyssynergia is specifically linked to anxiety, and a high proportion of patients with pelvic floor dyssynergia report a history of sexual abuse. This may be significant, since anxiety is known to be associated with chronically high levels of striated muscle tension—so much so that muscle relaxation training has frequently been used to treat anxiety disorders.

Treatment

Constipation has been more difficult to treat successfully than diarrhea or abdominal pain. The treatment should be individualized to the subtype of constipation present:

1. *Colonic inertia.* The first line of treatment is to increase dietary fiber up to at least 30 grams per day. Indigestible fiber binds more water in the stools to make them softer, and it increases stool volume. It is usually effective at doses of 30 grams or more daily, but a high-fiber diet is not very palatable, and compliance with therapy is poor. The second line of treatment is a laxative. Stimulant laxatives and enemas should be avoided because physiological tolerance to them develops rapidly, causing people to take larger and larger doses. Osmotic laxatives such as lactulose and sorbitol are preferable because they do not cause physiological tolerance. In extreme cases, the colon may be removed surgically and the terminal ilium connected to the rectum.

2. *Pelvic floor dyssynergia.* The preferred treatment is biofeedback training to teach relaxation of the pelvic floor muscles. This leads to significant clinical improvement in about 67% of cases. Simple habit training, in which the patient is instructed to sit on the toilet after one meal each day and to use an enema or laxative if no bowel movement occurs for 48 hours, is also effective in about 50% of patients with pelvic floor dyssynergia, and it is a less costly treatment to provide. Thus, it should normally be tried prior to biofeedback.

3. *Constipation-predominant IBS.* As noted above for IBS, education and reassurance, usually combined with a higher-fiber diet, are the first steps in treatment. For the abdominal pain associated with this type of constipation, a selective serotonin reuptake inhibitor may be recommended, although there are no placebo-controlled studies to support this recommendation.

FECAL INCONTINENCE

Definition

Fecal incontinence refers to any involuntary loss of stool from the rectum in an individual over the age of 3 years. Excluded from the definition are individuals who soil intentionally to obtain attention or to manipulate care providers, and individuals with rectal prolapse, who secrete mucus onto their undergarments from the exposed rectal lining.

Epidemiology

The prevalence of fecal incontinence in the U.S. adult population is 7.2% (for a breakdown by ages, see Figure 105.1). However, most of the overall group (6.9% prevalence) report that they only stain their underclothes or lose very small amounts. The most common cause of such minor soiling is IBS; 22% of patients with IBS report occasional fecal incontinence. Other causes of minor soiling include hemorrhoids and rectal prolapse, both of which may cause minor soiling by obstructing the closure of the anal sphincter.

Large-volume fecal incontinence has a prevalence of approximately 0.3% in adults. However, there is a strong association with age (see Figure 105.1). Large-volume incontinence occurs in 1.5% of children aged 7–9 years and in 1.2% of people over age 65, but its prevalence in young adults is less than 0.1%. The most common causes of fecal incontinence in the young and middle-aged are obstetrical trauma to the anal sphincters, resulting in a separation of the muscles, and pudendal nerve injuries. Pudendal nerve injuries may result from hemorrhoidectomy or other surgery to the anal canal and

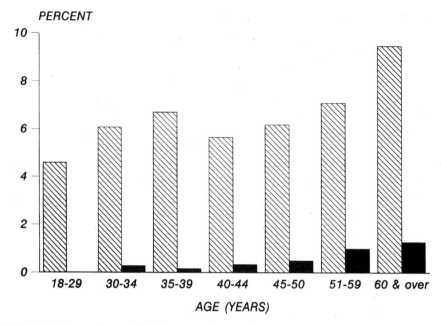

FIGURE 105.1. Prevalence of fecal incontinence at different ages, as reported by 5,400 community-dwelling U.S. adults. Striped bars show the percentage who reported that they had often leaked a small amount of stool (stained their underwear) in the last 3 months. Solid bars show the percentage who reported that they had often leaked 2 teaspoons or more of stool in the last 3 months. Adapted from Drossman et al. (1993). Copyright 1993 by Plenum Publishing Corp. Adapted by permission.

rectum, but a more common (although poorly documented) cause is a traction (stretch) injury to this nerve caused by repeated straining to defecate.

Epidemiological studies do not show the overall prevalence of fecal incontinence to be significantly greater in women than in men. However, sphincter muscle injuries are much more common in women because most of them occur during childbirth, and the minor soiling that occurs in association with diarrhea-predominant IBS is more common in women because IBS is more common in women.

Role of Psychological Factors

Psychological factors rarely contribute to the onset of fecal incontinence, but significant psychological distress and social withdrawal may occur as a consequence of fecal incontinence. Behavioral techniques are regarded as the treatment of choice for some types of fecal incontinence (see below), even though psychological factors rarely explain the development of fecal incontinence.

Treatment

The most common type of fecal incontinence in children is overflow incontinence, which occurs secondary to the accumulation of stool in the rectum. Habit training to teach children to defecate voluntarily at least every 2 days is effective in 65–85% of these youngsters, and the results are well maintained. Children with this type of fecal incontinence who do not benefit from habit training may benefit from biofeedback to teach them to relax the anal sphincter muscles when straining to defecate.

For fecal incontinence occurring secondary to pudendal nerve injury, biofeedback to improve the strength of the external anal sphincter is the treatment of choice and is effective in approximately 72% of patients. Unfortunately, for the type of fecal incontinence that is unique to women—namely, obstetrical injury to the anal sphincters—behavioral training techniques play a limited role; the preferred treatment for these patients is a surgical reconstruction of the sphincter muscles. However, biofeedback may be helpful under two circumstances. First, if the patient is a poor surgical risk, biofeedback should be tried (in combination with medical therapy to prevent loose stool). Second, if the surgery involves the transposition of another muscle (gracilis muscle or gluteal muscle) rather than a juxtaposition of the separated ends of the sphincter, the patient will have to relearn how to control this muscle for incontinence, and biofeedback may be beneficial in this process. The latter is a theoretical and not an established application of biofeedback.

GALLSTONES, GALLBLADDER DYSFUNCTION, AND SPHINCTER-OF-ODDI DYSFUNCTION

Definition

Gallstones are precipitations of solid pieces of cholesterol in the gallbladder, which cause pain when the gallbladder contracts or when the stones enter the bile duct. Gallbladder dysfunction refers to abnormalities in the contraction or relaxation of the gallbladder during filling and emptying, and sphincter-of-Oddi dysfunction refers to abnormalities in the tonic pressure or the phasic contractions of the sphincter of Oddi, which is the sphincter regulating the emptying of the common bile duct.

Epidemiology

Gallstones occur more frequently in women than in men, and sphincter-of-Oddi dysfunction (which is inferred when patients with a prior cholecystectomy continue to experience biliary cholic) is also more frequent in women than in men. Motility disorders of the gallbladder are also believed to be more common in women, although the series are too small to be certain. Among women, gallstones are more frequent in those who are premenopausal.

Etiological Mechanisms

Progesterone, and probably also estrogen, are believed to be responsible for the increased prevalence of cholecystic disease in women. The exact mechanisms by which this occurs are not known. Animal studies and muscle strip studies show that the motility of the gallbladder and the sphincter of Oddi are inhibited in the presence of progesterone. These studies suggest that the mechanism involves an interaction whereby progesterone and/or estrogen desensitize these smooth muscles to the excitatory effects of cholecystokinin and acetylcholine. Other investigators have proposed that estrogen increases the hepatic secretion of cholesterol. Gallstones are usually treated by removing the gallbladder together with the stones. However, an alternative technique is to snare the stones with a device passed into the bile duct from an endoscope or to make a small slit in the bile duct through an endoscope.

INTESTINAL ENDOMETRIOSIS

Definition

Endometriosis is defined as the presence of normal endometrial tissue outside the uterus. When it involves the gastrointestinal tract, symptoms may include constipation, diarrhea, rectal pain during defecation, and blood in the stools. In a small proportion of patients (2–18%), the bowel becomes partially obstructed.

Epidemiology

Endometriosis affects between 8% and 18% of women and is more common in nulliparous women of childbearing age. In about 5–37% of women with endometriosis, there is involvement of the gastrointestinal tract, and in 75–90% of cases of intestinal involvement, the rectum or sigmoid colon is the site of the endometriosis.

Diagnosis

The diagnosis of endometriosis as a cause of gastrointestinal symptoms is often delayed or missed, because the symptoms are similar to those of functional bowel disorders. There is not a reliable association of symptoms to the phase of the menstrual cycle, as was formerly thought. A barium enema, though nonspecific, appears to provide the greatest sensitivity for the diagnosis among noninvasive tests. The greatest specificity is achieved by laparoscopy or laparotomy. However, the diagnosis is usually only suspected when the presence of extraintestinal endometriosis is recognized.

Treatment

Effective therapies include exogenous hormones that suppress the estrogen–progesterone cycle (and induce menopause), ovariectomy, and bowel resection. Bowel resection is performed when there is significant bowel obstruction, and it is generally effective. It is important to recognize, however, that the majority of patients with intestinal endometriosis have minimal or no gastrointestinal symptoms and require no treatment.

FURTHER READING

Chen, A., & Huminer, D. (1991). The role of estrogen receptors in the development of gallstones and gallbladder cancer. *Medical Hypotheses, 36,* 259–260.
People who underwent cholecystectomy for gallstones had estrogen receptors and an abnormally high concentration of estrogen in their gallbladders, suggesting that estrogen influences the development of gallstones.

Drossman, D. A., Leserman, J., Nachman, G., Li, Z., Gluck, H., Toomey, T. C., & Mitchell, C. M. (1990). Sexual and physical abuse in women with functional or organic gastrointestinal disorders. *Annals of Internal Medicine, 113,* 828–833.
The first of a series of studies to show that women with functional gastrointestinal disorders are more likely than women with organic gastrointestinal disorders to report a history of sexual and/or physical abuse.

Drossman, D. A., Li, Z., Andruzzi, E., Temple, R. D., Tally, N. J., Thompson, W. G., Whitehead, W. E., Janssens, J., Funch-Jensen, P., Corazziari, E., Richter, J. E., & Koch, G. G. (1993). U.S. householder survey of functional gastrointestinal disorders: Prevalence, sociodemography, and health impact. *Digestive Diseases and Sciences, 38,* 1569–1580.
Postal survey of the prevalence of functional gastrointestinal disorders defined by international consensus criteria among 5,400 U.S. adults.

Enck, P. (1993). Biofeedback training in disordered defecation: A critical review. *Digestive Diseases and Sciences, 38,* 1953–1960.
Comprehensive review of published studies that used biofeedback to treat constipation related to pelvic floor dyssynergia.

Everhart, J. E., Go, V. L. W., Johannes, R. S., Fitzsimmons, S. C., Roth, H. P., & White, L. R. (1989). A longitudinal survey of self-reported bowel habits in the United States. *Digestive Diseases and Sciences, 34,* 1143–1162.
This study used two successive national health surveys of large random samples to characterize the prevalence and to identify demographic factors affecting the development of constipation.

Thompson, W. G., & the Working Team for Functional Bowel Disorders. (1994). Functional bowel disorders and functional abdominal pain. In D. A. Drossman, J. E. Richter, N. J. Talley, W. G. Thompson, E. Corazziari, & W. E. Whitehead (Eds.), *The functional gastrointestinal disorders: Diagnosis, pathophysiology, and treatment* (pp. 115–173). Boston: Little, Brown.
Report of an international consensus reached on the diagnostic criteria for IBS and related functional bowel disorders; it also contains a review of psychophysiology, epidemiology, and treatment of functional gastrointestinal disorders.

Whitehead, W. E., & Schuster, M. M. (1992). Irritable bowel syndrome. In S. J. Winawer (Ed.), *Management of gastrointestinal diseases* (Vol. 2, pp. 32.1–32.25). New York: Gower Medical.
Review of the pathophysiological basis of IBS and the effects of various treatments.

Zwas, F. R., & Lyon, D. T. (1991). Endometriosis: An important condition in clinical gastroenterology. *Digestive Diseases and Sciences, 36,* 353–364.
Review of the way in which endometriosis affects the gastrointestinal tract, the prevalence of endometriosis, and its treatment.

106

Headache

Edward B. Blanchard

*C*hronic benign headache (HA) is a widespread minor health problem; migraine HA, the more serious form, affects 17.6% of women between the ages of 12 and 80 in the United States in any one year. Migraine HA is present in women primarily from puberty through menopause, with an average prevalence of 25–30% during this time. Migraine HA continues to be present in about 10% of women throughout the eighth decade of life. During the young adult and middle years, women outnumber men about 3:1 in regard to HA complaints, with even higher ratios present in clinic (treatment-seeking) populations.

Migraine HA, the primary focus of this chapter, is an episodic, paroxysmal disorder characterized by throbbing pain and nausea, often accompanied by excessive sensitivity to light and sound, and occasionally accompanied by vomiting and mild confusion. Migraine HA tends to come on quickly and can last from 2–3 hours up to 2–3 days. Usually diagnosis can be reliably made by a primary care physician. Although psychologists can also make a reasonably reliable diagnosis by taking a careful history and perhaps making use of an HA diary, I strongly recommend that the psychologist work in close collaboration with a knowledgeable physician.

Standard treatment is probably over-the-counter (OTC) analgesic medication. When this does not bring adequate relief, which is often the case in migraine, one can progress to prescription drugs (analgesics, abortives, and prophylactics, including the new inject-able abortive, sumatriptan). For several reasons, nondrug treatment approaches to migraine HA and to chronic benign HA disorders have become fairly popular, especially among women. This may stem in part from a dislike of taking any medication, even

OTC analgesics, during the childbearing years for fear of inadvertent teratological effects; many women also dislike the side effects of the drugs.

NONDRUG TREATMENT OF BENIGN HEADACHE DISORDERS

Relaxation Training

The most frequently used form of relaxation training is some version of abbreviated progressive muscle relaxation. It has been shown to be effective with 40–60% of tension HA patients across several studies. With migraine HA and mixed migraine and tension HA, the results are more variable, with improvement rates ranging from 20% to 75%. Other forms of relaxation training that have been found useful with chronic HA include autogenic training and various passive, meditative forms of relaxation.

Biofeedback Training

Frontal electromyographic (EMG) feedback has been shown repeatedly to be of benefit to tension HA sufferers, with success rates of 30–80% across many studies. Thermal biofeedback, in which patients learn to warm the hands (engage in volitional peripheral vasodilation), has been shown to be very useful in managing migraine and mixed HAs. Again, success rates vary from about 30% to 80% across almost 20 published treatment trials. Thermal biofeedback is often combined with autogenic training and/or other forms of relaxation training.

Cognitive Stress Coping Therapy

Cognitive stress coping therapy was developed by Holroyd and has been shown to be very effective as a single therapy with tension HA. Adding it to relaxation training also yields a significant increment in benefit with tension HA. For vascular HAs (migraine and mixed) cognitive stress coping therapy adds nothing to standard thermal biofeedback and relaxation. The weight of evidence would indicate only a minor role at best for cognitive therapy with migraine HA.

Psychotherapy

There is no controlled research showing an advantage of psychotherapy over no treatment in the benign HA disorders. However, everyone who works with HA patients has seen patients for whom individual psychotherapy seems warranted.

General Comments

These various treatments are usually administered over 3–16 sessions spread over 6–8 weeks. The typical course of treatment is 8–12 sessions. Largely home-based treatment regimens have been found to be very effective. Beneficial results in terms of significant reductions in HA activity have been shown to be maintained as long as 5–6 years after treatment.

MENSTRUALLY RELATED MIGRAINE HEADACHE

A topic of particular relevance to women is menstrually related migraine HA. Questions of special concern that are emerging from the HA field are how to define this disorder and how to treat it, especially with the nondrug treatments discussed above. Clinicians and researchers in the field of headache have long been aware of potential connections between the onset of migraine HA and the phase of a woman's menstrual cycle. Everyone in this field has seen the prototypical female patient whose menstrual cycle shows great regularity and whose migraine HAs show a reliable relation to that cycle. Although these prototypical cases exist, investigators find less certainty once they begin to examine a series of women.

A difficulty with research in this area has been in defining what constitutes a menstrually related migraine HA. The various definitions used in the nondrug treatment studies addressing the responsivity of menstrually related migraine to treatment are summarized in Table 106.1. Three (or possibly four) different definitions have been used for menstrual migraine HA. In an attempt to bring some order to this confusing issue, Kim has examined the implications of the varying definitions for reports of treatment outcome.

Solbach and colleagues, using their definition of menstrual migraine HA, drew the inference that thermal biofeedback is ineffective with menstrual migraine. However, their inferential process is suspect. As noted in the table, they classified a woman as a menstrual migraineur if she had any menstrually related HA, thus making no distinction between menstrually related HAs and other migraine HAs in the same subject that were not menstrually related.

In their primary study, Solbach and colleagues found an advantage for thermal biofeedback versus two comparison treatments combined (EMG biofeedback and autogenic training). These results were based upon a sample that included 22 males and 31 women without menstrual migraine. When the same analyses were conducted on all of the HA activity for the 83 women with menstrually related migraine, no significant differences were found among the three treated groups and the control group. The investigators then concluded that treatment was ineffective for menstrual migraine, but effective for nonmenstrual migraine. This latter point was never tested. Moreover, no specific test of the effects of treatment on menstrually related versus menstrually unrelated HAs was made.

Gauthier and colleagues, using the same definition but distinguishing between kinds of HAs within the same patient, found significant efficacy of biofeedback treatments for menstrually related and unrelated HAs. In a comparison of HA patients with predominantly menstrual migraine (66% or more of HAs were menstrually related) to those with predominantly (66% or more) menstrually unrelated migraine HAs, significant effects of treatment (HA reduction) were found, but again no difference in efficacy was found based on HA type.

In our Study 1, Kim and I found significant reduction in HA activity with biofeedback treatments for both self-designated menstrual migraineurs and migraineurs whose HAs were not menstrually related, with no differential effect despite a total of 98 female subjects. In Study 2 (the within-subject comparison), there was again no differential effect of treatment on these women's menstrually related HAs and their menstrually unrelated HAs. Overall treatment effects were relatively weak in this latter study. However, Kim, defining menstrually related migraine HA on the basis both of HAs

TABLE 106.1. Definitions of Menstrual Migraine HA

Authors	Definition	Comments
Solbach, Sargent, & Coyne (1984)	"Menstrual migraine is defined . . . as any migraine HA which occurs 3 days prior to the menstrual flow, during the time of flow, or 3 days following."	A subject was classified as either having menstrual migraine or not. No distinction within menstrual migraineurs of HAs in target period versus rest of the month. Did not exclude subjects on oral contraceptives.
Gauthier, Fournier, & Roberge (1991)	Used Solbach et al. (1984) definition.	Compared menstrually related HAs to menstrually unrelated HAs in those with menstrual migraine. Also compared subjects with predominantly menstrual migraine to those whose migraines were not predominantly menstrual. Excluded subjects on oral contraceptives.
Szekely et al. (1986)	Menstrual HA was defined as "headache occurring regularly within plus or minus one week of day one of menstruation for a minimum of the past 6 consecutive months."	Included 2 patients with cluster HA and 4 with muscle contraction HA in total of 16. Excluded subjects on oral contraceptives.
Kim & Blanchard (1992)	Study 1: Subjects reported an association of HAs to menstrual cycle.	Lack of precise definition; relied on subjects' definition. Excluded subjects on oral contraceptives.
	Study 2: Subjects were asked which part of menstrual cycle HAs were most likely to occur during (e.g., premenstrual phase, actual menstruation, etc.) and this defined 1-week observation period.	Idiosyncratic definition of menstrual migraine for each subject. Excluded subjects on oral contraceptives.
Kim (1995)	Menstrual HAs were defined as HAs associated with declining levels of estrogen: the 3 days following ovulation, 3 days preceding day 1 of menstruation, and day 1 of menstruation plus next 7 days.	Defined two points in menstrual cycle: ovulation (from LH surge in urine) and onset of menstruation. Excluded subjects on oral contraceptives. Distinguished between menstrually related and other migraine HAs.

following ovulation (when estrogen levels are declining) and of HAs from the 3 days before onset of menstruation (when estrogen levels are also declining) through day 8, found a significant differential effect of thermal biofeedback on menstrually related migraine (43.7% reduction) versus menstrually unrelated migraine (60.7% reduction). Interestingly, the differential effect was not present when menstrually related migraine was defined in the manner of Solbach and colleagues or of Szekely and colleagues.

FURTHER READING

Blanchard, E. B. (1992). Psychological treatment of benign headache disorders. *Journal of Consulting and Clinical Psychology, 60,* 537–551.
A comprehensive review of the literature from 1982 to 1992 on psychological treatment of HA.

Diamond, S., & Dalessio, D. J. (1982). *The practicing physician's approach to headache* (3rd ed.). Baltimore: Williams & Wilkins.
A good, but simplified, description of medical approaches to the diagnoses and treatment of HA, designed for primary care physicians by two of the world's leading authorities.

Gauthier, J. G., Fournier, A., & Roberge, C. (1991). The differential effects of biofeedback in the treatment of menstrual and non-menstrual migraine. *Headache, 31,* 82–90.
A retrospective study of the effects of biofeedback on menstrually related migraine HA.

Holroyd, K. A., Andrasik, F., & Westbrook, T. (1977). Cognitive control of tension headache. *Cognitive Therapy and Research, 1,* 121–133.
Prospective study of cognitive therapy for tension type HA.

Kim, M. (1995). *Menstrually-related headaches and their responsiveness to non-pharmacological treatment.* Unpublished doctoral dissertation, State University of New York at Albany.
An unpublished dissertation studying menstrually related migraine, defined both by onset of ovulation and by onset of menses, which showed that nondrug treatment results are determined by the definition used for menstrual migraine.

Kim, M., & Blanchard, E. B. (1992). Two studies of the non-pharmacological treatment of menstrually-related migraine headache. *Headache, 32,* 197–202.
A report combining one retrospective study and one prospective study of the effects of biofeedback and relaxation on menstrually related migraine HA.

Solbach, P., Sargent, J., & Coyne, L. (1984). Menstrual migraine headache: Results of a controlled, experimental outcome study of non-drug treatments. *Headache, 24,* 75–78.
First retrospective study of the effects of biofeedback on menstrually related migraine HA; found no effects, but was probably flawed methodologically.

Stewart, W. F., Lipton, R. B., Celentano, D. D., & Reed, M. L. (1992). Prevalence of migraine headache in the United States. *Journal of the American Medical Association, 267,* 64–69.
Best available epidemiological data on migraine HA in the United States.

Szekely, B., Botwin, D., Eidelman, B. H., Becker, M., Elman, N., & Schemm, R. (1986). Non-pharmacological treatment of menstrual headache: Relaxation-biofeedback behavior therapy and person-centered insight therapy. *Headache, 26,* 86–92.
A prospective study of menstrually related HA.

107

HIV Infection

Jean L. Richardson

AIDS takes a toll on women that involves not solely a threat to health and life, but also a threat to dignity. HIV infection has different implications for women than for men, because of differences in the history of the disease in women, the biology of the disease in women, and psychosocial issues pertaining to women. These differences interfere with women's obtaining health care and with their obtaining support from others to meet the physical and emotional challenges of this disease.

HISTORY OF THE DISEASE IN WOMEN IN THE UNITED STATES

The story of HIV infection in women is a story of devaluation and isolation. Men with HIV were stigmatized because of the link between HIV and homosexuality, and the societal and institutional devaluation of homosexuality. However, among gay men with HIV in the early years of the 1980s, a natural support group had already banded together to achieve gay rights. This group was well positioned socially, economically, and politically to provide care for HIV/AIDS patients and to advocate for research dollars to study this disease. In contrast, HIV-infected women did not have such social support and were invisible and alone.

Those who have conducted support groups for HIV-infected women have reported that prior to entering these groups, most of the women had never met another woman with HIV. Most infected women assess HIV as a gay man's disease, and most social, health, and community services for persons with HIV are run by or primarily serve gay men. Only in recent years have clinics opened to serve infected mothers and children; however, infected women who do not have infected children may not be eligible for such clinics and are seen, often with great discomfort, in the "men's" clinic.

For women, the stigma associated with HIV infection may impose a heavy emotional burden. In one study, over 50% of women indicated that they thought their illness was a punishment, feared they would lose friends, and felt ashamed of the illness; over 40% feared losing a job or thought other people were uncomfortable being with them; and over 35% felt their families would reject them. Stigma and shame surround the diagnosis of HIV, especially because infected women are assumed to have done something of low moral character (i.e., promiscuity or drug use) to become infected. This stigma and shame are major barriers to women's seeking and receiving support and medical care.

Many women who are HIV-infected will choose not to disclose this information to others. Nondisclosure—whether it stems from fear of rejection, concerns about the sorrow that others will experience when they hear this news, or the lack of a reliable social support system even prior to the diagnosis—further enforces the isolation. One study found that 13% of infected women disclosed to no one, and 30% disclosed to only one person (most commonly to a lover, spouse, or friend).

Little attention was given to women with HIV until the transmission of HIV to infants focused attention on women and led to the initial consideration of infected women as "vectors." Much of the research funding with regard to women was concerned with how women could infect others through prostitution or pregnancy. It was not until 12 years into the epidemic that two women's cohort studies were funded by the Centers for Disease Control and Prevention (CDC) and the National Institutes of Health to examine the progression and manifestations of the disease in women, as well as women's psychological and social issues.

By the end of 1996, more than 85,000 U.S. women were reported to have AIDS. The incidence of AIDS is now increasing more rapidly among women than men, and is the fourth leading cause of death among women aged 25–44 years. In 1996, 20% of adults/adolescents with AIDS were women, as compared to 7% in 1985. Of the women reported with AIDS in 1996, 59% are African-American, 19% are Hispanic, 21% are non-Hispanic white, and 1% are other. In 1996, 34% of women with AIDS reported injection-drug use (IDU); 40% heterosexual contact with a partner known to be infected or at risk, 2% with transfusion and 24% with unknown risk. In the past (1994), of those with an unknown risk, 66% were reclassified as having heterosexual contact with an at-risk partner, and 27% had a history of IDU. Over the past 14 years the number of women infected through heterosexual contact has been increasing.

BIOLOGY OF THE DISEASE IN WOMEN, AND MEDICAL CARE FOR WOMEN

HIV disease does have different biological implications for women as compared to men. As evidence of this, the CDC revised the definition of AIDS in 1993 to include cervical cancer. Human papillomavirus and candida infections of the vagina and cervix are common manifestations for females.

Advances in the antiretroviral and antibacterial treatment of HIV infection have resulted in treatments that reduce the morbidity and extend the survival time of people with HIV disease. In 1987, zidovudine (or AZT) was recommended for HIV-seropositive individuals with CD4 cell counts below 200 ml, and in 1990 it was also recommended for those with CD4 cell counts between 200 ml and 500 ml. (CD4 cells are "helper" T cells, important in immunity.)

Several studies comparing HIV-infected men and women have suggested that women have shorter survival times than men do. It is not clear whether this is attributable to lack of HIV treatment or to gender related differences in HIV mortality. In two studies, women with AIDS had shorter survival than men; however, in both studies women were less likely than men to receive antiretroviral therapy, and in another study men were three times more likely to have been offered zidovudine than women. Data from two sites have shown that fewer than half the women with CD4 counts below 200 ml reported taking antiretroviral medicine.

It seems that less medical care may be obtained by women. The AIDS Cost and Services Utilization Survey, conducted in 1991, indicated that males with AIDS resulting from IDU were 20% more likely to be hospitalized than women; that the hospital cost for treating men was higher; and that men received more services. Melnick and colleagues showed that although women appeared to be healthier (significantly higher CD4 cell count) at study entry, they were more likely to die than were men. Surprisingly, among patients without a history of disease progression at study entry, death was the first event reported for more women than men (27.5% vs. 12.2%); the exact manifestations or conditions leading to death were unclear in many cases. These findings may reflect differences in access to health care, in levels of income or education, in life circumstances (49% of women and 27% of men had a history of IDU), or in social support.

PSYCHOSOCIAL ISSUES FOR WOMEN

Drug Use

As noted above, many of the cases of AIDS among women occur among those who have a history of IDU themselves, or those who have partners with a history of IDU. A high rate of HIV infection has also been documented among young adults in the inner city who smoke crack cocaine. Economic pressure to trade sex for drugs, money, or shelter is an underlying cause of sexual risk taking among young women. Drug-using networks may be especially unstable, causing greater possibilities for exposure and fostering risky behaviors (e.g., unsafe sex and needle sharing). For those offering services to HIV-infected women, the issues of substance use cannot be ignored. If infected women with IDU are to be maintained in health care and to be at less risk of infecting others, it is critical that they receive psychological and medical treatment for their IDU concurrently with their HIV treatment. It is even more important that they have a stable source of economic support; safe and private housing; and easy access to competent, nonjudgmental health care.

Issues Related to Children

The diagnosis of HIV infection is especially traumatic when it occurs during pregnancy. The threat to a woman's own life and that of her unborn baby is particularly stressful. IDU during pregnancy further complicates the medical picture for both the woman and the infant. The possibility of bearing an infected child, and the remorse and guilt that accompany that possibility, may weigh heavily on the minds of an infected pregnant woman. In addition, a woman with an infected child will need to obtain medical care and provide home care for the child during a period when she may be experiencing the onset of more serious complications of her own disease. This has raised concerns about whether HIV-infected women neglect their own care while attending to the care of their children. The role of women as caregivers for their uninfected and infected children, for their other family members, and perhaps for infected partners may cause such a high level of demand that the women do not seek out care for themselves. In recent years, the establishment of maternal and child clinics has allowed infected women to obtain care at the same place and time as their children, which improves their chances of obtaining care.

Clearly, women do transmit HIV to infants. In an attempt to control this, a prenatal zidovudine protocol was developed. A study of this protocol showed that prenatal zidovudine reduced the proportion of children infected at birth from 25.5% to 8.3%. Women obviously benefit from carrying and delivering healthy infants, as does society as a whole. However, the objective of delivering healthy infants has led to the suggestion that mandatory testing should take place during the prenatal period. Mandatory testing is seen by some as a legitimate protection of unborn children and by others as a major violation of women's constitutional right to privacy. Because testing is likely to be applied to women with known risks, it further stigmatizes and discriminates against select groups. Informing women that testing is available and that care is available for them and their children may be sufficient to persuade women to be tested. Should testing be undertaken without consent or education, it is less likely that the care provider will be seen as an ally or that the treatment plan will be followed.

Issues surrounding children are often the most painful. Women experience not only fears for their own health, but also great concerns about the traumatic impact on their children. Although women have reported unrelenting worries and even nightmares concerning the future of their infected and their uninfected children in the event of their own death, they often have done little to secure the legal assistance needed to establish their wishes for the long-term custody of their children. There are many reasons for this. Fear of loss of custody of their children is certainly high on the list of concerns. If women believe that by asking for assistance in planning they actually jeopardize their chances of keeping their children, they will probably not ask. In many cases the legal system has been a foe to them in the past, and asking this system for help is unlikely, especially as they become more ill. Moreover, there are usually financial barriers to obtaining legal help, and in many cases women are unclear themselves about who would be willing and able to provide care for their children. Because of these concerns, large numbers of children experience both the loss of their mothers and an unsettling period during which the courts, in the absence of any plans by the mothers, determine the best setting for the children.

Depression

Several studies have examined the prevalence of depressive symptomatology among HIV-infected populations. These studies suggest that depression is not a necessary consequence of the diagnosis of HIV per se, but is primarily related to progressive disease, lack of social support, and prior depressive episodes. However, because these studies have been most often conducted with gay men (who are often of high socioeconomic status), these results may not hold true for infected women.

Studies have also indicated that there is little difference between infected women and comparable controls with regard to depression. Some studies show that over 50% of HIV-positive *and* HIV-negative women score over specified cutoff points on depression inventories. Such rates of depressive symptomatology are extremely high. On the other hand, a group of infected women who were military medical beneficiaries did not show high levels of depression, and their levels were not elevated over those of comparable men. Taken together, these results suggest that not all of those who are HIV-infected also have problems with depression, although as physical effects increase, so does depression. Although findings thus far are speculative, the higher rates reported seem to occur among lower-socioeconomic-status individuals and individuals who are less likely to receive social support or to be in an HIV-supportive network. The high rates among women may reflect the fact that many infected women lead a life of abusive relationships, substance use, and hardship.

Domestic Violence

Domestic violence among HIV-infected women has recently been documented at Cook County Hospital in Chicago, where over 850 infected women have been enrolled in care. A small survey of 43 of these women in 1992 indicated that 35 (81%) had experienced physical abuse and 28% reported current physical abuse. In a subsequent survey of 72 women, 61% reported a history of domestic violence and 54% reported being sexually abused. Moreover, 2% of the deaths of HIV infected women that were non-HIV-related were due to domestic violence. Clearly, those who provide care for women with HIV need to be trained in appropriate methods to assess whether a woman is experiencing an abusive relationship, what the level of danger is to her (and possibly to her children), and what the appropriate referral and intervention may be.

In conclusion, it is fair to say that only in the past few years has attention been paid to the impact of HIV infection on the lives of women. In addressing the needs of women who are infected, the social circumstances, familial pressures and responsibilities, psychological impact, and medical manifestations are different than for infected men. These issues raise the importance of providing medical and community-based services specifically designed for women.

FURTHER READING

Centers for Disease Control and Prevention (CDC). (1995). Update: AIDS among women—United States, 1994. *Morbidity and Mortality Weekly Reports, 44,* 81–84.
Epidemiological data concerning the incidence and prevalence of AIDS in women.

Hellinger, F. J. (1993). The use of health services by women with HIV infection. *Health Services Research, 28,* 543–561.
Data from the first wave of the AIDS Cost and Services Utilization Study, documenting that women with AIDS receive less health care than men.

Melnick, S., Sherer, R., Louis, T. A., Hillman, D., Rodriquez, E. M., Lackman, C., Capps, L., Brown, L. S., Jr., Carlyn, M., Korvick, J. A., & Deyton, L., for the Terry Beirn Community Programs for Clinical Research on AIDS. (1994). Survival and disease progression according to gender of patients with HIV infection: The Terry Beirn Community Programs for Clinical Research on AIDS. *Journal of the American Medical Association, 272,* 1915–1921.
Study comparing disease progression and mortality in men versus women with HIV.

Minkoff, H., DeHovitz, J. A., & Duerr, A. (Eds.). (1995). *HIV infection in women.* New York: Raven Press.
Overview of medical, epidemiological, and service provision issues specific to women.

Pergami, A., Gala, C., Burgess, A., Durbano, F., Zanello, D., Riccio, M., Invernizzi, G., & Catalan, J. (1993). The psychosocial impact of HIV infection in women. *Journal of Psychosomatic Research, 37,* 687–696.
Study of current and past psychiatric morbidity and psychosocial problems of HIV-seropositive asymptomatic women.

Squire, C. (Ed.). *Women and AIDS: Psychological perspectives.* London: Sage.
Description of psychological factors related to HIV risk reduction, reproductive issues and HIV, and service provision.

108

Hormonal Influences on Epileptic Seizures

Marilyn Newsom

*P*aroxysmal disorders occur frequently in medicine. Attacks of angina and disturbances of heart rhythm occur paroxysmally, as do epileptic seizures, migraine headaches, and exacerbation of the symptoms of multiple sclerosis. An understanding of the factors that trigger the occurrence of paroxysmal events at a particular point in time is important to the effective management of such events. In the case of angina, the trigger is an inadequate blood supply to the heart. An understanding of this mechanism has led to a variety of effective treatments, including medical and surgical interventions and lifestyle changes.

The epileptic seizure is the epitome of the neurological paroxysmal disorder. The intermittent nature of epileptic seizures has been recognized for centuries, and for centuries physicians and others have theorized about the triggers responsible for this intermittency. This same question continues to be debated today, and in fact has been described as a "major problem in epileptology."

In modern-day neurology, many epileptics continue to experience at least an occasional seizure, in spite of dramatic improvements in the medical and surgical management of epilepsy. Although it is often possible to identify factors that trigger seizures, such as medical noncompliance, alcohol consumption, or sleep deprivation, many epileptics continue to experience seizures for which no apparent triggers can be identified.

Often, individuals whose seizures are poorly controlled experience "seizure clusters"—short periods of time with frequent seizures, separated by longer seizure-free intervals—and it has been suggested that these seizure clusters may be relatively refractory to control with antiepileptic drugs (AEDs). So in this group of individuals in particular, a search for triggering factors should be especially beneficial.

The clustering of epileptic seizures with menstruation in some female epileptics has been recognized by neurologists for well over 100 years. To this day, however, there is debate over the size of the group of women with menstrual seizures ("catamenial epilepsy," or CE) and over the physiological basis for CE.

664

INCIDENCE OF MENSTRUAL SEIZURES

Estimates of the incidence of CE range from 12% to 75% of women with epilepsy. There are several reasons for this wide range. First, seizures are most often self-reported, and the accuracy of self-reports of the frequency and timing of seizure has been questioned. Second, there are many types of seizures, and the different seizure types may have different triggers. A study that includes a range of seizure types may thus show a low correlation between seizures and hormonal changes, whereas a study including only one seizure type may show a higher correlation. And finally, there is little agreement about the definition of the perimenstrual period, with some studies including in this period of time the 4 days prior to and the 6 days following the onset of menstrual bleeding, and others including only the 2 days prior to and 4 days following the onset of bleeding. Clearly, some standardization of terminology would help to clarify the question of the incidence of CE.

THEORIES OF THE BASIS FOR SEIZURES

In recent years, several theories of the physiological basis for CE have been CE. Changes in sodium metabolism and in fluid retention were once felt to be responsible for various cyclic neurological disorders in women, including catamenial epilepsy. However, studies have failed to show a correlation between body weight (a measure of retained fluid) or sodium metabolism and the incidence of menstrual seizures. (It is interesting to note that in spite of this, the package insert for a commonly prescribed estrogen supplement still carries the warning that the product may lead to fluid retention, which "may make epilepsy worse"!)

A second potential explanation of the association between seizures and hormonal changes is based upon fluctuations in circulating levels of AEDs. Serum levels of AEDs are known to be influenced by the presence of certain other drugs and by other metabolic factors, such as changes in protein levels in the blood. An individual may have a narrow therapeutic range of AED levels, so that a slight reduction in AED level because of a hormonal change may result in loss of seizure control. One early study found no correlation between hormone concentration and AED levels in the blood of epileptic women; a more recent study has shown that blood levels of one AED (phenytoin) decrease more in the perimenstrual period in women with CE than they do in epileptic women who do not have CE. This very important point needs more study. If in fact menstrual seizures are triggered by a decline in circulating levels of an AED, menstrual seizures might be prevented by a premenstrual increase in dose of the AED. The observation that menstrual seizures, like other seizure clusters, may be pharmacoresistant is contrary to this theory.

In recent years, attention has focused on the direct effects of the sex hormones, estrogen and progesterone, and the role of fluctuating hormonal levels in altering seizure thresholds. Dramatic changes in the production of estrogen and progesterone occur during the course of a normal menstrual cycle. In the premenstrual period, when the seizure threshold in women with CE reaches its lowest level, there is a rapid drop in progesterone levels together with an increase in estrogen levels. The sex hormones are widely distributed in brain tissue. Although the influence of sex hormones on the hypothalamic–pituitary axis has long been appreciated, the precise role of these hormones in brain tissue outside the hypothalamic–pituitary axis is unclear. What seems clear is that estrogen and progesterone levels affect neuronal excitability.

Animal studies have demonstrated epileptogenic properties of estrogen and anticonvulsant properties of progesterone. Female rats with ovaries and pituitary glands surgically removed have seizure thresholds that are lowest when estrogen levels are highest, suggesting a direct effect of estrogen on brain tissue outside the hypothalamic–pituitary axis.

Early studies of electroencephalographic (EEG) patterns in epileptic women showed changes in background EEG rhythms that were correlated with phases of the menstrual cycle. In women with epilepsy, seizure frequency increases if estrogen is administered intravenously in the premenstrual period, and EEG epileptiform activity decreases when progesterone is administered intravenously. The EEG changes occur rapidly, suggesting a direct effect on neuronal excitability.

There is an accumulating body of evidence suggesting a direct hormonal effect on the excitability of brain tissue. The real proof of this theory rests on its applicability in a clinical setting. Can our understanding of the mechanism underlying CE lead to more effective treatment of CE? Although clinical evidence is limited, some research indicates that it may. Both high-dose progesterone and oral contraceptives suppress ovulation and show promise as treatments for CE. The hypothalamic hormone gonadotropin-releasing hormone (GnRH) is secreted as a part of a negative feedback loop that also involves the sex hormones. Administration of exogenous GnRH resulted in improved seizure control in 8 of 10 women with CE. Unfortunately, these treatments may be associated with significant side effects, including infertility, and are unlikely to represent ideal solutions for many women with CE.

CONCLUSION

There have been important advances in our understanding of the mechanism of CE in recent years, but much more must be done. Although CE is a relatively common disorder, affecting perhaps 8 of every 100,000 women, it has not played a prominent role in epilepsy research. It is hoped that with an awareness of health care issues unique to women, a greater research effort may be directed toward the understanding and treatment of CE.

FURTHER READING

Duncan, S., Read, C. L., & Brodie, M. J. (1993). How common is catamenial epilepsy? *Epilepsia, 34,* 827–831.
Study concluding that CE is uncommon.

Herzog, A. G. (1995). Progesterone therapy in women with complex partial and secondary generalized seizures. *Neurology, 45,* 1660–1662.
Report suggesting that oral progesterone may be effective in reducing CE in women with complex partial seizures or secondary generalized motor seizures.

Rosciszewska, D. (1987). Epilepsy and menstruation. In A. Hopkins (Ed.), *Epilepsy* (pp. 373–381). London: Chapman and Hall.
Review article.

109

Hypertension

Sylvia Wassertheil-Smoller

*H*ypertension is a major risk factor for stroke and heart disease among both men and women. Women tend to have lower prevalence rates of hypertension than men until age 55, similar rates at ages 55–74, and higher rates after age 75. Blacks have higher rates of hypertension than whites in both sexes.

Fortunately, hypertension is a condition that can be well treated and controlled in most people once it is identified. Progress has been made in the detection, treatment, and control of hypertension over the last two decades, but much remains to be done. Data from the third National Health and Nutrition Examinations Survey (NHANES III) indicated that only 21% of hypertension cases were under control. However, this was double the percentage under control two decades earlier, when only 11% of hypertensives had blood pressures below 140/90 mm Hg.

Blood pressure is a continuous variable, and risk of heart disease, stroke, or death increases with increasing levels of blood pressure. However, it is useful to speak of hypertensives as those persons whose blood pressure is above a specified cutoff point, in order to establish guidelines for treatment. The Joint National Committee on Detection, Evaluation, and Treatment of High Blood Pressure of the National Institutes of Health (NIH) has developed a classification scheme that is widely used to guide clinical decisions. This is shown in Table 109.1. Of course, a person cannot be classified by one measurement alone; thus, the committee's recommendations include confirmation of the blood pressure measurements within a time span dependent on the severity of the levels at screening. Mild hypertensives (those with systolic blood pressure of 140–159 mm Hg and/or diastolic pressure of 90–99 mm Hg) make up about 70% of the hypertensive population, and since nearly 35 million people are affected, mild hypertension presents the biggest public health problem. Mild hypertension should be treated.

There are many drugs available to treat high blood pressure, and mild hypertensives (or Stage 1 hypertensives) can usually have their blood pressure controlled with low doses of one drug. Persons with moderate or severe hypertension may need more than one drug to get their blood pressure under adequate control. Hypertension is a lifelong condition and requires lifelong treatment. Since all drugs have some side effects for some people,

TABLE 109.1. Blood Pressure Classification for Adults 18 Years or Older Not on Antihypertensive Medication

Hypertension[a]	Systolic (mm Hg)	Diastolic (mm Hg)	Follow-up recommendations[b]
Mild (Stage 1)	140–149	90–99	Confirm within 2 months
Moderate (Stage 2)	160–179	100–109	Refer to source of care within 1 month
Severe (Stage 3)	180–209	110–119	Refer to source of care within 1 week
Very severe (Stage 4)	≥ 210	≥ 120	Refer to source of care immediately

Note. National Institutes of Health (1993).
[a]Based on the average of two or more readings at each of two or more visits after an initial screening. Persons whose systolic and diastolic pressures fall in two different categories should be considered in the higher category.
[b]Follow-up after initial screening.

it would be desirable if nonpharmacological means were effective in lowering blood pressure. In fact, lifestyle modifications are the first steps recommended in the treatment of hypertension. If there is inadequate response to such modifications, then drug therapy must be initiated. The objective of the lifestyle modifications is to reduce overall cardiovascular risk, not just the high blood pressure. Thus, the Joint National Committee of the NIH recommends weight reduction, moderation of alcohol intake, regular physical activity, reduction of sodium intake, and cessation of smoking. The two primary dietary interventions that have received the most attention are weight reduction and sodium restriction.

WEIGHT REDUCTION

Overweight persons are more likely to have high blood pressure than those who are at desirable weight. Numerous studies have found that weight reduction lowers blood pressure. Adequate weight loss may be as effective as low-dose drug therapy with a beta-blocker or a diuretic, the two most commonly used drugs as a first step in the treatment of hypertension. Furthermore, when individuals on antihypertensive drugs reduce their weight, they may be able to take lower doses of the drugs. A 10-pound weight loss appears to be necessary for a significant antihypertensive effect for those not on drugs, and a 5-pound loss may be effective in combination with drug therapy. For those not on drugs, the percentage of weight lost is directly related to drop in blood pressure after age, race, sex, and baseline weight are controlled for.

In a planned and structured weight reduction intervention group, nearly 50% of people are able to achieve a 10-pound weight loss by 6 months. Of practical interest, however, is the long-term effect of weight loss. Anyone who has ever tried to diet knows that some or all of the weight lost is sooner or later (and usually sooner) regained. And, in fact, most studies do show considerable recidivism. Nevertheless, even after some weight has been regained, the long-term effects of weight loss on blood pressure continue to be beneficial—not only by lowering blood pressure, but also by lowering blood cholesterol and improving the cardiovascular risk profile. There are also benefits in terms of quality of life. Some studies have found that weight loss in hypertensive patients increases sexual functioning and sexual satisfaction.

It is important to note that women find it harder to lose weight than men, and that certain drugs also may impede weight reduction. Women on beta-blocker therapy lose less weight than those on no drugs and than those taking diuretics. Diuretics enhance weight loss, but some of such weight loss is attributable to decreasing water retention. The point is that weight reduction interventionists need to take into account the drugs patients are taking. If weight loss is slow, a health care provider would do well to prevent a patient from becoming discouraged to the point of giving up, by explaining the relationship between certain drugs and the ability to lose weight.

SODIUM RESTRICTION

The sodium story is not yet complete. Population studies have long shown that in societies with low sodium intake, people have lower blood pressure and also exhibit little rise in blood pressure with age, in contrast to the increase with age found in societies in which people have higher sodium intake. However, intervention studies have shown mixed results. Sodium intake is assessed either through dietary records or, more usually (and perhaps more accurately), through urinary sodium excretion which is a reflection of the intake and is measured in millimoles per day. The average sodium excretion in U.S. residents is about 150 mmol/day (or about 3,400 mg of sodium intake), with women having lower sodium intake then men. Multiple studies of short-term moderate sodium restriction to levels of less than 100 mmol per day (2,300 mg) have shown that systolic blood pressure can be reduced by about 5 mm Hg and diastolic pressure by about 3 mm Hg. Some studies, however, show little effect of sodium reduction on blood pressure unless the sodium is reduced to below a threshold of 70 mmol/day (equivalent to about 1,500 mg of sodium). Such a reduction can have a blood-pressure-lowering effect equivalent to that of low-dose drug therapy, but in free-living populations, reducing sodium is very difficult and may be hard to maintain below these threshold levels. The major sources of sodium in the U.S. diet, which constitute 40% of sodium intake, are bread and rolls, condiments and seasonings, and fast foods. Manufacturers will need to change the composition of such items before hypertensives can reasonably change their intake to levels necessary to reduce blood pressure meaningfully. On the other hand, achieving a daily intake equivalent to less than 100 mmol is feasible and is generally, though not universally, recommended. Fortunately, increasingly educated consumers have already led the food industry to lower both salt and fat in many products and to label the contents. However, recently there has been some evidence that for a general population, a low-salt diet does not protect against future mortality from cardiovascular disease. While a low-salt diet may lower blood pressure, this does not necessarily translate into better health outcomes since other factors may come into play.

There are some individuals who are particularly salt-sensitive, although it is generally not possible to identify them *a priori*. Some subgroups benefit from sodium restriction more than others. Women show greater short-term and long-term blood pressure response to sodium reduction, and so do less obese individuals. Generally, overweight hypertensives are not helped by sodium restriction alone and should undergo a program of weight reduction.

OTHER DIETARY FACTORS

Several other nutrients have been identified, mostly in epidemiological studies, as having a possible role in lowering blood pressure. These include a high intake of dietary potassium, dietary calcium, and dietary magnesium. At least one study has shown that a high potassium intake combined with a low sodium intake is effective in lowering blood pressure among persons with mild hypertension. A high potassium intake is associated with a lower risk of stroke. However, in a randomized trial of the prevention of hypertension among people who had high normal levels of blood pressure initially, it was found that supplements of magnesium, calcium, potassium, or fish oils were not effective in reducing blood pressure; nor was a program of stress management. Only weight reduction was effective in lowering both systolic and diastolic blood pressure, and sodium restriction was modestly effective. It has been shown that limiting alcohol intake to no more than two glasses of wine or 24 ounces of beer a day is beneficial with regard to blood pressure.

EXERCISE

The data on exercise and its long-term effects on blood pressure are sparse, but current evidence indicates that moderate physical activity, such as walking briskly for 30–45 minutes at least three times a week, may lower systolic blood pressure by about 10 mm Hg. Exercise is also helpful, and perhaps essential, in losing and maintaining weight.

BIRTH CONTROL PILLS AND HORMONE REPLACEMENT THERAPY

Women on birth control pills may have a slight increase in blood pressure. If hypertension develops, a woman should stop taking the pills after consulting with her doctor. Smoking is particularly dangerous for women taking oral contraceptives. All women should be encouraged not to smoke.

On average, women on hormone replacement therapy after menopause generally do not experience an increase in blood pressure. However, in some women there may be a marked increase in blood pressure with estrogen. Women who start hormone replacement therapy should have their blood pressure checked more frequently, to determine whether they are among the relatively few who experience such effects. It is also possible that women who take estrogen and progesterone cyclically may have lower blood pressure levels during the estrogen part of the cycle and somewhat higher levels during the progesterone phase.

ANTIHYPERTENSIVE DRUGS

If blood pressure is not controlled with lifestyle modifications, drug therapy needs to be initiated. Various drugs are now available. The first-step drugs recommended by experts are diuretics or beta-blockers, since they have been shown to reduce morbidity and mortality in randomized clinical trials. Beta-blockers tend to work better in white patients, and diuretics tend to work better in black patients. However, other classes of drugs, such as angiotensin-converting enzyme inhibitors, may be used as first-line drugs and have been shown to have some special beneficial effects. Currently, there is some controversy on the use of certain calcium channel blockers as first-line drugs for hypertension. Lifestyle modifications should be used concurrently with drug therapy, particularly since some of the drugs may adversely affect lipids, and this effect may be ameliorated by weight reduction.

ADHERENCE

Dietary and other lifestyle changes involve behavior modification techniques, which are best implemented by interventionists using psychological principles of behavior modification. Adherence is critical to the successful control of blood pressure. The following suggestions may aid clinicians in promoting adherence:

1. Educate patients about high blood pressure and its treatment, and emphasize the need for continued treatment.
2. If prescribing dietary modifications, encourage the use of dietitians, nutritional counselors, or established weight reduction programs.
3. Encourage self-monitoring of blood pressure, if possible.
4. If a patient is to be on drug therapy, try to use once-a-day dosages or to simplify the pill-taking regimen. Suggest ways to remember taking the pills.
5. Pay attention to reported side effects, and change drugs if necessary.
6. Provide feedback on blood pressure levels achieved.
7. Send reminders to ensure that patients keep their blood pressure appointments.

FURTHER READING

Cutler, J. A., Follmann, D., Elliott, P., & Suh, I. (1991). An overview of randomized trials of sodium reduction and blood pressure. *Hypertension, 17*(Suppl. I), I27–I33.
Randomized trials of sodium reduction indicate a blood-pressure-lowering effect of low-sodium diets.

Davis, B. R., Blaufox, M. D., Oberman, A., Wassertheil-Smoller, S., Zimbaldi, N., Cutler, J. A., Kirchner, K., & Langford, H. G. (1993). Reduction in long-term antihypertensive medication requirements: Effect of weight reduction by dietary intervention in overweight persons with mild hypertension. *Archives of Internal Medicine, 153,* 1773–1782.
Weight loss shows blood pressure benefits in the long term, even though some weight is regained.

National Institutes of Health (NIH). (1993, January). *Fifth Report of the Joint National Committee on Detection, Evaluation, and Treatment of High Blood Pressure* (DHHS Publication No. NIH 93-1088). Washington, DC: U.S. Government Printing Office.
The report provides guidelines for detection and treatment of hypertension.

SHEP Cooperative Research Group. (1991). Prevention of stroke by antihypertensive drug treatment in older persons with isolated systolic hypertension. *Journal of the American Medical Association, 265,* 3255–3264.
Persons with isolated systolic hypertension show a marked reduction in stroke with antihypertensive treatment.

Treatment of Mild Hypertension Research Group. (1991). The Treatment of Mild Hypertension Study: A randomized, placebo controlled trial of a nutritional–hygienic regimen along with various drug monotherapies. *Archives of Internal Medicine, 151,* 1413–1423.
Drug therapy is more effective in lowering blood pressure than nonpharmacological means, although weight reduction and to a smaller extent, sodium restriction, do lower blood pressure.

Trials of Hypertension Prevention Collaborative Research Group. (1992). The effects of nonpharmacologic interventions on blood pressure of persons with high normal levels: Results of the Trials of Hypertension Prevention, Phase I. *Journal of the American Medical Association, 267,* 1213–1220.
Supplements of magnesium, calcium, potassium, or fish oils are not effective in lowering blood pressure, nor is a program of stress reduction.

Wassertheil-Smoller, S., Blaufox, M. D., Oberman, A., Langford, H. G., Davis, B. R., & Wylie-Rosett, J., for the TAIM Study Group. (1992). The TAIM Study: Adequate weight loss alone and combined with drug therapy in the treatment of mild hypertension. *Archives of Internal Medicine, 152,* 131–136.
The study shows that a 10 pound weight loss may be equivalent to low-dose drug therapy in lowering blood pressure, and also potentiates the effects of drugs.

Wassertheil-Smoller, S., Oberman, A., Blaufox, M. D., Davis, B., & Langford, H. G. (1992). The Trial of Antihypertensive Interventions and Management (TAIM) Study: Final results with regard to blood pressure, cardiovascular risk, and quality of life. *American Journal of Hypertension, 5,* 37–44.
Weight reduction is more effective than sodium restriction in lowering blood pressure, and improves quality of life; sodium restriction in overweight individuals is not effective.

110

The Immune System

Henry N. Claman

*T*he major function of the immune system is to provide protection against damage from microbes (mainly bacteria), viruses, fungi, and parasites. We know this to be true because of two general situations in which the immune system is defective or damaged, so that the body cannot defend itself against microbes. First, in those rare instances in which the immune system fails to develop properly for genetic reasons, microbes that often cause disease but are not usually devastating (such as strep or staph) can become lethal. The second situation occurs in AIDS, where the immune system is itself the target of HIV. As the illness progresses, the immune system is damaged to the point that even seemingly inoffensive microbes such as *Pneumocystis carinii* (PC), which never bother people with normal immune systems, can produce a fatal illness—PC pneumonia.

Before going into details of the immune system, I should point out that a number of other protective barriers and mechanisms outside the immune system also shield us from pathogenic (disease-producing) organisms. These include the skin itself, saliva, and tears (which have antimicrobial activity). The lining of the gastrointestinal tract has various nonimmune strategies for protecting us from all the bacteria that normally live in the lumen of the gut. In the upper and lower respiratory tracts, we also have mechanisms protecting us from airborne microbes; these range from simple coughing and sneezing to sophisticated microscopic hairs within the bronchi, which sweep out undesired materials.

However, the immune system has a number of characteristics that are different from the functions of these barriers. The immune system has evolved to the point where it can specifically attack a microbe, where it can show specific memory, so that it can respond even more dramatically to a second assault by the same organism; and where it can be mobilized to reach the entire body even after a local assault. At the same time, it is crucial that the immune system only attack external agents and refrain from reacting against the body itself. In other words, the immune system must recognize and distinguish self from not-self. It must react against foreign (not-self) molecules, and ignore the self's molecules. If it gets deregulated and starts to react against the self's molecules, then autoimmunity ensues.

MECHANISMS

The machinery of the immune system basically inheres in a collection of cells called lymphocytes, and in their cell products, called antibodies and cytokines. There are two broad classes of lymphocytes. T lymphocytes arise in the thymus (located behind the breastbone); B lymphocytes are born mainly in the bone marrow. T cells and B cells exist together in various parts of the body, such as the blood, lymph nodes, spleen, tonsils, adenoids, lining of the gut, and respiratory tract.

The most difficult concept to understand is that each lymphocyte, T or B, is preprogrammed to respond to a specific microbial agent, even before that microbe approaches the body. Thus, we each have a small set of B cells (called a clone) able to make antibodies to poliovirus type III, and another clone of B cells able to make immune antibodies to the toxin produced by diphtheria bacilli. We have these B cells even if we never meet poliovirus or diphtheria bacilli. Antibodies are protein molecules made by B cells and are capable of circulating throughout the body through the blood and other body fluids. Antibodies are particularly effective in neutralizing viruses when they are outside body cells, and antibodies can also neutralize bacteria and bacterial toxins, which are also extracellular.

When poliovirus appears (either as a vaccine or as the natural, "wild type," infection), the antipolio clone of cells is activated, and it produces antibodies that are capable of neutralizing the virus. (At the same time, the clone of cells specific for making diphtheria antitoxin is not disturbed.) Furthermore, when this antipolio clone is activated, it produces additional copies of the same cells, thus enlarging the clone. If a further dose of polio appears, it will be disposed of even faster than was the first dose. This explains why some immunization programs include "booster" exposures for greater efficiency.

T lymphocytes are somewhat more subtle. They are more effective against viruses that have reached and invaded a body cell (where antibodies are kept out), and against foreign tissue and organ grafts. T cells also consist of small clones, each able to respond to specific foreign substances. For instance, each of us has a clone of T cells able to react against the PCP organism, and another clone of T cells able to react against a kidney graft from an unrelated donor. T cells either can carry out their activities themselves directly, or can secrete one or more soluble substances called lymphokines, which do the work. (T cells do not produce antibodies.)

Immune functions may be helpful or harmful, depending upon the situation. If damage is about to occur via invasion of a foreign harmful microbe, the immune system's function is beneficial. If the immune system is about to destroy a much-needed kidney or liver graft, its function in this respect will be detrimental. If something in the recognition system goes awry and the immune system begins to react against itself (which it should not), then autoimmunity exists.

ANTIBODY PRODUCTION AND SEXUAL STATUS

It is now quite clear that in experimental animals studies, females are better antibody producers than males. In brief, if two groups of genetically identical mice, one male and one female, are immunized with a standard dose of antigen (a specific stimulus for the immune system, such as tetanus toxoid), the females will make more antibodies than the males. The difference is not enormous, but it is quite real. Moreover, research has shown that this difference is indeed related to the female and male hormonal systems. Female mice that have had their ovaries removed, have been treated with testosterone, and are then immunized produce amounts of antibodies characteristic of males; similarly, castrated males treated with estrogens and then immunized produce the higher levels of antibodies seen in normal immunized females.

Two questions come to mind immediately. First, is the female "superiority" in making antibodies seen in humans as well? This really cannot be easily answered, as we are all so genetically diverse that even with large families to study, it would be difficult to answer the question. Second, is there a negative side to this "superiority in antibody production" in females? Does it relate to the fact that many autoimmune diseases, in which antibodies to the self (autoantibodies) are detrimental, are more common in women than in men? Again, this cannot be answered with certainty in humans, but in several mouse models of autoimmunity it does seem that the female predilection to disease is correlated with the female's ability to produce more autoantibodies than the male.

THE IMMUNOLOGICAL PARADOX OF PREGNANCY

How does a pregnant woman retain and nourish a fetus for 9 months when the fetus can be considered to be a "half-foreign tissue graft" because 50% of its genes come from the father? More specifically, how can the fetus thrive when a skin graft or a kidney graft from the father placed on the mother during pregnancy is rejected in less than 2 weeks without any damage to the baby? The answers are complex. This should not be surprising, because it is so very important for genetic diversity to be maintained in the population that more than one mechanism should be developed (in "fail-safe" terms) to permit or even encourage survival of offspring who are genetically different from their parents.

In ordinary pregnancy, the mother's B cells can make antibodies to the paternal antigens from the fetus, but special mechanisms have evolved to make sure that these antibodies do not cross the placenta to cause fetal damage. Conversely, there are complex mechanisms that prevent maternal T cells from ever reacting against paternal antigens from the fetus. Finally, there is an intriguing theory that some form of maternal immune response against the fetus actually fosters its development. Certainly, the animal husbandrists tell us that inbred matings (in which there is no genetic difference among mother, father, and offspring) produce smaller litters and more "runts" than do outbred matings. We still do not know details about the nature of any possible beneficial mechanisms that promote genetically disparate pregnancies.

FURTHER READING

Claman, H. N. (1987). The biology of the immune response. *Journal of the American Medical Association, 258,* 2834–2840.
An introductory article in an entire issue devoted to allergy and immunology.

Claman, H. N. (1993). *The immunology of human pregnancy.* Totowa, NJ: Humana Press.
Both this book and the 1987 article are written for physicians, but a fair amount can be understood by others.

Scientific American. (1993, September).
The entire issue is about immunology—basic and clinical.

111

Immunity and Behavior

Mark L. Laudenslager

The discipline of psychoneuroimmunology (PNI) suggests that the central nervous system (CNS), behavior (an obvious result of the activity of the CNS), and immune system regulation are highly interrelated. The field of PNI has grown by leaps and bounds over the last decade; unfortunately, in many instances PNI has largely neglected how these relationships might pose unique problems for women's health. It is well established that the immune response and its regulation represent an interesting example of sexual dimorphism. This dimorphism is likely to have important implications for the emerging field of PNI. The following overview is not intended to be either comprehensive or inclusive; rather, it indicates the state of the field of PNI as it relates to issues of direct relevance for women's health.

Two primary modes of communication exist between the CNS and the immune system: direct neural innervation of lymphoid organs by the sympathetic nervous system, and circulating humoral and neurotransmitter substances that are present in the blood and able to interact with circulating lymphocytes. It is now widely accepted that these communications are bidirectional. Just as behavioral factors may affect immune regulation, the immune response and its components may also affect behavior. For example, the rather unpleasant sensations of fatigue, altered sleep patterns, and impaired cognitive processing that accompany the flu are associated with immune mediators released in association with immunological activation during defense against the virus.

MORBIDITY AND MORTALITY IN MEN VERSUS WOMEN

The field of PNI has only begun to explore the important interactions of gender and immunity–behavior relationships. Women as a group live longer than men, but women report greater numbers of medical complaints for which they seek treatment. An important aspect of the apparent increased morbidity among women may simply be their greater sensitivity or willingness to report somatic complaints. Another potential contributor to the increased morbidity among women may be differences in immunoregulation related to female sex hormones.

Women are at far greater risk than men for autoimmune disorders. Autoimmune diseases reflect instances in which the immune system has failed to discriminate self from nonself and turns its activity against the self. Autoimmune processes such as systemic lupus erythematosus (SLE) (90% of cases), myasthenia gravis (75% of the cases), and multiple sclerosis (60% of cases) occur more frequently in women than in men. Men, on the other hand, are more likely to be affected by conditions that reflect CNS insults, such as dyslexia, seizure disorders, conduct disorder in childhood, schizophrenia, and severe mental retardation. These disorders have less clear or direct immune system origins.

In contrast to the apparent increased morbidity of infectious illnesses in women (though it is recognized that many hidden illnesses may go unreported among males), and the higher incidence of autoimmune diseases, women are often at far *lower* health risk after experiencing a significant psychosocial stressor. For example, men between the ages of 50 and 70 are at greater risk for all-cause mortality following loss of a spouse than are women of the same age. Gender differences in morbidity and mortality following loss are absent in both younger and older age groups, however; thus this is not a simple one-to-one relationship, but interacts significantly with age. In addition, one might ask whether women are more likely to attend to somatic complaints than men, and consequently to receive more timely medical care. Or perhaps other factors are present. It is well known that the presence of a social support network mitigates the negative consequences of many stressors; perhaps women may be more likely to be a part of and utilize a social support network than men. With changing trends in the use of social support by men, some of these gender differences may disappear, at least to the extent that social support mitigates the behavioral and physiological impacts of social stressors.

EFFECTS OF WOMEN'S MULTIPLE ROLES ON HEALTH

For women between the ages of 18 and 60, multiple roles (job and family responsibilities) represent a preeminent stressor. A recent U.S. Department of Labor survey, Working Women Count!, indicates that multiple roles are considered one of the greatest stressors for women in the labor force. Current stress models would suggest that the increase in stress levels associated with role overload would be associated with increased health problems; however, this may not be the case for some employed women. The impact of stress associated with employment is extraordinarily complicated for women in comparison to men. Little is definitely known as yet regarding the relationship of role overload and multiple roles to immune regulation for women. Nevertheless, discussion of some observations regarding the relationship of employment to other aspects of health helps document the complexity with which PNI is faced.

Support for the complexity of the relationship between women's multiple roles and their health is reflected in the observation that some employed women may be physically and mentally healthier than their *un*employed counterparts (note that a homemaker not seeking employment is distinguished from an *un*employed woman seeking employment). Role satisfaction, self-esteem, ability to maintain perspective, and a number of other factors have been suggested to contribute to these differences. If we disregard gender, the group with the best self-reported health scores consists of those who are employed, married, and parents. Men actually report fewer illness and health complaints than do women; however, this may reflect the reporting bias discussed earlier. Employment may preclude the ability to take a day off for a minor illness such as a cold, and this may inflate the reports of the unemployed group. If risk for cardiovascular disease is considered, a moderate amount of overtime is associated with a *reduced* risk for myocardial infarction (MI) in men, but with an *increased* risk for MI in women. Interestingly, when overtime hours (>40 hours/week) are compared between men and women, men consistently report more overtime hours than women in the same profession. These observations lend credence to a sex difference in impact of employment outside of the home.

A likely contributor to the greater impact of outside employment is the aforementioned role overload, particularly for women with children. When stress levels and health behaviors were assessed in mothers with very young children (between the ages of 2 and 11 months) who were employed full-time or were homemakers, the working mothers scored significantly higher on perceived stress than the homemakers. In addition to higher stress, the employed women reported fewer health-promoting behaviors. This may have been a choice to reduce the burdens of role overload; that is, the working women may have sacrificed health-promoting behaviors such as exercise in order to find additional time for other things. The relationship of such behaviors as adequate sleep, good nutrition, and exercise to immune function is well known.

SPECIFIC BEHAVIOR PATTERNS AND ILLNESS

The Type A behavior pattern, which is closely tied to the expression of anger, has been associated with increased risk for cardiovascular illness. When the characteristic of cynical hostility (e.g., "People are out to get me, and I intend to get them before they get me") was studied in medical students, cynically hostile male students had elevated serum cholesterol and reduced high-density lipoprotein (HDL) cholesterol, whereas their female counterparts showed the opposite pattern—lower cholesterol and higher HDL levels. Cynically hostile females were more likely to participate in routine exercise programs, whereas cynically hostile males tended to consume greater amounts of alcohol than males not rated cynically hostile. The contribution of health-promoting behaviors to stress–health relationships and potential gender interactions must be recognized and subjected to increased empirical attention. Similar research strategies in which immune regulation is the dependent variable do not presently exist.

There have been recent reports of a Type C personality pattern, which is associated with a greater risk for cancer. A Type C individual is characterized as unable to express emotions, particularly negative emotions; in contrast a Type A individual is quite likely to express negative emotions, particularly anger and hostility. Type C individuals are stoics who feel that they have little or no control in their world. The prognosis for cancer patients, both men and women, who possess this trait is typically poor. "Fatalism" is a similar behavior pattern associated with an expectancy for predetermined negative outcomes. This "fatalistic" pattern has also been associated with poor prognoses in individuals diagnosed with AIDS, a disease of the immune system. Other observations have indicated that the expression of both positive and negative emotions is associated with modulation of certain immune parameters. Do these styles simply represent different names for the same underlying concept and pathophysiology? Unfortunately, distinctions between the Type C pattern, fatalism, and pessimism on the one hand and the regulation of the immune system on the other, as well as their interactions with gender, have not been addressed directly.

THE ROLE OF SEX STEROIDS IN IMMUNE MODULATION

If we accept for the moment that the immune response can be modulated by emotional states (e.g., grief associated with loss), let us return to routes through which these interactions might occur. Obvious mediators in immune differences between men and women are the sex steroids. Sex steroids are well known to modulate immune function both *in vitro* (in the test tube) and *in vivo* (in the individual). A classic example of immune modulation by sex steroids occurs during pregnancy, which represents an important challenge for the immune system of the mother. Since the fetus is not isolated from maternal immune interactions, as was once thought, the fetus should be recognized as foreign by the immune system. Fortunately, a number of hormonal and immunological processes protect the fetus during pregnancy. It is worth noting that women with autoimmune disorders, such as rheumatoid arthritis (as many as 73% of patients), SLE (roughly 60% of patients), and allergies, experience remission during pregnancy. However, other women experience exacerbations in these diseases during pregnancy; this indicates the difficulties of disentangling the systems with which we are concerned.

The availability of strains of mice that demonstrate spontaneous autoimmune diseases similar to SLE has permitted further experimental investigation of the role of sex steroids in the pathophysiology of autoimmune diseases. In brief, treatment of SLE-prone female mice with the male sex steroid testosterone will delay or abolish the incidence of disease. Animal studies suggest that androgen deficiency, rather than estrogen availability, is critical in the development of many of these autoimmune processes. However, the use of sex steroids in treatment of autoimmune processes in humans has proven relatively ineffective. A "permissive" role for the sex steroids seems likely, as they seen not to be a necessary condition for the expression of the disease.

Immune Regulation and the Menstrual Cycle

What is the relationship between immune regulation and the menstrual cycle? The immune system is composed of a variety of different types of lymphocytes (white blood cells), including B cells (cells that produce antibodies) and T cells (cells with regulatory, recognition, and destructive functions). T cells can be further divided into several different subtypes (e.g., natural killer cells, helper T cells, suppressor T cells, and killer T cells). The investigation of the relative number of these various lymphocytes in peripheral blood has indicated some interesting relationships to plasma hormone level in females. For example, the number of these subtypes in peripheral blood is highly correlated with plasma hormone level, but there do not appear to be differential changes in these parameters associated with laboratory stressors at different times of the menstrual cycle. There may be menstrual fluctuations in these cell types in the absence of stressor exposure, although this is not uniformly accepted. Finally, patterns of lymphocyte cell types change from pre- to postmenopause.

Self-reported symptoms in both autoimmune and infectious illness also appear to vary with phases of the menstrual cycle. Individuals with rheumatoid arthritis report variations in symptom severity in association with menstrual phase. Symptoms of multiple sclerosis may worsen premenstrually for some women. In fact, many symptoms women describe as changing in conjunction with the menstrual cycle appear to be associated with immunological function. Respiratory, skin, gastrointestinal, and genitourinary infection symptoms tend to cluster during the perimenstrual phase as opposed to midcycle. However, when perceived stress and menstrual distress are controlled for, the effect of phase is eliminated. This suggests that a general relationship exists between distress and infectious symptoms and the menstrual cycle. A similar positive relationship among scores on depression scales, perceived stress and daily hassles, and self-reported illness symptoms has been noted in female medical students.

Infectious disease is associated with the growth of agents such as viruses, fungi, or bacteria. Immunological resistance in normally cycling women to *Candida albicans* (the infectious agent in recurrent vaginitis) is lowest during the luteal phase of the cycle, when progesterone levels in the plasma are highest. Isolation of *C. albicans* from vaginal swabs was greater from depressed subjects (82%) than from nondepressed controls (22%), suggesting the additional impact of emotional state on this relationship. In many studies, one must be cautious about self-reports of disease symptomatology, as these do not always correspond with verifiable infection or severity of infection. This fact does not, however, detract from the reality of the discomfort experienced by an individual.

Anovulatory women or women with irregular menstrual cycles were reported in one article to be at lower risk for breast cancer. This report argued that high levels of progesterone contribute to the increased risk for breast disease. Later, a controversial report suggested that breast tumor excision during the follicular phase (i.e., rising estrogen levels) in patients with cancer-positive axillary lymph nodes was associated with greater risk for cancer recurrence than was the removal of tumors at other times in the menstrual cycle. A more recent report with a smaller sample in which plasma hormone levels were available for verification of cycle phase indicated no relationship among menstrual phase, surgical removal of tumors, and prognosis for women with primary mammary carcinoma. In rodents, elevated estradiol levels and low progesterone levels in ovariectomized subjects, or implantation of tumors during the estrous phase (analogous to the follicular phase in humans, when estrogen levels are increasing), increased susceptibility to metastases of implanted mammary tumors. An important factor, often disregarded in the consideration of the influences of sex steroids on tumor metastases, is that sex steroids alter hemodynamics and peripheral blood flow. Changes in blood flow could directly affect the metastatic process, independently of an immunological mechanism.

Immune Regulation and Oral Contraceptives

It is not surprising to note that the use of oral contraceptives (OCs) is associated with changes in immune regulation. For example, both the numbers and activity of natural killer cells (immune cells partly responsible for control of viral infections and early control over tumor development) are reduced in healthy young women using OCs. Women using OCs also have a greater incidence of self-reported illness, such as gastrointestinal upset and common-cold-like symptoms. In contrast, use of OCs has been associated with an apparent delay or mitigation of autoimmune processes such as rheumatoid arthritis; however, OCs are ineffective in alleviating the symptoms once an autoimmune disease is diagnosed.

It is obvious that simple explanations of relationships between immune and hormonal regulation do not exist. The reader should also be aware of an important tenet in PNI: There are no single measures of immune function that reflect on the system as a whole. The immune system is well designed, with numerous redundancies; otherwise, we would require immediate medical care every time we experienced a mild upset. It is likely that long-term and chronic stressors place the immune system in greatest peril.

SUMMARY

In summary, sex steroid fluctuations associated with normal reproductive cycles may be associated with changes in immune system parameters, infectious disease incidence, symptom reporting, and autoimmune processes in women. A number of health behaviors may also contribute to reported gender differences (e.g., women may participate in healthier behavior patterns than men). Women do experience a number of stressors not generally experienced (or at least expressed) by men, such as role overload, that may contribute to their risk for disease. However, women as a group live longer than men. The causal processes contributing to the enhanced longevity of women remain as important challenges for the field of health psychology in general and PNI specifically.

FURTHER READING

Ader, R., Cohen, N., & Felten, D. (Eds.). (1991). *Psychoneuroimmunology.* New York: Academic Press.

An edited book containing reviews and technical chapters by leading researchers in the field of PNI. Topics covered include innervation of lymphoid tissue, hormone regulation of the immune response, and implications of PNI in HIV infection.

Glaser, R., & Kiecolt-Glaser, J. (Eds.). (1994). *Human stress and immunity.* New York: Academic Press.

An edited book with a primary focus on human studies of PNI; however, some animal research is included.

Grossman, C. (1991). Sex steroid regulation of autoimmunity. *Journal of Steroid Biochemistry and Molecular Biology, 40,* 649–659.

Technical review of the impact of sex steroids on autoimmune disease, written by one of the leaders in the field.

Gruman, J., & Chesney, M. (Eds.). (1995). Superhighways for disease [Special issue]. *Psychosomatic Medicine, 57,* 207–283.

Special journal issue that addresses a number of behavioral components of the health–behavior relationship, ranging from social support to PNI.

Maier, S. F., Watkins, L. R., & Fleshner, M. (1994). Psychoneuroimmunology: The interface between behavior, brain, and immunity. *American Psychologist, 49,* 1004–1017.

An excellent review of the brain–immune interactions that raises some interesting notions regarding the phenomenology of feeling sick.

Theorell, T. (1991). Psychosocial cardiovascular risks: On the double loads in women. *Psychotherapy and Psychosomatics, 55,* 81–89.

Discussion of the multiple roles of working women as they relate to health issues.

Wobbes, T., Thomas, C. M., Segers, M. F., Peer, P. G., Bruggink, E. D., & Beex, L. V. (1994). The phase of the menstrual cycle has no influence on the disease-free survival of patients with mammary carcinoma. *British Journal of Cancer, 69,* 599–600.

Article addressing earlier observations of the relationship between timing of mastectomy and menstrual phase.

112

Lupus

M. Karen Newell
Claire Coeshott

*T*he immune system functions to discriminate self from nonself. As Claman has described in his chapter of this volume, the immune cells provide protection from invading pathogens. In addition, the system provides an immune surveillance, so that if the self's tissues change (e.g., become altered), such changes are recognized and the tissues removed as though they were foreign. By definition, an autoimmune disease occurs when there is a breakdown in recognition and the immune system is no longer able to distinguish self from nonself. As a consequence, there is an attack on certain of the body's own tissues. Three major aspects of these events are discussed in this chapter. First, there is a greater frequency of autoimmune disease in women; second, the incidence of this disease is higher in people with particular genetic backgrounds; and third, stress and the endocrine system play a role in the incidence and amelioration of autoimmune disease.

The prototypical autoimmune diseases are systemic lupus erythematosus (SLE) and rheumatoid arthritis (RA). Because SLE reflects many of the features characteristic of autoimmunity, this chapter focuses primarily on SLE, but a brief discussion of RA is included at the conclusion. SLE is characterized by production of autoantibodies—that is, antibodies directed against the self's tissue—and by the consequent damage to multiple organ systems. The precise etiology of this disease is unknown. However, one frequently utilized model is that an environmental trigger acts upon a genetically susceptible individual, resulting first in manifestations that include increased levels of nonspecific antibodies, and later in a subset of autoantibodies to a defined set of the self's molecules (DNA, histones, etc.); the presence of these autoantibodies gives rise to a variety of pathologies.

CHARACTERISTICS AND PATHOLOGICAL MANIFESTATIONS OF LUPUS

Lupus means "wolf" in Latin, and *erythematosus* describes "redness." Lupus as a general rule is manifested in two forms: discoid (or cutaneous) lupus erythematosus or SLE.

Patients with the discoid type have skin involvement but normal internal organs. (Since the discoid form of lupus is not discussed further in this chapter, we will use "SLE" and "lupus" interchangeably hereafter.) SLE is classified as an autoimmune rheumatic disease and is a chronic inflammatory disease (i.e., it causes irritation with pain and swelling) that can affect virtually every part of the body. Nevertheless, patients for the most part experience symptoms in only a few target organs. Symptoms frequently associated with disease include arthralgia, fever, arthritis, skin rashes, anemia, kidney involvement, photosensitivity, hair loss, and mouth ulcers. Most patients will not experience all these symptoms, but rather a subset of them. Symptoms in most organs that will be affected will be evidenced in the first 2 years after diagnosis. The majority of lupus patients have skin and joint involvement and complain of aches, pain, and fatigue. To facilitate diagnosis in light of the variability in symptoms and nature of the disease, the American College of Rheumatology has compiled a list of criteria that includes the symptoms mentioned above, as well as blood tests to determine the presence of autoantibodies. Patients have to meet certain minimum requirements (usually 4 criteria from the list of 20) for a physician to be able to make a diagnosis of SLE.

GENDER AS A RISK FACTOR IN LUPUS AND AUTOIMMUNITY

The frequency of SLE is nine times greater in women than in men. Furthermore, it has been estimated that 1 in every 500 women is affected by the disease. These observations have led scientists to believe that sex hormones affect or influence certain factors in immunity. This notion is supported by the facts that the peak incidence of SLE occurs during the reproductive years and that the use of oral contraceptives can exacerbate the disease. There are certainly multiple factors in addition to sex hormones that contribute to the risk of developing the disease; these include a susceptible genetic background, environmental factors, abnormalities in B or T lymphocytes, and defective regulation of immune responsiveness. However, the strongest risk factor for the development of SLE is the female gender.

Much of the evidence for the influence of endocrine (gonadal) hormones on the immune system has been derived from observations supported clinically and scientifically. These include the fact that as a group men respond less well to a variety of foreign pathogens and succumb more readily than women to a variety of infections, in terms of both earlier onset and greater severity of a given infection. However, clinicians have noted for decades that women are more susceptible to autoimmune disease than men. Despite the clear evidence of gender-related differences in immune function, it was not until 1972 that the Arthritis Foundation issued a directive to seek an explanation for the "remarkable female to male ratio in systemic lupus." It is now apparent that one of the primary reasons for female susceptibility to SLE is increased immune responsiveness, particularly in antibody production. On the other hand, this increased immunocapacity may also account at least in part for the greater longevity of females on the whole.

LUPUS AND PREGNANCY

Once considered to be ill advised, pregnancy is now clearly an option available to women with SLE. Certain risks are of course associated with pregnancy in SLE patients, although most now appear to be clinically manageable. Studies of the relationship between SLE and pregnancy have shown that pregnancy can either affect lupus patients adversely or, in some cases, can have beneficial effects. In addition, miscarriage rates among lupus patients are high. A subgroup of autoantibodies, known as antiphospholipid antibodies, has been associated with these high miscarriage rates.

As the name suggests, antiphospholipid antibodies are directed predominantly against phospholipids, which make up the membranes of cells. These antibodies can cause recurrent fetal loss and are associated with thrombotic episodes, which can be manifested as fetal loss, stroke, or deep vein thrombosis. Simply stated, the antiphospholipid antibodies appear to promote problems related to clotting mechanisms. Some women who experience recurrent fetal loss have been found to have these antibodies without any other symptoms of lupus. This autoimmune disorder in the absence of other lupus symptoms may be a form of primary antiphospholipid syndrome.

SUSCEPTIBILITY IN GENETIC BACKGROUNDS

SLE frequently clusters in families, although for many years no classical pattern of inheritance was obvious. It was only after advances in studies of the genetics of the immune system and molecular biological techniques were made that the actual genetic markers became apparent. Over time, the clinical heterogeneity of the disease and a variety of disease subsets associated with different autoantibody subsets were recognized. Basic studies using mouse models, as well as clinical epidemiological studies, eventually made it possible to map at least one genetic contribution onto a cluster of gene products known as the major histocompatibility complex (MHC). However, it is important to note that, on the whole, SLE is highly complex and is now recognized to be multigenic.

Over 50 years ago, scientists discovered that certain molecules were centrally important in discrimination of self from nonself, especially for graft rejection. These molecules are expressed on all nucleated cells in the body and are termed the MHC. Perhaps, in retrospect, it is not surprising that the molecules allowing T cells to recognize and discriminate self from nonself are key elements in a disease characterized by failure of that function. In fact, increased frequencies of some of the molecules in the MHC complex (termed the human leukocyte antigen [HLA] complex in humans) correspond with expression of disease. The multiple genes of the MHC region are inherited in a Mendelian codominant fashion. That is, there is an equal contribution from each parent, and the type of MHC molecules expressed will represent a linked cluster of unique genes. In addition, hereditary deficiencies of a second group of molecules, the complement components, are found to increase disease susceptibility. These components also map genetically onto the MHC.

Understanding of the MHC's associations with SLE has closely followed the understanding of the structure and function of the MHC molecules themselves. MHC molecules have been categorized into subsets termed MHC Class I, which is expressed on all nucleated cells, and MHC Class II, which is generally expressed only on cells involved in immune function. The MHC contribution to SLE appears to come primarily from MHC Class II (or HLA Dr) molecules. These molecules play a particularly important role in the activation of $CD4^+$ T cells (a helper/inducer group of T cells). Antigens, presumably foreign pathogens, associated with MHC molecules are recognized and in that form by receptors on T cells. $CD4^+$ T cells become activated when the T cells recognize and respond to antigens associated with MHC Class II. When a T cell recognizes MHC Class II and antigen on a B lymphocyte, "help" is provided by the T cell, so that the B cell makes an antibody. Because autoantibody production is a primary characteristic of SLE, it is not surprising that part of the genetic basis for SLE has been mapped onto the MHC.

STRESS AND THE PSYCHOLOGY OF LUPUS

As discussed elsewhere in this volume (see especially Laudenslager's chapter), stress and psychological state influence the immune system and, as a consequence, autoimmune diseases such as SLE. Mental changes occurring in conjunction with other manifestations of SLE were first documented at least 100 years ago. More recently, it has become apparent that CNS involvement can occur as part of the disease process. Thus, psychological manifestations are involved in SLE in two ways: Stress itself may be a predisposing factor contributing to the onset of the disease, and CNS involvement and psychological manifestations may be part of the disease process. In addition, some of the drugs used to treat SLE can cause psychological symptoms. Finally, and not surprisingly, the patient's and family's concerns about the disease and the likely prognosis, and attempts to cope with varying symptoms, may cause depression and other problems of a psychological nature.

Psychiatric Manifestations

It is beyond the scope of this chapter to discuss in detail all psychiatric manifestations of SLE. However, it is reported that most patients with SLE do develop some neuropsychiatric problems, which range in severity from adjustment disorders (depression, withdrawal, etc.) to psychosis and personality disorders.

Recent work has examined the role of certain autoantibodies in the development of psychosis. These antibodies are specific for phosphoproteins associated with ribosomes in the cellular cytoplasm. Although there are no conclusive data showing that these autoantibodies cause psychiatric effects, they may serve as markers of lupus psychosis, and distinguish SLE-induced psychiatric disease from that caused by other processes. In one study, a patient with high levels of these antibodies in conjunction with severe psychosis was treated with a regimen of immunosuppressive drugs. Following treatment, both the antibody levels and the symptoms of psychosis were greatly decreased.

Other antibodies directed against neuronal components have been documented in SLE, and immune complexes (antibodies combined with their appropriate antigens) have been found deposited in the choroid plexus in the brain in much the same way as they are observed deposited in the kidneys in lupus nephritis. Thus, it is likely that at least some CNS involvement in lupus is a consequence of antibody activity and has a true pathological basis.

Adjustment of Lifestyle

The unpredictability of disease progression in SLE can make emotional and psychological adjustment particularly challenging. As mentioned earlier, the symptoms manifested by a particular patient during the first 2 years after diagnosis will in general predominate throughout the course of the illness. However, neither the patient nor the physician can predict the extent of episodes or the sites where the disease will strike next (kidney, skin, joints, etc.). Support from family members and/or close friends can be critical in a patient's ability to maintain a stable and optimistic attitude when faced with fluctuations in the severity and symptoms of the disease.

Again, it should be noted that some of the drugs used to treat SLE have been reported to cause or exacerbate psychiatric complications. In addition, other side effects of certain medications, though physical in nature, may require extensive psychological adjustment and/or lifestyle alteration. In particular, the weight gain associated with use of steroid therapy may negatively affect the patient's self-image. Coping mechanisms useful in such situations may include changes in diet, emphasizing good nutrition combined with lowered caloric intake; an exercise regimen compatible with disease symptomatology; and increased awareness that societal emphasis on a particular physical appearance (especially for women) as the desired norm does not in any way reflect the true value of a particular individual.

RHEUMATOID ARTHRITIS

Although the focus of this chapter has been on SLE as a prototype for autoimmune disease, RA is also a widespread, chronic inflammatory disease that affects women much more often than men. It is beyond the scope of this chapter to include an in-depth discussion of RA. However, it should be noted that this disease is also autoimmune in nature, and that its progressive nature can lead to joint destruction and varying degrees of incapacitation. The diagnostic factor of RA is rheumatoid factor, a complex of antibodies that binds to a portion of another antibody. In other words, rheumatoid factor is a different form of an autoantibody—an antibody against one's own antibodies. Although this disease is differentiated from lupus by the presence of rheumatoid factor and the manner in which joint involvement occurs, like lupus, it can be considered to be systemic in nature; it has many other features in common with lupus as well, including variability between patients and fluctuations in remissions and exacerbations. The cause of and cure for RA are not known, but treatments to manage the disease and control the inflammatory process are available (see Zautra's, Roth's, and Wisocki's chapters for details).

FURTHER READING

Aladjem, H. (1985). *Understanding lupus*. New York: Scribner's.
A good resource about SLE for the health care professional.

Lahita, R. G. (1992). *Systemic lupus erythematosus* (2nd ed.). Edinburgh: Churchill Livingstone.
A resource about SLE for the health care professional.

Moore, M. E., McGrory, C. H., & Rosenthal, R. S. (1991). *Learning about lupus: A user friendly guide*. Ardmore: Lupus Foundation of Delaware County.
Provides information for patients or for those who know patients with SLE.

Phillips, R. H. (1984). *Coping with lupus*. Wayne, NJ: Avery.
Provides information for patients or for those who know patients with SLE.

Rosinsky, L. J. (1990). *Lupus resource guide: For patients and professionals.* Bridgeport, CT: Lupus Network.
Provides information for patients or for those who know patients with SLE.

Schneebaum, A. B., Singleton, J. D., West, S. G., Blodgett, J. K., Allen, L. A., Cheronis, J. C., & Kotzin, B. K. (1991). Association of psychiatric manifestations with antibodies to ribosomal P proteins in systemic lupus erythematosus. *American Journal of Medicine, 90,* 54.
A resource about SLE for the health care professional.

Wallace, D. J., & Hahn, B. H. (Eds.). (1993). *Dubois lupus erythematosus* (4th ed.). Philadelphia: Lea & Febiger.
A good resource about lupus for the health care professional.

113

Multiple Sclerosis

Frederick W. Foley

PREVALENCE AND SYMPTOMS

There are between 150,000 and 300,000 individuals in the United States with a confirmed diagnosis of multiple sclerosis (MS), with the numbers of affected women almost double those of men. MS is a chronic multifocal central nervous system (CNS) disease in which myelin (the material that surrounds the axons of many nerve cells and acts as a sort of "insulation" for them) is selectively destroyed by immunocompetent cells and their products and replaced with astrocytic scar tissue. Although axons are largely spared in this process, the loss of nerve conduction secondary to myelin destruction results in a wide variety of symptoms, depending on where the lesions are formed. MS-related limitations may occur in walking, sight, touch, balance, coordination, speech, stamina, sexual function, bladder and/or bowel control, and cognitive function. These symptoms significantly affect a person's ability to engage in expected social roles, such as parenting and work.

The diagnosis of MS is generally made during the peak years of family and career formation (ages 20–50), and the disease has little or no impact on the lifespan. In contrast to its relatively benign impact on mortality, MS can be devastating in its disabling effects. According to the U.S. National Institute on Disability and Rehabilitation Research, persons with MS are more likely to need help in basic life activities than persons with any other chronic medical condition, including those with mental retardation, heart and cerebrovascular disease, cerebral palsy, blindness, rheumatoid arthritis, or emphysema, as well as lung, bronchial, or digestive cancers. In addition, women with MS are more likely to have greater activity limitations and need for assistance with basic life activities than men, although the reasons for this male–female difference are not known. In sum, the prevalence of MS is lower than many other chronic diseases in women (e.g., heart disease, breast cancer), but those affected are at much greater risk for becoming disabled and requiring assistance in activities of daily living.

THE NEUROENDOCRINE SYSTEM, DISEASE PATHOGENESIS, AND STRESS

The mechanisms involved in MS etiology and pathogenesis are thought to be primarily initiated by subpopulations of immunocompetent cells that become sensitized to myelin and oligodendrocyte (cells in the CNS that manufacture myelin) epitopes (molecular components of proteins and lipids on the surface of myelin or oligodendrocytes that "trigger" an immune response) in the CNS. The immunological cascade that ultimately results in inflammation and lesion formation in the microenvironment of the CNS is thought to be etiologically orchestrated by genetic vulnerability, a virus that is sequestered in CNS tissues, or both. Relatively little attention has been focused on the neuroendocrine system in MS etiology and pathogenesis, although a few studies have identified abnormalities in hypothalamic–pituitary–adrenal regulation of adrenal steroid production in MS. MS patients demonstrate hypercortisolism during periods of clinical stability and during exacerbation, show a blunted adrenocorticotropic hormone (ACTH) response to arginine vasopressin stimulation, demonstrate impaired cortisol suppression after dexamethasone administration during clinical exacerbations, and have enlarged adrenal glands on autopsy.

There is more striking evidence of neuroendocrine connection in the pathophysiology of experimental allergic encephalomyelitis (EAE), which is an accepted animal model of MS. The genetic susceptibility of EAE in different rat strains is linked not only to major histocompatibility complex (MHC) genes (i.e., genes that assist T cells in recognizing and attacking antigens), but also to non-MHC genes that determine neuroendocrine inhibition of the immune response. Production of adrenal steroids in response to antigenic challenge in part determines which species and strains are most vulnerable to contracting EAE. In chronic relapsing models of EAE, it is clear that increased corticosterone production is necessary for remissions to occur.

The experience of psychological stress can alter disease onset and course in EAE. The immunosuppressant effects of stress-related increases in corticosterone offer only a partial explanation, however. Stress reduces the severity of EAE, if it is applied at the time of antigen sensitization or early in the disease process, but may potentially worsen later-stage or well-established disease. However, the experimental strengths of evaluating cause and effect in a laboratory animal model are not as applicable in work with persons with MS. Because of various limitations in experimental studies published to date, it is not yet known whether stress affects MS pathogenesis or alters the disease course. Peripheral CD4+ (helper/inducer) and CD8+ (suppressor/cytotoxic) T-cell subpopulations are altered in drug-free distressed MS patients as compared to nondistressed MS patients with equivalent disability, but the linkage between these findings and the disease process is not yet known.

Of particular interest to women is the potential impact on MS of the physical and emotional stresses associated with pregnancy and childbirth. Several studies have been conducted on the effects of pregnancy and childbirth on MS. Pregnancy is associated with decreased risk of exacerbation, although there is increased exacerbation risk in the 6-month period following childbirth. Overall, there seems to be no reliable evidence reported to date that pregnancy and childbirth affect the long-term prognosis.

The mechanisms of change in pregnancy and postpartum exacerbation risk remain unclear. It has been observed anecdotally that self-reports of the intensity of MS symptoms vary during the menstrual cycle. Fluctuations in circulating sex hormone levels (especially estrogen) have been suspected as a possible causal factor, but little evidence has accrued until recently. Estradiol (E2) has been found recently to modulate the secretion of cytokines (soluble secretions of immunocompetent cells that regulate the immune response), in a complex fashion. IL-10 is a cytokine that strongly inhibits cell-mediated immune responses thought to be important in MS pathogenesis. E2 enhances IL-10 secretion by CD4+ T cells in dose-dependent fashion. In addition, E2 *inhibits* T-cell secretion of tumor necrosis factor (TNF) at high concentrations, and *enhances* its release at low concentrations. TNF has been implicated as one of the cytokines involved in MS demyelination.

COGNITIVE ASPECTS OF MULTIPLE SCLEROSIS

The prevalence of cognitive impairments in MS ranges from 43% in a large community sample to 55–59% in clinic samples. Neuropsychological studies have identified impairments as being more circumscribed than global; that is, deficits occur in verbal and visual memory function, although implicit memory (i.e., memory reflecting acquisition of skills without conscious awareness of explicit learning situations) seems intact. Specific deficits in speed of information processing, verbal fluency, complex attention, and/or executive function (i.e., systematic problem-solving ability) are impaired in approximately 20% or more of patients.

Cognitive impairments are not recognized universally by health care providers, even those who specialize in the diagnosis and treatment of MS. Neurologists may underestimate the prevalence of cognitive problems in MS by 10–20%, which may translate into a substantial proportion of clinic patients who do not receive counseling or cognitive rehabilitation for these problems. The underestimation of cognitive deficits may lead health care providers to make erroneous causal attributions regarding their patients' struggles in professional or family roles. Mislabeling cognitive impairments as "emotional problems" may further compromise an MS patient's ability to cope appropriately with symptoms. It is not known whether mislabeling cognitive impairments as "emotional" occurs with greater frequency among women with MS.

EMOTIONAL ASPECTS OF MULTIPLE SCLEROSIS

It has been observed since the late 19th century that MS is associated with affective disturbance. Since the mid-20th century, the euphoria, emotional lability, and depression sometimes seen in MS patients have been conceptualized in part as direct manifestations of the damage to the CNS. The psychological changes in MS have also been widely viewed as concomitants of the process of adjustment, in which an individual strives to adapt to and cope with the catastrophic stress imposed by a disabling illness.

MS has profound repercussions in patients' lives. An individual with MS frequently experiences major disruptions in school, work, and lifestyle; sexual functioning, family relationships, and friendships; ability to communicate and solve problems; and activities of daily living. It is not surprising that psychological distress and clinical depression are common, particularly during clinical exacerbations of the disease. The adjustment process in MS can probably best be viewed as a complex interaction of disease, psychological, and social-environmental factors.

Retrospective interviews examining the prevalence rates for a history of major depression in MS following the disease onset indicate that between 25% and 62%

of patients are at risk for this disorder. There is also epidemiological evidence for substantial suicide risk in the MS population, although it is not known what specific factors are associated with increased risk. The risk for major depression in MS is greater than that for the general population, persons with spinal cord injury, or those with amyotrophic lateral sclerosis. Prevalence estimates for a current major depressive episode among MS clinic patients range from 5% to 14%. In addition, the lifetime prevalence rates for bipolar disorder in MS clinic patients are estimated to be as high as 13–16%. However, the risk of mood disorders among the nonclinic (i.e., community) population has not been well studied, and the partial overlap of MS symptoms with those of both major depression and bipolar disorder (e.g., fatigue, difficulty concentrating, euphoria, affective lability, behavioral disinhibition, sleep disturbance) may lead to overestimation of prevalence rates. Research in women's health has revealed that women experience more difficulty than men in receiving accurate diagnoses of depression, although there have been no published studies to date on diagnostic accuracy in MS.

INTERVENTIONS TO ENHANCE EMOTIONAL ADJUSTMENT AND COPING

Ameliorating depression and assisting with adjustment are done via pharmacological, educational, and psychotherapeutic modalities. Among the most important factors in the treatment of psychological sequelae to MS are careful assessment, treatment, and education of patients about medical symptoms. Teaching patients effective self-management of fatigue, bladder incontinence, sexual dysfunction, spasticity, and other symptoms combats helplessness and demoralization, and aids in the ability to operationalize coping efforts. This can probably be done best in the context of multidisciplinary, comprehensive care; various members of the team can assess, treat, and educate patients and family members. In addition, comprehensive care allows all professionals on the MS treatment team to be educated about symptom management strategies and quality-of-life enhancement from differing professional perspectives. This serves to maximize detection of symptoms and to minimize professionals' and family members' misattributions regarding the patients' experiences, such as the tendency to mislabel MS-related fatigue and subtle cognitive impairments as reflecting affective or personality disturbance. Similarly, when major depression or other significant affective disturbance is present, it is more likely to be correctly identified and treated.

Prevalence rates of sexual dysfunction are roughly comparable in men and women with MS, ranging from approximately 40–90%. A great deal more research has been published on the etiology and treatment of sexual dysfunction in men with MS than women, and more treatment options are currently available for men. The most frequent sexual change reported by women is partial or total loss of libido (sexual desire). Until more research is done to investigate and treat this symptom, treatment options with carefully investigated outcomes are likely to remain limited. MS health care practitioners can help address this largely untreated symptom in women by: (1) educating themselves about sexuality and MS; (2) asking their female patients directly about sexual function; and (3) providing educational resources (available through Multiple Sclerosis Society Chapters) and appropriate professional referrals to women who are interested. Addressing sexual dysfunction represents an easier task for MS professionals that function within a multidisciplinary, comprehensive care environment.

Pharmacological management of depression in MS has been reported to ameliorate depressive symptoms to some extent, particularly in combination with psychotherapy. However, controlled psychopharmacological studies for other affective disturbances sometimes seen in MS, such as bipolar disorder, euphoria, and disturbances of emotional regulation, are notably absent from the literature.

The literature on psychological interventions in MS consists primarily of case reports and uncontrolled group studies. Most interventions described have been supportive or educational in nature. In general, these interventions seem to assist MS patients modestly in their psychosocial adjustment. Group psychodynamic therapy and individual cognitive-behavioral therapy have been successfully tested in MS populations in controlled clinical trials. Both are reported to improve affective outcomes, and individual cognitive-behavioral therapy has also been found to increase the variety of coping approaches patients engage in. Short-term orientation groups offered just after the diagnosis is made can help to provide basic information about MS and lay the groundwork for future communication and support. Couple groups and family counseling can help families deal with periodic role changes that may occur and can provide information and support.

RECOMMENDATIONS FOR ALTERING PSYCHOTHERAPEUTIC APPROACHES

The experience of MS affects the body and mind pervasively. These changes demand that psychotherapeutic practitioners modify their approaches while treating persons with MS. Symptoms that require mental health practitioners to modify their service delivery practices substantially include limitations in mobility and ambulation, spasticity, and cognitive dysfunction.

For cognitively impaired patients, educating the patients and family members as to the nature of the deficits and potential compensatory strategies can enhance family coping and planning. If memory function is affected, the use of a memory journal in which the patients can record between-session homework assignments and review the work they are doing in therapy can minimize discontinuity between therapy sessions. Audiotaping therapy sessions for use between sessions is a useful alteration for selected memory-impaired patients, particularly those with hand tremor or weakness that inhibits their use of writing in a memory journal. Sometimes spouses or other family members can be included in treatment to serve as "memory aids" regarding therapeutic assignments between sessions. If patients' planning ability or reasoning is impaired, psychotherapy can be aided by identifying interpersonal, affective, and behavioral "cues" that are associated with typical problem situations in which compromised reasoning or judgment is likely to manifest. These associated cues can be collaboratively generated by a therapist, patient, and family as a team to serve as signals to engage the patient in previously rehearsed problem-solving or coping behaviors. In sum, when cognition is impaired, psychotherapy methods should be altered in a variety of ways to enhance a patient's capacity to learn in therapy. Unfortunately, the efficacy of psychotherapy in cognitively impaired MS patients is not known at this time, because of the lack of controlled studies published to date.

Relaxation training approaches are commonly taught in MS as a means to enhance coping and ameliorate anxiety. Commonly utilized methods include progressive deep muscle relaxation (PDMR), autogenic training, and guided imagery. The symptoms of any particular patient may require the practitioner to modify these approaches. For example, PDMR is a procedure in which patients are instructed to alternate between tensing and relaxing large muscle groups in sequence. Since spasticity is a common symptom in MS, caution is advised in instructing patients in working with spastic muscles, as purposeful, strong muscle contractions may precipitate painful involuntary spasms. Similarly, patients with Lhermitte's sign (an electrical-like shock in the spine when the neck is tipped forward) need to be instructed in conducting PDMR to avoid inducing this painful symptom. In addition, sensory paresthesias and numbness may interfere with a patient's ability to detect levels of muscle tension accurately, which is required for successful learning of PDMR.

Autogenic or meditative relaxation approaches train patients to focus inwardly on a mantra or word silently repeated to themselves. If MS-related attention/concentration problems are present, however, this may be an enormously frustrating exercise for patients and thus may be contraindicated. Use of non-concentration meditation approaches, such as "mindfulness meditation" (meditation that welcomes distracting thoughts and tries to increase awareness of them), may be less frustrating for patients with attention impairments. Similarly, efforts to use imagery techniques may be frustrating for persons with visualization-related or constructional neuropsychological deficits. Recording patient-generated relaxation images on audiotape or videotape for daily practice at home may help compensate for mild to moderate deficits.

Coping effectively with MS-related changes requires patients to educate friends, family members, and employers about their MS-related experiences and any special needs they may have in order to perform their role functions as parent, spouse, or employee. This can represent a formidable challenge in communication skills, and can become even more difficult when cognitive problems are present. Communication skills training is an important adjunct to psychotherapy in working with persons with MS, particularly in those with attentional, verbal memory, and verbal fluency deficits. A number of difficult life problems enter the life of a family when MS is present; these require better-than-average family problem-solving and communication skills. Differences in preferred coping styles between spouses (e.g., seeking information and support from MS experts vs. minimizing awareness of the impact of MS and avoiding MS information) can contribute to marital distress and problem-solving difficulties if the partners both believe they have the "one right way" to cope.

Finally, limitations in mobility or ambulation may warrant a number of modifications. Telephone psychotherapy sessions can help maintain treatment continuity if transportation is unreliable, symptom exacerbations occur, or disabling fatigue is a factor. Therapists' usual prohibitions on touching patients may need to be altered if disabled MS patients need physical assistance in negotiating the office space or in transferring from their wheelchairs.

FURTHER READING

Fischer, J. S., Foley, F. W., Aikens, J. E., Ericson, G. D., Rao, S. M., & Shindell, S. (1994). What do we really know about cognitive dysfunction, affective disorders, and stress in multiple sclerosis? A practitioner's guide. *Journal of Neurologic Rehabilitation, 7*(5), 151–164.
The prevalence rates of neuropsychological deficits in MS have been better delineated than rates of affective disorders, and little is known about the impact of stress on MS pathogenesis.

Floyd, B. J. (1997). Problems in accurate medical diagnosis of depression in female patients. *Social Science and Medicine, 44*(3), 403–412.
Depression is commonly misdiagnosed in female patients, and medical conditions or treatments frequently produce symptoms or side effects that are confused with depression.

Gilmore, W., Weiner, L. P., & Correale, J. (1997). Effect of estradiol on cytokine secretion by proteolipid protein-specific T cell clones isolated from multiple sclerosis patients and normal control subjects. *Journal of Immunology, 158*(1), 446–451.
Estradiol is capable of modulating both pro-inflammatory and anti-inflammatory cytokine secretions of CD4+ T cells, and thus has the potential to influence the outcome of CD4+ T cell-mediated immune responses.

Foley, F. W., LaRocca, N. G., Kalb, R. C., Caruso, L. S., & Shnek, Z. (1993). Stress, multiple sclerosis, and everyday functioning: A review of the literature with implications for intervention. *Neurorehabilitation, 3*(4), 57–66.
Stress has been associated with increased risk for exacerbation in MS, but poor measurement, retrospective designs, small sample sizes, and limited understanding of possible physiological pathways make the meaning of research findings unclear.

Kalb, R. C. (Ed.). (1996). *Multiple sclerosis: The questions you have, the answers you need.* New York: Demos Vermande.
Edited text that includes chapters by MS experts on neurology, treatment issues, nursing care, physical therapy, occupational therapy, speech disorders, swallowing, cognition, psychosocial and emotional issues, sexuality, employment, insurance issues, fertility and pregnancy, and life planning.

LaPlante, M. P. (1991). *Disability risks of chronic illness and impairments* (Disability Statistics Report 2). Washington, DC: U. S. National Institute on Disability and Rehabilitation Research.
Chronic illnesses and impairments are compared in a national survey for risk of disability, with prevalence rates and activity limitations reported.

Mason, D. (1991). Genetic variation in the stress response: Susceptibility to experimental allergic encephalomyelitis and implications for human inflammatory disease. *Immunology Today, 12*(2), 57–60.
Susceptibility of animal species and strains to EAE is linked in part to hypothalamic–pituitary–adrenal (HPA) release of corticosterone in response to inflammatory immune products, and environmental stress clearly influences the disease via HPA-mediated corticosterone release.

Michelson, D., Stone, L., Galliven, E., Magiakou, M. A., Chrousos, G. P., Sternberg, E. M., & Gold, P. W. (1994). Multiple sclerosis is associated with alterations in hypothalamic–pituitary–adrenal axis function. *Journal of Clinical Endocrinology and Metabolism, 79*(3), 848–853.
Compared to matched controls, MS patients demonstrated higher plasma cortisol levels at baseline, normal plasma ACTH responses to ovine corticotropin-releasing hormone, and blunted ACTH response to arginine vasopressin stimulation, indicating mild increased HPA axis activity in MS.

Rao, S. M. (1995). Neuropsychology of multiple sclerosis. *Current Opinions in Neurology, 8*(3), 216–220.
Recent studies indicate that between 45% and 65% of MS patients have demonstrable neuropsychological deficits, which most frequently include changes on measures of recent memory, attention, and information-processing speed, executive functions, and visuospatial perception.

114

Pain

Richard J. Bodnar

K nowledge concerning the pathogenesis and treatment of pain has grown exponentially over the past 25 years. Research advances have included the identification of (1) specific pain transmission pathways in the central nervous system and peripherally released neurochemicals signaling pain; (2) descending neural pathways from the brain to the spinal cord that inhibit pain; (3) interactions between neurochemical systems to inhibit pain; and (4) identification of classes of endogenous peptides and receptors responsible for the actions of opiate analgesics. These advances have led to new therapies for treatment of chronic pain states, including electrode implantation and stimulation in the brain to alleviate chronic pain; peripheral transcutaneous electrical nerve stimulation; administration of analgesics directly into the spinal cord; patient-controlled analgesia; and coadministration of different classes of psychotropic drugs with opiates, to increase analgesic efficacy and decrease potential dependence. Finally, with the successful identification of opiate receptors, the potential exists to develop, via molecular techniques, highly selective probes for activating these receptors under chronic pain states.

SEX DIFFERENCES IN PAIN

Despite these developments, several outstanding issues still need to be addressed in the treatment of pain and the use of analgesics. One major issue is that of sex differences in the etiology of different states associated with pain. In addition to pain unique to labor and childbirth, women display a greater incidence of pain associated with arthritis, osteoporosis, myofacial neuralgias and causalgias, migraine headaches, and interstitial cystitis. Men show a greater incidence of pain associated with backache, cluster headaches, and cardiac conditions. In exploring sex differences in pain states, it is helpful to use Casey's dimensions of pain, including the sensory/discriminative, motivational/affective, and evaluative/cognitive dimensions. Interestingly, sex differences have been identified in human reactivity and responsivity to noxious stimuli (sensory/discriminative), in human emotional responses to pain and suffering (motivational/affective), and in the labeling and characterizing of pain states (evaluative/cognitive). However, research over the past 15 years has focused upon other aspects of sex differences and pain—namely, differential activation of selective pain-inhibitory systems, and differences in the magnitude, potency, and duration of analgesia as a function of gender, gonadal status, and presence of circulating gonadal hormones. These studies have primarily used rodents and have identified striking sex differences in the efficacy and ability to elicit analgesic responses. Since the sensory/discriminative aspects of reactivity to nociceptive (painful) stimuli have been the primary focus of study, this research illustrates some fundamental physical differences between male and female rodents in pain control, which have obvious clinical implications in treating human pain states.

INTRINSIC PAIN-INHIBITORY SYSTEMS

Over the past 25 years, specific neural pathways have been identified that, when activated, selectively inhibit incoming nociceptive (pain) signals without appreciably altering other somatic sensations. The periaqueductal gray region of the midbrain receives inputs from cortical, limbic (emotional), and striatal (motor) areas of the brain, as well as somatosensory inputs from the spinal cord. Neurons in the periaqueductal gray are activated by noxious somatosensory inputs, and these neurons in turn activate nuclei in the rostral ventromedial and ventrolateral medulla. Medullary neurons directly project to the dorsal horn of the spinal cord, where they specifically inhibit incoming nociceptive signals. This system retains a great deal of similarity as one progresses through the phylogenetic scale from rodents to primates. Strong correlations have been observed between the neurophysiological activation of this descending pain-inhibitory system and analgesia. This system's importance was underscored by the determination that analgesia occurs following either electrical stimulation of these nuclei or microinjections of minute (nanograms to micrograms) amounts of opiates. The discoveries of the opiate receptor and endogenous opioid peptides led to the subsequent findings that they were closely associated with this pain-inhibitory system at both supraspinal and spinal levels. This endogenous opioid system is quite complex, with three gene-related families of endogenous opioid peptides (e.g., endorphins, enkephalins, and dynorphins) and multiple opioid receptor subtypes (mu, delta, kappa, and epsilon). Although some sexual dimorphism has been observed either in levels of opioid receptors and peptides or in the neuroanatomical distribution of endogenous opioid peptides, the magnitude and location of such differences does not adequately describe the following sex differences in analgesic responsiveness.

SEX DIFFERENCES IN ANALGESIC RESPONSIVENESS

Pregnancy-Induced Analgesia

In assessing the functional significance of endogenous opioid peptides and receptors, several laboratories have attempted to determine environmental conditions that might trigger this analgesic system. One of these environmental conditions is unique to female animals: analgesia during pregnancy and parturition. Gintzler demonstrated that female rats over a 21-day pregnancy display a gradual decrease in responsiveness to aversive stimuli between 16 and 4 days prior to parturition, and an abrupt increase in pain thresholds 1–2 days before delivery. A parallel pattern of analgesic effects is also observed in human females as well. This analgesia is abolished if pregnant rats are treated with the opiate receptor antagonist naltrexone, indicating that pregnancy-induced analgesia is mediated by activation of the endogenous opioid system. Whereas the pituitary–adrenal stress axis is not involved in pregnancy-induced analgesia, the spinal cord is the primary site at which opioid modulation occurs through the release of dynorphin opioid peptides and activation of the kappa opioid receptor subtype. Combined increases of the ovarian hormones 17-beta-estradiol and progesterone constitute the means by which pregnancy-induced analgesia occurs, can induce pain threshold changes in pseudopregnant rats, and can modulate the levels of dynorphin in the spinal cord.

The relationship between pregnancy (particularly parturition) and the endogenous opioid system was further strengthened by the discovery of a placental opioid-enhancing factor (POEF) that is found in high concentrations of the amniotic fluid and placenta. Placentophagia, the ingestion of afterbirth materials in mammalian species from rodents to primates, accelerates the onset of maternal behavior. Ingestion of POEF also selectively increases opiate analgesia, pregnancy-induced analgesia, and other forms of analgesia sensitive to opiate antagonism, and relieves opiate withdrawal signs. Yet those forms of analgesia that are insensitive to opiate antagonism (see below) are unaffected by POEF ingestion, suggesting close neurochemical interactions between opioids and POEF. The active factor in POEF responsible for these synergistic effects has not been isolated. Although the relevance of placentophagia to humans during childbirth is anecdotal at best, the isolation of the active substance in POEF may provide for a natural substance that enhances analgesic efficacy.

Vaginal–Cervical Stimulation-Induced Analgesia

A second form of analgesia unique to females is that elicited following vaginal–cervical probing. It was initially found that cervical probing in rats blocked their withdrawal responses to noxious stimulation, and then demonstrated that self-stimulation of the anterior vaginal wall in human female volunteers raised detection and tolerance thresholds for painful cutaneous stimulation in humans. The analgesia in these volunteers was unrelated to either heart rate acceleration or stress. A functional role for this analgesic response has been supported by the observation of brief analgesia elicited by copulation in female rats. Intromission and ejaculation appear more important than mounting in eliciting this analgesia. Like pregnancy-induced analgesia, vaginal–cervical stimulation-induced analgesia is mediated at the level of the spinal cord, where it is dependent upon such neurochemicals as opioids, norepinephrine, serotonin, and glycine. Furthermore, the sensory innervation from the pelvic and hypogastric nerves, but not the pudendal nerve, is necessary for the full elicitation of both of these types of induced analgesia. Thus, copulation and ultimately reproduction elicit powerful pain-inhibitory responses across a number of species, indicating the adaptive significance of these responses.

Stress-Induced Analgesia

My laboratory at the City University of New York has been using acute exposure to stressors as a functional model for eliciting analgesic responses. Whereas some stressors (or parameters of a given stressor) produce analgesia by activating endogenous opioids, other stressors (or parameters of a given stressor) produce analgesia independently of this system. This dichotomy can be observed for analgesia elicited by cold-water swims; rats exposed to brief intermittent swims (10 seconds swimming, 10 seconds resting) over 6 minutes display an analgesic response that is cross-tolerant with morphine and blocked by general opiate antagonism, whereas rats exposed to a continuous swim over 3 minutes display an analgesic response that is insensitive to these manipulations. These "opioid" and "nonopioid" forms of stress-induced analgesia differ from each other both in terms of hormonal, anatomical, and neurochemical mediation; however, both forms of stress-induced analgesia are sensitive to sex differences. One of my former students, Romero, and I established that female rats displayed a lesser magnitude and shorter duration of both "opioid" and "nonopioid" forms of swim analgesia than male rats matched for either weight or age. Both forms of swim-induced analgesia were insensitive to estrous cycle changes in female rats. This pattern of decreased analgesic responsiveness was also observed in female rats following either restraint or brief exposure to a predator. Circulating gonadal hormones appeared responsible for the increased analgesic responsiveness following swims in male rats, since gonadectomy reduced their analgesic magnitude to that observed in females. Adult ovariectomy in female rats reduced swim-induced analgesia further. Steroid replacement therapy with testosterone, but not estradiol, reinstated swim analgesia to "normal" levels in male and female gonadectomized rats. Thus, male rats display a greater magnitude and duration of environmental analgesia than females, and these sex differences appear to be attributable to circulating adult gonadal hormones.

Opioid and Nonopioid Analgesia

The greater analgesia in male rats following stress may result from either a more intense experience of the stressors to elicit a greater analgesia or intrinsic sex differences in pain inhibition. The latter hypothesis was confirmed by another former student, Kepler, and me. Dose–response curves for central morphine analgesia were determined for male and female intact and gonadectomized rats. Male rats displayed maximal analgesia at central morphine doses of 5–10 µg, whereas female rats displayed only moderate analgesia at central morphine doses as high as 40 µg. Adult gonadectomy reduced central morphine analgesia in males and females to a lesser degree than stress-induced analgesia. Sex differences in analgesic responsiveness was also observed following central administration of a mu-selective opioid agonist, but was not observed for a delta-selective opioid agonist. Thus, the rank order of sex differences for opioid analgesia was as follows: morphine > mu agonist > delta agonist. The potent sex differences observed for morphine analgesia in rats may be due to differential metabolism of morphine into morphine-3-beta-glucuronide (which has no analgesic properties) and morphine-6-beta-glucuronide (which has intrinsic analgesic properties) in males and females. This latter effect should be explored further, because absorptive, kinetic, and metabolic factors could alter different degrees of analgesia in male and female pain patients. Finally, nonopioid analgesia elicited by drugs that stimulate receptors for the neurochemicals acetylcholine and norepinephrine is also subject to sex differences, with males displaying a larger effect than females. As in opioid analgesia, adult gonadectomy has far smaller effects upon the nonopioid analgesic response of each sex.

Age Factors

Other former students in my laboratory, Islam and Kramer, have demonstrated that sex differences can interact with aging to alter analgesic responsiveness. Male rats display an *increased* analgesic sensitivity to either morphine or stress as they progress through development, with older male rats (18–24 months, approximately equivalent to 55–70 years in humans) needing lower doses of morphine to produce an equivalent analgesic response. In contrast, female rats display a *decreased* analgesic sensitivity to either morphine or stress as a function of age, with older female rats needing higher doses of morphine to produce an equivalent analgesic response. The mechanisms of action of this interaction are unknown, but the implications of this interaction are of great potential clinical importance.

A "Female" Pain-Inhibitory System?

Liebeskind has proposed the existence of a novel, female-specific, estrogen-dependent pain-inhibitory mechanism. A "nonopioid" form of swim analgesia was blocked by an antagonist of excitatory amino acid receptors in male mice but not in female mice. If the female mice were ovariectomized, this excitatory amino acid antagonist was now effective in blocking this "nonopioid" analgesia. However, if the female mice were ovariectomized *and* received steroid replacement therapy with estrogen, the unique "female" pattern of insensitivity to the excitatory amino acid antagonist reemerged. These data indicate that circulating estrogen is acting upon a unique "female" pain-inhibitory system to mediate adaptive responses. It would be of interest to examine whether this system, which is activated during stress, is also activated during pregnancy.

CONCLUSIONS

This brief review has described some basic physiological and neurochemical mechanisms utilized by the body to inhibit pain, and has indicated that such mechanisms are subject to rather profound sex differences. These differences are neither motivational nor cognitive, but represent some basic physiological differences in responsiveness to noxious stimuli. In our continually evolving process in the treatment of pain, particularly chronic pain, it is imperative that clinicians appreciate these sex differences, and that treatments and therapies be established that will maximize the efficiency and potency of pain-inhibitory mechanisms for each sex.

FURTHER READING

Bodnar, R. J., Romero, M.-T., & Kramer, E. (1988). Organismic variables and pain-inhibition: Roles of gender and aging. *Brain Research Bulletin, 21,* 947–953.
Summarizes the roles of gender, gonadectomy, hormonal, and aging factors in the mediation of analgesic responses in animal research.

Casey, K. L. (Ed.). (1990). *Pain and central nervous system disease.* New York: Raven Press.
Summarizes recent neurological, psychiatric, neurosurgical, and physiological progress in chronic human pain states.

Gintzler, A. R. (1980). Endorphin mediated increases in pain threshold during pregnancy. *Science, 210,* 193–195.
A seminal article demonstrating that increased pain thresholds observed during paturition were mediated by the endogenous opioid system.

Mogil, J. S., Sternberg, J. S., Kest, B., Marek, P., & Liebeskind, J. C. (1993). Sex differences in the antagonism of non-opioid swim stress-induced analgesia: Effects of gonadectomy and estrogen replacement. *Pain, 53,* 17–25.
Identifies the existence of a separate, estrogen-dependent pain-inhibitory system in female rats.

115

Raynaud's Disease

Robert R. Freedman

*R*aynaud's disease is an episodic vasospastic disorder whose symptoms are provoked by cold and/or emotional stress. The attacks are characterized by color changes in the fingers and toes, consisting of pallor, cyanosis, and rubor (whiteness, blueness, and redness), although not necessarily in that order. The disorder is four times more common in women than in men, and its prevalence has been estimated to be roughly 5% of the female population in the United States.

The term "Raynaud's disease" refers to the primary form of the disorder, in which the attacks cannot be explained by an identifiable disease process, such as collagen vascular disease. When the symptoms occur secondarily to another disease, the term "Raynaud's phenomenon" is used. This chapter focuses mainly on the primary form of the disorder, because of its greater prevalence.

Reasons for the increased prevalence of Raynaud's disease in women are not known, but they may include gender differences in peripheral vascular function. In a study utilizing intra-arterial infusions of adrenergic drugs, we found that women had significantly smaller responses than men to compounds acting at alpha- and beta-adrenergic receptors, but not to neurally mediated stimuli or to non-receptor-mediated vasoactive drugs. These results, which suggest that the mechanisms regulating finger blood flow are fundamentally different in normal men and women, may eventually help explain gender differences in the occurrence of some vascular diseases.

ETIOLOGY

Although the cause of Raynaud's disease is unknown, two major theories have been advanced to explain it. Raynaud himself believed that excessive sympathetic nervous system activity causes an increased vasoconstrictive response to cold, while Lewis hypothesized that a "local fault" renders digital arteries hypersensitive to local cooling. Studies of plasma epinephrine and norepinephrine have not found consistently elevated levels in Raynaud's disease patients and therefore do not support Raynaud's theory. In addition, microelectrode recordings of skin nerve sympathetic activity found no differences between Raynaud's disease patients and control subjects during a variety of sympathetic stimuli.

Recent research has supported the theory of Lewis. We found no differences between primary Raynaud's disease patients and control subjects in their responses to sympathetic stimuli, such as reflex cooling or indirect heating. However, we did find that patients had significantly greater digital vasoconstrictive responses to intra-arterial alpha$_1$- and alpha$_2$-adrenergic agonists than did normal control subjects. These findings suggested that primary Raynaud's disease patients have increased peripheral vascular alpha$_1$- and alpha$_2$-adrenergic receptor sensitivity and/or density, compared with normal persons.

We then set out to determine the validity of Raynaud's hypothesis of excessive sympathetic activity. We studied 11 patients with primary Raynaud's disease and 10 patients with Raynaud's phenomenon and scleroderma. Two fingers on one hand were anesthetized with lidocaine, and the patients were placed in a 4°C room in order to induce attacks. The attacks were photographed with an automatic camera and subsequently scored by three "blind," independent raters. The frequency of attacks in nerve-blocked fingers was not significantly different from that in the corresponding intact fingers on the contralateral hand for either patient group. These findings clearly demonstrated that the vasospastic attacks of Raynaud's disease and phenomenon can be provoked without the involvement of efferent digital nerves; they thus argue against the etiological role of sympathetic hyperactivity.

These findings also raised the question of the triggering mechanism of the vasospastic attacks. Animal studies have demonstrated that peripheral vascular adrenergic receptors are thermally sensitive, and we sought to determine whether similar mechanisms might be involved in Raynaud's disease as well. We again utilized intra-arterial infusions of alpha$_1$- and alpha$_2$-adrenergic agonists while recording blood flow simultaneously in cooled and uncooled fingers. Cooling potentiated alpha$_2$-adrenergic vasoconstriction in the patients, but depressed this response in controls. Vasoconstrictive responses to the alpha$_1$-adrenergic agonist were not significantly affected by cooling, but were significantly greater in the cooled and uncooled fingers of the patients than in the corresponding fingers of the controls. These findings suggested that cold-induced sensitization of peripheral vascular alpha$_2$-adrenergic receptors constitutes the "local fault" through which cooling triggers the vasospastic attacks of Raynaud's disease.

Our most recent investigation confirms these findings. Here we utilized intra-arterial infusions of alpha$_1$- and alpha$_2$-adrenergic antagonists to determine whether these compounds would block the vasospastic attacks. We studied 24 patients with primary Raynaud's disease, who received intra-arterial infusions of one type of antagonist or the other, or both drugs together. After the infusion began, we rapidly decreased the temperature of the room from 23°C to 4°C, after which each patient held a beaker of ice water in both hands for 2-minute periods. The attacks were photographed and "blindly" scored as described above. We found that the alpha$_2$-adrenergic antagonist blocked virtually all of the vasospastic attacks in the infused fingers, whereas the alpha$_1$-adrenergic antagonist had no discernible effect. Furthermore, the combination of antagonists did not improve upon the results obtained with the alpha$_2$-adrenergic antagonist alone. These findings constitute strong evidence that the pathophysiological defect in primary Raynaud's disease lies in the thermosensitivity of peripheral vascular alpha$_2$-adrenergic receptors.

EMOTIONAL STRESS IN RAYNAUD'S DISEASE

Although the findings above argue against the etiological role of the sympathetic nervous system in Raynaud's disease attacks, they do not negate the role of emotional stress in the disorder. Anecdotal reports suggested that some Raynaud's attacks are provoked by emotional stress, and we studied this in the natural environment, using ambulatory monitoring. We recorded temperature, heart rate, and stress rating data in 32 patients with Raynaud's disease and 24 with Raynaud's phenomenon and scleroderma. In Raynaud's disease, about a third of the attacks appeared to be stress-related, as evidenced by increased stress ratings and heart rates. In contrast, cold temperatures alone were sufficient to provoke most of the attacks in Raynaud's phenomenon with scleroderma.

We then studied the role of stress in primary Raynaud's disease under controlled conditions in the laboratory. Thirty-two Raynaud's disease patients and 22 normal subjects listened to three tape-recorded scripts in the laboratory: a general stress script, a stress script specifically relevant to Raynaud's disease (lost gloves in a snowstorm), and a neutral script. The groups differed significantly only in their pattern of peripheral vascular responses to the specific stress script. Raynaud's disease patients vasoconstricted, whereas normal volunteers did not. Both groups vasoconstricted in response to the general stress script and showed no temperature in response to the neutral script. Thus, although local cooling can explain most of the attacks that occur in primary Raynaud's disease patients, emotional stress does play a role.

MEDICAL TREATMENT OF RAYNAUD'S DISEASE

Conservative medical treatment of Raynaud's disease has been mainly palliative, with patients instructed to stay warm, cover their hands, or move to a warmer climate. Sympathectomies have been employed in more severe cases, but have been generally ineffective because of the lack of etiological involvement of the sympathetic nervous system. Pharmacological treatment of Raynaud's disease has not been entirely satisfactory. Nifedipine is presently the drug of first choice for patients with primary Raynaud's disease. Nifedipine is a calcium slow-channel blocker that reduces the influx of calcium into cells, thereby decreasing vasoconstriction. Nifedipine has been demonstrated to decrease the frequency, duration, and intensity of vasospastic attacks in about two-thirds of the primary and secondary Raynaud's patients treated.

The most recent data show an average reduction in symptom frequency of about 45% with nifedipine. More recently, a slow-release form of nifedipine has become available;it should result in increased patient compliance, because it is taken only once a day. The most common side effects of nifedipine are headaches, hypotension, and flushing.

Since serotonergic vasoconstriction is also present in human fingers, ketanserin, a serotonergic antagonist, has been used with primary and secondary patients. However, a very large double-blind study of primary and secondary patients produced disappointing results. The reduction in attack frequency with ketanserin was only 34%, compared with a placebo rate of 18%. There were no changes in the severity or duration of vasospastic attacks. Moreover, there were no changes in finger blood flow measurements during cold or warm conditions.

BEHAVIORAL TREATMENT OF RAYNAUD'S DISEASE

Behavioral interventions for Raynaud's disease have attempted to elevate finger temperature and reduce symptoms through relaxation procedures (e.g., autogenic training) or through temperature biofeedback. In one early study, patients received either autogenic training alone or in combination with finger temperature biofeedback. Half the subjects served as a waiting-list control group and were then treated. Subjects as a whole showed improved responses to a cold-stress test, but the declines in attack frequencies (10–32%) were disappointing, and there were no group differences on any measure. A subsequent investigation of progressive relaxation, autogenic training, or a combination of the two found similar results.

Since the previous studies combined various behavioral treatments, we conducted a study in which temperature feedback alone was compared with autogenic training or frontalis electromyographic (EMG) feedback. We also wanted to enhance generalization of temperature biofeedback responses to the natural environment, so we tested a fourth procedure in which temperature feedback was given during mild cold stress to the finger. We found that patients who received temperature biofeedback alone or in combination with cold stress showed significant elevations in finger temperature during training and significant decreases in reported attack frequency the following winter (66.8% and 92.5%, respectively). These results were maintained at 2- and 3-year follow-up points. In contrast, patients who received autogenic training or EMG feedback showed declines in muscle tension, heart rate, and reported stress levels, but did not demonstrate finger temperature elevations or symptomatic improvement.

These results suggested to us that the vasodilation produced during finger temperature feedback is not mediated through decreased physiological arousal, but through a different mechanism. At that time, an active, beta-adrenergic, vasodilating mechanism was discovered in the human finger, and we sought to determine the possible involvement of this mechanism during temperature biofeedback. We studied 16 normal subjects and 18 patients with primary Raynaud's disease, and instructed them in either temperature biofeedback or autogenic training. In a subsequent session, we blocked the beta-adrenergic receptors in one hand with intra-arterial propranolol and left the other hand intact. Finger temperature and blood flow were measured in both hands. We found significant bilateral vasodilation before the propranolol infusion in the temperature feedback subjects. This vasodilation was then significantly reduced by propranolol in the infused but not the control hand. Similar effects were obtained in the Raynaud's patients and normal subjects. There were no significant blood flow changes at all in the patients or normal subjects who received autogenic training. The Raynaud's patients who received temperature biofeedback showed significant increases in finger temperature and capillary blood flow and significant declines in attack frequency (mean = 81%), which were maintained at 1- and 2-year follow-up periods. Thus, a beta-adrenergic mechanism is involved in feedback-induced vasodilation.

Since the only efferent vasomotor nerves in human fingers are adrenergic, this finding raised the question of whether feedback-induced vasodilation is neurally mediated. We therefore repeated these experiments while blocking the nerves in one finger with lidocaine. In two separate studies of normal subjects and a third study with primary Raynaud's patients, we found that feedback-induced vasodilation was not attenuated by nerve blockade, but again was reduced by propranolol. Thus the beta-adrenergic vasodilating mechanism of temperature biofeedback does not appear to be mediated through efferent digital nerves.

These findings then raised the question of whether changes in sympathetic nervous system activity as measured by plasma epinephrine and norepinephrine would occur during temperature biofeedback. We again studied primary Raynaud's disease patients and normal volunteers, who were randomly assigned to receive instruction in either finger temperature biofeedback or autogenic training. During the first and last treatment sessions, blood was continuously drawn from a vein on the back of one hand by means of a small pump and special nonclotting tubing. The pump was placed in an adjacent room so that the subject could not see the blood being withdrawn. Plasma catecholamine levels were subsequently analyzed by the HPLC-EC (high pressure liquid chromatography with electrochemical detection) method.

Significant temperature and blood flow increases were shown by temperature biofeedback patients but not by autogenic patients. However, there were no significant changes in plasma catecholamine levels for either group. Similar findings were obtained for the Raynaud's disease patients and the normal volunteers.

CONCLUSIONS

Work on the pathophysiology of Raynaud's disease indicates that the attacks are not caused by overactivity of the sympathetic nervous system, but probably by the hypersensitivity of peripheral vascular alpha$_2$-adrenergic receptors to cooling. Elevated catecholamine levels have not been consistently found in patients with primary Raynaud's disease, and the vasospastic attacks can be induced despite blockade of efferent digital nerves. Emotional stress may play a role in a minority of the attacks.

The results of temperature biofeedback treatment for primary Raynaud's disease are encouraging. Several controlled group outcome studies have shown that primary patients given temperature biofeedback alone reported declines in attack frequency ranging from 67% to 92%, which were maintained at 2- and 3-year follow-up points. We have found that feedback-induced vasodilation is not mediated through reductions in sympathetic nervous system activity, but rather through a beta-adrenergic mechanism. Further research should be conducted on the etiology of Raynaud's disease and on the efficacy and mechanisms of treatments for it.

FURTHER READING

Coffman, J. D. (1991). Raynaud's phenomenon. *Hypertension, 17,* 593–602.
A good review paper on the pathophysiology of Raynaud's phenomenon.

Freedman, R. R. (1991). Physiological mechanisms of temperature biofeedback. *Biofeedback and Self-Regulation, 16,* 95–115.
A review paper describing the physiological mechanisms of finger blood flow and their operation in temperature biofeedback.

Freedman, R. R., Mayes, M., Sabharwal, S., & Keegan, D. (1989). Induction of vasospastic attacks despite digital nerve block in Raynaud's disease and phenomenon. *Circulation, 80,* 859–862.
A laboratory study showing that Raynaud's attacks are not mediated through efferent digital nerves.

Freedman, R. R., Moten, J., Migaly, M., & Mayes, M. (1993). Cold-induced potentiation of α₂-adrenergic vasoconstriction in primary Raynaud's disease. *Arthritis and Rheumatism,* 36(5), 685–690.
A laboratory study showing that local cooling increases alpha₂-adrenergic vasoconstriction in Raynaud's disease patients but not in matched controls.

Freedman, R. R., Sabharwal, S., Ianni, P., Desai, N., Wenig, P., & Mayes, M. (1988). Non-neural ß-adrenergic vasodilating mechanism in temperature biofeedback. *Psychosomatic Medicine,* 50, 394–401.
A laboratory study showing that feedback-induced vasodilation is mediated in part through a non-neural, beta-adrenergic mechanism.

116

Respiratory Disorders

Mark H. Hermanoff

*T*he respiratory system includes the oral and nasal pharynx, the larynx, the tracheal and bronchial airways, and the lungs. With the exception of size, there are few obvious anatomical differences between the respiratory systems in women and men. There are, however, a number of important issues regarding women and lung disease. In addition, a number of respiratory conditions and illnesses are of particular concern to women. This chapter briefly reviews the issues that are of particular importance to women, and highlights those that require special attention.

SMOKING-INDUCED LUNG DISEASES

Smoking-induced lung disease has been recognized as a major public health issue for many years. Since the U.S. Surgeon General's first report on the health effects of smoking in 1964, there have been multiple reports linking smoking to a number of diseases. The effects of smoking-related health injury on women have been underestimated until recently. This may be because a smaller percentage of women than of men smoke, and women who do smoke tend to smoke fewer cigarettes than men. In addition, the overall incidence of smoking has fallen in both men and women since 1965. However, according to the National Health Interview Survey, the rate in all men fell from 41% to 29%, while in all women it fell only 5%, from 31% to 26%. Smoking rates have fallen faster in better-educated groups, but in recent years we have witnessed a disturbing rise in smoking rates among women with lower levels of education. It is also of great concern that teenage women continue to be added to the ranks of those who are addicted to cigarettes. There is a growing epidemic of smoking among teenage women, and this will have a long-term effect on the health of millions of women in the decades to come.

Lung Cancer

Cigarette smoke contains many known carcinogens and has been clearly linked to more than 90% of all lung cancers. A review of age-adjusted cancer mortality rates revealed a disturbing trend from 1930 to 1987. Uterine (cervix), gastric, and breast cancers were the leading causes of cancer deaths in women in 1930, whereas lung cancer caused only 2–3 deaths per 100,000 women. By 1962, however, the incidence of lung cancer in women began to skyrocket. Although medical screening programs and dietary changes have led to a marked decline in the rate of cervical and gastric cancer, the incidence of lung cancer has steadily risen in women. Since 1987, lung cancer has surpassed breast cancer as a killer of women, and is now the leading cause of cancer death in women. It is estimated that lung cancer will kill 66,000 women in 1997. These statistics are of even greater concern because the rate of increase in lung cancer deaths shows no signs of slowing.

In addition to active smoking, secondhand smoke or passive smoking is now recognized as a carcinogen by the Environmental Protection Agency. Approximately 12,000 deaths from lung cancer each year occur in patients who did not smoke. It has been estimated that between 2,500 and 8,400 of these deaths can be linked to exposure to secondhand smoke.

There are no known effective screening tests for lung cancer, and by the time most cases are diagnosed, the disease has progressed to a point where curative surgical excision is not possible and chemotherapy is far less effective. Although there have been some promising developments in the diagnosis and treatment of certain types of lung cancer, prevention remains by far the most effective tool in the fight against lung cancer.

Chronic Obstructive Pulmonary Disease

Chronic obstructive pulmonary disease (COPD) results from the progressive destruction of alveolar and distal bronchial wall structures. There is a loss of lung function, leading to progressive dyspnea, exercise intolerance, and (in many cases) ventilatory insufficiency, the institution of supplemental oxygen therapy, and death. Although inhaled bronchodilators provide some symptomatic relief, and many patients benefit from exercise and behavioral modification programs, the disease causes severe morbidity and mortality for thousands of women. Mortality statistics for 1993 revealed that more than 46,700 women died of COPD in that year, and thousands of women are diagnosed each year. There may be some degree of physician bias toward diagnosing older women with COPD as having asthma, although this point has not been studied in detail.

Most cases of COPD can be directly related to cigarette smoking. Female smokers should be informed that recent studies have found women to have a greater susceptibility to lung damage than men. Compared to men, lung function falls at a faster rate in female smokers, which may then lead to an earlier onset of symptoms and possible death. In COPD, as in lung cancer, a reduction in smoking rates would make a large difference in the health of thousands of women.

Smoking and Asthma

Asthma, like COPD, causes airway obstruction. Asthma involves bronchoconstriction and inflammation of the airways, which can be reversed in a large majority of patients (see below). Smoking exacerbates the symptoms of asthma, and only the most addicted asthmatic will continue to smoke in the face of severe asthma. A more pertinent issue for female smokers is that of pediatric asthma induced by maternal smoking. Recent studies have demonstrated a link between secondhand smoke (especially maternal smoking) and the development of asthma in children. There are a number of explanations for this trend. An increasing body of evidence supports the notion that maternal smoking can lead to the development of allergic disease and to recurrent respiratory tract infections in children. Both of these factors are known to increase the incidence of asthma. It is becoming clear that maternal smoking can cause detrimental health effects to a developing fetus as well as to a young child.

Smoking Cessation

It is clear from the discussion above that cigarette smoking is the most important cause of lung disease in women. Efforts to help women stop smoking and to prevent teenage smoking are critical to improving the health of millions. Programs to help prevent teenage women from smoking need to be initiated to help overcome the pressure from peers, the youth culture, and tobacco industry advertising.

Smoking cessation programs should incorporate both behavioral and medical therapies to initiate cessation and prevent relapse. Many of the behavioral techniques are discussed elsewhere in this text. Important components include goal setting, self-monitoring, and self-contracting. Other behavior modification options include stimulus control and aversion therapy. Medical interventions include nicotine replacement (gum and transdermal patches), and there has also been some research in the use of serotonin agonists, serotonin receptor antagonists, and tricyclic antidepressants. All studies have verified the importance of using behavior modification in conjunction with medical interventions. The use of nicotine replacement without some kind of behavior modification is almost always doomed to result in relapse.

ASTHMA

Asthma is a disease defined as reversible constriction and inflammation of the bronchial tubes. (For a more detailed discussion of asthma, see Schmaling's chapter in this volume.) In many patients, an allergic trigger from indoor or outdoor allergens can be determined; in other cases, various triggers (including viral or bacterial infections, chemical irritants, air pollution, cold air, or exercise) can exacerbate symptoms. There is also a group of patients who are sensitive to products containing aspirin or nonsteroidal anti-inflammatory drugs. The incidence of asthma has been rising, as has the death rate (more than 5,000 each year). Although asthma is more common in boys than in girls, this ratio is reversed in adulthood.

A number of issues in asthma are of particular importance to women. Many patients with moderate to severe asthma require intermittent or continuous treatment with systemic corticosteroids. Systemic (oral or intravenous) corticosteroids are clearly associated with osteoporosis when used over long periods of time. There are still no good treatments to prevent the onset of osteoporosis in patients exposed to high doses of corticosteroids, although estrogen replacement in postmenopausal women will slow the rate of bone loss. Inhaled corticosteroids to control asthma have enabled practitioners to reduce their reliance on oral steroids in many patients. Although there are still concerns that high doses of inhaled corticosteroids may increase the risk of osteoporosis, asthma can be controlled with lower doses in the majority of patients. Lower doses of inhaled corticosteroids have not been associated with the development of osteoporosis.

Asthma exacerbations associated with menses (premenstrual asthma) have been described. There are many very convincing case reports describing premenstrual asthma, but prospective studies have only been able to demonstrate a significant effect of menses on asthma when subjective measures are used. The etiology of premenstrual asthma is unknown, and no specific treatment, beyond the ones used for all asthmatics, has been proven to be efficacious. It is important for health care providers to be aware that some women can have exacerbations of their asthma associated with their menses, and that those with more severe disease will require more intensive treatment.

Asthmatics who are pregnant present a particular challenge to health care providers. During pregnancy about one-third of asthmatics will have more severe disease, whereas one-third will note an improvement in their asthma. The key to management of asthma during pregnancy is to keep the disease under control and to avoid exacerbations of asthma, which can lead to fetal hypoxemia. Details on the management of asthma during pregnancy are beyond the scope of this chapter.

Occupational and home/indoor exposures can act as a trigger for asthma as well as other pulmonary diseases. It is clear that certain indoor allergens, such as dust mites, cats, cockroaches, and certain molds, can be major triggers of asthma. Many occupations have also been associated with work-related asthma. Women need to be aware that a great many substances have been determined to trigger asthma. A careful occupational and environmental history by a health care provider can help determine whether an environmental trigger is responsible for a patient's asthma.

RESPIRATORY INFECTIONS

Respiratory infections can involve both the upper and lower respiratory tract, and range from laryngitis and sinusitis to bronchitis, pneumonia, and tuberculosis. Although there are no clear differences in either the incidence or severity of respiratory tract infections in women and men, a few important issues specifically apply to women.

The incidence of tuberculosis has been rising since 1985, and the medical profession's concern has been magnified by the emergence of multidrug-resistant strains that do not respond to medications presently available. With the number of women working in the health care field, the risk of occupational exposure to tuberculosis has been magnified in recent years. It is important for such women to be sure their employers provide adequate protection from exposure. The greatest risk comes from patients who have not yet been diagnosed and for whom no precautions have been taken to prevent the spread of this airborne disease. The incidence of tuberculosis in pregnant women has been rising in some larger cities, where the overall incidence of tuberculosis has risen markedly. Tuberculosis in pregnancy can progress at a much faster rate than usual.

It is possible to control the spread of tuberculosis with early diagnosis of the disease through skin testing with purified protein derivative of tuberculin; appropriate treatment of skin test converters; and the treatment of patients who have active disease with multiple drugs to which the organism may be susceptible. Details regarding the diagnosis and treatment of tuberculosis are beyond the scope of this chapter.

A group of atypical mycobacterial organisms related to tuberculosis is also a health concern in women. Atypical mycobacteria were once thought not to be a significant cause of pulmonary disease in humans, and in some individuals they are simply airway colonizers. However, it has recently become evident that atypical mycobacteria can cause progressive lung destruction in some patients. There appears to be an increased incidence of this disease in women (especially those living in the southeastern United States), as well as heavy smokers and patients with COPD or chronic lung disease. For reasons that are not clear, these patients have an increased prevalence of anatomical chest or lung abnormalities, such as pectus excavatum (exaggerated depression of the breastbone).

THROMBOEMBOLIC DISEASE

A venous thromboembolism (blood clot) in the veins of the legs or pelvis can migrate to the pulmonary circulation and cause a life-threatening pulmonary embolism. Once diagnosed, thromboembolic disease requires long-term treatment with anticoagulants. A number of circumstances put women at markedly increased risk for the formation of thromboembolic disease.

Pulmonary embolism is a major cause of maternal mortality during pregnancy and in the immediate postpartum period (it accounts for 11% of maternal deaths). Hypercoagulability during pregnancy can be increased by a number of factors, including increased serum clotting factors, decreased fibrinolytic factors, decreased venous tone in the lower extremities, and partial obstruction of the inferior vena cava by the enlarging uterus. Early diagnosis and treatment are important, but are complicated by the need to minimize radiation exposure to the developing fetus and the need to avoid the teratogenic effects of the oral anticoagulant coumadin. Long-term use of heparin (the alternative intravenous treatment for thromboembolic disease) is associated with the development of osteoporosis. Recognition of thromboembolic disease in pregnancy requires a high degree of clinical suspicion, and skilled management is called for once it is diagnosed.

Another important risk factor for thromboembolic disease in women is the combination of oral contraceptives and cigarette smoking. Because smoking markedly raises the risk of clotting in women, the use of oral contraception is relatively contraindicated in women who smoke. The risk of thromboembolic disease in women receiving postmenopausal estrogen replacement therapy has not been fully addressed. Although a few studies have not found an increased risk, the question requires further research.

OCCUPATIONAL PULMONARY DISEASE

Large numbers of women in the workplace, and an increase in the general awareness of occupational diseases, have made work-related lung injury an issue for women. Occupational lung disease can take many forms, including asthma, pulmonary fibrosis, occupational lung cancer, hypersensitivity pneumonitis, and pulmonary infections, as well as upper respiratory tract problems such as sinusitis. Occupational exposures associated with lung disease include exposures to organic and inorganic dusts, chemicals, carcinogens, and infectious agents. The most important aspect of occupational and environmental exposure is the need for health care providers to have some suspicion whenever a patient presents for treatment of a respiratory illness, and to take a complete occupational and environmental history.

OTHER PULMONARY DISORDERS OF SPECIAL INTEREST TO WOMEN

Primary Pulmonary Hypertension

Pulmonary hypertension is the development of increased blood pressure in the usually low-pressure pulmonary circulation. Typical symptoms of pulmonary hypertension include dyspnea, fatigue, chest pain, near-syncope, syncope, leg edema, and palpitations. Pulmonary hypertension can cause severe hypoxemia, heart failure, and death. In many instances, the etiology of pulmonary hypertension is known, but there is an idiopathic form known as primary pulmonary hypertension. For reasons that are not clear, more women than men develop this disorder (the ratio is approximately 1.7:1). Treatments for this disorder are limited, and the mortality rate remains high.

Connective Tissue Disease

The incidence of connective tissue diseases such as systemic lupus erythematosus (SLE) and scleroderma is increased in women. Some women with these disorders can go on to develop a wide range of lung diseases, including pleuritis, fibrosis, and restrictive lung disease. Although the other symptoms of these disorders are usually more apparent, the development of lung dysfunction can lead to significant disability.

FURTHER READING

American Thoracic Society. (1994). Treatment of tuberculosis and tuberculosis infection in adults and children. *American Journal of Respiratory and Critical Care Medicine, 149,* 1359–1374.
A detailed review of diagnosis and treatment of tuberculosis.

Bone, C. R., Higgins, W., Hurd, S. S., & Reynolds, H. Y. (1992). Research needs and opportunities related to the respiratory health of women. *American Review of Respiratory Disease, 146,* 528–535.
A review of respiratory diseases in women, and of research needs and available opportunities.

Cancer Statistics. (1997). *CA—Cancer Journal for Clinicians, 47,* 5–27.
Summary of cancer morbidity and mortality in the United States.

Chen, Y., Horne, S. L., & Dosman, J. A. (1991). Increased susceptibility to lung dysfunction in female smokers. *American Review of Respiratory Disease, 143,* 1224–1230.
Lung function declines at a faster rate for female than for male smokers.

Demers, C., & Ginsberg, J. S. (1992). Deep venous thrombosis and pulmonary embolism in pregnancy. *Clinics in Chest Medicine, 13*(4), 645–656.
A review of the association of deep venous thrombosis and pulmonary embolism in pregnancy.

Fielding, J. E., & Phenan, K. J. (1988). Health effects of involuntary smoking. *New England Journal of Medicine, 319,* 1452–1460.
A review of known effects of secondhand smoke.

Saleh, A. A., Dorey, L. G., Dombrowski, M. P., Ginsberg, K. A., Hirokawa, S., Kowalczyk, C., Hirata, J., Bottoms, S., Cotton, D. B., & Mammen, E. F. (1993). Thrombosis and hormone replacement therapy in postmenopausal women. *American Journal of Obstetrics and Gynecology, 169*(6), 1554–1557.
A study to determine the incidence of thrombosis in women treated with hormone replacement therapy.

Settipane, R. A., & Simon, R. A. (1989). Menstrual cycle and asthma. *Annals of Allergy, 63,* 373–378.
A review of asthma exacerbations with the menstrual cycle.

117

Syndrome X

Phyliss D. Sholinsky

Syndrome X is a cluster of metabolic cardiovascular risk factor abnormalities associated with insulin resistance that increase the risk of non-insulin-dependent diabetes mellitus (NIDDM) and coronary heart disease (CHD) in both men and women. These abnormalities include glucose intolerance, hypertriglyceridemia, low levels of high-density lipoprotein cholesterol (HDL-C), and possibly hypertension and abdominal obesity. The co-occurrence of multiple cardiovascular risk factors in some individuals has been recognized for many years. In the 1980s, evidence emerged indicating that hyperinsulinemia and insulin resistance might be the underlying causes for this phenomenon, which Reaven named "Syndrome X." The syndrome has been referred to by a multitude of other names, including the "insulin resistance syndrome," the "deadly quartet," the "deadly pentad," the "glucose intolerance/obesity/hypertension syndrome," and the "metabolic cardiovascular syndrome."

Reaven postulated that the cluster of risk factors associated with insulin resistance includes glucose intolerance, high plasma triglyceride, low HDL-C concentrations, and hypertension. Subsequently, others have reported that additional cardiovascular risk factors, such as abdominal obesity, are associated with insulin resistance and may also be considered components of Syndrome X. Unfortunately, a standard definition is currently lacking, and this complicates our understanding of the differences reported across studies.

Because the adverse metabolic profile associated with Syndrome X increases the risk of developing NIDDM and/or CHD, it is significant from a public health perspective. Syndrome X is especially important in women; although women develop CHD an average of 10 years later in life than men do, diabetes eliminates this apparent protective gender effect. In addition, diabetic women are at greater relative risk for CHD and cardiovascular death than diabetic men.

COMPONENTS OF THE SYNDROME

In September 1995, the National Heart, Lung, and Blood Institute held a workshop titled "The Metabolic Cardiovascular Risk Factor Clustering Syndrome," cochaired by Kannel and myself. Components of Syndrome X and its potential underlying determinants were discussed, as were methods to continue to study the syndrome in population studies. A summary of the workshop will be published in 1997. The candidate core components of Syndrome X, as well as several additional risk factors associated with the syndrome, are reviewed below. Results of studies focusing on women or on gender differences are highlighted.

Glucose Intolerance

Individuals with insulin resistance have a defect in insulin-mediated glucose uptake that may often go unrecognized before hyperglycemia and frank diabetes develop. During the prediabetic stage, the beta cells of the pancreas increase their secretion of insulin, resulting in compensatory hyperinsulinemia. Eventually the beta cells are unable to compensate, and glucose intolerance and hyperglycemia occur. Since the beta cells cannot sustain the insulin secretion, there is also effectively a drop in insulin levels from the hyperinsulinemic level. Normoglycemic relatives of NIDDM patients frequently have hyperinsulinemia or are insulin-resistant. Diabetics tend to have other cardiovascular disease (CVD) risk factor abnormalities considered part of Syndrome X, and they are at greater risk for CHD than nondiabetics. The risk of CVD has also been shown to increase progressively with increasing glucose levels.

The effects of the menstrual cycle and endogenous hormones on components of Syndrome X were studied in a subset of 260 women from the Baltimore Longitudinal Study of Aging, which is examining healthy individuals aged 22–89. No independent relationship was seen between menstrual cycle phase, or plasma level of estradiol or progesterone, and glucose tolerance. This finding was in agreement with several previous studies; however, others have reported a decline in glucose tolerance during the luteal phase, particularly in diabetic women, although the studies were small. The Baltimore Longitudinal Study investigators study concluded that the decreased glucose tolerance seen in their cohort was attributable to abdominal fatness and overall fatness, not to levels of endogenous sex hormones.

Numerous studies have shown the exogenous hormones of oral contraceptives to have an adverse effect on glucose tolerance, primarily demonstrated as increased 2-hour glucose levels in women taking formulations with high estrogens. However, current formulations of oral contraceptives consist of lower estrogen doses. Conflicting evidence exists for the effects of the conjugated estrogens used in postmenopausal hormone replacement therapy on glucose tolerance. Several studies have shown no differences in glucose levels between postmenopausal women undergoing hormone therapy and premenopausal women. However, another study in hormone-treated posthysterectomy patients found increased fasting glucose levels, compared to those of nonhormone-treated premenopausal women. These patients had gained weight during the study, which may account for the altered glucose metabolism independently from the therapy. Thus, overall, it appears that neither endogenous or exogenous hormones have a consistent effect on glucose levels. Hormone replacement therapy has been shown to improve the rest of the cardiovascular risk factor profile, though, and may prevent accumulation of abdominal fat postmenopausally.

Dyslipidemia

Insulin resistance and compensatory hyperinsulinemia also affect regulation of lipoprotein metabolism, most likely via effects on lipoprotein lipase activity. Insulin resistance is positively correlated with triglyceride concentrations and very-low-density lipoprotein triglyceride secretion rates in both normotriglyceridemic and hypertriglyceridemic people. Insulin resistance and plasma insulin are inversely correlated with HDL-C concentrations in healthy and obese individuals. Low HDL-C is considered to be less than 45 mg/dl in women and less than 35 mg/dl in men. In diabetic patients, the only lipid abnormalities consistently associated with CHD are hypertriglyceridemia and low HDL-C. CHD can occur in the absence of hypercholesterolemia in nondiabetics as well as in those with NIDDM, and thus dyslipidemia should not be ignored even when total plasma cholesterol and low-density lipoprotein cholesterol (LDL-C) levels are normal. The associations of insulin resistance with triglyceride and HDL-C may occur independently of overall obesity or abdominal obesity. However, weight loss can improve the levels of all three metabolic conditions, while carbohydrate overfeeding may worsen the levels, suggesting a more complicated relationship between insulin resistance and weight and obesity.

Hypertension

Hypertension has been associated with hyperinsulinemia and insulin resistance. This relationship has been seen in both obese and lean people, and in those individuals whose hypertension has been pharmacologically treated. Abnormalities of insulin resistance are also seen in normotensive first-degree relatives of hypertensive patients. However, most of these associations were found in groups of northern European origin. In African-Americans, Mexican-Americans, Nauruans, Native Americans of the Pima tribe, and Asians from India, only a weak association (if any) is usually observed between insulin resistance or hyperinsulinemia and hypertension. The inclusion of hypertension in the syndrome definition has thus been debatable.

Abdominal Obesity

The third National Health and Nutrition Examination Survey (NHANES III) has shown that the prevalence of obesity is increasing in the U.S. adult population for all race and gender groups examined. Both cardiovascular risk factors and insulin resistance are associated with overall obesity, which is commonly measured as body mass index (BMI) and is calculated as weight (in kilograms) divided by height (in square) squared. The inclusion of obesity in the definition or as an underlying determinant of Syndrome X, however, remains controversial. In some studies, associations of syndrome components are stronger or are seen only in lean individuals. In general, obese individuals are insulin-resistant and thin individuals are not; however, there are exceptions, implying the influence of other genetic or environmental factors on the relationship between overall obesity and insulin resistance.

Besides overall obesity, the distribution of body fat has been associated with cardiovascular risk factors and CVD. Abdominal obesity is often measured as the waist-to-hip ratio (WHR), calculated as the waist circumference (in centimeters) divided by the hip circumference (in centimeters). A larger ratio implies the "apple shape" of upper-body abdominal fat deposition commonly seen in men, whereas a smaller ratio indicates the "pear shape" of lower-body fat accumulation typically seen in women. When WHR is used, abdominal obesity is defined as 0.95 and above for men, and 0.85 and above for women. There is increasing evidence that abdominal obesity is a better predictor of NIDDM and CVD than overall obesity, and that it may be the more appropriate type of obesity to consider with Syndrome X.

In the Göteborg Population Study of 1,462 women, both WHR and BMI were univariately related to cardiovascular abnormalities. When both measures of obesity were included, WHR was more strongly related to the metabolic risk factors than BMI, and no independent contribution was made by BMI when WHR was already in the analysis. The Quebec City Study, whose subjects were healthy men and healthy premenopausal women, found differences in metabolic risk factors by gender that were not explained by controlling for body fat mass as assessed by underwater weighing. When both total fat and abdominal visceral fat (measured by computerized tomography, which is more accurate than WHR) were controlled for, most of the gender differences were accounted for; however, HDL-C remained significantly lower, and glucose levels significantly higher, in men than in women. In this study, for a given total fat mass, men had twice the amount of abdominal fat of women. In population-based studies, hyperinsulinemic women, although having more abdominal fat than normoinsulinemic women, still tend to exhibit relatively pear-shaped fat accumulation compared to men. Thus gender interaction complicates the relationship of Syndrome X components with obesity. A possible explanation is suggested by the study of 121 overweight postmenopausal women by Svendsen and colleagues, in which lower levels of sex-hormone-binding globulin levels were correlated with a higher proportion of abdominal fat. Other studies have also found reduced levels of sex-hormone-binding globulin or high free testosterone concentrations in abdominally obese women.

ADDITIONAL RISK FACTORS ASSOCIATED WITH SYNDROME X

Small, Dense Low-Density Lipoprotein Particles

Although neither hypercholesterolemia nor LDL-C concentration has been associated with Syndrome X, there is mounting evidence that small, dense LDL particle size may be another feature of the syndrome. The prevalence of dense LDL phenotype is approximately 30%, similar to the 20–25% estimated for Syndrome X. Normal subjects with the small, dense LDL phenotype are more insulin-resistant, glucose-intolerant, hyperinsulinemic, hypertensive, and hypertriglyceridemic than those without this phenotype, and have a lower HDL-C cholesterol concentration. Experiments have shown the size of the LDL particle to be inversely correlated with the degree of insulin resistance.

Apolipoprotein B

Much of the evidence for the association of apolipoprotein B (apo B) with Syndrome X follows that for the small, dense LDL phenotype, with which high levels of apo B are frequently associated. High plasma levels of LDL-apo B have been demonstrated in the presence of normal LDL concentrations, with insulin resistance, hypertriglyceridemia, and high plasma free fatty acids. The last of these may be involved in the regulation of apo

B. Apo B also has a strong genetic component and so insulin resistance may not cause high apo B, but may influence the genetic expression.

Hyperuricemia

Significant correlations exist between serum uric acid concentration and both insulin resistance and 2-hour insulin levels, even after adjustment for age, gender, BMI, and WHR. These associations have been found in normal, healthy individuals.

Plasminogen Activator Inhibitor 1

High levels of plasminogen activator inhibitor 1 (PAI-1) have been associated with recurrent myocardial infarction in younger men, most likely because of its actions impairing fibrinolysis. There is evidence that plasma insulin may be the most important regulator of PAI-1. Plasma insulin and PAI-1 levels have been found to be positively correlated in healthy individuals over a wide range of body weights. These associations are also seen in people with other components of Syndrome X, including those with hypertriglyceridemia, nondiabetic obese women, and patients with hypertension or glucose intolerance.

INTERVENTIONS

Interventions for Syndrome X vary according to whether only individual components of the syndrome, the combined conditions, or potential underlying determinants such as the insulin resistance are targeted. Also, the relationship of insulin resistance and Syndrome X components involves complex aspects of metabolic regulation that may be under genetic control, and thus not easy targets for intervention. For instance, there is likely to be genetic predisposition to the location of fat accumulation, and the phenotype of apo B is genetically determined. There may also be a genetic susceptibility to environmental factors that affect the Syndrome X components. However, intervention through physical activity, diet, weight loss, or pharmacology can ameliorate the insulin resistance and improve the adverse cardiovascular profile seen with Syndrome X.

Restriction of caloric intake and reduction in dietary fat have a positive effect on several components of Syndrome X, including obesity, hypertension, and glucose intolerance. Preliminary results suggest that caloric restriction may have beneficial effects independent of those following the resulting weight loss. Several studies have found gender differences in the changes seen in lipoprotein profiles after dietary change, corresponding to the diet composition. Physical activity has been shown to decrease triglyceride levels, to increase HDL-C levels, to reduce total body fat, and to have a beneficial effect on fat distribution. Physical activity has also been associated with lowering of blood pressure. In the Quebec City Study, substudies focusing on women have shown that regular (daily) brisk walking, although only a low-intensity exercise, can result in significant improvements in lipoprotein profiles and insulin resistance, even when overall weight losses are small or nonsignificant.

When diet and physical activity are insufficient to reduce the adverse cardiovascular profile of Syndrome X, medication may be necessary. Numerous antihypertensive, hypoglycemic, and lipid-lowering agents exist; however, these only target individual components of the syndrome. The other Syndrome X abnormalities should be assessed, and the treatment effects on these conditions should be considered. Drugs such as metformin target improvement in insulin resistance and show beneficial effects on some Syndrome X components. Studies are currently underway to evaluate the effects of troglitazone and other new thiazolidinedlione drugs on insulin resistance and Syndrome X.

Future studies should continue to explore the gender interactions in, and effects of hormones on, Syndrome X and its components. Prevention of abdominal fat accumulation and obesity and improvement of adverse cardiovascular profiles, through diet, physical activity, and pharmaceutical interventions, may have beneficial effects on Syndrome X and reduce the risk of CHD. Further elucidation of the underlying determinants may lead to new treatment or prevention strategies.

FURTHER READING

Busby, M. J., Bellantoni, M. F., Tobin, J. D., Muller, D. C., Kafonek, S. D., Blackman, M. R., & Andres, R. (1992). Glucose tolerance in women: The effects of age, body composition, and sex hormones. *Journal of the American Geriatrics Society, 40,* 497–502.
The effects of the menstrual cycle, endogenous hormones, and body fat distribution on glucose tolerance, a component of Syndrome X, were examined in a subset of 260 women from the Baltimore Longitudinal Study of Aging.

Després, J.-P., & Marette, A. (1994). Relation of components of insulin resistance syndrome to coronary disease risk. *Current Opinion in Lipidology, 5,* 274–289.
This annotated review discusses the etiology of insulin resistance, including genetic, biochemical, and environmental factors, and the interaction with other components of Syndrome X in relation to CHD and therapeutic approaches.

Hanson, M. J. S. (1994). Modifiable risk factors for coronary heart disease in women. *American Journal of Critical Care, 3,* 177–186.
This review of modifiable risk factors for CHD focused on the possible different mechanisms of these risk factors in women compared to men, as well as risk factors found only in women, including those related to menopause and oral contraceptive use.

Kuczmarski, R. J., Flegal, K. M., Campbell, S. M., & Johnson, C. L. (1994). Increasing prevalence of overweight among US adults: The National Health and Nutrition Examination Surveys, 1960 to 1991. *Journal of the American Medical Association, 272*(3), 205–211.
The trends in overweight prevalence and body mass index of the United States adult population are examined, using three surveys of the nationally representative NHANES, which cover a 30-year period.

Lapidus, L., Bengtsson, C., & Björntorp, P. (1994). The quantitative relationship between "the metabolic syndrome" and abdominal obesity in women. *Obesity Research, 2,* 372–377.
Measures of overall body fatness and abdominal obesity and their association with Syndrome X components were examined in 1,462 women from the Göteborg Population Study; stronger associations with abdominal obesity were found.

Lemieux, S., Després, J.-P., Moorjani, S., Nadeau, A., Thériault, G., Prud'homme, D., Tremblay, A., Bouchard, C., & Lupien, P. J. (1994). Are gender differences in cardiovascular disease risk factors explained by the level of visceral adipose tissue? *Diabetologia, 37,* 757–764.
Body fat distribution was assessed in the Quebec City Study population by means of underwater weighing and computerized tomography; it was found to explain many, but not all, of the gender differences in the metabolic risk factors measured.

Reaven, G. M. (1994). Syndrome X: 6 years later. *Journal of Internal Medicine, 236*(Suppl. 736), 13–22.

Syndrome X and its components are reviewed, updating progress in the years following Reaven's original 1988 publication defining the syndrome.

Svendsen, L. O., Hassager, C., & Christiansen C. (1993). Relationships and independence of body composition, sex hormones, fat distribution and other cardiovascular risk factors in overweight postmenopausal women. *International Journal of Obesity, 17,* 459–463.

The relationship among direct and indirect measures of body fat composition, sex hormones; and cardiovascular risk factors such as lipid and lipoprotein levels, cigarette use, and alcohol consumption were examined in 121 overweight postmenopausal women.

Section VIII

LINKAGES BETWEEN BEHAVIORAL, PSYCHOSOCIAL, AND PHYSICAL DISORDERS

118

Section Editor's Overview

Barbara G. Melamed

A common theme of the contributions to this section is that dysregulation of emotions can interfere with various aspects of a person's functioning, including intimacy, and occupational success, and (of particular interest here) physical well-being. Comorbidity of physical and psychiatric symptoms may drive an individual who is predisposed to biological depression or thought disorder beyond tolerable levels of comfort. As many as 50% of patients with diagnosable psychiatric conditions seek care in the general medical sector, because of the overlap between physical and psychological symptoms and the resulting fear of an impending medical crisis. Thus, unexplained feelings of weakness, lethargy, sleep difficulties, loss of appetite, uncomfortable fluctuations in weight, anxiety, or chest pain can lead individuals to perceive themselves as being in poor health. Over 16% of these patients report depression and anxiety to their primary care physicians. Unfortunately, major depressive disorder and anxiety disorders often fail to reach clinical threshold levels and go undiagnosed. Because of the stigma attached to mental (as opposed to physical) disorder, psychological referral is too often seen as a last resort. The patient feels dismissed or blamed, and the tendency to "shop" for another opinion can drive up the costs of medical care and often result in expensive and unnecessary diagnostic procedures. The responsiveness of the system to requests for diagnostic procedures inadvertently reinforces the patient's belief that a "real cause" will be found.

Women, who are more likely to seek medical care, receive more than 75% of all psychoactive drugs prescribed. Although these drugs may provide temporary relief, they often result in women's failure to consult mental health professionals to learn how to identify and deal with their problems. The "cure" is seen as the result of the medication and not of their own efforts. Paradoxical heightening of a woman's sense of ill feelings can often occur as a result of this polypharmacological approach, especially at certain points in the hormonal fluctuation cycle.

GENETIC VULNERABILITY VERSUS
ENVIRONMENTAL TRIGGERING: A TWO-AXIS MODEL

A model is postulated here that conceptualizes psychological/behavioral problems on two separate axes: (1) the extent to which they are associated with genetically linked predispositions, and (2) the extent to which symptom triggers are environmentally elicited. Individuals with schizophrenia are likely to have strong genetic vulnerabilities, which result in inflexible responses to both internal and external triggers when combined with poor prior coping resources (low or critical social support, few independent skills, and limited coping repertoires). Although individuals with borderline personality disorder may require long-term treatment to overcome the persistence of childhood inadequacies, they are less driven by biological urges. Depression and the anxiety disorders occur when predisposed individuals have a weak history of learned problem-solving abilities and are overwhelmed by the presence of multiple external triggers (e.g., comorbidity, life crises, daily hassles, disease onset, loss of job/spouse/house). In the case of agoraphobia, panic disorder, and depression, the internal cues themselves may lead to maladaptive coping (avoidance, denial, cognitive distortions). Therefore, individuals with these disorders need to learn to stay in the arousing environment, while distracting themselves from overvalued ideation (e.g., "Something terrible will happen") until the arousal dissipates without negative consequences.

For many of the problems and disorders described in this section, combined behavioral and pharmacological treatments may be most potent initially, with decreased reliance on medication as new skills are developed through behavioral rehearsal, assertiveness training, and modeling. For the more biologically driven disorders (e.g., schizophrenia, bipolar disorders), drug treatment must be considered primary to "quiet the waters" (reduce arousal or hyperreactive physiology) so that learning can take place. Whereas work- and role-related stresses can usually be resolved by recognizing conflicts and making decisions about their importance, rape victims suffering from posttraumatic stress disorder (PTSD) need to reexperience the loss of "safety" in a controlled environment (such as exposure with supportive counseling). In the middle of the continuum are the other anxiety disorders. For example, obsessive–compulsive disorder has mixed biological and environmental precipitants; these require simultaneous evocation of visceral reactivity while preventing escape or avoidance; in order to assist the individual in the reappraisal of somatic components as less threat-evoking.

FOUR BASIC QUESTIONS

The proposed model needs to explain four basic questions raised within the chapters in this section:

1. Why is the general prevalence of anxiety and mood disorders three times higher in women than in men?
2. Does having more than one psychiatric problem put women at greater risk for development of physical health problems?
3. Is actual biology or the *perception* of health more important in determining the outcome of treatment approaches?

4. What role can affect regulation play in our understanding of the course and/or treatment of psychological disturbances?

Male–Female Prevalence Differences

Why are the anxiety and mood disorders—the two most prominent groups of problems discussed in this section—likely to be found three times more frequently in women than in men? One reason is that there is a very different socialization process of emotional development and expression between the sexes. Goleman suggests that different schooling occurs between the sexes in learning about the regulation of emotions, with girls becoming adept at reading both verbal and nonverbal emotional signals and at expressing and communicating their feelings, and boys becoming adept at "minimizing emotions having to do with vulnerability, guilt, fear, and hurt." Failure to learn to interpret and monitor affects leads to feelings of helplessness, lack of control, and unpredictability in regard to both the external environment and the internal perception of one's emotional state. In addition, individuals who inherit a tendency toward cognitive, behavioral, or somatomotor problems may be predisposed to develop depression or bipolar disorders when exposed to inescapable stressors, particularly if they lack appropriate social skills. Learned avoidance may predominate in individuals with somewhat more flexible coping repertoires and may lead to the development of agoraphobia, panic disorder, or obsessive–compulsive disorder. The amelioration or exacerbation of problems with pharmacological approaches depends upon many factors, not the least of which involves the current nature of hormonal balance for women.

Linkage between Physical and Psychological Comorbidity

Although most of the disturbances described in this section are ones that are traditionally called "mental health problems," the comorbidity of such problems may enhance the likelihood that the biological system will be overwhelmed by a person's attempts at psychological regulation, and physical symptoms may occur. The ways people appraise or orient themselves toward stress may have a differential influence on immune function. In her chapter on psychoneuroimmunology in this section, Bower suggests that individuals who deny or minimize negative emotions or who inhibit the expression of these emotions show suppression of certain immune parameters. Although short-term expression of emotions may lead to transient decreases in certain immune parameters such as lymphocyte proliferation, more long-term or repeated emotional expression may be associated with positive changes in these and other immune measures. Social support has also been associated with immune enhancement. Perhaps individuals who express their own emotions to others, and allow others to express theirs, may take better care of themselves, comply with physicians' medical regimens, and reduce health-impairing habits such as drinking, non-nutritional eating, smoking, and lack of exercise.

Biology and the Perception of Health

Illness may progress to greater chronicity, and the symptoms themselves may become the problems when physical symptoms lack medical explanations. Thus, patients experiencing panic disorder or chronic fatigue syndrome (CFS) may fear a heart attack or paralysis.

The important concepts of uncertainty and/or uncontrollability must be integrated into this new conceptualization. As an example of uncertainty, women with CFS don't look sick, whereas sufferers from rheumatoid arthritis have swollen joints—obvious sources of pain. As an example of uncontrollability, a woman who is raped and develops PTSD suddenly loses all sense of safety and of invulnerability. Her enhanced vigilance in regard to physical symptoms may lead her to have a more negative perception of her health, to report more health problems, to have more doctors' visits per year, and to have more reproductive physiological illnesses. Trauma-related therapy focuses on giving her back some sense of control.

Affect Regulation and Emotional Disorders

In terms of the evolutionary significance of learning how to modulate emotion, one must consider the amygdala–cortical circuitry of the brain. If the organism can anticipate the emotions of others (verbally or nonverbally), it can set into action the appropriate fight–flight or quiescent vegetative response that is called for in its survival. Some of the cognitive behavioral approaches to psychotherapy have yielded structural and functional differences in this area of the brain, as measured by scanning devices. In each of the disorders and problems described in this section, there is a more or less hereditary defect that may be transmitted to the individual, who is likely to develop a low flexibility of emotional responding. It may be that too much or too little serotonin interferes with conscious control over the regulatory systems. It is postulated that individuals with schizophrenia and bipolar disorders have the least flexibility, with blunted emotion in the former and cyclic fluctuation in the latter controlling their responses. In depression and anxiety disorders, and to some extent borderline personality disorder, an interaction between the biological pattern and the influence of perceived threat cues the autonomic system's response. Individuals with stress-related disorders or disorders triggered by an acute precipitant (e.g., PTSD) modulate their visceral reaction based upon past experiences with the stressor, their current hormone cycle status, and to a lesser extent their biologically determined individual response stereotype. I now review each of the types of problems discussed in this section, to see how the two-axis model explains the occurrence of symptoms and effectiveness of treatment regimens in each case.

DISORDERS AND PROBLEMS DISCUSSED IN THIS SECTION

Anxiety Disorders

The anxiety disorders discussed by Bach, Weisberg, and Barlow—panic disorder, agoraphobia, generalized anxiety disorder, social phobia, and obsessive–compulsive disorder—are experienced three times more often in women than in men. Women tend to anticipate future harm when experiencing somatic symptoms. Thus, especially when negative affect is present, they are more likely to interpret heart palpitations, dizzy spells, and chest pain as indicating an impending heart attack. Panic symptoms may occur more often premenstrually, during or following pregnancy, or at menopause. Agoraphobia may develop as a way to ward off exposure to "unsafe" situations—those in which rapid escape is not possible, such as shopping malls, crowded places, and public transportation. When women are predisposed toward generalized anxiety, the anxiety is associated with such somatic symptoms as restlessness, fatigue, and muscle tension. In women well socialized to maintain relationships, the fear of negative scrutiny by others may lead to social anxiety; thus, a fear of looking crazy or of embarrassing themselves in public restricts their activities. Avoidance coping, rather than mastery of affect dysregulation, is likely to predominate in all of these cases. In obsessive–compulsive disorder, which may develop through biological predisposition, intrusive, unwanted fears, doubts, and sexual and aggressive thoughts lead to compulsive behaviors such as cleaning and washing rituals. These may be seen as attempts to neutralize the fear of acting out impulses, despite the patient's acknowledging the irrationality of these reactions. In some anxious individuals, particularly those who employ catastrophizing ideation or denial, the failure of defenses may lead to lethargy, immobilization, feelings of helplessness, misinterpretation of somatic symptoms, and ultimately to threshold diagnosis of a comorbid major depressive disorder (see "Depression," below). When depression is current, more negative thoughts lead to poor health perception and lack of coping responses.

When antianxiety and antidepressant medications are used, there is often a temporary remission of symptoms. Perhaps this dampening of physiological predominance allows a therapeutic intervention such as reexposure to sensations (as in flooding) or cognitive restructuring to assist the individual in developing new behavior repertoires. Unfortunately, many drugs are used in the absence of psychotherapy, or they may interfere with cognitive processing. When a patient attributes the reduction of anxiety to the medication rather than her own control, generalization does not occur when the patient is in other situations or when medication is withdrawn. Thus, approaches such as stress inoculation and *in vivo* desensitization give the individual an experience of control at a low dose of physiological arousal. Exposure or flooding is only effective if the patient can recognize the events, thoughts, and behaviors most likely to trigger the feelings of loss of control. It is necessary to maintain the patient's tolerance in face of these stressors without escape (e.g., as in response prevention, often used in obsessive–compulsive disorder), so that physiological habituation can occur. As Sanderson suggests in his chapter on panic disorder, the symptoms of panic may in fact be the results of a medical disorder. Thus, correct diagnosis and treatment may eliminate such sensations as heart palpitations, dizziness, and the like. This reassurance will allow patients to relabel their fear as recognition that medication to control symptoms is required.

Rape and Posttraumatic Stress Disorder

Although PTSD is classified in the official psychiatric nosology as an anxiety disorder, it is considered separately here because, unlike the anxiety disorders discussed above, it is precipitated by a single, overwhelming stressor. One such stressor, which is far more common among women than among men, is sexual violence; thus, Foa focuses in her chapter on PTSD resulting from rape. Rape is followed by a sense of helplessness and a loss of sense of security. A woman who has been raped can no longer take safety features of the environment for granted; she is no longer vulnerable. Her enhanced psychological vigilance is often accompanied by greater attention to physical symptoms. Because of a negative perception of their health, rape victims often report health problems and visit physicians much more frequently than nonvictims. In addition, because of the high prevalence of general bias against women in society and the tendency to blame rape victims for their experience in particular, these victims' psychological and physical problems are likely to be carried forward to new experiences and to be transmitted across generational lines. Mass media portrayals of victimization and abuse can reevoke incompletely extinguished memory schemas and can lead to avoidance and fear of close relationships. Foa's discussion of treatment provides suggestions for extinguishing such schemas.

Bipolar Disorders

Bipolar disorders, covered in the chapter by Miklowitz, are marked by extreme fluctuation between elation and depression; they are viewed as genetically transmitted and likely to have underpinnings of neurophysiological, neuroanatomical, and neuropsychological dysregulation. Women are more likely than men to show "rapid cycling," in which they experience four or more recurrences of mania, hypomania, or depression in 1 year. These mood disorders may in fact be hormonally influenced, as they predispose women to postpartum depression. Mood-regulating drugs are the primary choice for treatment. Educating a bipolar patient's family is a prerequisite for improving patient–family communication and generating problem-solving strategies to assure the patient's compliance with the medication regimen.

Depression is discussed in the chapters by McLean and Woody, Craighead and Vajk, and Allen and Schnyer. The extremely high rate of comorbidity with anxiety disorders (42–48%) in depressed women noted by Craighead and Vajk may be attributable to women's coping response styles: Men tend to cope with depression by self-medicating with alcohol, whereas women ruminate about their problems. A small percentage of women may resort to eating disorders, which can exacerbate depression. The self-defeating negative attitudes may lead further to isolation from other potentially supportive individuals. Marital discord and disruption may lead to depression, with higher rates of major depression in individuals who are separated or divorced than in those who are married or have never married. Although childhood sexual abuse is reportedly common among women reporting depression, other aspects of bias against women in society today, including role discrimination, harassment, and inequity of opportunity, may contribute to gender differences. Thus, poverty and loss of relationship support predispose women to recurrent depression, particularly where there is also a genetic predisposition for depression.

Borderline Personality Disorder

As Wagner notes in her chapter borderline personality disorder may occur when girls have been reared in situations where emotional neglect and lack of emotional synchrony by mothers have led to blunted emotional expression. Children reared in such an environment become hyperalert to the emotions of those around them, in what amounts to a posttraumatic vigilance to cues that have signaled threat, cruelty, and sadistic humiliation. Such children reach adulthood suffering from a poor sense of self accompanied by emotional ups and downs. What may appear to be a narcissistic orientation may in fact be a coverup for intense feelings of lack of self-worth.

Schizophrenia

In schizophrenia, as Lewine points out, genetic vulnerability has been proven. Women who suffer from schizophrenia have given up on the regulation of mood states and either show bizarre attention to external stimuli that they attempt to incorporate into their own bodily sensations (e.g., hallucinations and delusions), or exhibit catatonic internal concentration to the exclusion of environmental input. Hormonal fluctuations of estrogen may lead to delayed onset of symptoms and to greater susceptibility during life transitions such as menopause. The influence of estrogen on dopamine receptors and the disruption of neurotransmitters may result in disorganized thinking. The stronger hereditary nature of this disorder in women than in men, and women's greater sensitivity to medication, make it critical to evaluate polypharmacological approaches carefully; some medications may render a female schizophrenic even more susceptible to cognitive disorganization, accompanied by failure to comply with the treatment regimen. Childbearing creates special difficulties for schizophrenic mothers, who relate to their children as a function of their own desires. Thus, for example, they feed their children when they themselves are hungry.

Chronic Fatigue Syndrome and Chronic Pain

CFS and chronic pain are discussed in the chapters by myself and La Reche, respectively. Women may have a greater tendency because of their socialization to report fatigue or pain. Moreover, because of cultural differences in the acceptability of somatic versus psychological causes, fatigue or pain may be reported when indeed anxiety is present. When a patient experiences chronic pain or CFS, limitations in activity and lifestyle may follow. Thus anticipation of a repetitive cycle of pains associated with menstrual cycle variation, and degenerative changes in skeletal or muscular features, may set the way for conditioned pain or CFS experiences at different points in the life cycle. Temporo-mandibular disorder sufferers may not benefit from hormone treatment.

Stress-Related Disorders

As Pickering notes in his chapter on stress-related disorders, occupational stress as triggered by both actual and perceived role discrepancies has been shown to lead to autonomic dysregulation. The job strain of having a high-demand, low-control position increases the risk of coronary heart disease in both men and women (indeed, the effect is greater for men, though women are more likely to be in such jobs). Other work-related factors affecting women's health include worksite and occupation. For many women, there is also a role conflict between providing for children and satisfying their own job strivings; working women who have small children exhibit continued high blood pressure when they go home in the evening, whereas blood pressure falls in childless women and all men. Individuals who stay at home but would rather be at work show a similar dysfunctional stress reaction. Sex differences in social control itself have been shown, with husbands showing increases in angry, hostile displays and blood pressure, whereas wives showed little change while attempting to influence their husbands (see Stoney's chapter in Section VII of this volume). Synchronous physiological responses seem to produce the least conflict and may be what we think of as empathic responses. Other factors briefly considered by Pickering include bereavement, social support, and socioeconomic status.

CONCLUSION

In conclusion, it is evident that the perception of poor physical health or uncontrollability of symptoms often precipitates an individual's attention to stress-related somatic complaints that mimic disease, and often results in a visit to the physician. This then produces a cycle of reinforcement of the idea that there may be a biological determinant of the unpleasant feelings, which can easily be sorted out and treated by taking the right pill. Unfortunately, the interaction of physiological arousal and cognitive appraisal of feelings of controllability may be synergistic. In such cases, therapeutic strategies that allow for the management of arousal in the presence of conflicting situations and relationships have been shown to be more appropriate treatment approaches than reducing arousal through relaxation or hypnosis. In cases where heredity or predisposing personality features make individuals more resistant to short-term intervention, a more lengthy course of psychotherapy combined with pharmacotherapy and family psychoeducation is a necessity. Now that actual changes in the regulatory function of the amygdala–cortical structures have been linked to the use of cognitive behavioral psychotherapy, we should begin to see more collaborative relationships between physicians and psychologists.

FURTHER READING

Brody, L. R., & Hall, J. (1993). Gender and emotion. In M. Lewis & J. M. Haviland (Eds.), *Handbook of emotions.* New York: Guilford Press.
Goleman, D. (1995). *Emotional intelligence.* New York: Bantam Books.

119

Anxiety Disorders

Amy K. Bach
Risa B. Weisberg
David H. Barlow

Anxiety disorders are among the most frequently occurring mental disorders; 24.9% of all people develop a problem with anxiety at some point in their lifetime. The prevalence of anxiety disorders is particularly high for women; they sometimes occur as much as three times more often in women than in men. In addition, many of the physical symptoms of anxiety may feel similar to health problems. A woman experiencing heart palpitations, dizzy spells, and chest pain is likely to fear that she may have a cardiac condition, and thus to seek out general medical care rather than mental health care. Thus, knowledge of anxiety disorders is extremely important for anyone attending to the health care of women. The particular disorders we consider in this chapter are panic disorder, agoraphobia, generalized anxiety disorder, social phobia, and obsessive–compulsive disorder (OCD). (Panic disorder is discussed in more detail in Sanderson's chapter; Foa discusses another anxiety disorder—posttraumatic stress disorder resulting from rape—in her chapter.) Before we begin discussing specific disorders, however, let us clarify the difference between panic and anxiety.

PANIC AND ANXIETY

"Anxiety" is a mood state in which a person experiences negative affect and somatic symptoms of tension while apprehensively anticipating future danger or misfortune. Related to the state of anxiety is the experience of panic. Whereas anxiety appears to be a state of anticipation, panic is an alarm response that prepares the body to fend off immediate danger through fight or flight.

"Panic attacks" are defined as circumscribed periods of intense fear, during which time numerous symptoms are experienced. During a panic attack, people typically experience somatic symptoms such as heart palpitations, sweating, shaking, difficulty breathing, chest pain, and/or nausea. They may also experience cognitive symptoms such as fears of dying, going crazy, or losing control. Panic attacks frequently occur in the context of many different anxiety disorders. When one is assessing the nature of panic attacks, it is important to consider the relationship between the onset of the attack and the presence or absence of situational triggers. Unexpected panic attacks seem to occur "out of the blue," without any identifiable situational trigger. These attacks are required for the diagnosis of panic disorder. Situationally bound attacks occur when a situational trigger is present or anticipated. This type of panic attack occurs in many different anxiety disorders. An example is a woman with social phobia experiencing panic sensations in anticipation of a date.

Thus, the experience or complaint of panic attacks does not in and of itself indicate that a woman is suffering from panic disorder.

PANIC DISORDER

Panic disorder is more than twice as common among women as it is among men. The lifetime prevalence rates of panic disorder among women range from 2.1% to 5.0%, while those among men range from 1% to 2%.

Panic disorder is characterized by the occurrence of one or more unexpected panic attacks. Such attacks will seem to the individual to occur "out of the blue" rather than in response to a feared situation or stimulus. Following the unexpected panic, the person develops significant concerns about the experience or possible results of additional attacks. Alternatively, the person may deny such concerns but may change certain behaviors to avoid the risk of future panics. In panic disorder, therefore, the focus of anxiety is on the possible future occurrence of panic symptoms and their consequences. Just as someone with acrophobia fears heights, so does a person with panic disorder fear sensations such as heart palpitations and dizziness.

Panic symptoms may be influenced by certain phases of the female reproductive cycle. Symptoms may worsen for women during the premenstrum. In addition, symptoms may be affected by pregnancy. Some women report an improvement in their symptoms during pregnancy; others report a worsening; and still others experience no change. A more consistent finding has been that panic symptoms may worsen during the postpartum period.

Both psychological and pharmacological treatments have proven beneficial for people with panic disorder. One cognitive-behavioral intervention, developed over the past 10 years, has proven effective for more than 85% of patients. With the behavioral component, patients are taught to use diaphragmatic breathing rather than shallow chest breathing. Next, they are systematically exposed to the sensations they fear. They engage in exercises such as spinning in a chair, breathing through a straw, and running in place in order to elicit such symptoms as dizziness, shortness of breath, and heart palpitations. Repeated exposure to these symptoms reduces the associated anxiety. The cognitive component of treatment involves restructuring thoughts about the possible consequences of panic symptoms. Fears of having a heart attack, dying, going crazy, or being embarrassed during a panic attack are identified and challenged.

With respect to pharmacological treatments, both tricyclic antidepressants and benzodiazepines have proven beneficial. Research shows that approximately 60% of patients remain panic-free while on such medications. However, 20–50% of patients will relapse after discontinuing tricyclic antidepressants, and many will drop out of treatment because of the medications' side effects. Relapse will occur in nearly 90% of patients who discontinue benzodiazepines, though side effects are fewer and dropout rates are lower. Such high rates of relapse may be of particular concern for women during childbearing years. Discontinuation of benzodiazepines is often advised for women who are pregnant; the return of anxiety symptoms at that time can prove extremely distressing. In such cases, a psychosocial intervention may be the preferred treatment option. More recently, a new class of antidepressants—the selective serotonin reuptake inhibitors (SSRIs), such as fluoxetine and paroxetine—has demonstrated similar success rates to tricyclics, with fewer side effects.

AGORAPHOBIA

One complication that often results from panic disorder is the development of agoraphobia. The lifetime prevalence rate of agoraphobia ranges from 5.6% to 6.7%. It is estimated that 75% or more of those with agoraphobia are women. Some researchers have argued that the preponderance of this disorder among women results from a gender difference in coping strategies. In response to feelings of anxiety and panic, men may tend to consume alcohol rather than physically avoid their feared situations.

Agoraphobia refers to a fear of entering situations that may be difficult to escape from and that may not have help available if it is needed. This disorder most often results from the experience of panic attacks and a fear of their consequences; however, agoraphobia may also be associated with concerns about such symptoms as diarrhea, dizziness, or vomiting. People with agoraphobia often avoid situations such as shopping malls, driving, public transportation, small enclosed places, restaurants, and being far from home.

The treatment of agoraphobia involves *in vivo* exposure to the feared situations. It is estimated that 60–75% of patients will gain some benefit from this method. Antidepressants and benzodiazepines, as noted above, target the underlying anxiety and panic that lead to agoraphobic avoidance.

GENERALIZED ANXIETY DISORDER

Generalized anxiety disorder occurs in from 3.8% to 5.1% of the population over a lifetime. Like panic disorder, this anxiety disorder is twice as common among women as it is among men. The lifetime prevalence rates for women range from 4.95% to 6.6%, while those for men range from 2.4% to 3.6%.

Generalized anxiety disorder is characterized by excessive worry or anxiety about several activities or life events. The worry is hard to control and is associated with somatic symptoms such as restlessness, fatigue, and muscle tension. Although panic attacks may occur, they are typically cued by worries, unlike the unexpected panic attacks that characterize panic disorder.

Traditionally, both psychological and pharmacological treatments have had limited effects on generalized anxiety disorder. Such interventions have sometimes led to short-term improvements, but treatment gains have often been lost over time. Recently, more specialized psychosocial treatments have been designed. One such treatment involves helping patients to process, rather than avoid, the images and affect associated with their worries. A second treatment involves imaginal exposure to the feared scenarios that drive a person's worries. Although research is still in progress, it appears that these interventions may be more beneficial than those of the past. With respect to pharmacological treatments, benzodiazepines have traditionally been the drugs of choice. Research suggests that these drugs may bring about short-term improvement, but the benefits are often not maintained.

SOCIAL PHOBIA

Although social phobia is more common among women than among men, the gender difference is not as great as it is for panic disorder or generalized anxiety disorder. The lifetime prevalence rate for women ranges from 2.9% to 15.5%, while that for men ranges from 2.5% to 11.1%. Interestingly, among those who seek treatment for social phobia, the gender difference disappears. Traditionally, attributes such as shyness, inhibition, and a lack of assertiveness have been more acceptable for women, in both social and professional settings. It is perhaps for this reason that men appear more likely to seek help for such a problem. Social phobia is characterized by a strong, persisting fear of one or more situations in which the person may be scrutinized by others. A person with social phobia may experience panic attacks in response to social situations.

Both psychological and pharmacological treatments have proven beneficial for people with social phobia. Research shows that a form of cognitive-behavioral group treatment is effective. The treatment involves role-playing anxiety-provoking situations in front of other group members. This exercise serves as a behavioral exposure and allows for cognitive restructuring of interfering thoughts.

In terms of pharmacological treatment, antidepressants such as monoamine oxidase inhibitors have been found to reduce social anxiety. However, this class of drugs must be very carefully monitored because of possibly dangerous interactions with a number of foods. The SSRIs will most likely also prove effective with this disorder when properly evaluated.

OBSESSIVE–COMPULSIVE DISORDER

Recent studies suggest that OCD is more prevalent than was once thought. Data from the Epidemiologic Catchment Area study suggest that the lifetime prevalence rate in the general population is as high as 2.6%. OCD is only slightly more common among women than among men. The male-to-female ratio is approximately 1:1.1.

"Obsessions" have been defined as intrusive, unwanted mental events that cause distress or anxiety. Examples include fears of contamination, persistent doubting (e.g., whether a door is locked), fears of causing accidental harm to others, and distressing sexual thoughts (e.g., sexual activity with a child). A "compulsion" is a thought or behavior that is intended to neutralize distressing thoughts and relieve the associated anxiety or discomfort. Such behaviors often involve checking, counting, washing, internally repeating phrases or prayers, or adhering to certain rules. Research has suggested that checking behaviors are more common among men, whereas cleaning and washing rituals are more common among women.

For a person with OCD, obsessions and compulsions can be extremely distressing, time-consuming, and/or interfering. The person at some point realizes that such behaviors are unreasonable or excessive, but nevertheless has significant difficulty controlling them.

It appears that pregnancy and childbirth may significantly affect the course of OCD in women. As many as 69% of women with OCD have reported that the onset or worsening of their symptoms was related to some aspect of childbirth or pregnancy. In many of these cases, the focus of the obsessions and compulsions is a fear of harming the infant or unborn fetus. Such fears may cause women to avoid caring for their children.

The psychosocial treatment of choice for OCD involves exposure and response prevention. Patients repeatedly undergo either imaginal or *in vivo* exposure to the feared situations. During response prevention, patients abstain from performing compulsions. This abstinence provides them with evidence that their ritualistic behaviors are not necessary to prevent the feared outcomes. It is estimated that approximately 75% of patients benefit from this treatment.

Research has shown that antidepressants, particularly those acting rather specifically on the serotonergic neurotransmitter system, are of benefit to 30–60% of patients with OCD. Unfortunately, medications often have a limited effect, reducing symptoms by only 30–60%. Psychosocial treatments tend to produce more substantial and lasting changes, but are not readily available.

CONCLUSION

Anxiety disorders affect a large number of women. The symptoms these women suffer not only are distressing, but often cause much interference and have a profound effect on their families and close relationships.

Since many women experiencing anxiety problems first present to a primary care physician, pharmacotherapy is often the first treatment available to these patients. Many medications have proven to be quite effective in the alleviation of anxiety symptoms. However, pharmacotherapy may not be an attractive option for many women. As women have a larger proportion of body fat, their medication plasma levels may differ from those of men. As a result, women may be more susceptible to side effects. During pregnancy, medication may be particularly problematic. Benzodiazepines in particular have been reported to cause problems in this regard.

Specialized psychosocial treatments have also proven to be extremely effective, but have not heretofore been widely available. Fortunately, these treatments are now becoming more readily accessible to clinicians and patients. Over the past few years, much work has been done to increase the dissemination of effective psychological treatments, and treatment manuals, handbooks, and training courses are increasingly available.

FURTHER READING

American Psychiatric Association. (1994). *Diagnostic and statistical manual of mental disorders* (4th ed.). Washington, DC: Author.
The official classification manual for the anxiety (and other mental) disorders.

Barlow, D. H. (1988). *Anxiety and its disorders: The nature and treatment of anxiety and panic.* New York: Guilford Press.
Reviews theories of emotion and anxiety, and presents extensive information on the assessment, diagnosis, and treatment of each anxiety disorder.

Barlow, D. H. (Ed.). (1993). *Clinical handbook of psychological disorders* (2nd ed.). New York: Guilford Press.
Compilation of up-to-date treatment protocols for the anxiety disorders, as well as other commonly seen mental health difficulties.

Barlow, D. H., & Craske, M. G. (1994). *Mastery of your anxiety and panic II.* Albany, NY: Graywind.
Treatment manual for panic disorder. Designed for patients and therapists.

Craske, M. G., Barlow, D. H., & O'Leary, T. A. (1992). *Mastery of your anxiety and worry.* Albany, NY: Graywind.
Treatment manual for generalized anxiety disorder. Designed for patients and therapists.

Heimberg, R. G., Liebowitz, M. R., Hope, D. A., & Schneier, F. R. (Eds.). (1995). *Social phobia: Diagnosis, assessment, and treatment.* New York: Guilford Press.
Reviews theories of social phobia, as well as the most recent advances in the assessment, diagnosis, and treatment of the disorder.

Jenike, M. A., Baer, L., & Minichiello, W. E. (Eds.). (1990). *Obsessive–compulsive disorders: Theory and management* (2nd ed.). Chicago: Year Book Medical Publishers.
Comprehensive book that reviews theories of obsessive–compulsive disorder as well as research on the etiology, assessment, and treatment of the disorder.

Kessler, R. C., McGonagle, K. A., Shanyang, Z., Nelson, C. B., Hughes, M., Eshleman, S., Wittchen, H.-U., & Kendler, K. S. (1994). Lifetime and 12-month prevalence of DSM-III-R psychiatric disorders in the United States. *Archives of General Psychiatry, 51,* 8–19.
Based on the National Comorbidity Survey; presents prevalence rates of psychiatric disorders among noninstitutionalized citizens of the United States.

Magee, W. J., Eaton, W. W., Wittchen, H.-U., McGonagle, K. A., & Kessler, R. C. (1996). Agoraphobia, simple phobia, and social phobia in the national comorbidity survey. *Archives of General Psychiatry, 53,* 159–168.
Presents data on the prevalence, correlates, comorbidities, and impairments associated with phobias in the United States.

Robins, L. N., & Regier, D. A. (Eds.). (1991). *Psychiatric disorders in America: The Epidemiologic Catchment Area study.* New York: Free Press.
Based on a national, multisite study; presents community prevalence rates for various psychiatric disorders in the United States.

Steketee, G., & White, K. (1990). *When once is not enough: Help for obsessive compulsives.* Oakland, CA: New Harbinger.
Self-help book for the treatment of obsessive–compulsive disorder.

120

Panic Disorder

William C. Sanderson

EPIDEMIOLOGY AND COURSE

Panic disorder (PD) is a debilitating condition that is more common in females than in males. The overall prevalence of PD is 1.5%. However, approximately twice as many women as men suffer from PD, and nearly three-quarters of PD patients presenting for treatment are female. PD typically first strikes between late adolescence and early adulthood, although it can also begin in childhood and in later life. Although data on the course of PD are lacking, retrospective patient accounts indicate that PD appears to be a chronic condition that waxes and wanes in severity.

Unfortunately, the disorder's chronicity may be a result, in part, of the lack of appropriate treatment. Recent research has revealed that many patients—perhaps most—do not receive appropriate pharmacological or psychological treatment. The severity and chronic nature of PD result in a substantial decrease in quality of life. Consequences of PD include feelings of poor physical and emotional health, impaired social and marital functioning, financial dependency, and increased use of health services and hospital emergency services.

PSYCHOLOGICAL ASSESSMENT

As defined in the *Diagnostic and Statistical Manual of Mental Disorders* fourth edition (DSM-IV), the essential feature of PD is the experience of recurring, unpredictable panic attacks. A panic attack is defined as a discrete period of extreme fear or discomfort that develops suddenly, peaks within 10 minutes, and is accompanied by at least 4 of the following 13 somatic and cognitive symptoms: shortness of breath, dizziness, palpitations, trembling, sweating, a sensation of choking, nausea/gastrointestinal distress, depersonalization, numbness/tingling, flushes/chills, chest pain, fear of dying, and/or fear of going crazy or doing something uncontrolled. To warrant the diagnosis of PD in accordance with the DSM-IV, an individual must experience at least two unexpected panic attacks followed by at least 1 month of concern about having another panic attack. The frequency of attacks varies widely and ranges from several attacks each day to only a handful of attacks per year.

Perhaps the most disabling feature of PD is the development of agoraphobia, which affects approximately one-half of individuals diagnosed with PD. Agoraphobia is diagnosed three times as often in women as in men. The DSM-IV defines agoraphobia as the experience of anxiety in situations where a person might find escape difficult or might not find help immediately available in the event of the occurrence of a panic attack. Common agoraphobic situations include airplanes, buses, trains, elevators, being alone, being in a crowd of people, and so on. As a result of the anxiety experienced in these situations, individuals often develop phobic avoidance, resulting in a constricted lifestyle. The severity of agoraphobia may range from relatively mild (e.g., a person travels unaccompanied when necessary, but typically avoids traveling alone) to quite severe (e.g., a person is unable to leave home alone).

DIFFERENTIAL DIAGNOSIS OF PANIC DISORDER AND MEDICAL CONDITIONS

Although panic attacks are typically associated with PD, similar attacks can be a sign of an underlying medical condition. In particular, panic-like attacks are common features of hyperthyroidism, hypoglycemia, pheochromocytoma, and mitral valve prolapse (MVP). Thus, in order to make the diagnosis of PD, one must rule out potential medical conditions. This is of particular relevance to female PD patients, as several of these medical conditions occur more frequently in women than in men.

In the past, almost all patients with PD had been down a long road of medical evaluations until they finally arrived in a mental health professional's office. However, as a result of all of the information about PD in the popular media, increasing numbers of patients are diagnosing themselves and presenting directly to mental health professionals. Although this is beneficial, in that appropriate treatment can be implemented more quickly, *mental health clinicians are now responsible for ensuring that all patients have been medically evaluated.* Consequently, nonmedical clinicians treating PD patients should be familiar with potential medical aspects as well. Thus, the remainder of this chapter provides a brief overview of those medical disorders that may resemble PD.

Hyperthyroidism

Symptoms of hyperthyroidism result from excessive thyroid gland activity. Ninety-five percent of patients with hyperthyroidism report nervousness or episodic anxiety as their primary complaint. More than two-thirds report palpitations, tachycardia, and dyspnea (difficulty breathing)—common panic attack symptoms. Like PD, hyperthyroidism typically first occurs is between the ages of 20 and 40, and it is more common in females (1 in 1,000) than in males (1 in 3,000). Thyroid function tests are used to confirm the diagnosis. Several studies have suggested that hyperthyroidism is a commonly occurring comorbid disorder in females diagnosed with PD, although other studies have not supported this finding.

Hypoglycemia

Hypoglycemia is believed to be caused by excessive secretion of insulin after ingesting carbohydrates, resulting in a rapid decline of blood sugar. Symptoms of hypoglycemia occur 2–4 hours after meals. Common symptoms include headache, mental dullness, confusion, anxiety, irritability, sweating, palpitations, tremor, and hunger sensations. Research studies suggest that hypoglycemia is not a common comorbid condition associated with PD; still, it should be considered as a differential diagnosis, especially when (1) the attacks are typically related to meals, or (2) the attacks are accompanied by sensations of hunger. The 5-hour glucose tolerance test is used to confirm the diagnosis of hypoglycemia.

Pheochromocytomas

Pheochromocytomas are tumors of catecholamine-secreting tissues that result in the secretion of excessive amounts of adrenaline and noradrenaline. Pheochromocytoma is a relatively rare condition, occurring at a rate of 0.01%. This condition occurs most often in women between the ages of 20 and 50. Symptoms occur in episodes (paroxysmal attacks) lasting from several minutes to as long as a week. Headaches and hypertension are the most common symptoms, occurring in as many as 90% of patients. Other common symptoms include sweating, palpitations, shortness of breath, restlessness, and anxiety. Again, research studies suggest that pheochromocytoma is not a common comorbid condition associated with PD. However, it should be considered as a differential diagnosis, especially when (1) the attacks do not appear as frequently or as intensely as they typically do in PD patients; (2) the somatic symptoms are more prominent than the cognitive and affective symptoms (e.g., fear of dying, impending doom); and (3) no phobic symptoms are present. To confirm this medical diagnosis, plasma and urine catecholamines are measured, and radiological examinations are performed.

Mitral Valve Prolapse

MVP results from an alteration (sagging) in the connective tissue of the mitral valve of the heart. Symptoms of MVP include chest pain, dyspnea, tachycardia, palpitations, light-headedness, fainting, fatigue, and anxiety. Because different criteria are used for diagnosis of MVP, the estimated prevalence is quite variable; however, conservative estimates range between 4% and 7%. The rate of MVP is higher among women than among men, and MVP appears to be a function of age. Its prevalence in females during the third decade—a common age for the onset of PD—is as high as 17%. In almost all cases, the course of MVP is benign. Although there is still no "gold standard" for the diagnosis of MVP, it appears to be best confirmed by echocardiogram. Reviews of research studies on the relationship between MVP and PD suggest that there is no increased prevalence of panic among patients with MVP. Given the relatively common prevalence of MVP, it often does occur as a comorbid condition with PD; however, research has demonstrated that comorbid MVP does not affect the course or response to treatment of PD.

Other Disorders

In addition to the disorders discussed above, many other medical disorders, although perhaps not as common or similar to PD, must be considered in the differential diagnosis of PD. (Space limitations do not permit further elaboration here. For further details, see the 1990 discussion by Jacob and Lilenfeld.)

1. *Endocrine disorders.* Endocrine disorders appear to be the most common illnesses associated with medically produced anxiety and panic states. In addition to those discussed above (hyperthyroidism, hypoglycemia, and pheochromocytoma), other endocrine disorders to be considered are carcinoid syndrome, Cushing's syndrome, hypothyroidism, hypoparathyroidism, menopause, and premenstrual syndrome.

2. *Cardiovascular disorders.* Since cardiovascular symptoms are a cardinal feature of panic attacks, cardiovascular disorders must always be considered in the differential diagnosis of PD. In addition to MVP (discussed above), the following disorders should be considered: cardiac arrhythmias, congestive heart failure, coronary insufficiency, hypertension, and myocardial infarction.

3. *Respiratory disorders.* Dyspnea is a common feature of panic attacks, reported by almost all patients. As a result, respiratory disorders should be considered in the differential diagnosis of PD—specifically, asthma, chronic obstructive pulmonary disease, hyperventilation syndrome, and hypoxia.

4. *Neurological disorders.* Neurological disorders are associated with symptoms that are similar to PD. Temporal lobe seizures are commonly accompanied by intense feelings of fear, terror, and unreality, as well as autonomic symptoms. Therefore, seizures should always be considered in the differential diagnosis of PD. Other neurological disorders to be considered are collagen vascular disease, epilepsy, Huntington's disease, multiple sclerosis, organic brain syndromes, vestibular dysfunction, and Wilson's disease.

FURTHER READING

Asnis, G. M., & van Praag, H. M. (Eds.). (1995). *Panic disorder: Clinical, biological and treatment aspects.* New York: Wiley.
This book contains chapters on all aspects of PD—epidemiology, neurobiology, and biological and psychological treatment.

Hall, R. C. (1980). Anxiety. In R. C. Hall (Ed.), *Psychiatric presentation of medical illness* (pp. 13–35). New York: Spectrum.
This chapter discusses medical illnesses that may present with psychiatric symptoms.

Jacob, R. G., & Lilenfeld, S. O. (1990). Panic disorder: Diagnosis, medical assessment, and psychological assessment. In J. R. Walker, G. R. Norton, & C. A. Ross (Eds.), *Panic disorder and agoraphobia: A guide for the practitioner* (pp. 16–102). Pacific Grove, CA: Brooks/Cole.
This chapter details the assessment of PD, paying particular attention to differential diagnosis.

Katon, W. (1993). *Panic disorder in the medical setting* (DHHS Publication No. NIH 93-3482). Washington, DC: U.S. Government Printing Office.
This booklet reviews all areas of PD for general health care professionals.

McGinn, L. K., & Sanderson, W. C. (1995). The nature of panic disorder. *In Session: Psychotherapy in Practice, 1,* 7–19.
This chapter reviews the assessment, epidemiology, and psychological and biological theories of PD.

Raj, A., & Sheehan, D. V. (1987). Medical evaluation of panic attacks. *Journal of Clinical Psychiatry, 48,* 309–313.
This article reviews medical evaluations that should be conducted to rule out medical illness before a diagnosis of PD is made.

121

Rape and Posttraumatic Stress Disorder

Edna B. Foa

*I*n recent years, evidence has accumulated to indicate that many women experience multiple incidents of violence throughout their lifetimes and are at greater risk than men for being targets of sexual violence, during both childhood and adulthood. The problem is compounded by the fact that women are at greater risk than men for developing trauma-related psychopathology—that is, posttraumatic stress disorder (PTSD)—which is characterized by repeated reexperiencing, avoidance, emotional numbing, and heightened general arousal.

POSTRAPE PSYCHOLOGICAL PROBLEMS

In the largest epidemiological study to date of trauma prevalence and PTSD incidence among women, 69% of the sample reported experiencing at least one traumatic event during their lifetimes; 27% (one out of four women) had been victims of sexual assault, and 13% of completed rape. Thirty-two percent of the rape victims reported having had symptoms severe enough to meet criteria for lifetime PTSD, and 12.4% had current PTSD at the time of the interview. Thus, one out of four to five women in the United States (about 12 million) has been sexually assaulted at least once during her lifetime, and one-third of rape victims develop psychological difficulties severe enough to cause marked impairment in their daily functioning. In one out of eight victims, PTSD symptoms become chronic, lasting for years after the assault.

The picture emerging from prospective studies in which rape victims are interviewed within a short period after the trauma is even bleaker, because a large proportion of recent victims have psychological difficulties and are likely to remember their posttraumatic symptoms more accurately even after they have recovered. Indeed, prospective studies yield higher lifetime and current prevalence rates of PTSD than do retrospective studies. Rothbaum and colleagues assessed 64 female rape victims weekly for 3 months;

the first interview in each case took place within 2 weeks of the rape. Almost all victims (95%) met DSM-III-R symptom criteria for PTSD in the first interview; 1 month after the assault, 64% of the victims met criteria for PTSD, and 47% still had the disorder. These results were replicated in a second study. Thus, although postrape psychopathology decreases over time, many victims continue to be plagued by psychological difficulties.

POSTRAPE PHYSICAL PROBLEMS

Rape not only leads to psychological problems, but also causes health complications. Studies indicate that within 2 years of rape, female victims of rape have a more negative perception of their health, report more health problems, and engage in more negative health behaviors (e.g., lack of exercise, smoking), make more doctor visits per year, and have had more reproductive physiology illnesses than did nonassaulted women. Female crime victims (including rape victims) made twice the number of physician visits and incurred 2.5 times more outpatient costs than nonvictims. On the average, the doctor visits of victims increased by 15–24% during the year in which the crime occurred and increased by 31–56% in the year after, as compared to the 2 years before the crime. The degree of violence during the assault was related to the increase in visits to doctors.

TREATMENT AND PREVENTION OF POSTRAPE PSYCHOPATHOLOGY

Several types of psychological interventions have been suggested for rape victims, including brief dynamic psychotherapy, supportive counseling individually or in groups, pharmacotherapy, cognitive-behavioral therapy, and most recently eye movement desensitization and reprocessing (EMDR). Although some of these techniques are used routinely with rape victims, only a few controlled outcome studies have been conducted; these have tended to focus on the efficacy of cognitive-behavioral procedures, such as exposure and anxiety management techniques. Interestingly, the majority of studies on the efficacy of medication with PTSD were conducted on male war veterans, and the efficacy of pharmacological treatment for rape victims is as yet unknown.

Cognitive-Behavioral Therapy for Chronic PTSD

Several studies have examined female assault victims' responses to cognitive-behavioral treatment, including exposure to trauma reminders and anxiety management techniques. Exposure treatment involves helping patients confront their feared situations. It is designed to activate the trauma memories in order to modify pathological aspects of these memories. Obviously, the use of exposure techniques requires that a patient remember at least some details of the trauma and be aware of some of the stimuli that activate the trauma memory. Anxiety management training is used when anxiety pervades daily functioning. In this case the focus is not on fear activation as much as the management of fear, generally by teaching patients skills to control their anxiety. In PTSD, both specific fears and general chronic arousal are among the defining characteristics; therefore, both exposure and anxiety management training have been used.

Research Findings

In one study, anxiety management (also referred to as stress inoculation training or SIT), assertiveness training, and supportive counseling were all found to be modestly effective as compared to a wait-list control condition, but did not differ from one another. Two studies examined the comparative efficacy of treatments for women with chronic PTSD following rape or nonsexual assault. The treatment programs in the two studies were short—nine 90-minute sessions over 5 weeks. The first study showed that immediately after treatment, SIT and prolonged exposure (PE) were superior to supportive counseling and to a wait-list control in reducing PTSD. Specifically, 50% of women in the SIT condition and 40% in the PE condition lost the diagnosis of PTSD, whereas only 10% in the supportive counseling condition and none of the women on the wait-list lost the diagnosis. At follow-up, all treatments were effective. In the second study, which was completed recently, the efficacy of SIT, PE, and a combination of the two treatments was compared to that of a wait-list control condition. Of clients who received one of the three active treatments, 60–70% lost the diagnosis of PTSD and retained their gains overall. The PE-alone group showed superiority over the other two groups on a combined measure of PTSD, depression, and general anxiety. In contrast, none of the women in the wait-list control group lost the diagnosis of PTSD. A somewhat different cognitive-behavioral program called "cognitive processing therapy" was developed by Resick and Schnicke, and its efficacy was compared to a natural wait-list condition. Fifty percent of treated women showed improvement on PTSD measures, and this improvement was maintained over time. However, the lack of randomization in this study renders the results inconclusive.

The new technique called EMDR involves exposure along with saccadic eye movements. This technique has generated a lot of interest, but to date its efficacy is still unclear.

How to Implement Cognitive-Behavioral Therapy

When a clinician is presented with a rape victim, it is important that the clinician determine the client's diagnosis and target for treatment. Being a "rape victim" is not a psychological disorder. As noted earlier, the majority of victims show a natural decline of rape-related symptoms within 3 months after the assault, without intervention. Those who present for treatment may show a variety of disorders, with PTSD the most likely. Obviously, the specific presenting problem will determine the treatment prescribed.

Victims with PTSD seem not only to suffer from fear and reminders of the original trauma, but also to display fear and avoidance of the memory of the trauma itself. Therefore, exposure treatment with this population should focus on reexperiencing the original trauma via imaginal exposure. In this respect, imaginal exposure to the memory of the trauma is analogous to therapy with complicated bereavement, in which the patient is confronted with the painful memory. Anxiety management techniques have been described in detail in numerous sources, and therefore I do not elaborate on their application to PTSD here. During imaginal exposure, it is important to include physiological reactions ("My heart's pounding"), appraisals ("I know I'm really in trouble"), and threat-related thoughts ("He'll shoot me"), as well as detailed descriptions of what actually happened during the assault. The inclusion of all these stimuli and responses in imagery scenarios has been found to enhance emotional engagement, which is crucial for a successful outcome.

The idea of using exposure techniques with rape victims generated some controversy in the past; some experts claimed that women *should* be fearful of being raped, and that habituation to a rape experience is an inappropriate goal. At present, most experts seem to agree that the removal of excessive fear to reminders of the rape does not foster "recklessness," just as the decrease of pathological fear in a person with a height phobia does not prompt the person to jump off a cliff. The memory of the assault will never become neutral, but it need not remain intensely painful.

Programs for Prevention of Chronic PTSD

The concern with the high rate of chronic PTSD among individuals exposed to traumatic events has led to the implementation of critical-incident debriefing. Such programs are offered to emergency personnel and victims of natural disaster with increasing frequency, but their efficacy is largely unknown. Rape centers also offer crisis intervention immediately after sexual assault, and these programs tend to focus on supportive counseling and education about the legal and health issues related to assault. Again, although these programs are offered in many communities, they have not been subject to controlled investigations of their efficacy.

The first effort at evaluating a brief intervention program with rape victims failed to find differential reduction in clients' distress as compared to that of victims who underwent assessment only; both groups improved significantly with the passage of time after the rape. Methodological limitations, however, make these results inconclusive. In a controlled study, my colleagues and I compared the PTSD symptoms of recent assault victims (half of whom were victims of rape) who received a brief (four-session) cognitive-behavioral prevention program to those of victims who received assessment only. At 2 months after assault, 10% of the prevention group versus 70% of the control group met criteria for a diagnosis of PTSD.

CONCLUSION

Rape and other forms of sexual assault are very prevalent in U.S. society, according to epidemiological studies. Current figures on rape are likely to constitute an underestimation of the actual rates, because victims are reluctant to report rape to police and even to researchers. The psychological and physical consequences of rape are dismal and long-lasting. Fortunately, short-term psychological interventions that include cognitive-behavioral procedures are helpful to many victims. However, many health care professionals who work with rape victims are not familiar with these treatments, and disseminating this information is a challenge.

Although the brief program aimed at preventing chronic PTSD seems to be effective, it may be prohibitively costly to offer it to every victim, given the large number of trauma victims. Therefore, studies should focus on predictors of chronic PTSD, so that individuals at risk can be identified and treated. At present, we know that the severity of PTSD immediately after the assault is highly related to later severity. Thus, if resources are scarce, we should focus particularly on victims who manifest severe reactions to the trauma immediately after its occurrence.

FURTHER READING

Foa, E. B., Hearst, D. E., & Perry, K. J. (1995). The evaluation of a brief cognitive-behavioral program for the prevention of chronic PTSD in recent assault victims. *Journal of Consulting and Clinical Psychology, 63,* 90–96.
Evaluation of a brief program that aims to prevent assault victims from developing PTSD.

Foa, E. B., & Meadows, E. A. (1997). Psychosocial treatments for post-traumatic stress disorder: A critical review. In J. Spence, J. M. Darley, & D. J. Foss (Eds.), *Annual review of psychology* (Vol. 48, pp. 449–480). Palo Alto, CA: Annual Reviews.
A comparative review of studies that investigate treatment of PTSD.

Foa, E. B., Rothbaum, B. O., Riggs, D., & Murdock, T. (1991). Treatment of post-traumatic stress disorder in rape victims: A comparison between cognitive-behavioral procedures and counseling. *Journal of Consulting and Clinical Psychology, 59,* 715–723.
Study examining the efficacy of a cognitive-behavioral treatment program for rape or nonsexual assault victims.

Mitchell, J. T., & Dyregrov, A. (1993). Traumatic stress in disaster workers and emergency personnel: Prevention and intervention. In J. P. Wilson & B. Raphael (Eds.), *International handbook of traumatic stress syndromes* (pp. 905–914). New York: Plenum Press.
Overview of critical-incident debriefing programs offered to individuals exposed to traumatic events.

Resick, P. A., Jordan, C. G., Girelli, S. A., Hutter, C. K., & Marhoefer Dvorak, S. (1988). A comparative victim study of behavioral group therapy for sexual assault victims. *Behavior Therapy, 19,* 385–401.
A study comparing anxiety management, assertiveness training, supportive counseling and a wait-list control group for sexual assault victims.

Resick, P. A., & Schnicke, M. K. (1992). Cognitive processing therapy for sexual assault victims. *Journal of Consulting and Clinical Psychology, 60,* 748–756.
Description and evaluation of a cognitive-behavioral treatment program for sexual assault victims.

Resnick, H. S., Kilpatrick, D. G., Dansky, B. S., Saunders, B. E., & Best, C. L. (1993). Prevalence of civilian trauma and posttraumatic stress disorder in a representative national sample of women. *Journal of Consulting and Clinical Psychology, 61,* 984–991.
Epidemiological study of prevalence of trauma and PTSD.

Rothbaum, B. O., Foa, E. B., Riggs, D., Murdock, T., & Walsh, W. (1992). A prospective examination of post-traumatic stress disorder in rape victims. *Journal of Traumatic Stress, 5,* 455–475.
Study of rape victims interviewed several times during the year after the trauma, indicating prevalence of PTSD and associated problems.

Solomon, S. D., Gerrity, E. T., & Muff, A. M. (1992). Efficacy of treatments for posttraumatic stress disorder: An empirical review. *Journal of the American Medical Association, 268,* 633–638.
A general review of treatments for PTSD.

Waigandt, A., Wallace, D. L., Phelps, L., & Miller, D. A. (1990). The impact of sexual assault on physical health status. *Journal of Traumatic Stress, 3,* 93–102.
Health complications and illnesses that occur in the aftermath of sexual assault.

122

Bipolar Disorders

David J. Miklowitz

*B*ipolar disorders are recurrent mood disorders characterized by swings from states of severe depression to severe elation and overactivity (mania or hypomania). During depressive episodes, persons with bipolar disorders have low mood, loss of interests, fatigue, sleep disturbances, and suicidal ideas or behaviors. During manic episodes, they experience elated and/or irritable moods, increased energy and activity, a decreased need for sleep, "flight of ideas" and/or racing thoughts, impulsive behavior, and an inflated sense of self-worth. Hypomanic episodes involve milder forms of these symptoms or symptoms of shorter duration. Many bipolar patients also have comorbid psychotic symptoms (e.g., delusions or hallucinations) or comorbid substance use or anxiety disorders.

PREVALENCE AND COURSE

About 0.8% of the population have bipolar I disorder, characterized by swings from major depressive episodes to fully syndromal manic episodes or mixed episodes (episodes with both depressive and manic features). About 0.5% have bipolar II disorder, characterized by major depressive episodes and hypomanic episodes. Whereas bipolar I disorder affects both sexes with equal frequency, bipolar II disorder is more common among women than among men.

The first episode of a bipolar disorder is usually a manic (or hypomanic) episode in men and a depressive episode in women. Over the lifespan, women show a preponderance of depressive over manic/hypomanic episodes, whereas men show approximately equal frequencies of these mood states. Women are also much more likely than men to show "rapid-cycling" phases of illness, in which patients experience four or more recurrences of mania, hypomania, or depression in a single year. Moreover, there is some evidence—albeit inconclusive—that women are more likely than men to have mixed affective episodes, which tend to be difficult to treat pharmacologically.

Most forms of mood disorders predispose women to postpartum depression, and bipolar disorders are no exception. Furthermore, about 20% of pregnant bipolar women have postpartum recurrences of mania. In general, the postpartum period is a particularly high-risk interval for bipolar women.

GENETIC AND BIOLOGICAL FACTORS

Bipolar disorders are genetically transmitted illnesses. About 8% of the first-degree relatives of bipolar patients have bipolar disorders, and about 12% have major (unipolar) depression. Twin and adoption studies consistently support genetic transmission models. There is separate evidence for neurophysiological, neuroanatomical, and neuropsychological dysregulations in these disorders.

PSYCHOSOCIAL FACTORS

Both women and men experience a host of social and occupational dysfunctions as a consequence of having bipolar disorders, even when maintained on appropriate medications. In the 6 months after a major episode, about 57% of bipolar patients cannot maintain employment, and only 21% work at their expected level.

Special problems arise in the marriages of bipolar persons. Their rate of divorce is about two to three times that of the normal population. The marital interactions of bipolar couples appear to be more conflictual than those of normal couples, although not all studies have found this to be true. A woman married to a bipolar man often experiences an "emotional roller coaster" when attempting to cope with her husband's wide mood swings, fiscal irresponsibility, sexual impulsivity, and social/occupational dysfunction.

Bipolar women and men who reside in conflictual family or marital environments are at increased risk for recurrences. For example, patients who live with family members (parents or spouses) rated high in "expressed emotion" (i.e., showing high levels of criticism, hostility, or overprotectiveness regarding the patients) are about twice as likely to show recurrences over 9-month or 1-year follow-ups as those with family members rated low in expressed emotion. Patients who experience stressful life events (e.g., loss experiences) are also at increased risk for recurrences, especially during the periods immediately following these events. Various models have been proposed to explain these relationships, including the disruptive effects of life stress on the patients' daily routines and sleep–wake cycles.

PHARMACOLOGICAL TREATMENT

The "first-line offense" in treating bipolar symptoms is usually medication. In many patients, drug treatment is highly effective in controlling acute episodes and in preventing new episodes from occurring. Other patients continue to show "breakthrough" recurrences despite taking medication.

The type and dosage of medication recommended for a bipolar patient vary with the phase of the patient's disorder. Currently, the mood-regulating agents most frequently prescribed are lithium carbonate, divalproex sodium and carbamazepine. Mood-regulating agents are often supplemented with antipsychotic, antianxiety, and antidepressant medications. Electroconvulsive therapy is sometimes recommended for treatment-refractory patients.

All mood-regulating medications have side effects that may be disturbing to women. Lithium is associated with weight gain, physical tremors, nausea, diarrhea, rashes, frequent urination, and in some cases hair loss. Also, women appear to be more strongly affected than men by the antithyroid effects of lithium. Divalproex sodium is associated with a side effect profile that is possibly more benign than lithium's but may also include menstrual disturbances. When taking antidepressants, women may also be more likely than men to experience medication-induced mood cycling (e.g., shifting from depression to hypomania or mania, or beginning to cycle rapidly when taking an antidepressant).

Lithium and the other mood-regulating medications pose special hazards for pregnant bipolar women, especially if these are taken during the first trimester. Each of the major mood-stabilizing medications is associated with an increased prevalence of birth defects. For example, lithium increases the risk of congenital anomalies among offspring by two- to threefold. Furthermore, certain antidepressant medications increase the risk of miscarriage during the first trimester. Thus, unless willing to assume these risks, the pregnant bipolar patient may have only two options: to obtain regular psychotherapy and case management in lieu of medication, or, in the case of a severely ill patient, to undergo electroconvulsive therapy.

PSYCHOSOCIAL TREATMENT

There are new, although relatively untested, forms of psychotherapy available to persons with bipolar disorders. These therapies attempt to reduce the negative impact on the disorder of stressful family environments or disruptive life events. They are delivered in combination with medications during the postepisode stabilization and long-term maintenance phases of the disorders.

Michael Goldstein and I have developed a 9-month outpatient psychoeducational family therapy for bipolar disorders. This treatment consists of education for patients and families about bipolar disorders, and strategies for enhancing family communication and problem-solving. Ellen Frank and associates have adapted an individual modality, interpersonal psychotherapy of depression, to the special needs of a bipolar patient. Patients in this treatment learn new ways (1) to handle environmental stress and manage interpersonal relationships, and (2) to stabilize and regularize their daily routines and sleep–wake rhythms. These treatments, as well as other family and individually oriented therapies, are currently under empirical examination in randomized, controlled clinical trials.

CONCLUSION

Bipolar disorders are highly recurrent, often debilitating illnesses that affect approximately 1 in every 100 women. They are disorders with genetic, neurobiological, and psychosocial underpinnings. Bipolar patients clearly benefit from pharmacological treatments that reduce the risk and severity of recurrences; however, even patients taking appropriate medications continue to show recurrences. Women appear to be more at risk than men for developing certain severe forms of the disorders (e.g., rapid cycling).

Psychosocial treatments may be useful in combination with medications in further ameliorating the course of these disorders, as well as the negative psychosocial consequences of major affective episodes.

FURTHER READING

American Psychiatric Association. (1995). *Practice guideline for treatment of patients with bipolar disorder.* Washington, DC: Author.
This is a guide for the psychiatrist or psychologist to pharmacological and clinical management of the bipolar patient.

Cohen, L. S., Friedman, J. M., Jefferson, J. W., Johnson, E. M., & Weiner, M. L. (1994). A reevaluation of risk of *in utero* exposure to lithium. *Journal of the American Medical Association, 271,* 146–150.
An empirical study indicating that congenital anomalies affected 4–12% of the children of mothers treated with lithium during the early phases of pregnancy, compared with 2–4% of the children of untreated mothers.

Dion, G. L., Tohen, M., Anthony, W. A., & Waternaux, C. (1989). Symptoms and functioning of patients with bipolar disorder six months after hospitalization. *Hospital and Community Psychiatry, 39,* 652–656.
A 6-month follow-up of bipolar patients who had had an acute manic or depressive episode, focusing on their degree of occupational dysfunction.

Frank, E., Kupfer, D. J., Ehlers, C. L., Monk, T. H., Cornes, C., Carter, S., & Frankel, D. (1994). Interpersonal and social rhythm therapy for bipolar disorder: integrating interpersonal and behavioral approaches. *The Behavior Therapist, 17,* 143–149.
Describes a new individually oriented psychotherapy for bipolar disorders—an adaptation of interpersonal psychotherapy for depression.

Goodwin, F. K., & Jamison, K. R. (1990). *Manic–depressive illness.* New York: Oxford University Press.
A comprehensive textbook about the bipolar syndromes; the "bible" for investigators interested in these disorders.

Johnson, S. L., & Roberts, J. E. (1995). Life events and bipolar disorder: Implications from biological theories. *Psychological Bulletin, 117,* 434–449.
An overview of the research on life events and bipolar disorders, with emphasis on the various theoretical models that explain these stress–illness associations.

Leibenluft, E. (1996). Women with bipolar illness: Clinical and research issues. *American Journal of Psychiatry, 153,* 163–173.
An up-to-date critical review of the biological literature on gender differences in the course of bipolar disorders.

Miklowitz, D. J., & Goldstein, M. J. (1997). *Bipolar disorder: A family-focused treatment approach.* New York: Guilford Press.
Describes a new family psychoeducational treatment tailored to the needs of families of bipolar patients.

Miklowitz, D. J., Goldstein, M. J., Nuechterlein, K. H., Snyder, K. S., & Mintz, J. (1988). Family factors and the course of bipolar affective disorder. *Archives of General Psychiatry, 45,* 225–231.
A 9-month follow-up of recent-onset manic patients, suggesting that stressful family environments predispose patients to later mood disorder recurrences.

Powell, K. B., & Miklowitz, D. J. (1994). Frontal lobe dysfunction in the affective disorders. *Clinical Psychology Review, 14*(6), 525–546.
A review of the evidence suggesting frontal lobe dysfunction in the affective disorders (with an emphasis on bipolar disorders), including studies of neuropathology, neuropsychology, functional and structural neuroimaging, and electrophysiology.

Silverstone, T., & Romans-Clarkson, A. (1989). Bipolar affective disorder: Causes and prevention of relapse. *British Journal of Psychiatry, 154,* 321–335.
Presents an overview of research on factors that predict recurrences of bipolar disorders, as well as the efficacy of medications as preventive agents.

123

Depression

Peter McLean
Sheila Woody

*H*ealth care providers are generally aware that clinical depression is more common in women than in men. Although women seem to respond to treatment as well as men do, the increased risk for depression in women remains a serious problem. In response to this exigency, in 1987 the American Psychological Association formed a National Task Force on Women and Depression to identify the risk factors for and treatment needs of depressed women. This report (McGrath, Puryear, Keita, Strickland, & Felipe Russo, 1990) has been influential in its advocacy for investigation of gender-related causes of and solutions to depression in women. The present chapter highlights current research and promising trends in the understanding and treatment of depression in women.

PREVALENCE AND COURSE

The most stable finding in the study of depression is the gender difference in prevalence of clinical levels of depression, with women reporting a history of major depressive disorder at nearly twice the rate of men. Although the pattern of symptoms and subjective experience of depression are the same for women and men, the overall impact of depression may be more serious for women than for men. Some studies report an earlier age of onset of depression for women than for men; women frequently experience depression in midadolescence, whereas men more often are in their 20s before symptom onset. There is growing evidence that women experience more protracted episodes of depression, more recurrent depression, and more severe depression. Not only are women more likely to experience depression; anxiety disorders are also more prevalent among women, particularly the more serious anxiety disorders (e.g., panic disorder with agoraphobia). The increased incidence of these disorders is a likely contributor to the greater chronicity of depression experienced by women. When comorbid with depression, these anxiety disorders result in more severe symptoms and higher rates of relapse. Depression is also highly associated with physical disorders in women; conservative estimates are in the range of 50% overlap between physical disease and depressive disorders. (For a more detailed discussion of depression and comorbid disorders, see Craighead and Vajk's chapter.)

CAUSAL MECHANISMS

The search for a unique causal mechanism to explain the differential prevalence of depression between women and men has not yet yielded firm evidence. However, there is ample evidence that women and men experience different stressors, some of which may be related to the development of depression. Research into the interaction between depression and stressors for women has focused primarily on the reproductive life cycle and psychosocial factors.

Vulnerability to depression in women may include various stages of the reproductive cycle (puberty, the premenstrual period, and the postpartum period), as well as the period following abortion. Whether menopause increases risk for depression is now more uncertain, based on evidence from major community studies, which (contrary to clinical beliefs) indicate that sex differences in prevalence of depression may decline after about age 55. Previously, biochemical influences associated with these reproductive life cycle events or conditions were thought to be causally linked to depression. Evidence for this has been inconsistent, and most investigators adhere to a biopsychosocial model, wherein the role played by reproductive life cycle factors in causing depression in women can be explained in terms of both psychological and physical mediation.

In recent years much work has been done to identify psychosocial factors responsible for depression in women. Although the cognitive theory of depression links maladaptive cognitions (particularly about helplessness and hopelessness) to depression, there is no evidence that women's cognitive structure is different from that of men. There is some evidence that women derive self-esteem more from interpersonal interactions than men do, and that they are more prone than men to internalize stress, be less assertive, and be more dependent, as culturally prescribed. There is now consistent evidence that the 2:1 gender ratio in prevalence of depression can be significantly traced to social factors, including low social status, role strain, poverty, victimization, and differential power in marital relationships. Individually, these social factors have long been recognized as determining factors for women vulnerable to depression. What has only recently been appreciated is the extent to which women are exposed to these stressors and the increased toxicity of risk posed by these stressors when they are present in combined form. For example, victimization (e.g., rape, assault, incest), poverty, domestic role strain in terms of parenting/caregiver responsibilities, and relative social isolation frequently co-occur and interact. Furthermore, Hammen (1991) has shown that depression can be transmitted from one generation to the next by psychosocial means. Specifically, vulnerability to depression can be acquired by the children of depressed mothers (and presumably fathers) by means of negative interactions, such as criticism from and noninvolvement by depressed mothers. These negative interactions have been shown to contribute to negative self-concept, which in turn predicts future depression.

ASSESSMENT OF DEPRESSION IN WOMEN

Given the availability of treatment, there is a major public health challenge in the failure of practitioners to recognize clinical levels of depression and of depressed individuals to seek treatment. This problem disproportionately and adversely affects women. Community surveys in North America and Europe routinely find that approximately 70% of cases of clinical depression are untreated, and surveys have found that family physicians fail to recognize clinical levels of depression in 50% of their patients.

Traditional protocols for the assessment of clinical depression are not gender-specific. Primary focus has been placed on diagnostic determination, history of previous episodes, treatment history, and a review of lifestyle and stressors. A number of investigators have called for assessment of depression in women to be gender-sensitive, incorporating a full reproductive history, the meaning of gender membership for each patient over the lifespan, medical history, personality style, and full assessment of roles and stressors (e.g., Brown, 1986; McGrath et al., 1990). Determining the level of support or interference offered by the patient's social context is central to the establishment of treatment plans in the psychosocial treatment of depression. Similarly, the patient's functioning during periods of remission, or prior to the onset of the initial episode, is often key to the assessment of vulnerability and progress in depression. Functional assessment during full or partial remission enables the clinician to assess social, occupational, familial, cognitive, and other factors salient to a nondepressed lifestyle. This information can be used in treatment to help resolve an acute episode and to prevent relapse by improving overall quality of life. In cases of suspected depression in elderly women, a good differential diagnosis is essential, because systemic infections and other organic problems can masquerade as depression. Neuropsychological evaluation is the best ways to distinguish among Alzheimer's disease, other forms of dementia, and depression.

TREATMENT OF DEPRESSION IN WOMEN

Multiple studies have yielded no consensus on a treatment of choice in the care of depressed outpatients. The National Institute of Mental Health (NIMH) Treatment of Depression Collaborative Research Program (Elkin et al., 1989) reported treatment × severity interactions favoring pharmacotherapy for more depressed outpatients. However, this finding has not been supported by other investigations (e.g., McLean & Taylor, 1992). Furthermore, large treatment trials such as the NIMH study have consistently found that women and men respond equivalently to treatment of depression. This has largely been true for both psychological and pharmacological treatments, although women sometimes have a better treatment response to some antidepressant medications (e.g., monoamine oxidase inhibitors) than men do.

Two interesting developments, however, have shown promise in producing gender-specific response to treatment. The first involves matching patient characteristics (e.g., personality style, gender, depression history) with treatment (e.g., structure, individual vs. group format), along the lines recommended by Beutler and Clarkin (1990). There is now evidence that women do better in more highly structured treatments that feature problem solving, with an emphasis on a collaborative relationship with the therapist in order to achieve independence, self-mastery, and personal competence. This approach is common to cognitive-behavioral and interpersonal treatments of depression, and is less typical of psychodynamic and more open-ended, supportive psychotherapies. Since psychodynamic and supportive psychotherapies have not established efficacy in the treatment of depression beyond nonspecific treatment effects, it may be that the development of problem-solving skills is an "active ingredient" in cognitive-behavioral and interpersonal treatments of depression. Furthermore, there is evidence that women respond better in group therapy than in exclusively individual therapy, compared to men.

The second promising development in the treatment of depressed women involves couple therapy, which targets both the cognitive style of the depressed woman and the quality of marital interaction (Jacobson, Dobson, Fruzzetti, Schmaling, & Salusky, 1991; Koerner, Prince, & Jacobson, 1994). Major depression, by far the most frequent depressive disorder, is frequently reactive to marital distress, at least for depressed women. A significant inverse relationship between depression and marital satisfaction in women has been reported a number of times. Marital distress is also a predictor of relapse in depression following recovery from an acute episode. Studies of depressed women by Jacobson's group have found that treatment packages that target the quality of the marriage by reducing aversive behaviors (e.g., criticism, withdrawal, anger), and by improving facilitative interpersonal behaviors as well as depressive cognitions, act independently and provide the best overall result. Furthermore, high levels of a husband's facilitative behavior by the end of treatment predicted low levels of depression at a 1-year follow-up. These studies underscore the relationship between female depression and marital distress, and hold promise for integrated treatment approaches that target both. We are unaware of any studies in which depressed men and their marital interactions were targeted for treatment.

CONCLUSIONS

Not only is the prevalence of depression twice as great in women as in men, but the course of depressive episodes is more often severe, protracted, and recurrent in women. The pervasiveness of social factors that create vulnerabilities to depression in women, such as role strain, poverty, and victimization, has only recently been understood. Contemporary assessment of depression in women should include the assessment of potential reproductive life cycle triggers and conditions, as well as psychosocial factors salient to the onset and maintenance of depression. Treatment programs should be designed with a clear understanding of the problems particularly faced by women, including the need to care for children (often alone), as well as the special problems of spousal and sexual abuse.

Although gender has typically not been a significant predictor of treatment response, new findings indicate that depressed women respond relatively better in structured treatments with a problem-solving, skill-building focus, preferably in a group format. In the frequent case of marital distress, which leads to depression in the female partner, treatment packages that use cognitive-behavioral components to improve both the quality of marital relationship and the cognitive style of the depressed partner are the most promising. Finally, there is sufficient evidence available regarding the etiology of depression to warrant the development of prevention programs for young girls. We should intervene during adolescence to help young girls feel good about themselves, feel masterful, and develop good mood management strategies to carry them over the life course.

FURTHER READING

Beutler, L. E., & Clarkin, J. (1990). *Systematic treatment selection: Toward targeted therapeutic interventions.* New York: Brunner/Mazel.

Brown, L. S. (1986). Gender-role analysis: A neglected component of psychological assessment. *Psychotherapy, 23,* 243–248.

Elkin, I., Shea, T., Watkins, J. T., Imber, S. D., Sotsky, S. M., Collins, J. F., Glass, D. R., Pilkonis, P. A., Leber, W. R., Docherty, J. P., Fiester, S. J., & Perloff, M. B. (1989). National Institute of Mental Health Treatment of Depression Collaborative Research Program: General effectiveness of treatments. *Archives of General Psychiatry, 46,* 971–982.

Hammen, C. (1991). *Depression runs in families.* New York: Springer-Verlag.

Jacobson, N. S., Dobson, K., Fruzzetti, A. E., Schmaling, K. B., & Salusky, S. (1991). Marital therapy as a treatment for depression. *Journal of Consulting and Clinical Psychology, 59*(4), 547–557.

Koerner, K., Prince, S., & Jacobson, N. S. (1994). Enhancing the treatment and prevention of depression in women: The role of integrative behavioral couple therapy. *Behavior Therapy, 25,* 373–390.

McGrath, E., Puryear Keita, G., Strickland, B. R., & Felipe Russo, N. (Eds.). (1990). *Women and depression: Risk factors and treatment issues.* Washington, DC: American Psychological Association.

McLean, P. D., & Taylor, S. (1992). Severity of unipolar depression and choice of treatment. *Behaviour Research and Therapy, 30*(5), 443–451.

124

Depression and Comorbid Disorders

W. Edward Craighead
Fiona C. Vajk

*I*t is well established that women are diagnosed with unipolar major depression approximately twice as often as men. The Epidemiologic Catchment Area study by Regier, Burke, and Burke, a large-scale epidemiological study in five U.S. cities, found rates of lifetime major depression to be twice as high for women as for men. Another community epidemiology study by Blazer and colleagues found lifetime rates of major depression of 17.1% overall, with women reporting depression about twice as often as men. Results from community samples such as these demonstrate that the higher rate of clinical depression in women is not merely an artifact of greater help-seeking behavior or greater contact with psychiatric and health professionals among women, although in clinical settings women also receive a depression diagnosis about 2.5 times more often than men do.

Recent research has demonstrated that the comorbidity of other psychiatric diagnoses (especially those more common among women) with depression is common. The purpose of this chapter is to identify those clinical problems, as well as nonclinical problems in living, that co-occur with the presence of depression. Following the identification and description of these co-occurring problems, a brief discussion of the possible reasons for their comorbidity is presented. Finally, the clinical implications of the comorbidity of these problems with depression are presented.

CO-OCCURRENCE OF DEPRESSION WITH OTHER PSYCHIATRIC DIAGNOSES

Some researchers have reported that elevated rates of comorbidity may result from the increased risk of having any other psychiatric disorder once one psychiatric disorder is present, rather than from a unique relationship between any two particular disorders. On the other hand, even in the absence of a specific relationship between depression and a comorbid diagnosis, these disorders may frequently co-occur with major depression because of the high base rates of some disorders in women. In such cases, it is important for clinicians to be aware of likely comorbid diagnoses, particularly when the course of treatment will be affected by the presence of the comorbid disorder.

Perhaps the most frequent comorbid diagnosis with major depression is an anxiety disorder. In a sample of patients diagnosed with mood disorders, the diagnoses most commonly found to be comorbid with depression were anxiety disorders, particularly social phobia and generalized anxiety disorder. Forty-two percent of the patients with a principal diagnosis of major depression, and forty-eight percent of those with a principal diagnosis of dysthymia, were also diagnosed with an anxiety disorder. The comorbidity of depression and anxiety is especially important in women, given the relatively high base rates of both these diagnoses among them.

Eating disorders are also likely to be comorbid with major depression in women. In a population-based study of female twins by Walters and Kendler, anorexia nervosa was found to be frequently comorbid with major depression. Similarly, the rate of major depression in women with bulimia nervosa was more than double the rate of depression in women without bulimia nervosa. Thus depression may be a risk factor for the development of eating disorders in women. Because a common feature of eating disorders is guilt or shame in response to lapses in diet, and these emotions may be related to depression, it is also possible that depression may be partly caused by, or exacerbated by, a coexisting eating disorder.

Another consistent finding is that depression and substance use disorders frequently co-occur. Sanderson found that, among a sample of individuals in treatment for depressive disorders, 15% of those with major depression and 11% of those with dysthymia received additional diagnoses of substance abuse or dependence, most frequently involving the misuse of alcohol. Women with alcohol dependence were more likely than men to be diagnosed with depression prior to their misuse of alcohol; 31% of the women in a sample of alcoholic inpatients had a primary diagnosis of depression, versus 12% of the alcoholic men. Interestingly, this gender ratio for depression comorbid with alcoholism is the same 2.5:1 gender ratio found in nonalcoholic depressed patients.

Finally, Axis II personality disorders frequently co-occur with major depression. A review of the literature in this area indicates that approximately 35–65% of individuals with major depression also meet criteria for a personality disorder. Patients with comorbid depression and personality disorder are likely to respond more poorly to somatic treatment for depression and to receive lower levels of social support than depressed patients without a personality disorder, demonstrating the clinical importance of assessing Axis II comorbidity in depressed patients.

CO-OCCURRENCE OF DEPRESSION
WITH ASSOCIATED PROBLEMS IN LIVING

In addition to a greater risk of comorbid psychiatric diagnoses, women with major depression are likely to experience other problems in living related to their depressive diagnosis. Such problems may themselves be depression risk factors, tending to cause or exacerbate depressive symptoms; alternatively, many life problems may develop as a result of an individual's depression. It is important for clinicians to be aware of the potential for complicating problems to coexist with major depression, as such problems may interfere with functioning and with treatment.

Depression is associated with and preceded by marital discord in many cases of moderate to marked depression. Whatever the respective causes may be, there is a 50% overlap between marital discord and depression. It seems likely both that depression contributes to or exacerbates marital discord/dissatisfaction, and that marital discord contributes to or exacerbates depressive symptoms. It is also important to remember that both depression and marital problems may occur as a result of a third problem or disorder (e.g., financial difficulties).

Perhaps not surprisingly, divorce is also common among depressed women. Individuals who are separated or divorced have higher rates of major depression than those who are married or who have never married. In a population-based, 1-year longitudinal study, women who reported that they divorced or separated from their legal spouses during the study period were more likely to report a history of major depression than either the women who remained happily married or the women who remained unhappily married. In addition, women experiencing marital disruption were approximately three times more likely than happily married women to report a major depressive episode during that year (21% vs. 7%); this finding may apply more to women with a prior history of depression than to those without. It seems that marital discord or divorce is a frequent consequence of depression in women, but it is also a frequent precursor to depressive episodes.

Childhood sexual abuse and sexual abuse plus physical abuse ("dual abuse") are both more common among females than among males; a history of abuse in childhood is commonly associated with depression and anxiety, particularly in women. In fact, the gender difference in rates of child abuse may contribute significantly to the gender difference in depression. An estimate based on a review of several studies is that nearly 60% of depressed women report a history of childhood sexual abuse, whereas from 6.8% to 19% of women in the general population report a history of childhood sexual abuse. Childhood sexual abuse represents only one type of adverse experience; other traumatic experiences among women (including spousal abuse and adult rape) may be related to the greater proportion of cases of depression in women. In terms of treatment, it may be particularly important for clinicians to ask about and deal directly with childhood abuse; if, indeed, 60% of depressed women have a history of childhood abuse (as opposed to a 30% base rate among women), treatment that does not address this aspect of an individual's psychological profile may be of limited success in alleviating the depression or in improving long-term outcomes. On the other hand, it is important for clinicians to be aware of the demand characteristics of the therapeutic situation, and not to encourage or solicit inaccurate memories of abuse.

Not surprisingly, experiences of loss are strongly related to major depression. In a longitudinal study of women in the general population, depression was related to major losses throughout adulthood and to poor quality of ongoing social support. In addition, the onset of major depression was often immediately preceded by a severe loss event. Negative experiences throughout childhood also predicted later depression and were more common in children who had experienced the loss of one or both parents.

Poverty seems to be another important risk factor for major depression. In a community sample, poverty status—over and above the effects of gender, age, history of substance misuse, and subclinical depressive symptoms—was significantly related to the likelihood of a first-onset major depressive episode, representing an approximate doubling of risk for depression. Interestingly, in further analyses, this effect seems to be largely mediated by isolation from friends and family, suggesting that the social isolation and reduced social support associated with poverty may serve as a direct causal link to the development of depression.

PROPOSED EXPLANATIONS FOR THE COMORBIDITY OF DEPRESSION IN WOMEN

In support of the etiological role of life stressors in depression and co-occurring disorders, the community-based epidemiological study by Blazer and colleagues found that lower levels of education and lower income were risk factors for comorbid, but not pure, major depression. In other words, environmental stressors may lead both to symptoms of depression and to the co-occurrence of other psychiatric symptoms, such as anxiety or substance use disorders.

A related explanation for the comorbidity of certain disorders with depression is that the same types of adverse experiences in childhood or adolescence may predispose an individual to more than one disorder. For example, early negative experiences, including parental indifference and sexual and physical abuse, were found to predict higher rates of both depression and anxiety. Thus, common early experiences that play a role in the etiology of both disorders may partially explain why they tend to co-occur frequently.

A higher prevalence of both comorbid and pure major depression was found both for females and for homemakers, as opposed to those in other employment categories. This provides tentative support for the idea that the traditional social role of women may lead to higher rates of depression and other problems.

One reason for the comorbidity of depression and other disorders in women may be women's responses to their depressed moods. Women are more likely than men to ruminate about themselves, their emotions, and their problems in response to depressed mood. This ruminative style is related to longer-lasting and more intense depressed moods. It is possible that women who tend to ruminate about their depression will also be at greater risk for co-occurring disorders, especially anxiety disorders (of which such worry is a core characteristic), and problems such as marital discord. This dysfunctional ruminative style may be transmitted across generations, since women tend to adopt the affective styles modeled by their mothers; children of affectively disordered mothers are more likely than children of physically ill or normal mothers to show the depressive affective style characteristic of their mothers.

Finally, it is also possible that the comorbidity frequently observed between different disorders represents a common underlying biological vulnerability to both of the comorbid disorders. For example, in a population-based study of female twin pairs, genetic factors were found to be important in both major depression and generalized anxiety disorder, and these genetic factors were completely shared by the two disorders. Thus, the genetic influence on the development of major depression and generalized anxiety disorder may be the result of a common genetic vulnerability. It is also important to note that the 2.5:1 gender ratio, with women having higher rates of depression, emerges at or soon after the onset of puberty; this suggests that the gender differences may be at least partially rooted in biological dysregulations.

CLINICAL IMPLICATIONS

Although effective therapies for "pure" major depression are well developed and supported by empirical studies, the field has only begun to examine effective treatments for individuals with comorbid depression and other disorders. Initial research on the effects of comorbid disorders on the course and treatment of major depression indicates that comorbidity may be an important determinant of outcomes. This may partially be a function of the severity of depression, since patients with depression and another disorder may be more severely depressed than patients with pure depression. Preliminary evidence also indicates that depressed individuals with lifetime diagnoses of anxiety disorders or substance use disorders take longer to recover from their depressive episodes. Thus, women with comorbid depression are more resistant to treatment and more difficult to treat effectively than those suffering from depression alone.

Individuals with both major depression and an Axis II diagnosis may benefit more from therapies specifically designed for the treatment of personality disorders than from any of the standard therapies for major depression alone. Treatment for personality-disordered individuals tends to be longer, more intensive, and more challenging for the clinician. In addition, therapy with depressed patients comorbid for personality disorders may require a greater focus on changing the emotional components of disorders, as well as underlying schemas or deeply ingrained core beliefs—a difficult, time-intensive, and complex undertaking. Depressed patients with concurrent Axis II diagnoses also show poor treatment response to the standard somatic treatments for depression. Shorter, simpler treatments appear not to be effective for this comorbid population. Therefore, it is essential to take comorbid personality disorders into account when treating depressed patients.

Depressed women experiencing concurrent marital problems may need marital therapy instead of, or in addition to, individual cognitive, interpersonal, or somatic therapy. Prior research indicates that cognitive-behavior therapy for depressed women in discordant marriages is successful in alleviating depression, but does little to improve marital satisfaction. However, preliminary studies employing small samples have shown behavioral marital therapy to be effective in improving both depression and marital satisfaction for this group. Depressed women given marital therapy reported greater increases in marital satisfaction than did depressed women given either individual cognitive therapy or no therapy; in one of these studies, these differences remained 1 year later.

In summary, for an individual with comorbid depression and another disorder or problem, therapy that focuses solely on the depression may not have much impact on the individual's overall situation and general functioning. However, therapy that simultaneously addresses both the depression and comorbid problems or disorders may lead to better outcomes, both in terms of recovery from the depressive episode and in terms of preventing relapse or recurrence of the disorder being treated.

FURTHER READING

Andrade, L., Eaton, W. W., & Chilcoat, H. (1994). Lifetime comorbidity of panic attacks and major depression in a population-based study: Symptom profiles. *British Journal of Psychiatry, 165,* 363–369.
Epidemiological study showing a higher co-occurrence of depression and panic attacks than would be expected by chance.

Beach, S. R. H., Sandeen, E. E., & O'Leary, K. D. (1990). *Depression in marriage: A model for etiology and treatment*. New York: Guilford Press.
Book containing behavioral model of comorbid marital discord and depression, and method of treatment.

Blazer, D. G., Kessler, R. C., McGonagle, K. A., & Swartz, M. S. (1994). The prevalence and distribution of major depression in a national community sample: The National Comorbidity Survey. *American Journal of Psychiatry, 151*, 979–986.
National epidemiological study reporting rate and gender ratio of major depression in the United States.

Brown, G. W., Harris, T. O., & Eales, M. J. (1993). Aetiology of anxiety and depressive disorders in an inner-city population: 2. Comorbidity and adversity. *Psychological Medicine, 23*, 155–165.
Study showing that both early adverse experiences and recent adverse experiences raise the risk of depression in adult women.

Bruce, M. L., & Hoff, R. A. (1994). Social and physical health risk factors for first-onset major depressive disorder in a community sample. *Social Psychiatry and Psychiatric Epidemiology, 29*, 165–171.
Study showing that poverty, mediated by social isolation, is associated with greater risk for depression.

Bruce, M. L., & Kim, K. M. (1992). Differences in the effects of divorce on major depression in men and women. *American Journal of Psychiatry, 149*, 914–917.
Longitudinal, community-based study showing gender differences in the relationship between marital disruption and depression.

Craighead, W. E. (1991). Cognitive factors and classification issues in adolescent depression. *Journal of Youth and Adolescence, 20*, 309–324.
Review paper illustrating developmental pathways of comorbid depression and other disorders.

Craighead, W. E., Craighead, L. W., & Ilardi, S. S. (in press). Unipolar depression. In P. E. Nathan & J. M. Gorman (Eds.), *Treatments that work*. New York: Oxford University Press.
Succinct review of effective psychosocial treatments for depression.

Cutler, S. E., & Nolen-Hoeksema, S. (1991). Accounting for sex differences in depression through female victimization: Childhood sexual abuse. *Sex Roles, 24*, 425–438.
Review of the literature suggesting that sex differences in rates of childhood sexual abuse may contribute to the sex difference in depression.

Dunne, F. J., Galatopoulos, C., & Schipperheijn, J. M. (1993). Gender differences in psychiatric morbidity among alcohol misusers. *Comprehensive Psychiatry, 34*, 95–101.
Study of the gender differences in phenomenology of alcohol misuse, indicating that women had primary depression more often than men.

Hamilton, E. B., Jones, M., & Hammen, C. (1993). Maternal interaction style in affective disordered, physically ill, and normal women. *Family Process, 32*, 329–340.
Controlled study showing that children adopt depressed mothers' affective styles.

Ilardi, S. S., & Craighead, W. E. (1994–1995). Personality pathology and response to somatic treatments for major depression: A critical review. *Depression, 2*, 200–217.
Review demonstrating poor response to somatic treatment in depressed, personality-disordered patients.

Jacobson, N. S., Fruzzetti, A. E., Dobson, K., Whisman, M., & Hops, H. (1993). Couple therapy as a treatment for depression: II. The effects of relationship quality and therapy on depressive relapse. *Journal of Consulting and Clinical Psychology, 61*, 516–519.
Empirical study showing that improvement in marital satisfaction from marital therapy lasted over time.

Kendler, K. S., Neale, M. C., Kessler, R. C., Heath, A. C., & Eaves, L. J. (1992). Major depression and generalized anxiety disorder: Same genes, (partly) different environments? *Archives of General Psychiatry, 49,* 716–722.
Study of 1,033 pairs of female twins, showing that in women depression and generalized anxiety disorder share genetic factors, so that environment determines which of these disorders a vulnerable woman develops.

Kendler, K. S., MacLean, C., Neale, M., Kessler, R., Heath, A., & Eaves, L. (1991). The genetic epidemiology of bulimia nervosa. *American Journal of Psychiatry, 148,* 1627–1637.
Study of risk factors for bulimia nervosa, showing that bulimic women are depressed twice as often as nonbulimics.

Kessler, R. C., McGonagle, K. A., Swartz, M., Blazer, D. G., & Nelson, C. B. (1993). Sex and depression in the National Comorbidity Survey: I. Lifetime prevalence, chronicity and recurrence. *Journal of Affective Disorders, 29,* 85–96.
Epidemiological study showing that the sex difference in depression emerges at or soon after puberty.

Linehan, M. M., & Kehrer, C. A. (1993). Borderline personality disorder. In D. H. Barlow (Ed.), *Clinical handbook of psychological disorders* (2nd ed., pp. 396–441). New York: Guilford Press.
Chapter outlining the phenomenology and treatment of borderline personality disorder.

McLeod, J. D., Kessler, R. C., & Landis, K. R. (1992). Speed of recovery from major depressive episodes in a community sample of married men and women. *Journal of Abnormal Psychology, 101,* 277–286.
Survival analysis, studying time to recovery from a major depressive episode, which identifies several important predictors of recovery.

Nolen-Hoeksema, S. (1990). *Sex differences in depression.* Stanford, CA: Stanford University Press.
Excellent book on the phenomenon of, and possible explanations for, the sex difference in depression.

O'Leary, K. D., & Beach, S. R. H. (1990). Marital therapy: A viable treatment for depression and marital discord. *American Journal of Psychiatry, 147,* 183–186.
Controlled study showing that marital therapy improved both depression and marital satisfaction.

Regier, D. A., Burke, J. D., & Burke, K. C. (1990). Comorbidity of affective and anxiety disorders in the NIMH Epidemiologic Catchment Area program. In J. D. Maser & C. R. Cloninger (Eds.), *Comorbidity of mood and anxiety disorders* (pp. 113–122). Washington, DC: American Psychiatric Press.
Epidemiological study, in five U.S. communities, of depression and other psychiatric disorders.

Sanderson, W. C., Beck, A. T., & Beck, J. (1990). Syndrome comorbidity in patients with major depression or dysthymia: Prevalence and temporal relationships. *American Journal of Psychiatry, 147,* 1025–1028.
Empirical study showing that anxiety often co-occurs with major depression and dysthymia.

Walters, E. E., & Kendler, K. S. (1995). Anorexia nervosa and anorexic-like syndromes in a population-based female twin sample. *American Journal of Psychiatry, 152,* 64–71.
Study demonstrating that eating disorders are frequently comorbid with depression.

125

Depression and Acupuncture

John J. B. Allen
Rosa N. Schnyer

Severe depression is an unfortunately common condition, especially among women. A large-scale epidemiological study found that up to 21% of the population of the United States will experience severe depression at some point during life. Depression, however, is approximately twice as common in women as in men, with almost 5% of women meeting diagnostic criteria for major depression at any given time, and between 10% and 25% experiencing major depression at some point during their lives. The costs of major depression are substantial; in fact, they exceed those of other chronic diseases such as diabetes and hypertension in terms of personal distress, lost productivity, interpersonal problems, and suicide. A recent study estimated that these annual costs of depression in the United States exceed $40 billion.

DIAGNOSIS AND TREATMENT OF DEPRESSION
FROM THE WESTERN PSYCHIATRIC PERSPECTIVE

Major depression is diagnosed according to specific criteria outlined in the *Diagnostic and Statistical Manual of Mental Disorders*, fourth edition (DSM-IV). These diagnostic criteria specify that for a period of at least 2 weeks, for most of the day and nearly every day, a person must experience either depressed mood or a profound lack of interest in nearly everything. The diagnosis requires a total of at least five symptoms, with other symptoms occurring in conjunction with the depressed mood and/or lack of interest. These symptoms include change in weight or appetite, change in sleep pattern, change in basic activity level (appearing noticeably agitated or slowed down), a notable decrease in energy level, a decrease in the ability to concentrate, a feeling of being worthless, and thoughts of death or suicide. As these criteria would suggest, major depression can be quite disabling for those who suffer from it—interfering with their relationships, their jobs, and even their ability to care for themselves and those who depend on them. In addition to major depression, many more women suffer from depressive symptoms that, though falling short of meeting criteria for major depression, may significantly interfere with life satisfaction or the ability to work or relate to others. When the definition of depression is relaxed beyond the strict criteria for major depression, more than one in every five women report significant depressive symptoms at any point in time.

Depression is one of the more effectively treated psychiatric conditions. Various treatments are widely available for depression, including tricyclic antidepressant drugs (e.g., desipramine); the newer selective serotonin reuptake inhibitors (e.g., fluoxetine), which produce fewer side effects than the tricyclics; and psychotherapeutic treatments such as cognitive-behavioral therapy. Findings from a nationwide collaborative study reveal that among those depressed persons completing a psychological treatment or receiving drug treatment, 50–70% recover to the point of having few symptoms that significantly interfere with day-to-day living. Yet these treatments fail to provide lasting relief for a sizeable proportion of depressed persons. Almost one-third of the persons receiving these treatments will terminate therapy prior to its completion, citing factors such as dissatisfaction with their current treatment, their desire for another form of treatment, or intolerable side effects of their current treatment. When those persons who fail to complete treatment are taken into account, over half of all depressed persons who enter treatment fail to recover.

Even when it is treated, depression tends to recur. Without further treatment, one-fifth of previously recovered persons once again meet criteria for major depression 6 months after the completion of treatment, and nearly one-quarter will develop new depressive symptoms. A year and a half after treatment, over one-third of those persons who were remitted will relapse with full depression. A growing consensus among those who treat depression is that some form of continued maintenance treatment is necessary after recovery.

These statistics suggest that additional treatments may be welcomed by many persons with major depression. A recent survey of the U.S. population found that depression is one of the 10 most frequently reported medical problems for which persons seek treatment, and more individuals than not had sought alternative treatments (e.g., relaxation techniques, self-help groups) in addition to or instead of the medication or psychotherapeutic treatments mentioned previously. These findings suggest that current treatments may address only a part of the total symptom picture in depression, or that current treatments are insufficient for many depressed persons. New treatments may be welcomed as adjuncts to or substitutes for existing treatments, or as maintenance or preventive treatments following remission. Many researchers are actively investigating new treatments for depression, especially new and better drug treatments; other, "alternative" forms of treatment, however, have received comparatively little formal attention. Our experience, both clinically as well as in a controlled treatment study, suggests that acupuncture may prove an effective treatment for depression.

DIAGNOSIS AND TREATMENT OF DEPRESSION FROM THE PERSPECTIVE OF TRADITIONAL CHINESE MEDICINE

Chinese medicine does not focus on the diagnosis and treatment of disease, but rather on the detection of energetic imbalances. Therefore, strictly speaking, depression does not exist as a disease category in Chinese medicine. Because the patient is always considered as a totality of body and mind, physiological and psychological symptoms are equally important. In this way, Chinese medicine offers an alternative and complementary approach that integrates the physiological and psychological factors of depression.

Chinese medicine is based on the concept of "Qi" (pronounced "chee"), or vital energy, which represents the capacity of life to maintain and transform itself. Health is defined as the balance between "Yin" and "Yang," two complementary forces that represent the totality of the dynamic equilibrium. Yin and Yang have been described in detail by Ted Kaptchuk, who has written extensively about Chinese medicine. Yin, which is nourishing, grants individuals the qualities of rest, tranquility, and quiescence as well as the capacity to unfold gracefully, while being content, quiet, and mentally and physically present. When Yin is deficient, people lack the qualities of receptivity and contemplation and become easily agitated, unsettled, or nervously uneasy. Yang, which by contrast is activating, causes transformation and change, providing people with the capacity to engage life, to react, and to respond. When Yang is deficient, individuals find themselves paralyzed in fear, confused and indecisive, unable to express what they want, and hopeless.

The balance between Yin and Yang depends on the capacity of an organism to adapt to change; this balance is sustained by the proper circulation of Qi along energetic pathways or meridians. The meridians form a network that connects the surface of the body with internal organs. The organs in Chinese medicine are defined by their functions and interrelations, rather than by their structures or anatomical locations. They represent a complete set of functions that reflect energetic relationships among physiological and psychological events, and are referred to as "organ networks." Meridians and organ networks both work in pairs, with one Yin and one Yang function interconnected; each organ network is considered to have a Yin (storing, nourishing, cooling) component and a Yang (activating, protective, warming) component.

The experience of a disorder, the nature of its symptoms, and the protocol and outcome of the treatment are determined by the specific tendencies in every person toward either a relative deficiency (hypoactivity) or excess (hyperactivity) of either Yin or Yang. These tendencies, then, precipitate personal patterns of reaction. When this framework is applied to the traditional diagnostic criteria for major depression as it is defined in the DSM-IV, a person experiencing depressed mood with lethargy and weakness, decreased motivation, lack of appetite, and excessive desire to sleep would be understood as manifesting a pattern where Yin is predominant and Yang is deficient. On the other hand, if the person is experiencing irritability, anxiety, agitation, excessive appetite, and insomnia, this would reflect a pattern where the Yang is relatively excessive and Yin is deficient.

The relationship between Yin and Yang is further differentiated into stages that describe the process of change and that define the movement of Qi through the various organ functions; every stage or phase corresponds to a set of meridians and a set of organ networks, which in turn have physiological and psychological functions as well as specific emotions associated with each one of them. In assessing someone with depression, for example, it is important to determine which organ networks are affected and, in turn, whether the Yin or Yang functions of these organs are more involved. If someone with depression were experiencing the emotional and psychological symptoms of anger, irritability, and frustration, and the physical symptoms of headaches, painful periods, digestive disturbance, and insomnia, these symptoms would collectively point to an imbalance in the liver network.

Because all emotions are considered to be expressions of Qi, any emotion that finds no release through verbal expression or physical activity becomes stagnant, noxious energy that is not circulating properly. Most cases of depression will, at least in part, present Qi stagnation as a significant component. This stagnation of Qi combines with the predisposing factors of Yin or Yang, excess or deficiency in different organ networks, adding complexity to the energetic picture. In addition, Chinese medicine considers that emotional manifestations of an imbalance reflect, in particular, the condition of the "Shen"—the organizing force of the self, the emotional, mental, and expressive life of the individual that is supposed to be "housed" by the heart organ network. A person's response to the environment is determined by the health of the Shen; therefore, the lack of warmth to express life, joy, and fulfillment, or the confusion and agitation experienced during a major depressive episode, are manifestations of the heart's lost ability to enfold the Shen.

In sum, within the context of Chinese medicine, depression can be understood as a complex energetic reaction pattern that involves a predisposing tendency toward excess or deficiency of either Yin or Yang, combined with varying degrees of Qi stagnation and Shen disturbance. The question that Chinese medicine poses, then, is not only whether certain individuals are depressed, but how they are experiencing depression, and what precipitating factors—physical, psychological, and social—have contributed to their present condition. Chinese medicine provides a framework for understanding distinct symptom pictures and aims at developing a treatment approach based on the nature of each individual's experience of a disease. Furthermore, it offers a physiology that clearly links somatic and psychological symptoms, helping to close the gap between mind and body.

PRELIMINARY EVIDENCE ON THE EFFECTIVENESS OF ACUPUNCTURE AS A TREATMENT FOR DEPRESSION

Several reports from the former Soviet Union and from China suggest that acupuncture is an effective treatment for depression and other emotional disorders (listed as anxiety, hypochondria, neurasthenia, and obsessive–compulsive disorder). In addition, one study suggests that for a majority of persons with nonpsychotic depression—those who would be most likely to be seen in outpatient settings—acupuncture treatment was as effective as antidepressant medications. Several practitioners also report favorable results of treatment devised from their assessments of depression as an expression of a disharmony within the context of Chinese medicine.

Preliminary results from our ongoing controlled treatment study of major depression in women are similarly promising. In a sample of 24 women aged 18–45 with a diagnosis of major depression, we compared individually tailored acupuncture treatments for depression (specific treatments) both with a waiting-list control and with individually tailored treatments not designed to address depression specifically (nonspecific treatments). Women in all groups eventually received specific treatments. After the completion of specific treatments (pooled across all subjects), 71% of women experienced full remission from depression, whereas only 12% of women in the 8-week waiting-list condition had experienced full remission. Another 21% of women receiving acupuncture treatments (and 25% of those in the waiting-list group) experienced some lesser improvement (termed partial remission). Only 8% of women receiving specific treatments experienced no remission, compared with 63% of those in the waiting-list group. These rates of success compare favorably to the reported efficacy (50–70%) of existing drug and psychotherapeutic treatments. Moreover, in our study, only 12% of the women who initially began acupuncture treatments terminated them prior to completion (as compared with about one-third of persons undergoing traditional treatments). Definitive conclusions, however, await the completion of this study.

FUTURE DIRECTIONS

The existing data on the effectiveness of acupuncture as a treatment for depression are very promising. We caution that further research is required to corroborate these initial reports of a small number of depressed women with larger-scale studies. If additional research continues to show that acupuncture is an effective treatment for depression in women, it will then be important to address several additional issues. First, although acupuncture appears effective for major depression, its effectiveness needs to be determined for chronic depressions and long-lasting milder depressions (dysthymia). Second, the long-term prognosis of those women who respond to acupuncture treatment is not known at present. Therefore, future research can address whether the treatment gains are maintained or whether less frequent "maintenance" treatments are required after the initial set of treatments. Finally, and perhaps most importantly, future research is required to determine whether acupuncture can assist those who fail to respond to traditional treatments, and whether traditional treatments will assist those who fail to respond to acupuncture.

There is reason to be optimistic concerning the treatment of depression. Although at present many depressed persons do not fully benefit from treatment, many researchers are currently working in a variety of disciplines to develop and improve treatments for depression. The options available to depressed women will increase as research develops and refines psychotherapeutic interventions, pharmacological interventions, and other treatments such as acupuncture.

The challenges to those treating depression in women, however, are preventing the recurrence of depression in treated women and preventing initial episodes in women who have never experienced depression. Several studies now suggest the necessity of maintenance treatment to avoid further episodes of depression. Much research remains to be done in determining what constitutes effective maintenance treatment, whether such treatment consists of medication, psychotherapy, acupuncture, or other methods. Because the causes of depression are undoubtedly multifaceted, interventions that address those many causes may be required. If, through a combination of treatments, practitioners and researchers are better able to identify the interaction among physiological, psychological, and social factors involved in each person's depression, they may be better able to prevent depression or to prevent initial symptoms from progressing to the point of a full syndrome of major depression. Acupuncture can contribute in this area by providing a framework for understanding distinct symptom pictures and by offering the ability to treat distinct patterns with individually tailored treatments.

FURTHER READING

American Psychiatric Association. (1994). *Diagnostic and statistical manual of mental disorders* (4th ed.). Washington, DC: Author.
The comprehensive listing of diagnosable mental disorders, with descriptions for each.

Beinfield, H., & Korngold, E. (1991). *Between heaven and earth: A guide to Chinese medicine.* New York: Ballantine Books.
A comprehensive introduction to Chinese medicine as a framework for understanding the human body and mind in illness and in health, including images that help the nonpractitioner grasp the challenging concepts.

Eisenberg, D. M., Kessler, R. C., Foster, C., Norlock, F. E., Calkins, D. R., & Delbanco, T. L. (1993). Unconventional medicine in the United States: Prevalence, costs, and patterns of use. *New England Journal of Medicine, 328,* 246–252.
Details about the frequency of use of alternative treatments for the most common conditions, including depression.

Elkin, I., Shea, T., Watkins, J. T., Imber, S. D., Sotsky, S. M., Collins, J. F., Glass, D. R., Pilkonis, P. A., Leber, W. R., Docherty, J. P., Fiester, S. J., & Perloff, M. B. (1989). National Institute of Mental Health Treatment of Depression Collaborative Research Program: General effectiveness of treatments. *Archives of General Psychiatry, 46,* 971–982.
Summary of a large-scale treatment study for depression, involving both psychotherapy and drug treatments.

Hirshfield, R. M. A., & Schatzberg, A. F. (1994). Long-term management of depression. *American Journal of Medicine, 97*(Suppl. 6A), 33S–38S.
Statistics and suggestions concerning the treatment of depression after the initial episode has been treated.

Kaptchuk, T. J. (1983). *The web that has no weaver: Understanding Chinese medicine.* New York: Congdon & Weed.
A concise yet thorough overview of the principles of Chinese medicine, with special emphasis on the interaction between signs and symptoms to create an energetic "pattern of disharmony."

Kessler, R. C., McGonagle, K. A., Zhao, S., Nelson, C. B., Hughes, M., Eschleman, S., Wittchen, H. U., & Kendler, K. S. (1994). Lifetime and 12-month prevalence of DSM-III-R psychiatric disorders in the United States. *Archives of General Psychiatry, 51,* 8–19.
Summarizes a large-scale epidemiological study of psychiatric disorders, including depression, detailing the incidence and co-occurrence of various disorders.

Linde, K., Ramirez, G., Mulrow, C. D., Pauls, A., Weidenhammer, W., & Melchart, D. (1996). St. John's wort for depression—an overview and meta-analysis of randomized clinical trials. British Medical Journal, 313, 253–258.
A recently published meta-analysis of randomized trials of hypericum in treating mild to moderately severe depressive disorder, which concluded that the herb was significantly superior to placebo, and appeared comparably effective to standard antidepressants while producing fewer side effects.

Seem, M. (1987). *Bodymind energetics: Towards a dynamic model of health.* Rochester, VT: Thorsons.
An exploration of acupuncture theory as the "missing link" in explaining the relationship between somatic and psychological events, postulating an energetic framework that aims at closing the gap between soma and psyche.

Shea, T., Elkin, I., Imber, S. D., Sotsky, S. M., Watkins, J. T., Collins, J. F., Pilkonis, P. A., Beckham, E., Glass, D. R., Dolan, R. T., & Perloff, M. B. (1992). Course of depressive symptoms over follow-up: Findings from the National Institute of Mental Health Treatment of Depression Collaborative Research Program. *Archives of General Psychiatry, 49,* 782–787.
Summary of the longer-term outcomes from the large-scale treatment study for depression, involving both psychotherapy and drug treatments.

126

Borderline
Personality Disorder

Amy W. Wagner

At some point, virtually all health care providers will encounter individuals who meet criteria for borderline personality disorder (BPD). Epidemiological studies, as reported in Widiger and Weissman (1991), estimate that 11% of psychiatric outpatients and 15–20% of psychiatric inpatients meet criteria for BPD. Because they tend to have a variety of comorbid medical problems, as well as to engage in medically high-risk behavior and self-injurious behavior, individuals with BPD frequently present to medical settings as well. Despite the relatively high prevalence of BPD, it remains one of the most misunderstood and misused psychiatric diagnostic classifications. The purpose of this chapter is to provide a very broad overview of BPD, highlighting current knowledge on the etiology, course, and treatment of this disorder.

"ON THE BORDERLINE OF WHAT?"

Some of the misunderstandings surrounding the BPD diagnosis stem from the term "borderline" itself. First introduced by Stern in 1938, the term was initially used to describe a group of patients who did not fit into the then-standard psychiatric categories of "neurotic" or "psychotic." Unlike the "neurotics," these patients did not generally improve with common psychoanalytic practices, yet they also did not display the more extremely disturbed behaviors of the "psychotics." Thus, they were viewed as falling on the "border" between the neurotics and psychotics. Then, through the early work of several other psychoanalytic theorists, the behaviors of the "borderline" individual were more systematically categorized. BPD became a formal psychiatric diagnosis in 1980.

DIAGNOSTIC CRITERIA

With more extensive clinical observation and research, the criteria for BPD have evolved over time. Currently, as described in the fourth edition of the *Diagnostic and Statistical Manual of Mental Disorders* (DSM-IV), BPD refers to a far-reaching pattern of instability and dysregulation, affecting the domains of behavior, cognition, emotion, and interpersonal functioning. The criteria for BPD include affective lability, problems with anger, chaotic relationships, fears of abandonment, problems with sense of self, sense of emptiness, self-injurious behavior, impulsive behavior, dissociative behavior, and paranoid ideation. The criteria for BPD have been changed slightly in the DSM-IV from the DSM-III-R by changing the wording of some of the criteria and adding criterion 9, which covers dissociative symptoms and paranoid ideation. To receive the diagnosis of BPD, an individual must meet five of the nine criteria, and these must be "characteristic" of the person's long-term functioning. BPD is diagnosed much more frequently among women, with recent research suggesting that approximately 76% of borderline individuals are women.

Although not diagnostic in itself, one of the cardinal features of BPD is parasuicidal behavior, defined as any intentional, acute, self-injurious behavior. This can include actual suicide attempts in which the intent is to die and the result is medically serious or lethal, or behavior with little or no intent to die, such as cutting, burning, overdosing, head banging, suicide ideation, and suicide threats. It has been estimated that 69–75% of individuals with BPD engage in (chronic) parasuicidal behavior. Therefore, individuals with BPD often present for medical as well as psychological services.

Nonetheless, it is becoming widely recognized that BPD is a heterogeneous disorder. For example, some people with this diagnosis are fairly high-functioning; they are capable of maintaining jobs and forming relationships, and rarely (if ever) require psychiatric hospitalizations. Others with the BPD diagnosis, however, may be unemployed for extended periods, are socially isolated or in and out of chaotic relationships, are chronically suicidal, and require multiple psychiatric hospitalizations. This heterogeneity has led some researchers to suggest that there may be subtypes of BPD, based on the severity of symptomatology and on particular constellations of symptoms. Future research may lead to official subtypings of BPD.

Furthermore, it is not uncommon for the same individual to appear extremely competent at some times and in some situations, and extremely dysfunctional at other times. This perception seems to be related to *actual* fluctuations in competencies, based on context and on a BPD person's current emotional state. Linehan has labeled this characteristic the "apparently competent person" syndrome. This characteristic can be confusing both to health care providers and to BPD individuals themselves, and may be related to the (usually inaccurate) perception that these individuals sometimes have "exaggerated" or "malingering" symptomatology.

COMORBID DIAGNOSES

The heterogeneous presentation of the borderline individual may be partly related to the wide variety of psychological diagnoses that often coexist with BPD. The most common comorbid diagnoses among individuals with BPD include major depressive disorder, dysthymia, substance abuse and dependence, eating disorders (anorexia nervosa and bulimia nervosa), somatization disorder, dissociative identity disorder, and other personality disorders (including histrionic, dependent, avoidant, and schizotypal). Although there may be a nonspecific genetic relationship between BPD and these disorders (e.g., temperamental vulnerability), extensive research has failed to support direct genetic relationships. It is more likely that these different disorders share similar environmental etiologies.

Recent attention has been given to the high rates of posttraumatic stress disorder (PTSD) diagnosed among individuals with BPD. This, combined with recent research that indicates high rates of childhood trauma among individuals with BPD (described below), has led some to attempt to reconceptualize BPD as a posttraumatic syndrome. Nonetheless, only about one-third of the individuals with BPD meet criteria for PTSD, and a substantial proportion of individuals with BPD deny histories of trauma. Therefore, BPD and PTSD appear to be distinct disorders that frequently co-occur, most likely because of similar environmental (i.e., traumatic) etiologies.

ETIOLOGY: BIOSOCIAL THEORY

Clinicians and researchers of most theoretical orientations generally believe that BPD is caused by a combination of biological and environmental factors. One of the best-articulated theories of the etiology of BPD is Linehan's biosocial theory. Guided by learning, developmental, and biological psychology, as well as by research on emotion, Linehan proposes that BPD arises from a combination of biologically based difficulties in the processing of emotions (i.e., in the perception of, reaction to, and modulation of emotion) with an environment that is inherently and severely "invalidating" in nature (described below). The result of the combined biological vulnerability and invalidating environment is a pervasive disruption of the emotion regulation system. Linehan views all problematic behaviors of the borderline individual as related to emotion dysregulation or as (dysfunctional) attempts at modulating emotions.

The factors that lead to the biological vulnerability in BPD are probably varied, including genetic influences, harmful intrauterine events, and environmental events during development that alter the brain and nervous system. The genetic influences on the development of BPD appear to be nonspecific. For example, although first-degree relatives of individuals with BPD have higher rates of BPD than the general population, they also have higher rates of mood disorders, such as depression. There is no consistent evidence that BPD is *directly* genetically transmitted. Possible intrauterine contributors to emotional vulnerability include malnutrition, substance misuse, and environmental stress; however, no studies have yet examined the rates of these factors in the mothers of BPD individuals. Related to environmental contributors to biological vulnerability, recent studies have shown that extreme environmental events can actually modify neurological development. In particular, extreme stress has been shown to alter and compromise the limbic system, which has been directly implicated in the effective regulation of emotions. Thus, it is likely that there are multiple biological contributors to the development of BPD.

Again, Linehan's biosocial theory states that BPD develops when this emotional vulnerability is coupled with an invalidating environment. An invalidating environment is one that consistently communicates to a child that her (or his) reactions and perceptions are not appropriate or valid. Often a child's communication of private experiences (i.e., thoughts and feelings) meets with extreme, erratic, inappropriate, or neglectful reactions from caregivers. The result is that the child never really learns how to understand or regulate her (or his) own emotional experiences. This, combined with a biologically based predisposition to a vulnerability to emotions, leads to the systemic and pervasive emotion dysregulation characteristic of BPD.

Although the invalidating environment can take many forms, Linehan asserts that childhood sexual abuse represents the prototypic invalidating experience. Rates of childhood sexual abuse among outpatients and inpatients with BPD range from 40% to 86%, compared to 22–34% of those without the BPD diagnosis. This has led many researchers to suggest that childhood sexual abuse is directly related to the development of BPD. However, it should be stressed that a substantial proportion of borderline individuals deny histories of sexual abuse, and that many people who have experienced childhood sexual abuse do not develop BPD. It appears that many of the characteristics of childhood sexual abuse are extremely invalidating, and *can* thus lead to the development of BPD when combined with biological vulnerability. Other childhood experiences can be similarly invalidating, and in fact individuals with BPD also report higher rates of physical abuse, neglect, and separation from caregivers than do other psychiatric patient groups.[1]

COURSE

The course of BPD is variable, depending in part on the type and quality of treatment received. In general, however, improvements are slow, and individuals often continue to meet criteria for BPD for many years. In a thorough review of follow-up studies to date, Linehan and Heard report that 60–70% of borderline individuals continue to meet criteria 2–3 years after an index assessment. The rates drop slightly, although not dramatically, 4–7 years later. In a recent study by Links and colleagues, using a prospective design and in-person interviews, 47% of the original sample of borderline individuals still met criteria 7 years later. In two 15-year follow-up studies by McGlashan and Paris and colleagues, rates of individuals who still met BPD criteria at follow-up ranged from 25% to 44%. Rates of remittance have been higher among adolescents diagnosed with BPD; one study by Garnet and colleagues found that only 33% of 21 patients aged 17–19 met criteria after 2 years. However, the application of the BPD diagnosis to adolescents is questionable and is not recommended by the DSM-IV.

It is estimated that approximately 10% of all BPD individuals will eventually succeed in committing suicide. Even higher rates have been reported for individuals who meet eight or more of the BPD criteria. One of the strongest predictors of eventual suicide is the presence of past parasuicidal behavior. Therefore, although parasuicidal behavior is frequently not medically serious, the potential dangerousness and lethality of parasuicidal behavior among borderline individuals should not be minimized.

---

[1]Because of the high rate of childhood sexual abuse among individuals with BPD, a number of comorbid medical problems associated with this type of abuse, such as chronic pelvic pain, pain during sexual intercourse, pelvic inflammatory disease, breast disease, yeast infections, complicated pregnancies, premenstrual syndrome, and gastrointestinal problems, are common in this population as well.

TREATMENT

BPD has been commonly treated by both pharmacotherapy and psychotherapy. A number of controlled clinical trials have been conducted to examine the efficacy of pharmacotherapy for the treatment of BPD. Targeting the *symptoms* of BPD, these studies have generally focused on neuroleptics (antipsychotics), antidepressants, and anti-anxiety agents. Low doses of neuroleptic medications have been found to improve cognitive processes and psychotic symptoms (e.g., paranoia, hallucinations, derealization, depersonalization), impulsivity, and affective problems, particularly for individuals with more severe symptoms. However, few replication studies exist, and some studies contradict these findings.

Depressed mood in BPD individuals has shown improvement in some trials of tricyclic antidepressants (TCAs) and monoamine oxidase inhibitors (MAOIs). Again, the findings across studies are mixed, with some studies reporting no effects, and some reporting a "paradoxical" worsening of depression symptoms and suicidal thinking on the medications. The side effects of TCAs and MAOIs are compounded by the risk of possible overdose by borderline individuals. Both classes of medications are highly lethal when ingested in large quantities. The selective serotonin reuptake inhibitors (SSRIs) are less harmful antidepressants in overdose situations. Although few studies exist, initial investigations suggest that fluoxetine in particular may lead to improvements in depression, impulsivity, psychoticism, and hostility. The potential danger of overdose even on the SSRIs should not be dismissed, however.

Finally, attempts have been made to manage the anxiety symptoms of BPD with benzodiazepines. In the few studies conducted, improvements have been reported for anxiety, hostility, sleep problems, suspiciousness, and other cognitive disturbances. However, the benzodiazepines have also been found to lead to worsening of symptoms, particularly disinhibition of responses and behavioral dyscontrol. Individuals on these medications have shown increases in parasuicidal and violent behavior. These findings on the efficacy of pharmacotherapy for BPD led Soloff to conclude that the effects are "modest" at best, and that when pharmacotherapy is used, it should be done in conjunction with psychotherapy.

Unfortunately, there have been few randomized, controlled outcome studies on the efficacy of psychotherapy for BPD. Although the majority of the literature on BPD has been provided by clinicians from psychoanalytic or psychodynamic orientations, reports on the effectiveness of these approaches have been supported by case studies or uncontrolled outcome studies only.

The majority of randomized, controlled psychotherapy outcome studies have been on cognitive-behavioral approaches to the treatment of BPD, and here the results are promising. In particular, Linehan's dialectical behavior therapy (DBT) was shown to be superior to "treatment as usual" (TAU) in the community in a randomized, controlled design. Subjects were assigned to either 1 year of DBT (individual psychotherapy and group skills training) or TAU. After 1 year of outpatient psychotherapy, DBT subjects had fewer parasuicides, less medically severe parasuicides, higher treatment retention, fewer psychiatric hospital days, less anger, higher social functioning, and higher global functioning. Linehan and Heard also found DBT to be more cost-effective than TAU. Similar findings have been reported for inpatient applications of DBT.

Turner also demonstrated the efficacy of cognitive-behavioral therapy in a randomized, controlled study of "dynamic cognitive-behavior" therapy compared to "supportive" individual therapy. After 6 months after the end of treatment, and again at 6 months post treatment, the cognitive-behavior subjects had less parasuicide, anger, depression, and anxiety than the control subjects, as well as better ratings on overall psychopathology.

In 1995 Munroe-Blum and Marziali conducted a controlled, randomized trial comparing the efficacy of a short-term (25-session) "interpersonal" group psychotherapy to that of individual psychodynamic therapy. No differences were found between the two groups on the major outcome variables; however, combined, all subjects showed significant improvement on most outcome variables. Given the cost-effectiveness of group therapy, these results support the use of interpersonal group therapy over individual psychodynamic therapy for BPD. Nonetheless, since the two groups did not differ from each other, it is difficult to know how these improvements compare to naturally occurring change over time or to cognitive-behavioral approaches.

CONCLUDING REMARKS

In summary, the conceptualization and understanding of BPD have changed considerably since Stern's original formulation in 1938. With this understanding have come refinements and new developments in the treatment of BPD. To date, the research supports cognitive-behavioral approaches for the treatment of BPD, and there is mounting evidence that some pharmacotherapy, when well monitored, can be effective in symptom reduction as well. Because of the developmental and biological etiology of BPD, however, it should be emphasized that change is slow even with cognitive-behavioral approaches. Future studies are clearly needed to continue improving and evaluating our approaches to BPD.

FURTHER READING

American Psychiatric Association. (1994). *Diagnostic and statistical manual of mental disorders* (4th ed.). Washington, DC: Author.
The official psychiatric classification manual; source for the formal criteria for BPD.

Brinkley, J. R. (1993). Pharmacotherapy of borderline states. *Psychiatric Clinics of North America, 16,* 853–884.
This article provides a comprehensive review of current studies evaluating efficacy of pharmacotherapy for the treatment of BPD.

Garnet, K. E., Levy, K. N., Mattanah, J. J., Edell, W. S., & McGlashan, T. H. (1994). Borderline personality disorder in adolescents: Ubiquitous or specific? *American Journal of Psychiatry, 151,* 1380–1382.
This study examined the stability of BPD criteria among 21 adolescents over a 2-year time period, and concluded that the diagnosis has low stability over time in this age group.

Linehan, M. M. (1993). *Cognitive-behavioral treatment of borderline personality disorder.* New York: Guilford Press.
This book is Linehan's comprehensive treatment manual for DBT; in it, she also describes her theoretical formulation of BPD.

Linehan, M. M. (1993). *Skills training manual for treatment of borderline personality disorder.* New York: Guilford Press.
This workbook outlines and provides the materials for the skills training module of Linehan's DBT.

Linehan, M. M., Armstrong, H. E., Suarez, A., Allmon, D., & Heard, H. L. (1991). Cognitive-behavioral treatment of chronically parasuicidal borderline patients. *Archives of General Psychiatry, 48,* 1060–1064.
This article presents the first outcome data demonstrating the efficacy of DBT—specifically in reducing parasuidical behavior, psychiatric hospitalizations, and anger—in a randomized, controlled study.

Linehan, M. M., & Heard, H. L. (in press). BPD: Costs, course, and treatment outcomes. In N. Miller (Ed.), *The cost effectiveness of psychotherapy: A guide for practitioners, researchers, and policy-makers.* New York: Oxford Press.
This chapter provides a comprehensive review of BPD, highlighting the short- and long-term cost of services for this disorder, and the relative cost-effectiveness of DBT.

Linehan, M. M., Tutek, D. A., Heard, H. L., & Armstrong, H. E. (1994). Cognitive behavioral treatment for chronically suicidal borderline patients: Interpersonal outcomes. *American Journal of Psychiatry, 151,* 1771–1776.
This article presents additional data demonstrating the efficacy of DBT in improving social and global functioning in a randomized, controlled study.

Links, P. S., Heslegrave, R. J., Mitton, J. E., van Reekum, R., & Patrick, J. (1995). Borderline psychopathology and recurrences of clinical disorders. *Journal of Nervous and Mental Disease, 183,* 582–586.
This study improved on previous longitudinal investigations on the course of BPD by using a prospective design and in-person interviews. Almost half of the sample continued to meet full diagnostic criteria after a 7-year time period.

McGlashan, T. H. (1992). The longitudinal profile of borderline personality disorder: Contributions from the Chestnut Lodge follow-up study. In D. Silver & M. Rosenbluth (Eds.), *Handbook of borderline disorders* (pp. 53–83). Madison, CT: International Universities Press.
This chapter reviews findings related to the long-term course of BPD.

Munroe-Blum, H., & Marziali, E. (1995). A controlled trial of short-term group treatment for borderline personality disorder. *Journal of Personality Disorders, 9,* 190–198.
This article presents outcome data from a study comparing interpersonal group therapy to individual psychodynamic therapy. Results indicated that both therapies were equally effective in reducing a number of key problematic behaviors.

Paris, J., Brown, R., & Nowlis, D. (1987). Long-term follow-up of borderline patients in a general hospital. *Comprehensive Psychiatry, 28,* 530–535.
This study reports the diagnostic course of a sample of 100 individuals with the borderline diagnosis over a 15-year period.

Soloff, P. H. (1989). Psychopharmacologic therapies in borderline personality disorder. In A. Tasman, R. E. Hales, & A. J. Frances (Eds.), *Review of psychiatry* (Vol. 8, pp. 65–83). Washington, DC: American Psychiatric Press.
This chapter provides a comprehensive review of current studies conducted prior to 1989, evaluating efficacy of pharmacotherapy for the treatment of BPD.

Soloff, P. H. (1994). Is there any drug treatment of choice for the borderline patient? *Acta Psychiatrica Scandinavica, 89*(Suppl. 379), 50–55.
This article provides a comprehensive review of more recent studies evaluating efficacy of pharmacotherapy for the treatment of BPD.

Stern, A. (1938). Psychoanalytic investigation and therapy in the borderline group of neuroses. *Psychoanalytic Quarterly, 7,* 467–489.
One of the initial conceptualizations of "borderline" patients, influential in later classifications of BPD.

Turner, R. M. (1993, November). *Dynamic cognitive-behavior therapy for borderline personality disorder*. Paper presented at the 27th Annual Convention of the Association for Advancement of Behavior Therapy, Atlanta, GA.

This paper presents outcome data from a randomized, controlled study comparing "dynamic cognitive-behavior" therapy to supportive therapy. The former was more effective in reducing negative affect and psychopathology.

Wagner, A. W., & Linehan, M. M. (1996). A biosocial perspective on the relationship of childhood sexual abuse, suicidal behavior, and borderline personality disorder. In M. Zanarini (Ed.), *The role of sexual abuse in the etiology of borderline personality disorder* (pp. 203–223). Washington, DC: American Psychiatric Press.

This chapter overviews Linehan's biosocial theory of the etiology of BPD, highlighting the role of childhood sexual abuse in the development of this disorder.

Widiger, T. A., & Weissman, M. M. (1991). Epidemiology of borderline personality disorder. Special section: Borderline personality disorder. *Hospital and Community Psychiatry, 42,* 1015–1021.

Summarizes epidemiological data on the prevalence of borderline personality disorder in both community and psychiatric settings.

127

Schizophrenia

Richard R. J. Lewine

Schizophrenia is a psychiatric disorder that has a devastating impact on the sufferer's mental, emotional, and interpersonal life, independent of that individual's sex. Why then, in the face of the many commonalities between female and male schizophrenia patients, examine sex differences—in particular, those aspects of the disorder that may be specific to women? There are two reasons. First, there is now considerable evidence that schizophrenia has a different timing and biological context in men than in women, and that these differences have both etiological and treatment implications. Second, there are general women's health issues (largely focused on reproductive functions) that are both often overlooked in the treatment of, and create special problems for, the woman with schizophrenia.

THE FEMALE SCHIZOPHRENIA PATIENT

Although schizophrenia is often thought of as a disorder of adolescence, the period of greatest risk for first hospitalization in women is between the ages of 25 and 34 (onset of first symptoms has been estimated to occur approximately 4 years earlier). There is a second high-risk period following menopause. In contrast, risk of schizophrenia onset peaks between 15 and 24 years for men, with a steady decline over the remainder of the lifespan.

Although the primary schizophrenia symptoms of thought disorganization, hallucinations, and delusions are comparable in the two sexes, women appear to retain much more emotional responsiveness and more often have mood disorder in the clinical picture than do men. One effect of these disturbances is to interfere with personal relationships, as reflected in lower marriage rates among individuals with schizophrenia than in the general population. Given that schizophrenia often erupts during the years of courtship, this may not seem surprising. However, whereas women are clearly affected by age of onset (the later the onset of schizophrenia, the more likely they are to marry), men very rarely marry, independent of the disorder's onset age. It has been variously estimated that up to approximately 50% of women with schizophrenia marry. Fertility rates, estimated in early studies to be significantly lower in both men and women than in the general population, appear to be increasing for women but remain low for men. The implications for women are discussed below.

ETIOLOGY OF SCHIZOPHRENIA

Though schizophrenia has long been thought to have a genetic component, it has recently been suggested that heredity plays a stronger role in the development of schizophrenia in women than in men. In contrast, there is strong evidence of more frequent brain damage or anomaly, perhaps linked to impaired fetal neurodevelopment (secondary to either pregnancy and birth complications or second-trimester exposure to a toxin such as a flu virus), in men than in women.

Differences in the timing of peak risk periods for women and men have led to the hypothesis that estrogen may serve to delay the onset of or buffer the effects of schizophrenia. Specifically, it is well established that women reach biological maturity (puberty) about 2 years earlier than men; this is accompanied by very large increases in the level of estrogen. In turn, this early exposure to high levels of estrogen may underlie the later onset of schizophrenia in women than in men. That women experience a second schizophrenia risk period postmenopausally, when estrogen levels drop again, is consistent with such a view, as are scattered animal studies demonstrating the influence of estrogen on dopamine (excessive levels of this neurotransmitter may be associated with hallucinations, delusions, and disorganized thought).

TREATMENT WITH MEDICATIONS

As a group, women are more sensitive to antipsychotic medications than are men. That is, less medicine is required to achieve a given level of treatment response in women than in men, even when sex differences in body weight are taken into account. This may be attributable to differences between the sexes in the biochemical processing of the antipsychotic medications. Similarly, women will often experience subjective changes in response to smaller dose changes than will men. Women (especially if older) are also at higher risk than men for the development of tardive dyskinesia, an involuntary movement disorder that can be a side effect of antipsychotic medications. The major hormonal changes women experience—such as with pregnancy, over the menstrual cycle, or in menopause—can dramatically alter the physiological environment in which medications are administered, and hence the need to vary medication dose accordingly. Stewart and Robinson point out, for example, that the significant increase in body water content during pregnancy may lead to lower drug serum concentrations than in nonpregnant women. To complicate matters, the antipsychotic medications can in turn alter a woman's hormonal environment, resulting in extreme cases in amenorrhea.

Equally problematic is the frequent use of polypharmacy regimens (i.e., treatment with more than one psychoactive medication at a time) with women. Some of this may be appropriate, as women are more likely than men to have major affective disorder accompany the schizophrenia. Some, however, may be attributable to the general tendency to polypharmacy in the delivery of health services to women. It is important, therefore, that medication review be thorough and regular.

SEXUALITY AND SCHIZOPHRENIA

Because it is frequently assumed that schizophrenia interferes completely with interpersonal relationships, many clinicians do not explore their patients' sexual lives. This can be particularly disastrous for women, who, despite schizophrenia, often remain quite sexually active. It has been estimated in various surveys that up to 75% of female schizophrenia patients have been sexually active within the past 3 months of the survey. In addition, these women's high rates of cocaine abuse and dependence, and their frequent exchange of sex for drugs, increase their chances of contracting a sexually transmitted disease. Issues of safe sex and the use of contraceptives should therefore be routinely addressed in treatment. Unfortunately, the cognitive disorganization characteristic of schizophrenia often makes thoughtful and safe sexual practices difficult.

PREGNANCY

Pregnancy raises difficult ethical and practical concerns for a woman with schizophrenia. As 50–60% of the pregnancies of schizophrenic women are unplanned, one of the first issues is that of family planning and the use of contraceptives. This issue usually receives very little attention, and success in contraceptive use is rare. Nevertheless, open and direct discussion is necessary. Once a woman is pregnant, there is the problem of medication. Although there are scattered anecdotal reports that pregnancy in schizophrenia is often accompanied by symptom remission, there are many mothers-to-be who require continued medication to keep the psychotic disorder under control.

Although the use of antipsychotic medications does not appear to cause genetic or structural damage to the fetus, there are documented reversible effects, such as extrapyramidal symptoms, jaundice, intestinal obstruction, respiratory depression, and behavioral abnormalities. Furthermore, the mother herself is subject to orthostatic hypotension, tachycardia, decreased gastrointestinal motility, and lower seizure thresholds (which increase the risk of eclampsia), all of which complicate the pregnancy.

It may seem that medication in such a situation would naturally be discontinued. The risk is that medication discontinuation may lead to the return of the psychosis, in which the mother herself may become a risk to the fetus—through, for example, her psychotic denial of her pregnancy and/or her failure to care properly for herself and her developing baby. The decision to continue or discontinue medication is, practically speaking, complex and demands detailed knowledge of the patient's course of illness and the individual features of her psychosis that need to be resolved.

It is generally agreed that the period of highest risk to the fetus is 4–10 weeks after conception, during which time antipsychotic medications should be discontinued. When medications are used, the high-potency ones such as haloperidol are preferable to the low-potency ones, as the former are usually associated with fewer and less severe extrapyramidal symptoms.

More generally, psychosis can interfere seriously with a woman's obtaining appropriate pre- and perinatal care. In the most extreme instances, a woman with schizophrenia may deny altogether that she is pregnant (denial may occur in as many as 35% of psychotic pregnant women). A woman who denies her pregnancy will fail to institute the dietary and lifestyle changes necessary for optimal development of the fetus. Even in the absence of denial, the disorganization of thought and behavior that accompanies schizophrenia can compromise a woman's ability to care for both herself and the fetus.

MOTHERING

Pregnancy and motherhood under the best of conditions involve massive adjustments involving body image, dependence versus independence, nurturance of others, and concerns about the ability to care properly for another person. This is especially salient for those with schizophrenia, who already are uncertain about their ability to care for themselves, let alone someone else who is totally dependent. The reality of this concern is reflected in the fact that about 60% of schizophrenic mothers lose custody of (although not necessarily contact with) their offspring, with custody often assumed by other family members. As a caretaker, the schizophrenic mother is often unable to take the child's perspective; in extreme instances, there is little or no psychological boundary between the two. The mother will relate to the child as a function of her own desires, rather than to the child's needs. For example, if a mother is hungry, she might feed the baby. Clinicians need to be aware of how medications may affect caretaking. Since the antipsychotics often cause lethargy or drowsiness, medication should be taken in the evening only, rather than splitting the dose between morning and evening. Otherwise, the morning dose can lead to side effects that interfere with caretaking.

CONCLUSION

The differences between female and male schizophrenia patients are more than academic. Medication dosing as a function of hormonal status, sexuality, discontinuation of medication during pregnancy, and mothering are issues that must be addressed when treating the female schizophrenia patient. Despite growing sensitivity to such issues, an anecdote provides a fitting note on which to end. A neuroendocrinologist colleague of mine was recently asked what effect lithium has on estrogens. After reviewing the current literature (and finding only a few references to estrogen's effect on lithium), he concluded that very little was known about the effect of lithium on estrogens. When the questioner expressed surprise that such a fundamental fact was not known, the neuroendocrinologist replied that it was not at all surprising and reflected "a general lack of interest in the reproductive functions of psychiatric patients."

FURTHER READING

Goldstein, J., Faraone, S., Chen, W., Toomiczenko, G., & Tsuang, M. (1991). Gender differences in the familial transmission of schizophrenia. *British Journal of Psychiatry, 161*, 1185–1198. Empirical study that suggests familial transmission of schizophrenia plays a stronger role in women than men.

Lewine, R. R. J. (1988). Gender and schizophrenia. In M. Tsuang & J. Simpson (Eds.), *Handbook of schizophrenia: Vol. 3. Nosology, epidemiology and genetics* (pp. 379–398). Amsterdam: Elsevier. A review of sex differences in the epidemiology and clinical presentation of schizophrenia.

Mowbray, C. T., Oyserman, D., Zemencuk, J., & Ross, S. R. (1995). Motherhood for women with serious mental illness: Pregnancy, childbirth, and the postpartum. *American Journal of Orthopsychiatry, 65,* 21–38.
A review of the meaning of childbearing for, and the parenting problems experienced by, mothers with schizophrenia.

Stewart, D. E., & Robinson, G. E. (1993). Psychotropic drugs and electroconvulsive therapy during pregnancy and lactation. In D. E. Stewart & N. L. Stotland (Eds.), *Psychological aspects of women's health care: The interface between psychiatry and gynecology* (pp. 71–95). Washington, DC: American Psychiatric Press.
A review of the use of psychoactive medication and electroconvulsive therapy during pregnancy and lactation, including practical guidelines.

128

Chronic Fatigue Syndrome

Barbara G. Melamed

*T*he most significant controversy surrounding chronic fatigue syndrome (CFS) is whether it is a disease or a factitious complaint. It has been vehemently argued that CFS may be a return to neurasthenia (an older conceptualization of a psychoneurotic disorder largely experienced by middle-class white women). Case definitions have recently been refined to reflect that there are many subtypes of the syndrome. CFS is characterized by severe, disabling fatigue and a combination of symptoms, including self-reported impairments in concentration and short-term memory, sleep disturbances, and musculoskeletal pain. At present the diagnosis of CFS can be made only after alternate medical and psychiatric causes of chronic fatiguing illness have been excluded. No pathognomonic signs or diagnostic tests have been validated in scientific studies. No definitive treatments exist for CFS, but various symptom-focused treatments have been used to some benefit. Symptom-focused treatments include amitriptyline for sleep disturbances; fluoxetine for mood disorder; anti-inflammatory agents; muscle relaxants; mild, low-dose tranquilizers; cognitive-behavioral treatments; immunotherapy for augmentation of natural killer cells; and nutritional approaches.

PREVALENCE AND COURSE OF ILLNESS

The prevalence of CFS in the population that comes for treatment is less than 1%; however, community studies reveal a higher incidence of 12%. Patients with CFS average about 23 visits to their primary health care providers in the course of a single year. Women are three times as likely to receive this diagnosis as men. Gender-related differences are varied, with women showing more tender lymph nodes, fibromyalgia, and lower physical functioning; in contrast, men show more pharyngeal inflammation and a higher lifetime prevalence of alcohol misuse. Some persons affected by CFS improve with time, but most remain functionally impaired for years.

Current recommendations for diagnosing CFS include a complete physical examination; a mental status examination to screen for abnormalities in intellectual function, mood, memory, and personality; and laboratory screening tests to rule out other disorders. A National Institute of Mental Health study suggested that CFS patients could be grouped into four meaningful clusters, based on the following symptoms: (1) severe fatigue following an acute illness, appearing in an individual with no previous physical or psychological problems; (2) signs and symptoms of an acute infection; (3) severe and persistent headache and/or myalgia; and (4) an abrupt change in cognitive function or appearance of a new mood disorder.

THEORIES OF ETIOLOGY

Psychological Factors

Fatigue is a common symptom in many different syndromes and occurs in 24% of primary care patients. The psychological similarities of patients with CFS, fibromyalgia, and multiple chemical sensitivities are greater than their differences. The anxiety and depression that accompany CFS are more likely to be consequences than causes of the disorder.

Viral Pathogens

Prospective studies conducted in primary care patients, such as a 1995 study by Wessely and colleagues, revealed that the strongest predictor of postinfectious fatigue was fatigue assessed before and at the time of clinical infection. There have been some epidemic outbreaks of CFS associated with "sick building syndrome," hospital environments, and school settings; these have precipitated beliefs that environmental or infectious agents may play a role in precipitating this syndrome.

Immune and Central Nervous System Disorders

No consistent evidence has been found for either immune markers or dysregulation of the central nervous system in CFS, although several researchers are vigorously investigating the impairment of activation of the hypothalamic–pituitary–adrenal axis.

Muscle and Physiological Changes

A carefully conducted study by Edwards and colleagues compared morphological changes in patients with CFS or muscle pain to those in normal volunteers, and evaluated the changes by electron microscopy; no consistent correlation was found between symptoms and changes in chemistry or features of the muscle fibers. The CFS patients did report higher perceived exertion scores than did the volunteers.

Sleep and/or Cognitive Disturbances

It has been found that in patients with CFS but without depressive disorders, there are more cognitive impairments than in patients with concurrent depression. There seems to be a problem in information acquisition, especially in the auditory channel. Sleep dysfunction is commonly reported in fibromyalgia patients.

Interactions of Factors

It is possible that there may be special vulnerability factors in patients' personalities before a viral illness, but that the disorder is released by the viral illness. Abnormal illness behavior may be maintained by stigmatization, as well as by social reinforcement factors such as spouse support and disability incentives.

THERAPEUTIC STRATEGIES WITH EMPIRICAL VALIDITY

Cognitive Therapies

In a 1994 study, Friedberg and Krupp assigned CFS patients to one of three conditions cognitive-behavioral treatment for CFS, cognitive-behavioral treatment for primary depression, and a no-treatment control condition. The investigators found that there were no significant changes in stress-related symptoms or fatigue severity, although there was a subset of CFS patients with cognitive-related depressive symptomatology that tended to respond favorably.

Psychopharmacology

Studies have shown that various antidepressants have been found useful for patients with CFS or fibromyalgia, even at lower doses than those used in major depression. The more serotonergic treatments (e.g., clomipramine) seem more successful in alleviating pain than depression, whereas catecholaminergic agents (e.g., maprotiline, bupropion) seem particularly effective for depression.

Immunotherapy

High-dose intravenous immunoglobulin leads to improvement in depressive symptoms and immune markers. Researchers have found that immunological status and depression are not correlated at the onset, which suggests that depression may occur secondary to the illness.

Nutritional Approaches

Numerous studies show that adequate vitamins and minerals, especially folic acid and zinc, are critical for proper immune function. Teitelbaum also recommends various vitamin (A, B_6, B_{12}, C, and E), iron, and magnesium as supplements to a normally healthy diet.

Predictors of Recovery

Prolonged disability is predicted in patients who initially report more than eight medically unexplained physical symptoms (not overlapping with those for CFS), have a lifetime history of dysthymic disorder, have had chronic fatigue for more than 1½ years, have fewer than 16 years of formal education, and are older than 38 years of age. Patients diagnosed in primary care settings rather than hospital settings are more likely to recover. These patients are less likely to attribute their symptoms to wholly physical causes, including viruses, as opposed to social or psychological factors. Thus, identification and management of persistent fatigue in primary care may prevent the secondary disabilities seen in patients with CFS. Unfortunately, point prevalence is low, making it unlikely that many patients will be diagnosed, particularly if the diagnostician does not believe in the existence of this syndrome.

In a longitudinal study, Wilson and colleagues found that assignment of a primary psychiatric diagnosis at follow-up, and the strength of the belief at entry to the trials that a physical disease process explained all symptoms, predicted poor outcome. Age of onset, duration of illness, premorbid psychiatric diagnoses, and cell-mediated immune function did not predict outcome.

FUTURE DIRECTIONS

Given the nature of this syndrome, a comprehensive and integrated approach to the study of CFS, including psychological, physiological, and medical indices, needs to be developed and refined. Prospective studies should be undertaken in subgroups of patients with physical illnesses where the chance of developing CFS is high (e.g., mononucleosis or Lyme disease), or those with a history of psychiatric diagnoses (especially major depression, panic disorder, or substance abuse or dependence). The findings of studies employing genetic and imaging techniques can play a role in uncovering the etiology of this uncertain illness. Meanwhile, doctors should proceed in a manner that conveys concern, supports adaptive function, and avoids inadvertently reinforcing dysfunctional illness behavior and disability. At the present time, CFS should be thought of as an interaction of premorbid factors (psychological and immunological factors), environmental trigger factors (viral pathogens), and enhancing factors (emotional responses to illness).

FURTHER READING

Bates, D. W., Schmitt, W., Buchwald, D., Warfe, N. C., Lee, J., Thoyer, E., Kornish, R. J., & Komaroff, A. L. (1993). Prevalence of fatigue and chronic fatigue syndrome in primary care practice. *Annals of Internal Medicine, 153*, 2759–2765.
A point prevalence study of CFS meeting U.S., British, and Australian criteria. Point prevalence was very low, varying from 0.3 to 1.0%.

Buchwald, D., & Garrity, D. (1994). Comparison of patients with chronic fatigue syndrome, fibromyalgia and multiple chemical sensitivities. *Annals of Internal Medicine, 158*, 2759–2765.
Buchwald, D., Pearlman, T., Kith, P., & Schmaling, K. (1994). Gender differences in patients with chronic fatigue syndrome. *Journal of General Internal Medicine, 9*, 397–401.
A prospective study.

Clark, M. R., Katon, W., Russo, J., Kith, P., Sintay, M., & Buchwald, D. (1995). Chronic fatigue: Risk factors for symptom persistence in a 2½ year follow-up study. *American Journal of Medicine, 98*, 187–195.
A discriminant function using five variables correctly classified 78% who had recovered and 74% with persistent symptoms.

DeLuca, J., Johnson, S. K., & Natelson, B. H. (1993). Information processing efficiency in chronic fatigue syndrome and multiple sclerosis. *Archives of Neurology, 50*, 301–304.

Demitrack, M. A. (1991). Evidence for impaired activation of the hypothalamic–pituitary–adrenal axis in patients with CFS. *Journal of Clinical Endocrinology and Metabolism, 73*, 1224–1234.

Edwards, R. H., Gibson, H., Clague, J. E., & Helliwell, T. (1993). Muscle histopathology and physiology in chronic fatigue syndrome. *Ciba Foundation Symposium, 173*, 102–117.

Fukada, K., et al. (1994). Chronic fatigue syndrome: A comprehensive approach to its definition and study. *Annals of Internal Medicine.*

Friedberg, F., & Krupp, L. B. (1994). A comparison of cognitive behavioral treatment for chronic fatigue syndrome and primary depression. *Clinical Infectious Diseases, 18*(Suppl.), S105–S110.

Hickie, I., Lloyd, A., & Wakefield, D. (1992). Immunological and psychological dysfunction in patients receiving immunotherapy for chronic fatigue syndrome. *Australian and New Zealand Journal of Psychiatry, 26*, 249–256.
Double-blind, placebo-controlled prospective study showing that only patients receiving active immunotherapy demonstrated a consistent pattern of correlations between improvement in depressive symptoms and markers of cell-mediated immunity.

Levine, P. H., Jacobson, D., Pocinki, A. G., Cheney, P., Peterson, D., Connelly, R., Robinson, S. M., Ablashi, D. V., Salahuddin, S. Z., et al. (1992). Clinical, epidemiological, and virological studies in four clusters of chronic fatigue syndrome. *Annals of Internal Medicine, 152*, 1611–1616.

McDonald, E., David, A. S., Pelosi, A. J., & Mann, A. H. (1993). Chronic fatigue in primary care attenders. *Psychological Medicine, 23*, 987–998.

Pawlikowska, T., Chalder, T., Hirsch, S. R., Wallace, P., Wright, D. J., & Wessely, S. C. (1994). Population based study of fatigue and psychological distress. *British Medical Journal, 308*, 763–766.

Teitelbaum, J. (1995). *From fatigued to fantastic.* Annapolis, MD: Deva Press.

Wessely, S., Chalder, T., Hirsch, J. S., Pawlikowska, T., Wallace, P., & Wright, D. J. (1995). Postinfectious fatigue: Prospective cohort study in primary care. *Lancet, 345*, 1333–1338.

Wilson, A., Hickie, I., Lloyd, A., Hadzi-Pavlowic, D., Boughton, C., Dwyer, J., & Wakefield, D. (1994). Longitudinal study of outcome of chronic fatigue syndrome. *British Medical Journal, 308*, 756–759.
A longitudinal study of patients who were originally assessed at a university hospital referral center.

129

Chronic Pain

Linda LeResche

Are women more sensitive to pain than men are? Do women cope with pain better than men do? Are men or women more likely to experience chronic pain? Although these questions are related, the subtle distinctions among them are important and reflect the fact that gender may influence the experience of pain in a variety of ways. Examination of cultural stereotypes would suggest that women may be more sensitive to all sorts of physical sensations (including pain) than men, and may be more likely to seek care for pain from health care providers, but may tolerate and cope with pain more effectively than men do. To what extent are these stereotypes borne out by research? Because the investigation of gender and pain is a young and growing field, it does not yet provide clear and comprehensive data on these questions. However, it is apparent that while the existing scientific literature appears to provide support for some of the cultural stereotypes, it also offers evidence that contradicts many of these notions.

Animal research, reviewed in Bodnar's chapter in Section VII of this volume, indicates significant sex differences in the pain modulation systems of rodents. It is certainly reasonable to suppose that similar differences exist in humans. Human psychophysiological studies suggest that women are, on average, somewhat more sensitive to pain than men are. Whether the sources of these differences are biological or psychosocial remains unclear. In addition, the limited age and cultural distributions of the subjects in these studies, the artificiality of the stimuli used, and the conditions for reporting pain in some experiments raise doubts as to whether these studies are generalizable to clinical pain, and in particular whether they are relevant to chronic pain conditions.

The International Association for the Study of Pain defines pain as "an unpleasant sensory and emotional experience associated with actual or potential tissue damage or defined in terms of such damage." Thus, pain is essentially a subjective experience, accessible to researchers primarily through the self-report and nonverbal behavior of patients and research subjects. Pain is also widely acknowledged to be a multidimensional experience, with biological, psychological, and social components.

Based on these perspectives, Dworkin, Von Korff, and I have proposed a model of chronic pain that is useful for structuring both research investigations and clinical interventions in persons with pain. In the context of studying gender and pain, the model suggests that gender differences are possible at several levels:

1. Males and females may differ in the anatomical structures or physiological mechanisms involved in nociception (pain neurotransmission and pain neuro-modulation).
2. It may be that the perceptual apparatus or the perceptual styles of men and women are different.
3. Men and women may also differ in their cognitive and emotional experiences of pain and in their pain coping mechanisms.
4. Pain behaviors, including the propensity to report pain, may differ for the two sexes.
5. The social roles of men and women are different; these roles may present different risks for developing and maintaining pain, as well as different roles for persons in pain within the context of the family, the workplace, the social welfare system, and the health care delivery system.

These perspectives are useful not only in trying to understand the existing body of research on gender and pain, but also in formulating hypotheses to be investigated in future studies.

Chronic pain is variously defined as pain that lasts more than 3 (or, alternatively, more than 6) months; pain that persists past the time of healing; or pain that is associated with the emergence of "chronic pain behaviors," including significant activity limitation and excessive use of medications and health care services. Much of the research on chronic pain has been conducted in multidisciplinary pain centers with patients who are likely to meet this last definition and to experience significant life disruption because of pain. This chapter defines chronic pain much more broadly to include persons with the most common and persistent nonmalignant pain conditions, including back pain, headache, temporomandibular disorder (TMD) pain, joint pain, abdominal pain, and chest pain. Although some people experience only a single episode of these conditions and others experience pain on a daily basis, these pain problems typically run a chronic, recurrent course, with several episodes occurring over a period of years.

AGE, GENDER, AND THE PREVALENCE OF CHRONIC PAIN

Prevalence is the epidemiological statistic that measures the proportion of the population with a specific condition at a particular point in time. In investigating pain in the context of women's health, it is essential to examine the prevalence of pain across the life cycle, because factors influencing pain may vary with age and stage of life as well as with gender. Different clinical pain conditions show different prevalence patterns in the population across the life cycle, and these age patterns, coupled with gender differences, can provide important clues as to risk factors influencing the onset or maintenance of pain. It is informative to consider how the age and gender distributions of different pain conditions vary, and to compare these prevalence patterns to major biological, psychological, and social milestones in the lives of males and females (e.g., puberty, marriage, employment, child rearing, menopause, retirement).

Examples of common pain conditions for which age and gender prevalence patterns are clear are discussed below. Although a cross-cultural perspective on these issues would add greatly to our understanding of possible pain mechanisms, epidemiological data on pain at present come primarily from Western Europe and North America. It is also beyond the scope of this chapter to review the epidemiology of pain in children, although an understanding of which gender differences in pain are present in childhood and which emerge later in life could certainly help illuminate biological, psychological, and social influences on chronic pain.

Certain chronic pain conditions are, of course, confined to women, as they are based in anatomical structures or physiological processes found only in females. These pain conditions include pelvic inflammatory disease, menstrual pain, and premenstrual related pain symptoms outside the pelvic region (e.g., breast pain). According to Unruh's comprehensive review, 75% of all girls experience some menstrual pain by late adolescence; severity of pain is highest among women in late adolescence and the young adult years. The 1985 Nuprin Pain Report estimated 75 million work days were lost annually in the U.S. because of menstrual or premenstrual pain.

Other pain problems, such as neck pain, joint pain, and fibromyalgia (a condition involving muscle pain and palpation tenderness at multiple body sites), are more prevalent in women than in men throughout adulthood. For example, the male: female prevalence ratio for neck pain averages about 1:1.5. In addition, the prevalence of all these conditions increases with age in both sexes. This pattern suggests that these pain conditions are influenced not only by a higher level of pain sensitivity (or a greater willingness to report pain) in women throughout adulthood, but also by some other factor or factors that increase with age. These influences may be biological (e.g., degenerative changes), psychological (e.g., changes in coping strategies), and/or social (e.g., changes in rewards for the expression of pain). At present, there is little research to suggest which of these factors may be operating in such conditions.

Still other pain conditions exhibit a pattern of higher prevalence in women throughout the adult years (about 1.5–1.8 times the male rate), but prevalence slowly declines with age. One such condition is common tension-type headache; abdominal pain probably also fits this pattern. Since these pain conditions are thought to be significantly influenced by responses to stress, the age and gender pattern suggests that stressors common to young women should be investigated as possible risk factors for these conditions. Similarly, from a public health perspective, intervention research should be targeted at young women if the social and economic impacts of these very common pain conditions are to be reduced.

In contrast, some pain conditions that are more common in women than in men show a bell-shaped curve across the adult life span, peaking in the reproductive years. These conditions include migraine headache, with a ratio of about 3.5 women to every man, and TMD pain, which is roughly twice as prevalent in women as in men. It is interesting that both of these conditions are rather uncommon before puberty. This pattern would suggest that either hormonal or psychosocial factors tied to women's lifestyles would be good candidates for investigation as possible risk factors.

It is now apparent that female reproductive hormones can play a role in migraine headache, although the specific mechanism of action remains unclear. Because of the similar prevalence pattern for TMD pain, we investigated the possibility that hormones may increase the risk of developing musculoskeletal pain in the temporomandibular region. Our study examined postmenopausal hormone use among TMD cases and controls in a health maintenance organization. Results indicated that use of estrogen, but not progestins, significantly increases the odds of having TMD pain, and that the risk appears dose-related. This initial investigation needs to be followed up with further research. However, it provides a clear example of how examination of the prevalence patterns of pain can generate research hypotheses.

Whereas the age- and gender-specific prevalence patterns for the pain conditions just discussed are rather consistent, the patterns for other conditions, including chest pain and back pain, are less clear and vary from study to study. These pain conditions may be more strongly linked to occupational and cultural factors than to gender. Finally, of course, there are conditions that appear to be more common in men than in women at all ages (e.g., cluster headache).

Little research has examined the question of the differential impact of chronic pain on men and women. However, some studies have found that women are more likely to experience significant pain-related interference with life activities than men with comparable pain conditions are. More research is needed to confirm this finding, and, if it is verified, to identify those factors that place women at greater risk for pain-related disability.

MANAGEMENT OF CHRONIC PAIN

Because pain is a multidimensional phenomenon, strategies for pain management can be implemented at several levels, ranging from pharmacological interventions to interrupt nociceptive processes to cognitive-behavioral strategies aimed at modification of pain behaviors and maladaptive cognitions. As with other chronic conditions, active patient participation is an essential element for effective management of chronic pain. Undoubtedly, the vast majority of chronic pain episodes are handled through self-care. In a smaller percentage of episodes, patients present to primary care providers. Finally, a highly selected group of patients reach specialty centers or multidisciplinary pain clinics. As noted earlier, almost all research on management of chronic pain has focused on this last patient group.

In the 1970s, Fordyce introduced the application of operant conditioning principles to the management of chronic pain in multidisciplinary treatment centers. In addition to the medical, nursing, physical, and occupational therapy components of these programs, pain clinics today overwhelmingly employ cognitive-behavioral approaches that continue to include operant therapies as a significant component. Recent clinical trials indicate that behavioral interventions are generally superior to usual (medical) treatment controls in improving pain, decreasing chronic pain behaviors and disability, and increasing activity levels among patients in multidisciplinary pain programs. A major research question currently under investigation is whether less intensive interventions based on cognitive-behavioral principles can be effective for the management of pain in primary care settings and for enhancing self-care for chronic pain.

CONCLUSIONS

A review of the epidemiological research on chronic pain indicates higher prevalence rates in women than in men for a number of pain conditions, including migraine and tension-type headache, TMD pain, abdominal pain, neck pain, and fibromyalgia. However, because the age-specific patterns for these conditions differ, the observed female predominance is not likely to be attributable to a single, simple mechanism. Anatomical, physiological, perceptual, cognitive, emotional, behavioral, and social factors can all influence the experience of pain; consequently, interventions for pain can be targeted at any of these factors. The most effective management approaches for disabling chronic pain at present employ cognitive-behavioral principles. Further research is needed to delineate specific risk factors for chronic pain associated with female gender, and to develop and evaluate effective primary care and self-care strategies for the most common chronic pain conditions.

FURTHER READING

Dworkin, S. F., Von Korff, M. R., & LeResche, L. (1992). Epidemiologic studies of chronic pain: A dynamic–ecologic perspective. *Annals of Behavioral Medicine, 14,* 3–11.
Presents a theoretical model for the study of chronic pain, suggesting that chronic pain results from the interaction over time of nociception, pain perception, pain appraisal, pain behavior, and social roles for chronic pain and illness.

Fillingim, R. B., & Maixner, W. (1995). Gender differences in response to noxious stimuli. *Pain Forum, 4,* 209–221. (See also commentaries on this article in the same issue.)
Summarizes the literature on gender differences in response to experimental pain stimuli, and postulates a psychophysiological model to explain observed differences.

Fordyce, W. E. (1976). *Behavioral methods in chronic pain and illness.* St. Louis, MO: C.V. Mosby.
Classic monograph outlining the application of behavioral principles to the evaluation and treatment of chronic pain and illness.

Louis Harris and Associates. (1985). *The Nuprin pain report.* New York: Author.
Reports a survey of the U.S. population concerning the prevalence and severity of different kinds of pain, demographics of pain sufferers, impact of pain, ways people cope with pain, relationship between pain and stress and use of health care for pain.

Task Force of Taxonomy, International Association for the Study of Pain. (1994). *Classification of chronic pain* (2nd ed.; H. Merskey & N. Bogduk, Eds.) Seattle: IASP Press.
Provides descriptions of chronic pain syndromes and definitions of pain terms.

Turk, D. C., & Melzack, R. (Eds.). (1992). *Handbook of pain assessment.* New York: Guilford Press.
Provides and evaluates methods for assessing pain by means of clinical, behavioral, self-report, and psychophysiological approaches.

Turner, J., & Romano, J. (1990). Cognitive-behavioral therapy. In J. J. Bonica, C. R. Chapman, W. E. Fordyce, & J. D. Loeser (Eds.), *The management of pain in clinical practice* (2nd ed., pp. 1711–1721). Philadelphia: Lea & Febiger.
Reviews the principles of cognitive-behavioral therapy, the techniques employed, and their efficacy for a range of chronic pain conditions.

Unruh, A. M. (1996). Gender variations in clinical pain experience. *Pain, 65,* 123–167.
Comprehensive review of gender-specific prevalence of various pain conditions, as well as gender variations in use of health care for pain and the relationship of psychological factors to pain.

Von Korff, M., Dworkin, S. F., LeResche, L., & Kruger, A. (1988). An epidemiologic comparison of pain complaints. *Pain, 32,* 173–183.
Uses results of a survey of a large health maintenance organization population to compare the age- and gender-specific prevalence, intensity, temporal dimensions, psychological distress, treatment seeking, and activity limitation associated with five common chronic pain conditions.

130

Sleep and Sleep Disorders

Suzanne L. Woodward

We all understand the benefits of a good night's sleep. Approximately a third of our lives are spent sleeping. We organize our time for work and play, and even our society, in order to meet the demands of sleep. It is therefore not surprising that trouble sleeping for a few nights, weeks, months, or years can affect our health, our jobs, and almost every aspect of our lives. It has been estimated that 40 million U.S. residents suffer from chronic complaints of sleep and wakefulness, and that an additional 20–30 million experience intermittent sleep-related problems. Considering these figures, it is amazing how few people actually consult their physicians about problems during sleep, leaving many of these problems undiagnosed and therefore untreated.

BASIC FACTS

Sleep research has come a long way since 1935 when Loomis and colleagues described stages of sleep characterized by distinct electroencephalographic (EEG) patterns. There are two distinct kinds of sleep: non-rapid-eye-movement (non-REM) sleep, and rapid-eye-movement (REM) sleep. These phases of sleep are as different from each other as they are from waking, and can be measured by polysomnography. Non-REM sleep has four stages (Stages 1–4), which together constitute close to 80% of a night's sleep. Stage 1 is the transition between wakefulness and sleep. A mixed voltage pattern replaces the rhythmic alpha activity seen when eyes are closed, and people feel drowsy. Reaction to outside stimuli is decreased, and although mentation may occur, it is no longer based in reality. Although short dreams may develop, many people feel that they are still awake during Stage 1 sleep.

Stage 2 sleep is considered to be the first true stage of sleep and consists of a moderately low-voltage background EEG with sleep spindles and K complexes. Heart rate and respiration are slower and more regular than in Stage 1, and thoughts are short and fragmented.

793

Slow-wave sleep consists of Stages 3 and 4, and is distinguished by the presence of slow delta waves (as the name indicates). Heart and respiration rates are very slow and regular during this deeper stage of sleep.

About 70–100 minutes after sleep onset, the REM sleep period begins. The EEG pattern is similar to that of Stage 1 sleep, except that sawtooth waves are often seen. Rapid eye movements occur in REM sleep (as the term suggests) and there is an active inhibition of muscle activity. Most people report vivid dreaming during REM sleep, and heart and respiration rates are increased and irregular. REM sleep alternates with non-REM sleep at about 90–100 minute intervals in adults. A typical sleep cycle consists of a sequential merging of Stages 1 through 4, which then reverses and is followed by the first REM period. A normal sleep pattern consists of three to five such cycles. As the night goes on, the amounts of Stages 3 and 4 decrease, and the proportion of REM sleep tends to increase.

SLEEP DISORDERS

The American Sleep Disorders Association has published a diagnostic classification of sleep and arousal disorders, including: disorders of initiating and maintaining sleep (insomnia), disorders of excessive daytime sleepiness (hypersomnia), and behavior disorders occurring during sleep (parasomnias). Clinical polysomnography is used to confirm and diagnose these clinical sleep syndromes.

Insomnia

Insomnia—difficulty in either falling asleep or staying asleep—is the most common sleep-related complaint encountered in the general population. Generally women, the elderly, and shift workers report higher rates of difficulty with sleep. In addition, depression, chronic medical illness, recent life stress, and alcohol use all contribute to an increased incidence of insomnia.

This interplay of factors results in the perception that sleep is inadequate or abnormal. During the night these symptoms include difficulty initiating sleep, frequent awakenings during the night, a short sleep time, and nonrestorative sleep. Daytime symptoms of disturbed sleep (such as fatigue, daytime sleepiness, memory problems, anxiety, or even depression) also need to be considered in order to determine whether poor sleep is actually causing disturbed daytime functioning, or whether a psychological disorder such as depression is primary and the sleep disturbance is secondary.

A good initial step in evaluating someone with insomnia is consideration of the duration of the complaint. Both transient and short-term insomnia last less than 3 weeks and are usually situational; that is, they are related to an emotional problem, excitement, a schedule change such as jet lag, or a shift work change. Chronic insomnia lasts for more than 3 weeks and begins with a clear precipitating event, but as the person deals with the resulting poor sleep, a maladaptive response to sleep disruption or inappropriate sleep habits may develop and maintain the insomnia even after the precipitating factor has disappeared. When chronic insomnia develops as a result of perpetuating factors or somatized tension, it is best treated with behavioral techniques. The use of sleep logs, the practice of good sleep hygiene (e.g., reducing caffeine use; reserving the bedroom for sleep, not work; and avoiding clock watching), and a review of medication use are beneficial.

Stimulus control therapy was designed to promote the association of the bedroom with sleep rather than with frustration, anxiety, or wakefulness. Patients are told to go to bed only when sleepy; to reserve the bed only for sleeping and sex; and, if unable to sleep, to get out of bed and do something relaxing until they feel sleepy again. Frequent contact with the therapist is necessary to encourage patients through the initial stages until proper associations are developed.

Sleep restriction therapy involves asking insomniacs to spend the same amount of time in bed as they report actually sleeping, but never less than 4 hours. The therapist computes each patient's moving average over 5 days from reports left on an answering machine of daily sleep time. When the average sleep efficiency reaches at least 85%, time in bed is increased by 30-minute increments. Although this technique involves initial sleep deprivation, the improvement in sleep quality can be significant.

In addition to the above behavioral treatment regimes, training in relaxation has also been shown to help with insomnia. These have been detailed nicely by Hauri and Linde in an excellent book, *No More Sleepless Nights*. Regardless of the type of therapy, relaxation therapy—progressive muscle relaxation, meditation, self-hypnosis, or electromyographic biofeedback—the technique must be overlearned, preferably in the daytime to avoid performance anxiety.

A common cause of insomnia, particularly in the elderly, is nocturnal myoclonus (periodic limb movements in sleep). Patients are often unaware of this disorder, which consists of repetitive muscle contractions, usually of the lower leg. These movements occur in rhythmic series throughout the sleep period and can result in arousals and complaints of disturbed or unrefreshing sleep.

Unlike insomnia, which has many causes, a complaint of hypersomnia—excessive daytime sleepiness—is usually caused by either narcolepsy or excessive obstructive sleep apnea.

Narcolepsy

Since the etiology of narcolepsy is not clear, treatment is directed at the relief of symptoms. The primary symptom of narcolepsy is excessive daytime sleepiness. In addition to sleepiness, auxiliary symptoms include cataplexy, hypnogogic hallucinations, and sleep paralysis. These auxiliary symptoms are considered to be manifestations of REM sleep intruding into wakefulness and contribute to the diagnosis. Cataplexy is a sudden loss of muscle tone, usually triggered by an emotional event. A hypnogogic hallucination is a vivid dream-like image occurring at sleep onset. Sleep paralysis is a total paralysis of voluntary muscles when falling asleep or waking up. Short naps taken during the day and stimulant medication can help relieve symptoms and allow a more normal lifestyle.

Obstructive Sleep Apnea

Obstructive sleep apnea is the other common cause of daytime sleepiness, and can be life-threatening. In sleep apnea, an obstruction of the airway occurs during sleep and is terminated by an arousal from sleep. Apneas and the accompanied arousals can occur numerous times during sleep, leading to the complaint of daytime sleepiness. Sleep apnea syndrome is also associated with increased risk of automobile accidents and with increased cardiovascular morbidity and mortality. The typical apnea sufferer is an obese, middle-aged male who snores. Apnea is much less common in women than in men until after the age of menopause. Naps are usually nonrestorative, and patients often complain of morning headaches, memory problems, and morning irritability. A clinical polysomnogram is helpful in assessing the frequency and severity of obstructive sleep apnea and in determining treatment protocols, which can range from weight loss to tracheostomy.

Parasomnias

Behaviors or movements that occur during sleep or are exacerbated by sleep are called parasomnias. It is estimated that 5% of the general population suffers from some clinically significant parasomnia. Among the most common parasomnias are sleepwalking, night terrors, and REM sleep behavior disorder.

Sleepwalking is more common in children than in adults, and usually occurs in the first third of the night during slow-wave sleep. Episodes last 15 seconds to 30 minutes, and recall is sketchy the next day. Frequent sleepwalking in adults is more serious than in children, since it is more often associated with dangerous activity. Night terrors, also called pavor nocturnus, are characterized by an arousal from slow-wave sleep. Like sleepwalking, night terrors are more common in children than in adults. A night terror consists of an arousal along with agitation, sweating, and tachycardia. The patient looks terrified, often emits piercing screams, and is usually inconsolable. Night terrors can be differentiated from nightmares by the time of night and stage of sleep during which they occur. Recall of a nightmare during REM sleep is often vivid and detailed, whereas night terrors are rarely associated with morning awareness of the event. Occasionally, adults may experience both night terrors and nightmares, usually in response to stress. REM sleep behavior disorder occurs during REM sleep and is complex, often dangerous behavior sometimes associated with dream-like thoughts and images. Patients who complain of disturbed sleep, injuries to themselves or bed partners, or vivid, unpleasant dreams should be evaluated. REM sleep behavior disorder usually occurs in the middle-aged or elderly, and a systematic evaluation needs to be conducted to eliminate seizure activity and verify REM sleep muscle activity. In most people, REM sleep is accompanied by limited muscle movement, but in this disorder muscle tone is preserved during some or all of REM sleep.

The fact that diagnosis of sleep disorders is often difficult reflects the numerous causes of poor sleep. However, research in this field of sleep medicine is expanding every day.

SLEEP AND WOMEN

Sleep complaints increase with age and are twice as prevalent among women of all ages than men. Most of what we know about sleep is based on studies with male subjects. In fact, about 75% of all sleep research has been conducted with men. Recently, more researchers have been taking gender into consideration; these studies provide a better look at sleep and sleep disorders in women.

Hormones may set women up for special problems during sleep. Women of childbearing age report more difficulty with sleep during certain phases of the menstrual cycle. There is some evidence suggesting that the regular fluctuations of gonadal hormone levels during the menstrual cycle may be related to recurrent insomnia, particularly in women who experience mood and other physical symptoms characteristic of the premenstrual syndrome. In addition, the elevated body temperature in the postovulary phase of the menstrual cycle may disrupt sleep stages and structure, as measured by REM sleep latency. However, a clear relationship between sleep disturbance and the menstrual cycle has not been established. It is possible that mood may affect sleep as much as or more than the menstrual cycle does.

Mood disorders occur in both men and women, but the incidence is higher in women. Depression is not the everyday "blues" that we all experience on occasion, but a persistent disturbance of mood that has a strong impact on daily functioning. Sleep disturbances, such as difficulty falling asleep, trouble maintaining sleep, and early-morning awakenings, are associated with major depressive disorder and in some cases may occur prior to an actual depressive episode. Research into the link between changes in sleep and depression indicates that treatment of sleep disturbances may help improve the course and management of depression.

Seasonal affective disorder is a disorder of mood that occurs during the winter months and is also diagnosed more frequently in women than in men. Seasonal affective disorder is thought to affect sleep–wake rhythms; symptoms include diminished energy and oversleeping. Bright-light treatment either at night or in the morning is believed to be helpful in reducing symptoms, but more studies are needed in order to determine the mechanism behind the antidepressant effect of bright-light treatment.

Reports of daytime fatigue and poor sleep during pregnancy are not new. What is new is that researchers are encouraging physicians to take sleep complaints during pregnancy more seriously. The high levels of progesterone during pregnancy may contribute to the feelings of tiredness that women may experience during pregnancy. Progesterone has also been shown to increase body temperature and to speed breathing, as well as to act on the smooth muscle of the urinary tract to cause frequent urination, which is potentially disruptive to sleep. Sleep disruption can begin as early as the third month of pregnancy and can persist at least 8 months into the postpartum period. The need for attention to pregnancy-related sleep disruption is emphasized by the fact that the mood alterations often accompanying complaints of poor sleep both during and after pregnancy may constitute a risk factor for postpartum depression.

Unfortunately, problems with sleep do not cease when menopause arrives. Complaints of disturbed sleep, daytime fatigue, and mood lability increase during the climacteric—the transition phase in women from the reproductive stage of life to the nonreproductive stage of life, which includes menopause. Hot flashes are the most common symptom of the climacteric and are experienced by the majority of women. Hot flashes consist of intense feelings of heat, sweating, and (in some women) rapid heart rate and feelings of suffocation. They can occur frequently during both the day and night; those that occur during sleep almost always cause awakening. When nighttime hot flashes are particularly severe, they are called "night sweats" and may necessitate a change of nightclothes and bed linen. Even when hot flashes are relatively mild or do not occur at all, menopausal women still exhibit some signs of sleep disruption. On average, a menopausal woman's sleep is disrupted by brief arousals every 8 minutes if she is experiencing hot flashes and every 18 minutes if she is not. In addition to arousals from sleep, the thermoregulatory effects of hot flashes have the potential to alter sleep stage by increasing slow-wave sleep. Hot flashes and associated sleep disruption can continue for 5 years or more if untreated, so it is not surprising that complaints of insomnia are increased during the menopausal period.

The treatment most usually suggested for menopausal symptoms is hormone replacement therapy (HRT). HRT, either estrogen alone or a combination of estrogen and progesterone, is effective in alleviating hot flashes as well as other menopausal symptoms. However, HRT is often contraindicated, leaving some women with little relief of symptoms that may disturb sleep. Following the basic sleep hygiene, suggestions described earlier in this chapter may help prevent the insomnia caused by menopausal symptoms from progressing to chronic insomnia that continues even when symptoms abate. Sleeping in a room with a thermoneutral temperature or even a slightly cool temperature may help. Cotton nightclothes and control of one side of the electric blanket may help as well.

As women age, their susceptibility to respiratory disturbance during sleep begins to increase. In fact, severe apnea, which (as noted earlier) consists of frequent brief episodes of breathing cessation during sleep, has been found to increase the mortality rate among women in nursing homes. There is a strong prevalence of sleep-related respiratory disturbance in men throughout life. In women, the incidence of disordered breathing during sleep is very low before the age of 50, but increases dramatically following menopause. The estimated prevalence of sleep-related breathing disturbance in middle-aged women is reported to be 9%, much higher than previously expected among women. Suspicion of apnea or even heavy snoring should be evaluated.

Any sleep disturbances severe enough to affect the quality of a woman's life deserve attention. A good night's sleep is something every woman needs and deserves.

FURTHER READING

Ford, D. E., & Komerow, D. B. (1989). Epidemiologic study of sleep disturbances and psychiatric disorders: An opportunity for prevention? *Journal of the American Medical Association, 262,* 1479–1484.
The overlooked danger of sleep-related breathing syndromes in older women.

Hauri, P., & Linde, S. (1991). *No more sleepless nights.* New York: Wiley.
An excellent book on diagnosis and treatment of sleep problems; relevant to both patients and primary care professionals.

Lee, K. A., & DeJoseph, J. F. (1992). Sleep disturbances, vitality, and fatigue among a select group of employed childbearing women. *Birth, 19,* 208–213.
How working women cope with sleep problems during pregnancy.

Lee, K. A., Shaver, J. R., Giblin, E. C., & Woods, N. F. (1990). Sleep patterns related to menstrual cycle phase and premenstrual affective disorders. *Sleep, 3,* 403–409.
A good insight into menstrual-related sleep problems.

Loomis, A. L., Harvey, E. N., & Hobart, G. (1935). Further observations on the potential rhythms of the cerebral cortex during sleep. *Science, 82,* 198–200.
A background article on the initial scientific discoveries related to sleep.

National Commission on Sleep Disorders Research. (1994). *Wake up, America: A national sleep alert* (Vol. 2). Washington, DC: Author.
Comprehensive classification of sleep disorders, and implications for future health policy and research.

Woodward, S., & Freedman, R. R. (1994). The thermoregulatory effects of menopausal hot flashes on sleep. *Sleep, 17,* 497–450.
A good review of the relationship between menopausal symptoms and sleep complaints.

131

Psychoneuroimmunology

Julienne E. Bower

*P*sychoneuroimmunology (PNI) is the study of interactions between psychological states, the brain, and the immune system. This field of research developed from studies indicating that the immune system, once thought to be relatively autonomous, is linked to the central nervous system and can be altered by certain psychological states and traits. The primary psychological factors that have been examined in human PNI resesarch include stress, mood, and social support. At this point there is compelling evidence that both acute and chronic stressors, and both major and more commonplace life events, are associated with changes in the human immune system. In addition, mood states, particularly depression, and the presence and quality of social relationships have been linked to alterations in immune status.

Of course, individuals may cope with stressful events in a number of different ways. For example, they may express their emotions about the event, seek help with the problem, and/or try to deny the reality of the experience. In addition, individuals may have different perceptions of the event and its meaning for their lives. Although these coping and appraisal processes are known to affect psychological adjustment following a stressful experience, PNI researchers have only recently begun to consider how these processes affect the immune system's response to stress. The influence of coping and appraisal on the stressor–immunity relationship is particularly important to understand because these processes have the potential to be modified. Although stressors can never be eliminated from life, people can learn different ways to view and respond to them which may have beneficial effects on the immune system and, potentially, on physical health. This chapter reviews human studies that have provided some insights into the association between coping and appraisal processes and immunity, with an emphasis on those studies that have included female subjects and have utilized experimental or longitudinal designs.

THE IMMUNE SYSTEM

The purpose of the immune system is to defend the body against disease-causing microorganisms and tumors. (See Claman's and Laudenslager's chapters in Section VII of this volume for further descriptions of this system and its functioning.) The immune system is made up of three types of immune cells, lymphocytes, phagocytes, and auxiliary cells, each of which plays a particular role in the immune response. Lymphocytes include natural killer (NK) cells, B cells, and T cells, which are further differentiated into T helper (CD4) and T cytotoxic (CD8) cells. NK cells destroy virally infected cells and certain types of tumors, while B cells and T cells attack bacteria, viruses, parasites, and fungi. Phagocytes include monocytes, neutrophils, and eosinophils, which are involved in the phagocytosis or destruction of invading microorganisms.

Both the number and the activity of immune cells are assessed in PNI research. Common enumerative assays include counting the number of different types of immune cells in the peripheral blood and measuring the amounts of substances produced by immune cells, such as antibodies. Common functional assays include measuring the ability of lymphocytes to divide or proliferate in response to foreign substances, called antigens, and the ability of NK cells to kill tumor cells. An increase in the number or activity of most immune parameters is interpreted as a positive change or enhancement of immune function.

Although these measures are presumed to reflect the functional capacity of the immune system, their actual relevance for physical health has not been determined in most cases. The changes in these immune parameters found in PNI research are usually quite small and fall within the normal range, and the health consequences of these types of small changes in healthy populations have rarely been investigated. Thus, any link between these immune changes and disease vulnerability is, in most cases, hypothetical. The best evidence for a link between immune changes and physical health comes from studies that examine immune parameters known to be relevant for a particular disease, such as studies that examine immunological markers of HIV progression (e.g., CD4 T cell decline) among HIV-positive individuals.

COPING

"Coping" can be defined broadly as any emotional, cognitive, or behavioral response to stress that is directed toward resolving the stressful situation and/or regulating one's emotional response to it. PNI research has primarily focused on coping strategies that involve emotion regulation, although a few studies have examined other types of coping.

Emotion Regulation

The way in which one regulates one's emotions is thought to be important for both psychological and physical health. In particular, "repression" or failure to express negative emotions has been associated with the onset and progression of cancer, although this is a controversial area. These findings have stimulated interest in the association between emotion regulation and immune function, as some investigators have hypothesized that any negative health effects of repression may be mediated by the immune system.

There is evidence to suggest that the inhibition of emotional experience or expression has a negative impact on immunocompetence. In studies examining the association between personality styles and immune status, a repressive style has been associated with decreased monocyte counts and elevated antibody titres to the Epstein–Barr virus (EBV). (Unlike most immune measures, higher levels of antibody to EBV and other latent viruses are interpreted as a poorer immune response, because they suggest that the immune system has less control over viral replication.) Similarly, an experimental study found that individuals who did not disclose emotional material on a laboratory task had elevated antibody titres to EBV. These findings suggest that individuals who deny or minimize negative emotions, or who inhibit the expression of these emotions, show suppression of certain immune parameters.

If inhibiting one's emotions is associated with immune suppression, what effect does expressing one's emotions have on the immune system? Experimental mood induction studies have found that short-term expression of negative and positive emotions is associated with changes in certain immune parameters, providing evidence for a link between emotional expression and immunity. Another series of studies has examined the immune effects of emotional expression about traumatic events, or emotional disclosure. In this paradigm, subjects are asked to write or talk about their thoughts and feelings about a traumatic past experience once a day for several consecutive days. Compared to subjects who are asked to write about trivial topics, subjects who write about traumatic events show increased lymphocyte proliferation, decreased antibody titres to EBV (indicating greater immunological control), and increased antibody response to a hepatitis B vaccine (indicating greater immunological protection). These findings are consistent with research on social support and immunity, which indicates that marital disruption and loneliness are associated with immune suppression. To the extent that supportive relationships provide a forum for emotional disclosure, these findings suggest that the lack of an outlet for this type of expression has a negative impact on immune function.

It has been hypothesized that the positive immunological effects of emotional disclosure are related to the increased understanding and acceptance that often result from this process. The idea that the cognitive outcome of a stressful event, such as understanding or meaning, may be associated with immune changes was supported in a study of HIV-positive men who had recently lost a close friend or partner to AIDS. Men who were able to find some positive meaning from the bereavement experience showed less rapid decline of CD4 T cells in the 2–3 years following the loss, indicating slower disease progression over that period than men who did not find meaning. In addition, men who found meaning showed lower rates of AIDS-related mortality over an extended follow-up period.

Overall, the research on emotion regulation and immunity supports the hypothesis that inhibition of emotional experience or expression is associated with immune suppression, whereas emotional expression, at least about traumatic events, is associated with immune enhancement. The health consequences of these changes in healthy individuals have not been determined, although one study that assessed physical health outcomes found that emotional disclosure was associated with fewer health center visits. The immune effects of emotion regulation were consistent for men and women in those studies that included both sexes and reported gender effects.

Other Coping Strategies

Only a few other coping strategies have been assessed in PNI research. "Active coping," including planning, seeking instrumental and emotional support, and positive reinterpretation, was associated with increases in NK cell activity among HIV-positive gay men in one study. Another study conducted with HIV-positive men found that "denial coping," or attempting to deny the reality of a stressful event, was associated with decreases in number of CD4 T cells and in lymphocyte proliferation after 1 year. From these limited findings, it appears that active coping may be associated with enhancement of certain immune parameters among HIV-positive gay men, whereas denial coping may lead to suppression of certain immune parameters among this group.

APPRAISAL

"Appraisal" can be defined as the process of evaluating the significance of an event for one's well-being. This may include an evaluation of one's ability to control and cope with the event, and of the meaning of the event for one's self-esteem, goals, and future. Several types of appraisal processes have been examined in PNI studies, although there is still very little research in this area.

Appraisals of stressor controllability, or how controllable one perceives a stressor to be, have been associated with immune status in two experimental studies. The results of these studies suggest that subjects who perceive that they have little or no control over an acute stressor show declines in certain immune parameters, compared to subjects who perceive that they do have control. Self-appraisals have also been associated with immune changes in an experimental study in which subjects exposed to more negative self-evaluations showed decreased NK cell activity.

Appraisals of the future have also been linked to changes in immune status. A recent longitudinal study examined the association between one type of future appraisal, expectancies about future health, and immune changes among HIV-positive gay men. Men with more negative expectancies about their future health who had also been bereaved in the last year showed immunological evidence of more rapid disease progression, including more rapid loss of CD4 T cells, a greater decrease in lymphocyte proliferation, and a greater increase in several markers of immune activation (associated with more rapid destruction of CD4 T cells). In two companion studies, negative expectancies about future health were associated with decreased survival time among gay men with AIDS and with increased symptoms of HIV infection among previously asymptomatic HIV-positive men.

Overall, there appears to be some evidence for an association between specific types of appraisal and immune outcomes. In particular, negative appraisals of oneself, of a stressor's controllability, and of one's future health have been associated with decreases in certain immune parameters. There is some evidence that negative appraisals of future health or "fatalism" may also be associated with disease progression, at least among HIV-positive gay men. Because the majority of studies in this area were conducted with men, the generalizability of these findings to women is unclear.

PSYCHOSOCIAL INTERVENTIONS

If how one copes with and appraises a stressful event are associated with changes in immune status, interventions that attempt to change coping and appraisal processes may also have immune effects. Interest in the association between psychosocial interventions and immunity was sparked by a landmark study conducted by Spiegel and his colleagues, in which breast cancer patients who participated in group therapy for 1 year lived significantly longer than patients in the control group.

Several studies have investigated the association between participation in cognitive-behavioral interventions and immune status. These interventions have typically included health education, enhancement of illness-related problem-solving skills, and psychological support. Cognitive-behavioral group therapy was associated with positive changes in a number of immune parameters among recently diagnosed cancer patients (increases in number and activity of NK cells) and HIV-positive gay men who were notified of their serostatus during the intervention (increases in CD4 T cells, increases in NK cells, and decreases in antibody titre to two latent viruses). However, no immune changes were found in a study conducted with HIV-positive men in which the intervention was conducted some time after serostatus notification.

Relaxation interventions have also been linked to changes in immune status. Older adults showed increases in NK cell activity and decreases in antibody titres to the latent herpes simplex virus (indicating greater immunological control) following participation in a relaxation intervention. Medical students have also shown immune benefits following participation in relaxation interventions, specifically increases in CD4 T cells and increases in lymphocyte proliferation, although these changes were associated with the frequency of relaxation practice rather than with the intervention itself in one report.

Overall, the results of these studies suggest that certain psychosocial interventions may have a positive effect on immune status. This effect, however, is not uniform and may depend on the timing of the intervention (e.g., before or soon after diagnosis with a serious illness) as well as on the degree of involvement in the treatment (e.g., frequent practice of treatment skills). Whether treatment-related immune changes are associated with improvements in disease onset, progression, or survival is still unclear, although one follow-up study conducted with cancer patients did find that participation in cognitive-behavioral group therapy was associated with better survival rates 6 years later. It has been suggested that participation in psychosocial interventions may be most beneficial for individuals who are already immune impaired, as the relatively small immune changes seen following treatment are unlikely to have health consequences in a healthy population. In those studies that included both men and women, no gender differences were reported, suggesting that any immune benefits of treatment extend to both men and women.

GENDER DIFFERENCES IN IMMUNITY AND IMMUNE RESPONSES TO STRESS

There is consistent evidence to suggest that women and men differ in their baseline levels of immune function. Women appear to be more immunologically reactive than men, as indicated by higher antibody levels, higher primary and secondary responses to a number of antigens, higher rates of graft rejection, and higher rates of autoimmune diseases. These differences may be attributable to differences in sex hormones, which have been linked to the immune system in both animals and humans. Immune cells have been shown to bear receptors for sex hormones, and changes in these hormones caused by gonadectomy, sex hormone replacement therapy, or pregnancy have been associated with changes in immune status.

Given gender differences in immunity, it might be expected that men and women would differ in their immune responses to stress. However, the few PNI studies conducted with all-female samples have found stress-related immune changes similar to those reported in studies including both women and men. For example, both bereavement and unemployment were associated with immune suppression in studies conducted with women only, consistent with the literature on chronic stress and immunity. Acute stress has also been associated with similar immune changes among both women and men. One study did find that women were more likely to show negative immunological changes in response to hostile or negative marital interactions than men, indicating that the extent of the immune system's response to certain types of stress may vary by gender, even though the direction of the effect is the same. In terms of gender differences in the association between coping and appraisal processes and immune function, none of the studies described earlier reported any differences between women and men. Many of these studies were conducted in all-male samples, however, limiting the generalizability of the results to women.

CONCLUSION

It is important to recognize that the small size of this literature and the diversity of measures and methodologies used limit the conclusions that can be drawn at this time. In particular, the findings of the nonexperimental studies included here should be interpreted with caution, as these studies often do not control for behaviors known to affect immune function nor do they allow determinations about the directionality or causality of the relationships found. Despite these qualifications, the evidence reviewed in this chapter suggests that how one perceives and copes with stress may indeed have an impact on the immune system. The interactions between coping, appraisal, and immunity require more consideration in future research, as they may guide the development of interventions to improve both psychological and immunological adjustment to stressful life events.

FURTHER READING

Ader, R., Felten, D. L., & Cohen, N. (Eds.). (1991). *Psychoneuroimmunology* (2nd ed.). New York: Academic Press.
Very detailed and comprehensive review of recent research in PNI, including a chapter on sex hormones and immune function.

Baum, A., & Grunberg, N. E. (1991). Gender, stress, and health. *Health Psychology, 10,* 80–85.
Review article highlighting important issues in gender and health, including gender differences in immune function.

Fawzy, R. E., Kemeny, M. E., Fawzy, N. W., Elashoff, R., Morton, D., Cousins, N., & Fahey, J. L. (1990). A structured psychiatric intervention for cancer patients: Changes over time in immunological measures. *Archives of General Psychiatry, 47,* 729–735.
Intervention study demonstrating association between participation in cognitive-behavioral group therapy and changes in mood, coping, and immunity among cancer patients. Follow-up study found that patients who participated in group therapy lived significantly longer than patients in the control group.

Glaser, R., & Kiecolt-Glaser, J. K. (Eds.). (1994). *Handbook of human stress and immunity.* New York: Academic Press.
Thorough review of the literature on stress and immune function in humans.

Goleman, D., & Gurin, J. (Eds.). (1993). *Mind/body medicine: How to use your mind for better health*. New York: Consumer Reports Books.
Excellent overview of PNI and other research on psychology and health; appropriate for all readers.

Maier, S. F., Watkins, L. R., & Fleshner, M. (1994). Psychoneuroimmunology: The interface between behavior, brain, and immunity. *American Psychologist, 49*, 1004–1017.
Review article, written for psychologists, providing a broad overview of research in PNI.

Pennebaker, J. W., Kiecolt-Glaser, J. K., & Glaser, R. (1988). Disclosure of traumas and immune function: Health implications for psychotherapy. *Journal of Consulting and Clinical Psychology, 56*, 239–245.
One of the first studies to demonstrate an association between emotional disclosure and immune function.

Sieber, W. J., Rodin, J., Larson, L., Ortega, S., & Cummings, N. (1992). Modulation of human natural killer cell activity by exposure to uncontrollable stress. *Brain, Behavior, and Immunity, 6*, 141–156.
Interesting experimental study showing an association between appraisals of control and immune function.

Spiegel, D., Bloom, J. R., Kraemer, H. C., & Gottheil, E. (1989). Effect of psychosocial treatment on survival of patients with metastatic breast cancer. *Lancet, ii*, 888–891.
Landmark study that found that breast cancer patients who participated in weekly supportive group therapy lived significantly longer than patients in the control group.

132

Stress-Related Disorders

Thomas G. Pickering

Most of the research into the consequences of chronic environmental stress for human disease has been conducted with men, but there is increasing interest in how these influences affect women. A popular but almost certainly mythical view is that one reason men are at higher risk of heart disease than women is that they go out into the world and face the slings and arrows of outrageous fortune, while women enjoy the protected environment of the home. The past half-century has witnessed an enormous change in all Westernized societies, as women have entered the work force, without at the same time giving up their traditional child-rearing roles. The lower mortality that women enjoy from coronary heart disease—a condition that is usually considered one of the outcomes of chronic stress by the public, if not by physicians—does not appear to have been adversely affected by their entry into the work force in the 1970s and 1980s. Nevertheless, many women seem to be unaware of the fact that cardiovascular disease is the leading cause of death and accounts for many more deaths than cancer. Furthermore, the dramatic decline in the death rate seen in men over the past 20 years has not been paralleled in women. The two major sources of stress for most people are their work and/or their home lives; these are considered separately below. Other factors considered briefly are bereavement, social support, and socioeconomic status.

OCCUPATIONAL STRESS

Although women now constitute about 45% of the employed population, there is a remarkable persistence of segregation of the sexes in different occupations. Only 11% of women were in managerial and professional specialties, according to a 1987 report; moreover, 98% of secretaries are women, as compared to 3% of operators, fabricators, and laborers. This type of segregation by gender is found even in Sweden, which is certainly one of the most advanced countries in terms of equalization of opportunities for men and women. Even there, women have fewer jobs to choose from, and have less control over their work than men. One of the few studies with prospective data on the effects of work on women's health is the Framingham Heart Study, where it was found that although employed women complained of more daily stress and marital dissatisfaction than housewives, their incidence of coronary heart disease was the same. Possible exceptions to this are single working women with children, who may be at increased risk compared with other women. The group at highest risk appears to consist of women clerical workers with major domestic responsibilities and a restrictive psychosocial work environment.

This apparent absence of any long-term effects on cardiovascular health does not mean that there is no price to be paid for the transition from the home to the workplace. Studies done in Framingham in the 1970s and 1980s that compared housewives and employed women found more Type A behavior, more reports of daily stress, and more marital dissatisfaction in the employed women. The two most widely studied stress-related factors that could adversely affect cardiovascular health are the type A behavior pattern and hostility. However, virtually all of the research on the prognostic significance of these related factors has been done in men, and so far as can be estimated, they are probably of less pathogenic significance in women.

Another variable, which has been less extensively studied, is job strain. It differs in a fundamental way from hostility, in that it is focused more on the environment in which the individual is situated than on his or her personality. The model has two components: "decision latitude," or control, and "psychological workload," or demand. Several studies, nearly all of which have been conducted in men, have shown that people employed in high-strain jobs—defined as those that combine high demands and low control—are at increased risk of developing coronary heart disease. Again, however such data as exist suggest that the effect sizes are stronger in men than in women. In one of the largest surveys of Swedish data relating psychosocial variables to coronary heart disease, it was found that in men (particularly those in blue-collar jobs), the combination of high demands, low control, and low social support increased the risk of coronary heart disease by a factor of more than seven; in women, the trend was still present but not statistically significant. Job strain has been shown to be related to blood pressure in men, most consistently when the latter is measured by ambulatory monitoring. It appears that men in high-strain jobs have higher pressures not only while they are at work, but also while they are at home and during sleep. Our own work has so far found no relationship between job strain and blood pressure in women, even though women were more likely to be in high-strain jobs.

Light et al. used two measures to evaluate occupational stress in a biracial group of working men and women. The first was job status, which was based on the job title, and the second was what they called "high-effort coping." This was assessed by means of a measure called the John Henryism Active Coping Scale, high scores on which have been related to blood pressure in black men. Women who had high-status jobs requiring high-effort coping had higher diastolic pressures while at work than other women.

The place of employment may also be an important factor. In a survey of women employed by four large corporations, it was found that the single most important predictor of blood pressure status was the company they worked at; this ranked higher than more typical risk factors, including obesity, age, and family history of hypertension.

The prevalence of hypertension was markedly higher at one company than at the other three, and this was true for managers, clerical workers, and blue-collar workers. This could not be accounted for by any of the conventional risk factors, but the authors commented that workers at this particular company appeared to be under greater than ordinary performance pressures. In a survey of seven New York organizations, we found that both worksite and occupation were significantly related to blood pressure, with clerical workers having higher pressures than managers.

In a study of male and female managers and clerical workers employed at a Volvo plant in Sweden, Frankenhaueser et al. found that the female managers reported more conflict between the demands of their work and their home life than the other three groups. In addition, their blood pressure remained high when they returned home, and their norepinephrine excretion increased, in marked contrast to male managers, whose blood pressure and norepinephrine excretion both dropped markedly at 5 P.M. We have also observed that the blood pressure usually remains elevated in women who have small children when they go home in the evening, whereas in childless women and in men (regardless of whether or not they have children), it falls.

DOMESTIC STRESS

In a series of studies of blood pressure and related variables in healthy normotensive women employed mostly in clerical jobs, we have classified the subjects according to whether they perceived their work or their home life to be greater sources of stress. About 60% of women considered their jobs to be more stressful, and 40% their home lives. Not surprisingly, the latter subjects were significantly more likely to have young children; more surprisingly, they were also more likely to be black. The "work-stressed" women had average systolic pressures 8 mm Hg higher than the "home-stressed" women during working hours, whereas at home the blood pressures were similar in the two groups, because the home-stressed women showed less of a fall in blood pressure after going home than the work-stressed women did.

Women with unhappy marriages, or those who are recently divorced or separated, have been reported to have a higher prevalence of depression and impaired immune responses when compared to women with stable marriages. In another study, healthy former spouses (i.e., widowed, divorced, or separated) under the age of 45 were found to have higher total and low-density lipoprotein cholesterol levels than married women of the same age. No differences were found in older women.

BEREAVEMENT

Although it is well established that men who have lost a spouse are at increased risk of mortality than those who are still married, the data for women are less consistent. However, Jones found that for 6 months following bereavement there was a peak in all-cause mortality in women, but not in men. There was no clear effect of bereavement on ischemic heart disease mortality. One of the most striking pieces of evidence on the effects of bereavement comes from a study of women dying suddenly of atherosclerotic heart disease, who were found to be six times more likely than the controls to have experienced the death of a significant other in the 6 months preceding death.

SOCIAL SUPPORT

Lack of social support is becoming increasingly recognized as a major risk factor for cardiovascular and other forms of disease. Women with the fewest sources of support (including marriage, friends, church, and other social groups) have been reported to have nearly three times the risk for mortality that those with the most sources of support have. For men this ratio may be somewhat lower. The effects of social support can be demonstrated in laboratory studies, which have shown that cardiovascular reactivity to a stressful task can be reduced by the presence of a friend. This applies to both sexes.

There are two general theories as to how social support might operate. The first has been termed the "direct effects" model, and assumes that support has a beneficial effect at all levels of stress. The second, called the "buffering" model, assumes that support is only protective at high levels of stress. The two models are not mutually exclusive, and in a study designed to discriminate between them, in which subjects were exposed to two levels of stress with and without an associate present, we found evidence to support both mechanisms. In an ambulatory monitoring study of college students monitored during a normal campus day, Linden et al. found that a high level of social support was associated with low ambulatory systolic pressures in women, but not in men. In men, high pressures were associated with self-deception and hostility.

SOCIOECONOMIC STATUS

Low social class seems to be an independent risk factor for coronary heart disease in women, just as it is in men. One of the predictors of hypertension in working women is a low personal income.

CONCLUSIONS

The evidence that chronic environmental stress can adversely affect people's physical as well as mental health is suggestive if not conclusive. For women, as for men, coronary heart disease is the single most important cause of death, but such evidence as exists suggests that neither hostility nor job strain—two factors thought to be important in men—is a significant risk factor. One of the striking differences between men and women is that women are now potentially exposed to more environmental stressors than men, in that they are now in the work force in similar numbers but at a generally lower level, without at the same time having given up their domestic work. Despite this, there is no firm evidence that this has had any adverse effects on women's health.

FURTHER READING

Frankenhaueser, M., Lundberg, U., Fredrikson, M., Melin, B., Tuomisto, M., & Myrstren, A.-L. (1989). Stress on and off the job as related to sex and occupational status in white-collar workers. *Journal of Organizational Behavior, 10,* 321–346.
A classic study of occupational and domestic stress in women managers and clerical workers in a Swedish Volvo plant.

Haynes, S., & Feinlieb, M. (1980). Women, work, and coronary heart disease: Prospective findings from the Framingham Heart Study. *American Journal of Public Health, 70,* 133–144.
A report from the Framingham Heart Study, noting that working women reported more symptoms of emotional distress than men or housewives, but did not have more coronary heart disease.

Haynes, S., Feinlieb, M., & Kannel, W. (1980). The relationship of psychological factors to coronary heart disease in the Framingham Study (Part III). *American Journal of Epidemiology, 111,* 37–58.
Another report from the Framingham Study, examining the relationship between Type A behavior and heart disease in men and women.

House, J. S., Landis, K. R., & Umberson, D. (1988). Social relationships and health. *Science, 241,* 54–545.
A comprehensive review of the relationship between social support and health.

Jones, D. R. (1987). Heart disease mortality following widowhood: Some results from the OPCS longitudinal study. *Journal of Psychosomatic Research, 31,* 325–335.
A report indicating that recently widowed women showed increased mortality.

La Rosa, J. H. (1988). Women, work, and health: Employment as a risk factor for coronary heart disease. *American Journal of Obstetrics and Gynecology, 158,* 1597–1602.
A review concluding that working women are generally healthier than housewives or unemployed women.

Light, K. C., Brownley, K. A., Turner, J. R., Hinderliter, A. L., Girdler, S. S., Sherwood, A., & Anderson, N. B. (1995). Job status and high-effort coping influence work blood pressure in women and blacks. *Hypertension, 25,* 554–559.
A study finding that women who had achieved high job status requiring high-effort coping were likely to show an increase in blood pressure.

Linden, W., Chambers, L., Maurice, J., & Lenz, J. W. (1993). Sex differences in social support, self-deception, hostility, and ambulatory cardiovascular activity. *Health Psychology, 12,* 376–380.
A study of psychosocial influences on ambulatory blood pressure, in which social support appeared to be of more importance in women than in men.

Schlussel, Y. R., Schnall, P. L., Zimbler, M., Warren, K., & Pickering, T. G. (1990). The effect of work environments on blood pressure: Evidence from seven New York organizations. *Journal of Hypertension, 8,* 679–685.
A survey of blood pressure in different worksites.

Schnall, P. L., Landsbergis, P. A., & Baker, D. (1994). Job strain and cardiovascular disease. *Annual Review of Public Health, 15,* 381–411.
A comprehensive review of the evidence relating job strain and heart disease.

Section IX

GENDER, CULTURE, AND HEALTH

133

Section Editors' Overview

Amy W. Helstrom
Elaine A. Blechman

*T*he relationship between gender and health is a central topic of this volume. This section considers the complex interactions among health, gender, economic and social status, and ethnicity. Chapters in this section examine not only differences but commonalities of ethnicity, social roles, and culture across disorders and conditions and across health-promoting interventions. The section includes chapters on the implications for health of membership in diverse ethnic groups (African-American, Asian-American, Hispanic-American, Native American), and occupancy of diverse social roles (lesbian woman, woman physician, woman patient).

The section that opens this book focuses on life course perspectives. Stages of the life course provide experiences shared by women, regardless of class or culture. Middle-aged women of all income groups and ethnicities, for example, have a common stock of life experiences that unite them and influence their status in the health care delivery system. This closing section deals with experiences that seemingly divide rather than unite women. Only a small segment of women in the United States will experience the unique health implications of status as a lesbian or Latina woman. Experiences that seem at first glance to divide women, upon closer inspection really do unite us. Like it or not, every woman in her lifetime will have an equal opportunity, as Westkott points out in her chapter, to be marginalized, devalued, and sexualized. Every woman struggles, knowingly or not, with constraints on her well-being that are imposed by the general culture, by the circumstances of her upbringing, and by her own internalized (and rarely conscious) self-derogation. As Westkott's chapter suggests, a woman's ability to care for her own physical and psychological health depends to a great extent upon what her family and culture of origin have taught her about her self-worth.

In McNair's chapter, she shows that African-American women have significantly higher rates of mortality from heart disease, lung cancer, breast cancer, diabetes, and AIDS than European-American women, as well as a higher overall mortality rate. Socioeconomic and behavioral influences work independently and interactively to affect the quality and type of care an African-American woman receives. As McNair points out, many circumstances of African-American women's health are poorly understood, including the reason for the higher incidence of low-birthweight babies among wealthy African-American women than among European-American women.

The chapter on Asian-American women's health, by Helstrom, Coffey, and Jorgannathan, notes both the relative paucity of research on this large and fast-growing ethnic group (most such research to date has been done in the state of California) and the fact that Asian-American women underutilize both mental and physical health services. The reasons for this underutilization include language and financial barriers, cultural views of mental health and illness, and cultural views of women and sexuality. Helstrom and her colleagues stress Asian-American women's need for health services that are affordable, accessible, culturally appropriate, and provided in their native languages, as well as for facilities that create an environment of trust, confidence, and reassurance.

Woodward's chapter on Hispanic women and health care emphasizes Hispanic women's barriers to health care. These barriers, Woodward contends, are both financial (lack of insurance coverage) and nonfinancial (lack of available and accessible services); some nonfinancial barriers are also intimately linked to Hispanic culture. Language and geographical location can influence a Hispanic woman's decision to pursue health care and her access to the care she needs.

Baines discusses Native American women's health and health care. Among Native American females, the leading causes of death are cardiovascular disease, malignant neoplasms, accidents, diabetes, cerebrovascular disease, chronic liver disease and cirrhosis, pneumonia and influenza, and kidney diseases. Baines notes that many of these diseases are related to socioeconomic and cultural factors. Inadequate access to health care, combined with Native American women's approach to health care, have an impact on their health outcomes.

Reflecting available research findings regarding lesbians, Perry and O'Hanlan focus on the larger identity and relationship issues, rather than on specific issues affecting health status and access to health care (e.g., the process of "coming out" to health care providers). In surveys, the majority of lesbians report committed, monogamous, long-term relationships, although some also describe codependency and various forms of relationship instability. Lesbians report less sexual dysfunction than heterosexual women but more domestic violence than has thus far been recognized. The continuing prohibition of same-sex marriages is unsettling to many lesbians who desire what the marriage ideal offers, but lesbians often form "families of choice," and an increasing number are having children (in addition to children they may have from previous marriages or relationships). The chapter concludes with a brief look at aging lesbians, whose needs may best be met by homosexual retirement communities that extend the "family of choice" concept into old age.

In her chapter on physician gender and physician–patient interaction, Bertakis discusses the ways in which women's health care is affected by the gender of the physician. As Bertakis points out, the impact of gender on the medical field has increased with the growth in the number of women graduating from medical school. This "feminization" of the field has resulted in more humanistic care. Although earlier findings that female physicians spend more time with patients than physicians do are now believed to reflect methodological flaws in these studies, practice styles do differ between male and female physicians in that females provide more preventive services than males do. In addition, communication styles differ, with female physicians placing greater emphasis on psychosocial issues and concerns. As a result, patients express more satisfaction with female than with male physicians.

This book on women's health is opened by a section on life course perspectives and closed by a section on cultural, ethnic, and social roles. As the organization of this book suggests, we believe that human health and well-being are functions of developmental and ecological contexts. We are certain that this book will prove useful to readers seeking new knowledge relevant to their own and others' suboptimal health. We are hopeful that this book will prove inspiring to readers seeking new ways to promote optimal health among women through social action.

134

Culture and Women's Health

Marcia Westkott

> Our whole civilization is a masculine civilization. The State,
> the laws, morality, religion, and the sciences are the creation of
> men. . . . If we are clear about the extent to which all our be-
> ing, thinking , and doing conform to these masculine stand-
> ards, we can see how difficult it is for the individual man and
> also for the individual woman really to shake off this mode of
> thought.
>
> —*Karen Horney*

Why is an understanding of culture important to women's health? Culture is a matrix of beliefs, values, and norms that inform, give meaning to, and regulate experience. No individual act, no matter how private, is excluded from cultural influence. Naturally, women's health is affected by cultural beliefs, values, and norms about women and "femininity." When Karen Horney wrote about "masculine civilization" over 70 years ago, she was referring to the presumption within Western culture of male superiority and female inferiority. The cultural beliefs and practices that presume female inferiority permeate the social context in which girls and women are devalued as a matter of normal, everyday routine. "No matter how much the individual woman may be treasured as a mother or as a lover," Horney wrote, "it is always the male who will be considered more valuable on human and spiritual grounds." Female devaluation suffuses the atmosphere in which female character develops: "In actual fact a girl is exposed from birth onward to the suggestion—inevitable, whether conveyed brutally or delicately—of her inferiority." Women are impressed with the belief in their own inferiority, and they act on this belief, "adapting themselves to the wishes of men and . . . [feeling] as if their adaptation were their true nature."

Despite the political and economic changes that have occurred over the past 70 years, the idea of male superiority and female inferiority has persisted. Social scientists have documented the ways in which gender inequality has affected girls and women from all cultural backgrounds, races, and ethnicities. Although Karen Horney's words may appear a bit dated, her work offers a useful theoretical perspective for understanding how

816

cultural forms become internalized as psychological constructs. More specifically, she provides a framework for explaining the ways in which presumptions of female inferiority (regardless of their specific cultural expression) are mediated by family psychodynamics and internalized as a conflicted character structure. This inner conflict (and the cultural values and psychodynamics that produce it) threatens women's psychological health, and often their physical health as well.

Two abiding themes thread their way through the various cultural manifestations of the idea of female inferiority: sexualization and devaluation. The idea that women should be sexually pleasing objects for male desire is a traditional one among various ethnic and racial groups. In the 20th-century United States, the expectation that a woman's chief concern is to make herself an attractive mate for a man has been termed the "heterosexual imperative" by historian Mary Ryan. This expectation has fostered women's obsessive concern with making their bodies into the proper objects for male approval and with expressing "normal" heterosexuality in terms of subservience. Thus, women are not only expected to be heterosexual, but also to express their heterosexuality (i.e., their normality) in seductive, alluringly compliant behaviors. Attractiveness, male approval, and ulti- mately marriage are viewed as the necessary signs of normality. In this pursuit, a woman is expected to outshine all other women in attempting to conform to a narrowly defined and unattainable standard of beauty—most often expressed in terms of European-Ameri- can women's features. It is an expectation that fosters competition and envy among women, suspicion of female independence, and an obsessive attention to the needs and judgments of men.

Devaluation is also lodged in the belief in women's inferiority. Contemporary social scientists have documented the ways in which the presumption of women's inferior abilities informs the labor market, politics, social organization, interpersonal relations—in short, the ways masculine civilization continues to create a second-class status for women of all races and ethnicities. One ability, however, is viewed as women's uniquely superior quality: nurturing others. But, interestingly, this quality is used to justify women's subordination in other spheres. Women are expected to care for others—men and children—and their own needs are presumed to have a secondary priority. Indeed, their own needs are expected to be realized through serving others. Embedded in this expectation of female altruism is a male sense of entitlement to nurturing and care, which is best embodied in the idea of the motherly wife.

Psychodynamics within the family convey these wider cultural values through patterns specific to particular class and racial groups. Some of these behaviors may be blatant, but others may be more subtle. For example, parents who are overly concerned with having "successful" or "normal" children are especially likely to reproduce stereo- typically gendered behavior in their offspring. In these circumstances, children are treated as narcissistic extensions of the parents rather than as beings who are valued for themselves. Their authentic needs are denied as they are treated as objects that are expected to fulfill stereotypically gendered ideals, all in the name of what is "best" for them.

A female child's sexualization within the family can be conveyed either brutally, as in incest, or more subtly, through flirtatious sexual advances. A sexually seductive father, for example, may flirt with the bounds of propriety through sexual teasing, flirting, courting, joking, innuendo, caresses, exhibition, spying, and sexually tinged concern with a girl's appearance. This kind of sexual dominance is conveyed as if it were normal, unintentional, and thus consistent with the ordinary routines of everyday life.

Devaluation is conveyed in what Karen Horney called "the thousand little daily experiences of a child," where a girl learns that she is less valued than a boy. Contemporary writers have recorded this phenomenon in a variety of cultures: the Chicana who sees that it is always her brother who receives her mother's attention; the Caribbean-American who learns that asserting herself is unladylike, the Italian-American who is not sent to college because she is a girl; the Jewish youngster who is silenced by her father's demand for attention. Fundamental to the devaluation of a girl's aspirations and abilities is the "nurturing imperative"—the expectation that a female should transform her own needs into meeting the needs of others. When this gender expectation is combined with generational power differences within families, the result is a reversal of nurturing, in which girls are expected to attend to the needs of those adults who should be caring for them. Becoming a confidant to or empathizing with an unhappy parent, restricting her own needs in order to relieve a parent of that task, and submitting to sexual advances are examples of ways in which this reversal of nurturing can inform parent–daughter relationships.

Sexualization and devaluation mirror and reinforce each other. If a girl learns through being sexualized that she is an object to be used for men's purposes and pleasures, she learns that lesson again from the limits placed on her efforts to become a self-directed human being. Through sexualization, her desire is transformed into desirability; through devaluation, her own needs are resculpted into a wish to be valued through meeting the needs of others. In both instances, a woman is treated as an object. Devaluation of her competence and needs confirms her sense of herself as only a sexualized object, and sexualizing encounters erode her sense of herself as a human being with independent agency and personal competence.

The theoretical link between culture and psyche in Horney's theory is the category of safety. "Safety" refers to the conditions that caretakers must create in order for the satisfaction of needs to take place. The theoretical primacy of safety assumes that an infant is not just a bundle of drives, but a vulnerable being, dependent upon adult protection and care.

Unfortunately, the psychodynamics of sexualization and devaluation—even when they are carried out with the best of intentions—create danger, not safety. A female child's responses to these experiences are fear and anger. Fear is an understandable reaction to sexualizing and devaluing conditions that the child cannot control. Powerless and devalued, she feels weak, helpless, and worthless. At the same time, however, she protests through anger. But because female anger is culturally unacceptable, and because it implicitly criticizes devaluing and sexualizing adults, a girl's anger intensifies the possibility of danger. Thus, out of a fear of reprisal or loss of whatever love and safety are available, the child's anger is deflected, turned back upon itself. In this process of reaction formation, the feared parent is admired, and the child becomes the object of her own hostility. According to Horney, this "shift from true rebellion to untrue admiration" serves to diffuse the conflict and thus to promote safety.

In this process, however, the conflict is internalized as a characterological split. On the one hand, turning anger against the self creates self-contempt—a feeling of being unworthy and thus deserving of further sexualizing and devaluing treatment. On the other hand, the attempt to find safety through conforming to the behaviors that the sexualizing and devaluing experiences elicit creates a defense against danger. The expectations for self-abnegating and sexualized femininity are internalized as a defensive "proud" or idealized self. Exhibiting these behaviors and embracing their attendant feelings are rewarded, and thus these become the major defenses against both self-contempt and social disapproval. Hence, the idealized self becomes the inner critic that demands adherence to the "shoulds" of a perfectionistic, culturally stereotypical definition for female appearance and behavior. Through this mechanism, compulsory femininity is compulsively pursued.

The idealized self both masks and sustains the underlying self-contempt. In order to escape feelings of worthlessness, a woman who is caught in this inner conflict will attempt to live up to the perfectionistic demands of the idealized self. Moments of achieving the ideals can bring temporary pride, but cannot be sustained. Failure deepens her self-loathing. Her attempts to live up to the unrealistic standards of stereotypical femininity thus keep her on a seesaw of pride and self-hatred. The combination of defensive perfectionism and inevitable shortcomings serves to make anger against herself an enduring feature of her character.

The anger can sabotage the very behaviors that the idealized self demands. It can seep through as martyrdom when others do not fully appreciate a woman's caretaking. It can be experienced as a continuing depression that accompanies self-sacrifice in an intimate relationship. It can be released in begrudging envy and grinding resentment of those for whom a woman "responsible." It can be expressed in compulsive eating, resulting in image-defeating weight gain. And it can be conveyed in an attitude of vindictiveness toward others. In short, anger at trying to live up to the proud self's internalized gendered ideals continually threatens to undermine a woman's efforts to become perfectly feminine. The prohibition against expressing anger directly, however, keeps her experience of it hidden, indirect, passive–aggressive, and ultimately turned against herself.

Women suffer psychologically from the cultural bias against them. The idealized self internalizes these biases as self-expectations and makes the inner world a battleground between the desire for self-realization and the demand for gendered conformity. The cultural demands are not always consistent, and in fact are often contradictory. The socially prescribed roles as lover, wife, mother, and worker, for example, can call for widely opposing behaviors. Moreover, different groups of women are subjected to different sets of conflicting ideals. Women of color, living in two racial/ethnic worlds, are forced to negotiate competing sets of cultural ideals as well as to attempt to withstand the internalization of both sexist and racist values. The heterosexual imperative, while forcing heterosexual women into a subservient heterosexuality, places lesbians and bisexual women in the position of questioning their own desires and internalizing homophobic self-definitions. Feminist therapy begins with the recognition that women's psychological conflict is informed by limiting and psychologically harmful cultural values, beliefs, and norms. It seeks to undo the internalized definitions of what a woman should be, in order to illuminate and expand her actual possibilities.

FURTHER READING

Anzaldua, G. (Ed.). (1990). *Making face, making soul, haciendo caras: Creative and critical perspectives by feminists of color*. San Francisco: aunt lute books.
A collection of writings by contemporary women of color about breaking through idealized images.

Herman, J. (1981). *Father–daughter incest*. Cambridge, MA: Harvard University Press.

A study of 40 incest victims that examines the phenomenon of incest within the cultural context of the patriarchal society.

Horney, K. (1967). The flight from womanhood: The masculinity complex in women as viewed by men and women. In H. Kelman (Ed.), *Feminine psychology* (pp. 54–70). New York: Norton. (Original work published 1926)
One of Horney's earliest published essays, which takes issue with Freud's ideas on feminine psychology.

Kaschak, E. (1992). *Engendered lives: A new psychology of women's experience.* New York: Basic Books.
A contemporary analysis of the effects of sexism on women's psychological development.

Lott, B. E. (1981). *Becoming a woman: The socialization of gender.* Springfield, IL: Charles C. Thomas.
A comprehensive survey and analysis of the patterns of gender discrimination and their psychological effects on female development

Ryan, M. (1983). *Womanhood in America: From colonial times to the present* (3rd ed.). New York: Franklin Watts.
A synthesis of the major strands of the history of women in the United States.

Westkott, M. (1986). *The feminist legacy of Karen Horney.* New Haven, CT: Yale University Press.
An elaboration of the ideas presented in this chapter.

Williams, C. (1993). The psychology of women. In J. Wetzel, M. L. Espenlaub, M. A. Hagen, A. B. McElhiney, & C. B. Williams (Eds.), *Women's studies: Thinking women.* Dubuque, IA: Kendell/Hunt.
A review of the contemporary issues and scholarship on the psychology of women, drawing attention to differences between white women and women of color.

135

African-American Women's Health

Lily D. McNair
George W. Roberts

*T*he health of African-American women is closely tied to their social position in the United States. Health indices such as lowered life expectancy and higher death rates for selected diseases reflect one facet of this group's marginal status in U.S. society. For every major disease category, mortality rates for African-American women are higher than those for European-American women. This pattern also holds for African-American men, who fare considerably worse than European-American men on all health indices. These consistent racial disparities have been well documented over the years, and have been associated with socioeconomic status (SES). In this chapter, we discuss the role of both socioeconomic and behavioral factors in the poorer health of African-American women, and consider ways of improving these women's health status. First, however, we discuss health indices at greater length.

AFRICAN-AMERICAN WOMEN'S HEALTH STATUS

Comparative data are presented here that highlight the persistent disparities between African-American and European-American women's health. An examination of life expectancy and mortality rates for leading causes of death provides one means of describing the current state of African-American women's health.

Life Expectancy

Life expectancy at birth is not only an indicator of health, but also a marker for living standards within societies. Life expectancy for African-American women in 1994 was

73.8 years, compared to 79.5 years for European-American women. This gap in the life expectancies of these two groups has widened in recent years, from 5.6 years in 1980 to 6.1 years in 1994.

Mortality Rates for Leading Causes of Death

On the basis of age-adjusted mortality rates in 1992, the leading causes of death for African-American women are heart disease, lung cancer, breast cancer, diabetes, and AIDS. African-American women's rates for all of these diseases (as indicated in Table 135.1) are significantly higher than those for European-American women. The number of deaths from heart disease is especially striking (162.4 deaths per 100,000 for African-American women, compared to 98.1 deaths per 100,000 for European-American women).

African-American women's rates of mortality from breast cancer are particularly significant, in light of the low incidence of breast cancer in this group. African-American women's survival rate (62%, as opposed to 70% for European-American women) reflects a number of factors, ranging from later detection to differences in estrogen metabolism and dietary habits.

African-American women's rates of death from diabetes and HIV/AIDS are also comparatively high. African-American women die of diabetes at almost three times the rate of European-American women; for deaths related to HIV infection, African-American women's mortality rate is over eight times greater. In 1991, HIV infection was the third leading cause of death for African-American women aged 25–44 years. Furthermore, African-American women accounted for 55% of all women with AIDS.

Reproductive Health Issues

Similar to life expectancy, infant mortality rates are indicators of the general health status of women, as well as the overall standard of life in a particular culture or country. The mortality rate for African-American women's infants in 1992 was 2.4 times the rate for European-American women's infants (16.8 vs. 6.9 per 100,000).

"Maternal mortality" refers to mothers' deaths associated with childbirth. Not surprisingly, maternal mortality rates are also higher among African-American women than among European-American women. In 1990, the maternal mortality ratio (number of maternal deaths per 100,000 live births) was 3.3 times greater for African-American women than for European-American women.

TABLE 135.1. Age-Adjusted Mortality Rates (per 100,000) for Leading Causes of Death in African-American and European-American Women, 1992

Cause	African-American	European-American
Heart disease	162.4	98.1
Lung cancer	28.5	27.4
Breast cancer	27.0	21.7
Diabetes	25.8	9.6
AIDS	14.3	1.6

Note. The data are from the National Center for Health Statistics (1995).

INFLUENCES ON AFRICAN-AMERICAN WOMEN'S HEALTH

Socioeconomic Influences

There is an inverse relationship between SES and health, with lower SES being associated with higher rates of morbidity and mortality. For African-American women, this relationship is moderated by the influences of ethnicity and gender, which have been associated with variations in SES. The SES of African-Americans tends to be lower than that of European-Americans, and women's SES is generally lower than men's. Thus, African-American women are particularly vulnerable to the negative effects of SES on health.

The diseases that cause death for African-American women at higher rates than for European-American women are also the diseases often linked to lower SES (e.g., diabetes, lung disease, cerebrovascular disease, and cirrhosis of the liver). Even HIV/AIDS, which was once primarily associated with homosexuality, has a strong socioeconomic determination. Groups that are currently experiencing the greatest risk for contracting HIV (through either sex or injection drug use) are groups that tend to be economically vulnerable: poor men and women; prostitutes; and youths living in high-risk social environments.

Behavioral Influences

In addition to socioeconomic influences, risk behaviors such as substance use, unprotected sex with multiple partners, overeating, and physical inactivity also influence negative health outcomes for African-American women. In fact, an examination of risk behaviors may offer an understanding of mechanisms by which socioeconomic influences are exerted upon health. For example, in a national survey of risk factors for chronic disease, better-educated African-American and European-American respondents (those with more than 12 years of schooling) reported fewer of these risk factors than their less educated counterparts. African-American women were more likely than European-American women to have less than 12 years of schooling, and to report higher rates of obesity and physical inactivity.

Health-related behaviors may also act independently of SES. The finding that African-American women are more likely than European-American women to have poor reproductive health outcomes, regardless of SES, is a case in point. African-American women at all educational and income levels have disproportionately higher numbers of preterm and low-birthweight infants than do European-American women of similar education and income. Several factors have been hypothesized to explain this perplexing finding, including behaviors linked to substance use and seeking prenatal care. Although their effects on reproductive health outcomes have been shown, these factors fail to explain why well-educated, more affluent African-American mothers give birth to infants with very low weights at rates that are virtually identical to those of poor European-American women.

The impact of racism on health is less well understood. Although its effects have been hypothesized for some time, there has been little research documenting the processes through which racism influences negative health outcomes. Racism reflects differences between groups that result from the systematic distribution of socioeconomic resources on the basis of race. Therefore, systematic health differences between African-American and European-American women may also be explained by disparate race-related experiences.

Racism can have an adverse impact on health through a variety of differential effects on lifestyles, risk behaviors, access to health care, help-seeking patterns, quality of care, and environmental conditions. Persistent inequities in access to medical care, and consistent gaps in medical insurability between African-Americans and European-Americans, are race-related outcomes that have obvious implications for health.

Influenced by SES and race/ethnicity, psychosocial factors also affect health-related behaviors, and thus ultimately play a role in African-American women's high morbidity and mortality rates. Factors such as stress and coping, risk perception, and gender role orientation may offer an understanding of behavioral etiology and antecedents. The powerful role of stress in moderating the relationship between behavior and health is well acknowledged. As an example, African-American women's coping with race- and economic-related stress can have deleterious effects on their health. James suggests that an active coping orientation among African-Americans, which he terms "John Henryism," may be in part responsible for high rates of hypertension among low-income African-American men and women. Similarly, Geronimus posits the "weathering hypothesis" as an explanation for African-American women's negative health status; "weathering" is defined as a consequence of cumulative stress resulting from discrimination.

IMPROVING THE HEALTH OF AFRICAN-AMERICAN WOMEN

In light of the foregoing discussion, several recommendations relating to improving the health status of African-American women are warranted. Rather than focusing on changing behavior at the individual level, these recommendations acknowledge the validity of social, economic, and cultural influences on health.

Health care providers need to be knowledgeable about the specific socioeconomic and behavioral risk factors for African-American women's negative health outcomes. For example, the increased level of stress these women face—precipated by employment difficulties, and aggravated by the "daily hassles" of constant race- and gender-based discrimination—can lower their probability of engaging in health-promoting behaviors. Interventions targeted solely at the individual level are unlikely to be effective by themselves in such cases. Social-level interventions may increase the likelihood that behavioral change will be initiated and maintained.

Improving the status of African-American women's health entails improving the conditions of their lives on critical socioeconomic and political fronts. Health care policy addressing inequities in access to care and insurance coverage, for example, will be a necessary step toward ameliorating the negative health status of African-American women. Relatedly, public health efforts targeting improved housing and neighborhood conditions, and increased opportunities for education and employment, will all contribute to improving the quality of life for African-American women. Culturally relevant prevention and intervention strategies for African-American women should be developed with the participatory input of the groups they are meant to serve. Such programs should conceptualize health problems as social problems in need of comprehensive strategies for altering the social conditions contributing to the negative health status of African-American women.

FURTHER READING

Geronimus, A. T. (1992). The weathering hypothesis and the health of African-American women and infants: Evidence and speculations. *Ethnicity and Disease, 2,* 207–221.
The relationship between discrimination and health is examined by Geronimus, who hypothesizes that cumulative stress resulting from discrimination ("weathering") negatively influences the health of African-American women and their children.

James, S. A. (1994). John Henryism and the health of African Americans. *Culture, Medicine and Psychiatry, 18,* 163–182.
Examines the development of an active, problem-focused coping style, termed "John Henryism," in African-Americans. ("John Henryism" refers to the legendary African-American who collapsed and died after outperforming a mechanical driller.) The relationship between this coping style and negative health consequences is discussed.

National Center for Health Statistics. (1995). *Health, United States.* Hyattsville, MD: Public Health Service.
A comprehensive documentation of health statistics for Americans, highlighting major trends in health status.

136

Asian-American Women's Health

Amy W. Helstrom
Colleen Coffey
Priya Jorgannathan

Asian-Americans (including Pacific islanders) are, in terms of percentage increase, the fastest-growing ethnic group in the United States. The 1990 U.S. census enumerated a population of 3.7 million Asian-American women. With a current total Asian-American population of 7.3 million, projections are that by the year 2020 this number will rise to 20 million. The term "Asian-American" covers more than 50 different ethnic groups. An average of 65.6% of all Asian-Americans living in the United States are foreign-born, and an average of 75% of Asian-Americans speak a language other than English at home, choosing from one of more than 30 different Asian languages. These statistics reveal a growing need for a large number of low-cost health care options geared toward the diverse needs of Asian-American women.

For the purposes of this chapter, we have relied heavily on recent surveys conducted throughout California, where there is a strong movement toward specialized care for Asian-American women. The state of California, with a 2.8 million Asian-American population, has benefited from the National Asian Women's Health Organization, located in San Francisco, which has implemented several programs; these include the South Asian Women's Health Project, the Asian Health Services Organization, the Statewide Resources Handbook for Asian Women and Girls, the Reproductive Health Empowerment Project, and the Asian American Donor Program. California also has the National Research Center on Asian American Mental Health, a research program based at the University of California at Los Angeles (UCLA). As do women of each ethnic group, Asian-American women need specific kinds of prevention and intervention strategies to promote their mental and physical well-being, growth, and development. This chapter reviews what we currently know about their health and health care needs, and examines the specific health care Asian-American women require.

THE CURRENT STATE OF RESEARCH

Serious research on the mental and physical health of Asian-Americans began less than two decades ago, and there is still a serious lack of empirical information about the health status of this group. In regard to mental health in particular, a prevailing myth has been that Asian-Americans are extraordinarily well adjusted; this myth was based on earlier statistics that revealed relatively low divorce rates, high socioeconomic and educational attainments, and low rates of social deviance such as crime. However, researchers are now uncovering evidence that the previous statistics were simply underestimates, reflecting the low numbers of Asian-Americans utilizing mental health services. Fortunately, several recent studies have been done by the Asian Health Services Organization in California, including a Chinese behavioral risk factor survey conducted in 1989 that has been published, and a more recent Korean community behavioral risk factor survey that has not yet been published (Chinese study, *n* = 300, and Korean study, *n* = 650). In addition, research by the Centers for Disease Control and Prevention, and various other national studies, have contributed to our understanding of the status of Asian-American women's health and their health behaviors.

PREVENTIVE HEALTH ISSUES

Recent research has consistently demonstrated that Asian-Americans tend to underutilize mainstream mental health services and are more likely to do so than are African-Americans, American Indians, Hispanic-Americans, and European-Americans. Asian-American women also consistently underutilize preventive medical health services, including Pap smears and breast exams, and consistently do not seek advice concerning health issues (e.g., pregnancy or hepatitis) until they require immediate or emergency assistance.

Gynecological Exams

Forty-five percent of the Chinese women surveyed by the Asian Health Services Organization had never had a Pap smear, and 35% of the Korean women had never had a Pap smear. By contrast, 5% of all adult women in California had never had a Pap smear. This is consistent with Asian women's lower survival rates for cervical cancer; the national data base indicates that breast, lung, and cervical cancers are by far the most commonly occurring cancers among Asian-American women. One study of Vietnamese women found that over half of the women had never had Pap smears. Another on Chinese-American women found that only 18% had annual pelvic exams. Cervical cancer is considered, if identified early enough, an entirely "curable" cancer, yet the mortality rates related to cervical cancer for Asian women are particularly high. This points to issues of utilization, access, or some other reasons why these women are not understanding the need to get this kind of preventive care.

Breast Exams

Asian women have low survival rates for detected breast cancer. Of all the cancers that showed up in Asian women in the state of California during 1991–1992, 30% were breast cancer. Again, that is a much higher proportion of that kind of morbidity (and mortality as well) than is really necessary, given the various kinds of breast cancer screenings available, including breast self-exams, clinical exams, and mammography. To judge from the results of the Chinese and Korean surveys, very few Asian women make use of such screenings. Twenty-eight percent of the Chinese women and 43% of the Korean women surveyed had never had a clinical breast exam, compared to 16% of women in the general California population. Seventy-five percent of the Chinese women and 33% of the Korean women never did breast self-exams, compared to only 9% of California's general adult female population. As for mammographies, 68% of Chinese women and 59% of Korean women had never had a mammography, compared to 51% of women in the general California population. The Centers for Disease Control and Prevention also report that mammography rates are low among Asian-American women over 40 throughout the United States. Among Chinese, Vietnamese, Hawaiian, and other Asian and Pacific islander women, over 50% of women have never had a mammography, as compared to 30% of European-American women. Again, it becomes evident that there are significant differences in the use of cancer screening and prevention techniques between Asian-American women and the general population.

Abortion, Birth Control, and Prenatal Care

A national reproductive health poll found that one-third of Asian-American women said that they did not know where to obtain an abortion. As for birth control, over half of the 600 Asian-Americans responding to a recent national sexuality survey reported not using contraception or protection regularly, even though they were not planning a pregnancy. In terms of pregnancy care, research reveals that at least one-third of Vietnamese, Laotian, and Cambodian women receive no first-trimester prenatal care.

Disease Prevention

Hepatitis B has been well documented as a major health problem among all Asian-American populations; it is a particular concern because of the major mode of transmission, which is from mother to child. Hepatitis B is five times more prevalent in Asian-Americans than in the general population. However, because hepatitis B has a very low incidence rate in the mainstream population, a person who goes to a mainstream provider of care or a mainstream physician will not be routinely screened for hepatitis. The same is true for thalassemia, a genetic condition that is carried in about 10% of Chinese people and about 40% of Southeast Asians, but rarely shows up in the mainstream population. These conditions, if not screened for, can result in very significant negative outcomes; hepatitis B is a precursor to liver cancer, and thalassemia can result in a stillbirth.

BARRIERS TO HEALTH CARE

Why are Asian-American women underutilizing health services? There are several reasons.

Views of Mental Health and Illness

In regard to mental health care, research conducted at UCLA's National Research Center on Asian American Mental Health (established in 1988) has theorized that underutilization of services and subsequent underreporting of mental health problems can be attributed in part to culturally biased views of mental health and illness, which result in shame and stigma's being attached to using mental health facilities. Consequently, Asian-Americans avoid or delay using such services until symptoms become very pronounced and families or other forms of support are unable to assist.

Language

In the Asian Health Services organization surveys, a high percentage of women were found to suffer from language barriers; 87% of the Chinese respondents and 57% of the Korean respondents spoke little or no English. According to the 1990 U.S. census, over 50% of all Asians in Oakland, California are categorized as "linguistically isolated." This access barrier makes it virtually impossible for Asian-American women to receive much-needed health care. Approximately 4 to 5 million Asian-Americans living in the United States do not speak English.

Measures are now being taken to provide health care in various Asian-American languages. The Asian Health Services Organization provides services in nine different Asian languages. Full language access is provided at all points of contact. In addition, the organization has started a "language bank," which is a service to which health facilities subscribe that provides medical interpretation services 16 hours a day in Chinese and Vietnamese (as well as Farsi and Spanish).

Insurance Coverage

Seventy-three percent of all the Korean respondents and 35% of all the Chinese respondents to the surveys described above did not have health insurance. Among those aged 45–65, 65% had no health insurance. Compare these rates to the general California no-insurance rate of about 19–20%. As a direct result, 25% of the Chinese women and 18% of the Korean women had never had a routine checkup during their U.S. residency. (The average length of time that most of the respondents had been in the United States was approximately 11 years for the Chinese, and a little less for the Korean.) This compares to 4% of California women who had never had one. Of all Asian and Pacific islander families headed by women, 22%, almost a quarter, are below the poverty level. Only 51% of nonelderly Asian and Pacific islander women in California have employment-based insurance, as compared to 65% of European-American (non-Hispanic) women. Because of this general lack of health insurance, Asian-American women often do not employ preventive health tactics.

With the legislation recently initiated by the U.S. Congress, it could become even more difficult for these vulnerable Asian women and their families to gain access to much-needed health services. In 1995, a House and Senate Conference Committee in Congress completed a reform bill that targets legal immigrants for denial of public assistance benefits. If this bill becomes law, about 4 in 10 Asian persons in the United States will be excluded from receiving any public assistance that is federally based. This includes community health centers, public health programs, welfare, and food stamps.

Views of Women and Sexuality

Asian-American women's underutilization of health care services can also be attributed in part to a cultural norm that places a strong emphasis on silence on topics of sexuality. This silence is taught to Asian-American women at a very young age, along with several other assumptions about sexuality, which are to be accepted without question or conversation. These assumptions include that sex only occurs within the confines of heterosexual, marital relationships, primarily for the goal of reproduction; that sex is a duty that women perform for their husbands; and that there are different standards for sexual conduct for men and women. The problem with these assumptions is that they ignore the realities of women's sexuality, which include both good components (consensual, responsible, and pleasurable sex between partners, both heterosexual and homosexual) and bad components (violence, sexual abuse, infection, unwanted pregnancy, and unsafe abortions) that need to be openly addressed and understood. Women's bodies are constantly changing and going through cycles that need continual monitoring and understanding. The assumption that women's sexuality is only related to reproduction does not encourage any monitoring, fosters a negative view of utilizing health care services, and thus has severe health and social consequences.

As an adjunct to this sexual silence for women is a devaluing of sexual health that Asian-American women have been experiencing for generations. According to Beckie Masaki, executive director and cofounder of the Asian Women's Shelter in California, Western society has continually objectified Asian-American women through the pornography industry and the global trafficking of women as "mail-order brides." Immigrant and refugee Asian women face sexual stereotypes of being "exotic and willing to please," along with the fallacy that their role is solely to please their partners. Such sexual stereotypes have prohibited these women from feeling that it is necessary for them to take care of their bodies, as well as helping to perpetuate continued domestic violence.

Asian women confront many of the same patterns of domestic violence that other women do, but there are some additional experiences that Asian women in the United States face. The first is isolation. All battered women are isolated, but for many Asian-American battered women this isolation is extreme. The extended family is a link to survival for many Asian women living in the United States, and when domestic violence exists, the extended family is often no longer available for support. Sadly, but often, an extended family actually contributes to the violent behavior and isolates a woman from any potential family support. Another issue is silence. Asian-American women are bound by the myth that all Asians take care of themselves, that they do not use social services, and that the problem of domestic violence does not even exist in their community. The shame and stigma associated with use of mental health services (see above) can inhibit women from getting the support and information they need.

THE FUTURE OF ASIAN-AMERICAN WOMEN'S HEALTH CARE

Asian-American women need and deserve health services that address the specific issues of their culture, so that they may educate themselves and live healthy and happy lives.

Asian-American women's health is now being examined in the context of their culture—their daily lives, their psychological states, and their cultural and social behaviors. They need facilities that provide services in their native languages; facilities that create an atmosphere of trust and confidence, allowing Asian-American women a chance to speak openly and honestly; and facilities that ensure a supportive community network's reassurance that they are not alone in their concerns, and that it is acceptable to seek out preventive care.

As an example of efforts in the area of mental health, a study conducted at UCLA examined the importance of an ethnic and gender match between therapists and Asian-American women clients. Fujino and colleagues analyzed over 1,000 Asian-American women who received mental health services at Los Angeles County facilities in the mid-1980s, to determine the effects of match on client's satisfaction (i.e., premature termination, length of treatment), therapists' assessment of client's initial functioning (i.e., diagnosis and ratings of general functioning at admission), and treatment outcome (i.e., general functioning at discharge after controlling for initial functioning). The findings indicated that ethnic and/or gender match conditions were significantly associated with reduced premature termination, increased treatment duration, and ratings of higher functioning at admission, in comparison to the no-match condition.

Researchers also emphasize the need to provide good-quality reproductive and sexual health services that are affordable, accessible, and culturally appropriate for Asian-American women of all ages. The work that needs to be done is to change the standards of care, to change policies, and to recognize that certain populations need to be screened for certain kinds of conditions. Services should include the full range of contraceptive methods; safe and legal abortions; pregnancy care, including pre- and postnatal care; safe delivery; nutrition and child health; sexually transmitted disease prevention, screening, and treatment, including voluntary screening and care for HIV/AIDS; gynecological care, including screening for breast and cervical cancer; health counseling and information on sexuality, relationships, and gender; and, finally, referral systems for other health problems. We also need to continue and expand our current research on the needs of the Asian-American population and on the individual and social meanings attached to gender roles and expectations within Asian-American culture.

Finally, there is a need for community-based peer education, in which Asian-American women can learn about preventive strategies and facilities within their own environment; ideally, this should instigate open communication about sexuality and health not just among Asian-American women, but among all family members. Many times the mainstream U.S. values of individualism and independence do not make a lot of sense to Asian women, who have grown up putting the community before the individual and putting their families before themselves. It is necessary not to deny the importance of community, but to help them learn how to incorporate self-care with family care. This can happen through community-based peer education, which can include early prevention through practical skills and building a network of support. The studies described earlier have taken important steps toward our understanding of Asian-American women's health care. This increased knowledge will assist health care providers in creating appropriate health care for Asian-American women. Expanding this solid base to a national level will help Asian-American women maintain healthy bodies and minds.

FURTHER READING

Fujino, D. C., Okazaki, S., & Young, K. (1994). Asian-American women in the mental health system: An examination of ethnic and gender match between therapist and client. *Journal of Community Psychology, 22,* 164–176.

This empirical article reports a study of 1,000 Asian-American women who received mental health services at Los Angeles County facilities in the mid-1980s. The study found that ethnic and/or gender match conditions were significantly associated with reduced premature termination, increased treatment duration, and ratings of higher functioning at admission in comparison to the no-match condition.

National Asian Women's Health Organization. (1995). *Coming together, moving strong, mobilizing an Asian women's health movement: Proceedings from the First National Asian Women's Health Conference.* San Francisco: Author.

This booklet summarizes the speeches presented at this health conference, and provides an insightful rendition of personal stories and struggles in improving health care facilities for Asian-American women.

Sue, S., Nakamura, C. Y., Chung, R. C., & Yee-Bradbury, C. (1994). Mental health research on Asian Americans. *Journal of Community Psychology, 22,* 61–68.

This review article considers the problems and issues associated with the ethnic diversity in the United States. The authors discuss the culture of Asian-Americans and their specific health needs. They also address types of prevention and intervention strategies that can be used to promote the well-being, growth, and development of individuals from diverse ethnic groups.

Zane, N., Hatanaka, H., Park, S. S., & Akutsu, P. (1994). Ethnic-specific mental health services: Evaluation of the parallel approach for Asian-American clients. *Journal of Community Psychology, 22,* 68–81.

This empirical article reviews a study that examined parallel services for Asian-American outpatients with respect to client characteristics, types of services utilized, and service effectiveness. Their findings strongly suggest that for most Asian-American groups, equitable care and service effectiveness can be achieved through the use of ethnic-specific services.

137

Hispanic Women and Health Care[1]

Albert M. Woodward

*T*he Hispanic-American population,[2] the second largest and one of the fastest-growing minority populations in the United States, faces barriers in its access to health care. "Access" refers to entrance into the health care system. Factors that can facilitate or impede entrance into the health care system include personal accessibility or acceptability, availability of comprehensive services, and sufficient amounts of services to meet needs. Since it is difficult to measure these factors, analysts often study outcomes of the process of accessing health care services and tie these outcomes to the factors under study. Examples of outcomes include comparative rates of service utilization and health outcomes between the group under study and a larger, comparison population.

FINANCIAL BARRIERS TO HEALTH CARE ACCESS

One of the first factors or determinants of access is the availability of insurance coverage (private health insurance or public subsidy) for health services. In the absence of such coverage, the individual faces a barrier to health care access. The national reports on

---

[1]This chapter was written by Albert M. Woodward. No official support or endorsement by the Substance Abuse and Mental Health Services Administration or the U.S. Department of Health and Human Services is intended or should be inferred.

[2]In this chapter, the terms "Hispanic" and "Hispanic-American" are used in the sense that the U.S. government uses them. That is, persons of Hispanic origin or descent are considered to include those who classify themselves in one of the specific Hispanic origin categories on government questionnaires (e.g., Mexican, Puerto Rican, or Cuban), as well as those who note that they are of "other" Hispanic origin (e.g., from Spanish-speaking parts of the Caribbean other than Puerto Rico). Terms for other ethnic groups, such as "black" and "white," are also used in the U.S. government's sense.

health insurance coverage contain data on persons of Hispanic origin but do not separate coverage by gender. If it is assumed that coverage between the genders for Hispanics is roughly equivalent to that between the genders for all persons in the United States, then it is possible to compare Hispanics (and, by assumption, Hispanic women) against other groups in terms of coverage.

Statistics from the National Center for Health Statistics (NCHS) for coverage for 1994 show that 81% of all U.S. men and 83% of all U.S. women had coverage. Women were only insignificantly more likely than men to have coverage. The statistics by race and Hispanic origin, however, show that Hispanics (and, by assumption, Hispanic women) had much less coverage. Whereas 82% of blacks and 88% of whites had coverage, only 71.8% of Hispanics had coverage. According to the NCHS, in 1994 Hispanic persons were more than twice as likely as white persons to have no coverage (33% vs. 17%). Another source states that more than 7 million Hispanics, or 39%, are without health insurance coverage. The implication of these statistics for access of Hispanic women to health care is clear: As a group, they are more likely to face a barrier to entry because of lack of insurance coverage. This barrier is heightened for the half of those Hispanic women-headed families that are below the poverty level.

NONFINANCIAL BARRIERS TO HEALTH CARE ACCESS

Nonfinancial barriers can compound the financial barriers to health care access. Among the nonfinancial barriers, geographic location and institutional barriers are particularly significant. Migrant farm workers (many of whom are Hispanic) risk not getting access to care when needed, because they usually do not have health care providers nearby. When they do seek care, too often it is at hospital outpatient and emergency departments. In addition, there are institutional barriers tied to sociocultural barriers. For example, Hispanic women have the added burden of overcoming institutional cultural differences and language problems that most other women do not have.[3] Cultural factors, such as nationality, language, heritage, ethnicity, and religion, are meshed with socioeconomic factors, such as education, occupation, and income level. The extent to which Hispanic women have achieved cultural assimilation affects their ability to get access to care.

EFFECTS OF BARRIERS TO ACCESS

The effects of both financial and nonfinancial barriers can be measured by differences in utilization of health services. Hispanic women share many of the same differences in underutilization as Hispanic men and children, but their gender creates some special characteristics and outcomes. For example, there is a body of research showing that Hispanics use fewer mental health services in proportion to need for such services, and Hispanic women can be differentiated in certain aspects of this underutilization. Hispanic women underuse outpatient mental health services in comparison with white women and

---

[3]They share these language and cultural barriers with other groups of women for whom English is a foreign language (e.g., Asian women), but Hispanic women constitute by far the largest of such groups.

at rates comparable to those of black women, even after socioeconomic and epidemiological variables are controlled for. This is part of a general problem of mental health service access faced by Hispanics and the uninsured. Hispanic women, however, appear to face added barriers in the form of gender-related cultural factors that impede seeking mental health treatment. For example, a network of family support and institutional sensitivity is important in reducing the psychosocial problems accompanying pregnancy in low-income Hispanic women.

Barriers to access should also adversely affect women in the two areas that only they experience—childbearing and health conditions specific to women. However, the data on underutilization of services and the related outcomes of infant births and deaths suggest that the relation between barriers and outcomes is not a simple one. In 1991, the percentage of live infants of low birthweight for Hispanics was similar to that for whites, and much lower than those for black, American Indian, and Alaska Native women, even when marital status and prenatal care were examined. That is, even though Hispanic women were less likely to receive prenatal care and more likely to be unmarried, the percentage of low-birthweight infants for Hispanic women, with exceptions for certain subpopulations, was comparable to that for white women and much lower than those for the other groups mentioned. There are similar data for infant deaths per 1,000 live births: Hispanic infant deaths were lower, excepting certain subpopulations, than in most other racial/ethnic groups. In this area, at least for most Hispanic women, birth and infant outcomes do not appear to be related solely to service utilization (i.e., prenatal care). Tables 137.1 and 137.2 provide more detailed data on live births and deaths, respectively.

There are a large number of site-specific studies offering a variety of reasons for these comparative outcomes, but there is no substantive congruence among these reasons. The studies suggest that for the specific Hispanic populations studied, the availability of health insurance coverage and ability to pay for care are important predictors of care—perhaps more important than factors of acculturation. At a national level these reasons are not as compelling, because Hispanics as a group have lower insurance coverage in comparison to whites, as well as lower income (and hence less ability to pay), but their outcomes as measured by low-birthweight infants and infant deaths are not substantially different from those of whites.

TABLE 137.1. Data on U.S. Live Births by Mothers' Ethnic Groups

Ethnic origin of mothers	% low birthweight infants	% births to unmarried mothers	% of mothers receiving prenatal care
White	6.0	23.6	81.8
American Indian/ Alaskan Native	6.4	55.8	63.4
Black	13.3	68.7	66.0
Mexican American	5.8	37.0	64.8
Cuban	6.2	21.0	88.9
Central/South American	5.9	45.2	68.7
Puerto Rican	9.2	59.4	70.0

Note. This table is based on 1993 data. Low birthweight is less than 2,500 grams. For prenatal care, percentages are based on live births for which the trimester when prenatal care began was the first. The data are from the National Center for Health Statistics (1996).

TABLE 137.2. Data on U.S. Infant Deaths by Mothers' Ethnic Groups

Ethnic origin of mothers	Infant deaths per 1,000 live births
All mothers	9.0
White	7.4
Black	17.1
American Indian/Alaskan Native	12.6
Hispanic origin (total)	7.6
Mexican American	7.2
Puerto Rican	10.4
Cuban	6.2
Central/South American	6.6
Other and unknown Hispanic	8.2

Note. This table is based on data for the birth cohort of 1989–1991. This item was included in birth certificate records of 49 states and the District of Columbia. The data are from the National Center for Health Statistics (1996).

The findings about access to treatment for cervical and breast cancer detection and treatment suggest a variety of explanations. According to the National Health Interview Survey (NHIS) data, among older Hispanic women 93.2% had not had a mammogram, whereas comparable rates were 83.5% of older black women and 75.0% of older white women. Both cervical and breast cancer are preventable through early detection, appropriate intervention, and adequate follow-up. Income to pay for care and the presence of health insurance are factors cited in access to detection and treatment. Other factors that influence access include a belief that health outcomes are under individual control; the quality of outreach among poor, inner-city women; and English-language ability.

Access to care also affects detection and treatment for those health conditions often associated with behavioral influences. Hispanic women appear to have special problems in gaining access to care for these conditions. For example, hypertension and associated cardiovascular problems occur frequently among Hispanic women. Interestingly, however, according to the NCHS, there were 271 deaths per 100,000 resident population for Hispanic women age 45 and over, compared with 395 for all women during 1989–1991. Lack of understanding about a particular behavioral condition and the associated health risks is an important barrier in seeking care, especially when combined with other factors, such as no regular place of health care, lower income and education, and not being married. This finding suggests that commonly cited determinants of access are insufficient by themselves to explain outcomes for these conditions, but are linked to a knowledge of behavioral conditions and risks.

In the area of smoking and tobacco use, Hispanic women are proportionately less likely to smoke than Hispanic men, who (like other minority males) tend to smoke proportionately more than white males, especially in comparison with whites' higher incomes. The reasons for this particular difference are unknown. The National Household Survey on Drug Abuse shows that fewer Hispanic women reported in 1995 ever using illicit drugs (19.0%) than Hispanic men (30.6%), white women (32.9%), or black women (23.2%). The same prevalence rate patterns are observed by Rouse and colleagues with respect to alcohol use. These lower prevalence rates for Hispanic women are reflected in gender proportions by race/ethnicity in publicly funded substance use treatment: 22.7% of Hispanics in treatment are women, versus 28.4% of women of all races/ethnicities. This suggests that Hispanic women may not face special barriers to access to substance use treatment.

For diseases in which sexual behavior frequently plays a role—for example, sexually transmitted diseases (STDs), AIDS, and intravenous drug use (IVDU) associated with both STD and AIDS—there is a paucity of knowledge about these conditions among Hispanic women. It *is* known that HIV disproportionately affects Hispanic women: Although Hispanic women account for 20.4% of the reported female AIDS cases, they constitute only 8.6% of the U.S. female population, according to March 1993 Centers for Disease Control and Prevention data. The causes for their higher rates of pneumonia from IVDU and proportionately shorter lifespans after the diagnosis of AIDS are not well known. Some site-specific studies, such as that by Melnick and colleagues, show that access to appropriate screening and to family planning services (whether through a physician or through a clinic) is an important determinant of disease incidence and outcome.

CONCLUSIONS

There are numerous financial and nonfinancial barriers to health care access for Hispanic women. Financial barriers are tied either to income or to the availability and adequacy of health insurance. Nonfinancial barriers include many factors, from individuals' knowledge and education to cultural, locational, and institutional factors. Some studies, such as that by Davis and colleagues, have found that environmental conditions such as family and church supports affect access. These barriers have been explained by a variety of reasons, many of which are interconnected. There is no general explanation for the effects of Hispanic women's barriers to health care access, however, and there are unexpected results in the areas of low-birthweight infants and infant deaths. In sum, it is clear that for most health conditions availability and sufficient quantity of service are determined by health insurance coverage or public payment and sufficient income, but they are also importantly influenced by cultural and institutional factors.

FURTHER READING

Aday, L., & Andersen, R. (1975). *Development of indices of access to medical care.* Ann Arbor, MI: Health Administration Press.
This source provides the definition and attributes of "access" that are still perhaps the most widely used on the subject.

Bundek, N., Marks, G., & Richardson, J. (1993). Role of health locus of control beliefs in cancer screening of elderly Hispanic women. *Health Psychology, 12*(3), 193–199.
This study found that beliefs about one's ability to control one's health had a correlation to health behavior, including cancer screening.

Chen, V. (1993). Smoking and the health gap in minorities. *Annals of Epidemiology, 3*(2), 159–164.
This article reports the adverse effects on minority populations of increased advertising and product promotion by tobacco companies.

Davis, D., et al. (1994). The urban church and cancer control: A source of social influence in minority communities. *Public Health Reports, 109*(4), 500–506.
A total of 1,012 women between the ages of 21 and 89 years attended educational sessions about cancer screening in 63 churches in Los Angeles. Forty-four percent were found either to have no screening or no screening prior to 2 years of the study.

Ginzberg, E. (1991). Access to health care for Hispanics. *Journal of the American Medical Association, 265*(2), 238–241.
This source is a thorough analysis and statistical report of the determinants of Hispanics' access to care.

Lewin-Epstein, N. (1991). Determinants of regular source of care in black, Mexican, Puerto Rican, and non-Hispanic white populations. *Medical Care, 29*(6), 543–557.
This article examines the determinants of the regular source of care, and shows disparities among different ethnic groups.

Melnick, S., et al. (1994). Survival and disease progression according to gender of patients with HIV infection. The Terry-Beirn Community Programs for Clinical Research on AIDS. *Journal of the American Medical Association, 272*(4), 1915–1921.
In this comparative study of 768 women and 3,779 men, HIV-infected women were at increased risk of death but not disease progression in comparison with HIV-infected men. These findings suggest that women have less access to care than men.

National Center for Health Statistics. (1996). *Health, United States 1995* (DHHS Publication No. [PHS] 96-1232). Hyattsville, MD: U.S. Public Health Service.
Source for many health statistics, including those on infant births and death.

Padgett, D., Patrick, C., Burns, B., & Schlesinger, H. (1994). Women and outpatient mental health services: Use by black, Hispanic, and white women in a national insured population. *Journal of Mental Health Administration, 21*(4), 347–360.
This article reveals that black and Hispanic women in a federal insured group had lower service use than white women, even after a number of variables were controlled for.

Rouse, B., Carter, J., & Rodriguez-Andrew, S. (1995). Race/ethnicity and other sociocultural influences on alcoholism treatment for women. In M. Galanter (Ed.), *Recent developments in alcoholism: Vol. 12. Women and alcoholism* (pp. 343–367). New York: Plenum Press.
This chapter examines the interrelated effects of cultural and socioeconomic variables on health outcomes and service use, but it is focused on alcoholism and its treatment.

Rudolph, A., Kahan, V., & Bordeu, M. (1993). Cervical cancer prevention project for inner city black and Latina women. *Public Health Reports, 108*(2), 156–160.
A report on a proposed intervention in Boston to improve screening and follow-up for treatment of women who lack cervical cancer treatment services.

Short, K. (1992). *Health insurance coverage: 1987–1990. Selected data from the Survey of Income and Program Participation* (Current Population Reports, Household Economic Studies, Series P-70, No. 29). Washington, DC: U.S. Bureau of the Census.
This source is a comprehensive study of health insurance coverage for selected groups in the United States over selected years by selected population.

Substance Abuse and Mental Health Services Administration. (1996). *National Household Survey on Drug Abuse: Population estimates 1995* (DHHS Publication No. [SMA] 96-3095). Rockville, MD: Office of Applied Studies, Substance Abuse and Mental Health Services Administration.
Source of national statistics on the Survey, conducted annually among the general U.S. civilian non-institutionalized population age 12 and over. The Survey is designed to produce drug and alcohol use incidence and prevalence estimates.

Zayas, L., & Busch-Rossnagel, N. (1992). Pregnant Hispanic women: A mental health study. *Families in Society, 73*(9), 515–521.
This study of 86 low-income, pregnant Hispanic women found that improved screening and intervention services, as well as the network of support, were important to these women.

138

Native American
Women and Health Care

David R. Baines

*T*he term "Native American" refers to American Indians and Alaska Natives. Alaska has three separate aboriginal groups: Indians, Eskimos, and Aleuts. American Indian and Alaska Native populations make up less than 1% of the U.S. population. In the 1990 census, there were about 1.7 million American Indians and Alaska Natives. They come from over 500 federally recognized tribes, each with its own language, traditions, and culture. Approximately one-third live on reservations or federal trust lands, one-half live in urban settings, and the rest live on rural nontrust land. Twenty-nine percent of Native American families live in poverty. The unemployment rate is twice the national average. Educational attainment is dismal: Only 31% of American Indian adults have finished high school, and only 7% have a college degree. The population is young, with a median age of 23 years (compared to 32 for the U.S. population of all races); this is attributable to a high birth rate and the fact that 37% of deaths occur before age 45.

In Native American females, the leading cause of death is cardiovascular disease, followed by malignant neoplasms, accidents, diabetes, cerebrovascular disease (primarily stroke), chronic liver disease and cirrhosis, pneumonia and influenza, and kidney diseases. There is quite a range of rates in the different geographic regions; for instance, accidents are the leading cause of death in Alaska, and heart disease is more prevalent in the northern plains than in the southwestern United States. The leading cause of outpatient visits by Native American females is prenatal care, followed by upper respiratory infections/common colds, diabetes mellitus, otitis media, and hypertension. Teen pregnancy, sexually transmitted diseases, and AIDS are other health issues of importance.

PREVENTABLE CAUSES OF MORTALITY AND MORBIDITY

Most of the causes of mortality and morbidity in Native American women can be significantly reduced by prevention programs and strategies and by behavioral changes in the population. It is beyond the scope of this chapter to go into each area in depth, but selected areas and strategies are discussed.

Tobacco Abuse/Dependence

Traditionally, tobacco was used in ceremonies. Stories from various tribed tell how the Creator gave tobacco to the tribes to help their prayers ascend to Him. Nonceremonial use of tobacco occurs in 42–70% of the American Indian population; the rates are highest in the northern plains and lowest in the southwestern United States. Some traditional spiritual leaders believe that recreational use of tobacco is a misuse of a sacred substance, and that this is why harm comes to those who use it in this manner. There has been a resurgence of interest in traditional ways, so this belief can be utilized in community campaigns to reduce the rate of smoking and use of smokeless tobacco. Tobacco certainly has a significant role in cardiovascular disease, cancer, cerebrovascular disease, pneumonia, upper respiratory infection, low birthweight in infants, and sudden infant death syndromes.

Alcohol Abuse/Dependence

It is widely accepted by professionals and laypeople alike that alcohol has had a very negative impact in Native American communities. It certainly has a significant role in accidents, intentional and unintentional injuries, liver disease, and fetal alcohol syndrome. Traditional Western treatments for alcoholism have been largely unsuccessful in Native American communities. Treatment centers that integrate traditional Native American beliefs and ceremonies have better success rates. This involves working with traditional spiritual leaders, who can have positive impacts in many other areas, especially depression and other drug addictions.

Obesity

Obesity is a problem in all U.S. populations, but Native American communities have some of the highest rates in the country. Obesity has a role in cardiovascular disease, diabetes, cerebrovascular disease, and hypertension. Sedentary lifestyles and increased fat and refined sugar in the diet have brought about high rates of obesity in a population in which it was nonexistent prior to contact with European cultures. Utilizing registered dietitians and other health educators to implement community programs, especially in the schools, has been effective; unfortunately, this has not been widely implemented. Dietary changes must be accompanied by physical activity programs to maximize the chances for success.

Inadequate Access to Care

In this time of federal and state budget cuts, the problem of inadequate access to health care will probably become much worse. The Indian Health Service, and the rural and inner-city settings where most Native Americans reside, have inadequate health personnel resources. This means that patients must wait longer to be seen, and that their illnesses are often more advanced because of this delay. Utilizing physician assistants, community health representatives, and nurse practitioners can help, but until Congress and U.S.

society in general develop enough of a social conscience to fund these programs adequately, it will continue to be a major reason why there are differences in health outcomes among populations.

NATIVE AMERICAN CULTURE

Some selected areas of Native American culture are covered briefly here, as its influence (both actual and potential) on health care in Native American women is immense. Understanding patients' beliefs is critical to providing good care for them. Unfortunately, cultural sensitivity has not been stressed in medical education. Improving this aspect of training would have a tremendously beneficial effect in the care provided to all people, not just Native Americans, in the United States.

In the traditional Native American belief system, health is not just the absence of disease but the state of harmony—harmony with oneself (mind, body, and spirit), harmony with others, and harmony with one's surroundings or environment. When this harmony is broken, disease is allowed in. Traditional medicine seeks to reinstate harmony, thus healing from the inside, whereas Western medicine treats the symptoms with pills, thus healing from the outside. These two methods can be viewed as compatible, since the goal of both is a healthy patient.

Native American cultural norms are very different from those of mainstream U.S. society. For instance, eye contact during an interview means that a clinician does not trust a patient, because looking in the eye is done to see whether a person is telling the truth. It has nothing to do with self-confidence. Moreover, Indians are group-oriented, seeing themselves as part of a family, community, and tribe; the individual is not the center of the universe, as in Western culture. It is most important in Western society to have individual goals and to seek personal perfection. This is different from Native societies' orientation toward group goals, such as world peace. Clinicians treating Native American patients should remember how these patients view themselves and should involve their families as much as possible. For example, a patient with newly diagnosed diabetes is usually reluctant to change her diet, as it will affect the whole family. She would rather not change her diet than inconvenience the family. It can be pointed out that the other family members have an increased risk of developing diabetes, and that the diet is therefore beneficial for all family members; the focus is thus on group—not individual—benefits. Western medical care providers often view Native American patients as not being motivated enough to care for themselves, but this is often because self-care is presented as having selfish, individual benefits and not family-oriented, group benefits.

Native Americans are also very community-oriented. Programs that involve the blessing of tribal leaders and involve community members are more effective than programs that focus on individual patients. A Native group in Canada, the Alkali Lake Band, had a grassroots community campaign against alcoholism and virtually eliminated it in the community, despite no assistance from health care providers or clergy.

Traditionally, the women were the social leaders who held families together. Many tribes were matriarchal, in that one's clan membership was passed down from one's mother. Women could be traditional spiritual leaders, but since most of their lives were focused on creating and nurturing their families, the majority of spiritual leaders were (and are) male. This does not detract from the respect and position women have Native American society.

The massive forces that traditional cultures have faced—the loss of culture, lowered self-esteem and hope, lack of career opportunities, and lack of good role models who have successfully bridged two worlds—have led to high rates of domestic violence, suicide, and self-destructive behaviors. Support from community leaders, federal and state support, and health care providers who understand Native American culture can significantly improve the health of the First Americans.

FURTHER READING

Aiken, L. P. (1990). *Two cultures meet: Pathways for American Indians to medicine.* Garrett Park, MD: Garrett Park Press.
Good comparison of how the American Indian and mainstream U.S. cultures view healing.

Coulehan, J. L. (1980). Navajo Indian medicine: Implications for healing. *Journal of Family Practice, 10*(1), 55–61.
Basic overview for dealing with Indian patients.

Hammerschlag, C. A. (1988). *The dancing healers: A doctor's journey of healing with native Americans.* San Francisco: Harper & Row.
Excellent short book on a non-Indian's learning and living Indian culture and healing.

Lang, R. S. (1992). Special health problems of Native Americans. In R. S. Lang (Ed.), *Principles and practice of clinical preventive medicine* (pp. 729–738). St. Louis, MO: C. V. Mosby.
Excellent overview of Indian health problems and cultural aspects of healing.

Orlandi, M. O. (Ed.). (1992). *Cultural competence for evaluators: A guide for alcohol and other drug abuse prevention practitioners working with ethnic/racial communities* (DHHS Publication No. ADM-92-1884). Washington, DC: U.S. Government Printing Office.

U.S. Department of Health and Human Services. (1996). *Trends in Indian health* (Department of Health and Human Services, Indian Health Services, Office of Planning, Evaluation, and Legislation. Division of Program Statistics). Rockville, MD: Author.
Statistics on Indian health problems.

139

Lesbian Health

Melissa J. Perry
Katherine A. O'Hanlan

Many of the issues relating to lesbians and their relationships affect the physical health status of lesbians, such as the process of "coming out" to health care providers and the common assumptions of heterosexuality that lesbians experience in health care settings. Other sexual orientation and relationship issues unique to lesbians are also an integral part of general lesbian health, including relationship issues around commitment, power sharing, codependency and instability; sexuality and forging sexual identities, and child rearing decisions. These larger relationship and identity issues are explored in this chapter.

COMMITMENT AND POWER SHARING IN LESBIAN RELATIONSHIPS

Despite the prohibition against same-sex marriage, which denies lesbians the essential ability to form socially legitimate relationships and the subsequent legal, financial, and psychological perquisites of heterosexual marriage, many lesbians are observed to be in long-term relationships. Several misconceptions abound regarding the ability of lesbians to form committed and stable involvements. In 1970, researchers from the Kinsey Institute surveyed lesbians between the ages of 36 and 45, and found that 82% of the women were living with a partner. More recently, the Michigan Lesbian Survey, the National Lesbian Health Care Survey, and the Black Women's Relationships Project reported that 60–65% of lesbian respondents were in typically monogamous, committed long-term relationships. A 1991 survey of gay and lesbian couples revealed that 75% of lesbian couples shared their income, 88% had held a wedding ceremony or similar type of ritual celebrating their union, 91% were monogamous, only 7% had broken their relationship agreements, and 92% were committed to their partners for life.

Power sharing in lesbian relationships was investigated by a survey of 70 lesbian couples, which demonstrated that arrangements could not be explained by the usual variables of age, income, education, and asset differences between partners. Egalitarianism was considered the ideal in most relationships, and the stereotypic notion of "butch–femme" role playing was not observed. In another study, relational satisfaction was observed to relate more strongly to essential qualities of the relationship itself than to an individual partner's attitudes or assets, with greatest satisfaction associated with equality of involvement and shared power in the relationship. Some research studies have reported that lesbians typically begin to self-identify as homosexual and engage in homosexual sex at a later age than gay men self-identify and become sexually active, although both genders experience same-sex attraction at a similar early age. Lesbians more often become aware of their orientation first in the context of an emotional relationship, whereas gay men more often recognize their homosexuality in the context of a sexual encounter. In fact, 78% of lesbians in one survey revealed that their first same-sex sexual/romantic relationship had grown out of a previously established friendship with another woman. Similarly, friendship has been found to be an important maintenance factor lesbians' current relationships, with 77% describing their current lovers as their closest friends.

CODEPENDENCY AND INSTABILITY IN RELATIONSHIPS

Intimacy in lesbian relationships can be so intense that some lesbians lose their own sense of themselves and their sense of boundaries. In fact, some degree of stress in a lesbian dyad may stem from difficulties in maintaining a sense of self. Codependency occurs in a lesbian relationship when a woman's desires to be in a partnered relationship are pathologically and unreasonably pursued. Such merger or fusion problems in relationships and identity can result in clinical dysfunction and require therapy. Intimacy in such relationships can usually be restored by the partners' creating some distance between them, maintaining their personal space, and focusing on individual autonomy.

Lesbian women and heterosexual women have much in common in their relational offerings, but may experience a significant difference in their partners' response to such offerings. In a study using a questionnaire based on a cost–reward investment model, it was observed that women, whether lesbian or heterosexual, reported both investing more in their relationships and having greater commitment to maintaining their relationships than either heterosexual or homosexual men. In addition, females reported more often than males that relationship costs were more strongly related to satisfaction and commitment. Relational satisfaction was associated with higher levels of rewards and lower levels of costs. Relational commitment was associated with greater satisfaction and greater investments, but poorer quality with regard to alternatives. All heterosexuals reported both greater costs and marginally greater investments in their relationships. Interestingly, this cost–reward investment model effectively predicted satisfaction and commitment for all four groups of respondents. The authors concluded that gender was a more important predictor of the relationship behaviors explored in this study than was sexual orientation.

In a survey of 34 couples, homosexual women demonstrated greater interpersonal dependency, compatibility, and intimacy in their intimate relationships. In contrast, heterosexual women evidenced more positive dispositions toward sexual fantasy, stronger sexual desire, greater sexual assertiveness, and higher frequencies of sexual activity.

In an interview report with eight African-American lesbians, preference for primary relationship partners was clearly expressed for other lesbians of African-American descent, even though most had previously a relationship with a European-American woman. Cultural differences reported by these women caused relationship conflicts that were not easily or eagerly dealt with, reflecting the complexity of interacting influences of ethnicity, orientation, and external and internalized homophobia.

Relationship instability in lesbian couples can also occur because of the common relational conflicts observed in all couples, but it can be compounded by effects of several sources of cultural homophobia: "coming-out" issues, self-concept issues, and the absence of wedding traditions and marital role models. In particular, lesbians who did not hide their homosexuality were more likely to report satisfaction with their relationships, according to a questionnaire comparing "closeted" and "out" lesbian and gay men. This suggests that internalized homophobia manifesting as self-doubt and shame may make some lesbians doubt their ability to form any relationship at all.

LESBIAN SEXUALITY

The rate of anorgasmia is low for both heterosexual and lesbian women (12% vs. 3%, respectively). Most lesbians report higher rates of regular orgasm than most heterosexual women do. This is probably because the preponderance of lesbian sexual activity entails manual (digital and especially oral) stimulation of the clitoris. It is estimated that only 30% of heterosexual women experience orgasm regularly from intercourse alone; the majority require additional oral or manual stimulation of the clitoris. Some lesbians theorize that they have the added benefit of heightened knowledge of desirable sexual activity, given the similarity of their genital anatomy. Masters and Johnson reported that lesbian couples seemed less goal-oriented and had better communication during sexual activity than heterosexual couples. Although it is apparent that sexual dysfunction occurs in the lesbian population, it appears to occur less frequently than among heterosexual women. The Kinsey Institute researchers reported that 10% of lesbians in their sample reported some dysfunction, whereas a Seattle survey of heterosexual women revealed a 63% incidence of self-reported dysfunction.

LESBIAN DOMESTIC VIOLENCE

Although there is growing awareness in human service and medical communities concerning domestic violence among heterosexuals, there is little awareness that domestic violence also occurs in lesbian relationships. The National Lesbian Health Care Survey reported that 11% of lesbians had been victims of violence committed by their lesbian partners. Victims and perpetrators are more likely to experience violence in the context of alcohol or other substance use. Such substance use often perpetuates a cycle of denial and continuing violence.

LESBIAN FAMILIES

Once a person's basic physical survival needs for food, shelter, and safety are met, then the individual naturally seeks to fulfill higher needs, such as intimacy and, for some, procreation. With this in mind, it is not unreasonable to expect lesbians and gay men to desire marriage and even children when their relationships reach a point of mutual satisfaction, intimacy, and commitment. For many lesbians, the absence of a legal right to marry each other is unsettling. Recalling the 1967 Supreme Court case of *Loving v. Virginia,* in which it was ultimately decided that citizens should not be denied the right to marriage on the basis of the physical condition of the color of their loved ones' skin, most lesbians believe they should not be denied the right to marriage because of the physical condition of their loved ones' gender.

Some individuals worry that legal marriage for gays and lesbians might "endorse homosexuality," possibly resulting in higher numbers of homosexuals. Some are worried about the erosion of "traditional family values" and other threats posed to the ideal of the nuclear family. In fact, an actual "conversion" to homosexuality does not occur, and the term does not accurately describe the process of "coming out" or determining one's sexual orientation. Instead, for many, there is a natural evolution of the self into more honest and full expression. No scientific basis supports the idea that marriage would be devalued if such a right were to be extended to people who desire what the marriage ideal offers: a monogamous, long-term, mutually supportive, committed relationship. The effect of the denial of marriage to lesbians touches the very core of human satisfaction for many. Such discrimination in legal rights is deeply corrosive to the self-concept of many lesbians and precludes the fulfillment of their natural psychosocial needs.

The "Family of Choice"

The definition of "family" for a lesbian couple is more likely to involve creation of a network of close friends as a "family of choice," especially if the partners' families of origin have rejected them. The most frequent sources of support for lesbians in a survey of couples were, in order of frequency, friends, partners, genetic family members, and coworkers. A very diverse picture has emerged in lesbian conceptions of family. Lesbians in a relationship may incorporate their previous partners and children from those relationships, each other's family of choice, and their children into their "familial network."

Children in Lesbian Households

There are a variety of ways in which lesbians can become parents. For example, many lesbians have children from previous marriages. Many lesbians in relationships inseminate themselves, using either known or unknown donors' sperm. Some lesbians have reported in surveys that they would have sex with a man in order to become pregnant, either with his permission or without it. Adoption and foster parenting are used by many lesbians, but these routes can be very costly and lengthy, and are also legally reversible to varying extents in many states. Some states' adoption laws, as well as some adoption clinics, refuse to allow lesbians to adopt.

Impregnation with sperm donated by friends or unsuspecting men leaves custody questions unanswered and may result in a legitimate paternity suit by a sperm donor.

This route is also riskier in terms of sexually transmitted diseases such as HIV. Use of banked sperm confers legal protection in cases of disputed custody and significantly reduces the likelihood of infection. For these reasons, it is recommended that lesbians desiring insemination employ the services of an established sperm bank. Obstetricians/gynecologists and midwives can provide the safest environment for insemination and subsequent delivery. It should be noted that physicians providing insemination services can provide valuable advice by familiarizing themselves with some of the medico-legal issues pertinent to lesbian clients.

In one study of 35 lesbians who had delivered a child in the past 5 years, most had conceived through donor insemination, and all had sought care within the first 16 weeks of pregnancy, with 89% participating in childbirth classes and 80% breastfeeding for 6 months or longer. All of the lesbian mothers had obtained obstetrical care from physicians or midwives, with 91% disclosing their relationships to their care providers. Most of the women reported being very satisfied with their obstetrical experiences.

Studies of the children in lesbian households provide useful information about the effects of lifelong exposure of children to homosexuals and to information about homosexuality. There are concerns that children in lesbian households, of which there are an estimated 6–14 million in the United States, may develop differently and will be psychologically maladjusted as compared to their peers. Such concerns derive from the false perception of lesbians as abnormal and immoral, even though this thinking has been strongly repudiated by the American Psychiatric Association, the American Psychological Association, and the American Medical Association. In a study of 269 cases of child molestation, between 0% and 3.1% of children identified adults who were homosexual as their abusers; the vast majority of those abusers were males. Given that current estimates of the prevalence of both male and female homosexuals in the general community are 3–6%, homosexuals are therefore no more likely to abuse children than heterosexuals.

Patterson reviewed studies of over 300 children (aged 5–17) raised in gay and lesbian households, and concluded that the children's gender identity developed no differently from that of children raised in heterosexual households. No differences in femininity or other sex role behavior were observed in female offspring studied at ages 6–9, ages 10–20, and ages 21–44. Patterson also reviewed studies examining other psychological differences in the children of lesbian parents and found no significant difference in self-concept, locus of control, moral judgment, or intelligence. Indeed, in one study, children of lesbians appeared to have a greater sense of well-being. Another finding was that rates of homosexuality among the children with lesbian parents were similar to those of the offspring of heterosexual parents. Most psychiatrists believe that sexual orientation is not influenced by parents' behavior or orientation; rather, as individuals mature, they become more aware of their own basic innate feelings, more comfortable owning them, and later more comfortable acting upon them.

Although 5% of the children in the studies reviewed by Patterson were taunted by their peers because of their parents' sexual orientation, two studies have suggested that children fare better when they are told about their parents' orientation in early childhood rather than later, when their mothers are psychologically healthy, and when their biological fathers are accepting rather than homophobic. In a study using the California Psychological Inventory, correlates of psychological health for lesbian mothers were openness to their employers, ex-husbands, and children; having a lesbian community; and involvement in feminist activism.

AGING LESBIANS

Age, poverty, and health issues can all render older lesbian invisible. For aging lesbians, acceptance of the aging process and high levels of life satisfaction are associated with connection to and activity in the lesbian community. Because most older lesbians continue to prefer the companionship of other lesbians, usually within 10 years of their own age, it is important to provide a safe environment for older lesbian patients by educating nursing home attendants and nursing personnel. In one survey, most lesbians over 60 stated that they would prefer an intergenerational homosexual retirement community. This type of context would be a logical extension of the diverse family units that lesbians already tend to construct through their social networks. Such retirement communities are likely to provide support to both the health needs and affiliation needs of aging lesbians while at the same time providing an extended "family of choice" of the sort that many lesbians prefer.

FURTHER READING

Bradford, J., Ryan, C., & Rothblum, E. D. (1994). National Lesbian Health Care Survey: Implications for mental health care. *Journal of Consulting and Clinical Psychology, 62*(2), 228–242.
A study of 1,925 lesbians, the most comprehensive study of U.S. lesbians to date.

Cabaj, R. (1988). Gay and lesbian couples: Lessons on human intimacy. *Psychiatric Annals, 18*(1), 21–25.
A thoughtful discussion of the challenges that gays and lesbians face in forging fulfilling relationships.

Kaufman, P. A., Harrison, E., & Hyde, M. L. (1984). Distancing for intimacy in lesbian relationships. *American Journal of Psychiatry, 141*(4), 530–533.
Describes the dynamics of closely merged lesbian relationships and outlines therapeutic avenues for change.

Kehoe, M. (1988). Lesbians over 60 speak for themselves. *Journal of Homosexuality, 16*(3–4) I–III.
Reports findings of a nationwide survey of 100 lesbians 60+ exploring careers, families, and relationships.

Masters, W., & Johnson, V. (1979). *Homosexuality in perspective.* Boston: Little, Brown & Company.
Although dated, this work still provides important insight for understanding lesbian relationships.

Patterson, C. J. (1992). Children of lesbian and gay parents. *Child Development, 63*(5), 1025–1042.
A review of the studies of over 300 children on the developmental effects of growing up in gay and lesbian families. Documents that children of gay and lesbian parents are not greatly distinguishable from children of heterosexual couples in their psychological development.

140

Physician Gender and Physician–Patient Interaction

Klea D. Bertakis

*I*nterest in the impact of gender on the delivery of medical care has risen in parallel with the growth in the number of women in medicine. In fact, the percentage of women graduating from medical school increased from 13.4% to 40% between 1975 and 1997. This expanding population of female physicians makes it increasingly important to evaluate whether physician gender influences patient care. It has been suggested that greater numbers of women physicians may lead to a "feminization" of the medical field, which will result in a greater emphasis on humanistic care. However, there is a paucity of data in this area. Previous studies comparing male and female physicians have often suffered from methodological flaws, which limit their ability to give definitive answers as to how physician gender affects practice style. Confounding variables such as patient gender and health status have not been controlled for in the majority of these studies. Despite their flaws, however, they do provide evidence for differences in the way men and women practice medicine.

AMOUNT OF TIME SPENT WITH PATIENTS

One apparent difference is the amount of time male and female physicians spend with their patients. It has been demonstrated that women physicians have longer visits with them. Data from the National Ambulatory Medical Care Survey showed that female physicians report averaging almost 5 minutes more per patient than male physicians (23.5 vs. 18.7 minutes). Furthermore, women physicians spend more time with female than with male patients. Similar results were found in a more recent study done at 11 primary care sites across the United States, with women physicians averaging 22.9 minutes per medical visit, compared to 20.3 minutes for male physicians. However, the difference between male and female physicians in length of time spent with patients may be related to the gender distribution and health status of patients seen. Women physicians tend to see more female patients, and female patients are less healthy and have longer visits than male patients. In addition, a larger percentage of younger patients are making their first appointments to see women physicians, and initial visits are significantly longer than established patients' return visits.

PRACTICE STYLES

Practice style differences in the way physicians behave and communicate with their patients also seem to be related to physician gender. One area of striking dissimilarity between male and female physician practice styles has been detected in the area of preventive services. Women physicians have been found to provide more preventive services, such as Papanicolaou (Pap) smears and breast examinations. It has just been noted that a larger number of young patients see female physicians; this may in part explain why female practitioners focus more on preventive care. It has also been suggested that physician gender is relevant to preventive care, because it is easier to accomplish breast and cervical screening with gender concordance between physician and patient. Others have proposed that female physicians may be more attentive to preventive care because of their perceptions of their own susceptibility to cancer. However, some researchers have failed to find any significant difference between gender-congruent and gender-incongruent patient encounters in the performance of breast, genitourinary, and rectal examinations. In another study, hospital location, rather than physician gender, was strongly associated with differences in cancer screening behavior. Despite these conflicting findings, gender appears to be a contributing, although still not fully understood, factor in the delivery of preventive services. Thus the notion that gender plays an important role in determining behavior in the physician–patient interaction cannot be ignored.

There is also evidence pointing to differences in the ways male and female physicians communicate with their patients. Analyses of audiotapes of physician–patient communication have demonstrated that male physicians are more imposing and presumptuous (giving more advice and interpretation), whereas female physicians are more attentive and nondirective (giving more subjective and objective information and acknowledgments). Others have found that, compared to male physicians, female physicians engage in more positive talk, partnership building, question asking, and information giving. They also tend to smile and nod in agreement more often, inviting further communication.

Practice style differences are also supported by the relationship of physician gender to patient satisfaction with the medical encounter. One study examining this association found that patients seeing female physicians were significantly more satisfied. This higher satisfaction with female physicians was particularly pronounced among female patients. In another study, there was no difference between male and female physicians in the mean patient satisfaction rating of their total patient populations; however, female patients expressed greater satisfaction with their female physicians than did patients in any other gender pairing of patients and physicians. Indeed, female patients have shown a preference for female physicians, whereas the male patient population continues to express a preference for male physicians. This demonstrates that patients are often more comfortable with a physician of the same sex.

POTENTIAL EFFECTS OF PHYSICIAN GENDER

In their review of the potential effects of physician gender on the physician–patient relationship, Weisman and Teitelbaum suggest that gender may affect the relationship in three ways: gender differences among physicians, particularly with regard to sex role attitudes; differences in patient expectations of male and female physicians; and differences in status levels between the patient and physician in opposite-sex, as opposed to same-sex, physician–patient dyads. In order to allow independent assessment of the effects of physician and patient gender, they recommend that researchers analyzing the physician–patient relationship should study initial visits with same-sex and opposite-sex dyads.

Although such careful planning can eliminate one critical confounding factor, an additional factor cannot be ignored: The health status of patients affects physician–patient interactions. Better health is related to a greater portion of the medical encounter's being spent on physical examination and chatting, and a smaller portion of the visit on history taking. Thus, it is also imperative to measure and control for the patient's health status, in order to permit a valid analysis of the influence of physician gender on the medical visit.

A CONTROLLED STUDY

In a recent study at the University of California at Davis, my colleagues and I sought to clarify issues surrounding physician gender and physician–patient interaction. Since it has been previously shown that physician practice style is dependent on patient health status, on the length of the physician–patient relationship, and on the practice setting, these factors were controlled for while the impact of physician gender on the medical encounter was measured. New patients were randomly assigned to male and female primary care physicians. Their initial medical encounters were videotaped and evaluated, and the Davis Observation Code (DOC) was used to assess physician practice style. The DOC records the occurrence or nonoccurrence of 20 clinically relevant behaviors (such as preventive services, discussions of family information, and history taking) during successive 15-second observation intervals. Patient health status was evaluated before the visit by means of the Medical Outcomes Study Short-Form General Health Survey. Patient satisfaction with medical care was measured via a patient satisfaction questionnaire administered after the patient was seen by the physician.

Contrary to prior studies, our study found only a small and statistically insignificant difference between male and female physicians in the total time spent with their patients during these initial visits. This diminished even further when patient gender and health status were controlled for. The results of prior studies were most likely confounded by the failure to recognize the different patient mixes of male and female physicians. Controlling for type of visit (initial vs. return visit), patient gender, and health status eliminated previously measured differences in visit length.

The study did find, however, that female physicians devoted significantly more time to discussing family medical and social information. This included the current functioning of each patient's family, as well as that of unrelated but significant individuals from his or her social group or workplace. Male physicians devoted significantly more time to history taking, in which a patient gave details related to the current complaint or previous illnesses. (It should be noted, parenthetically, that prolonged history taking has previously been shown to result in a decrease in patient satisfaction.) Thus, the female physicians demonstrated a greater interest in their patients' social milieus and the psychosocial issues affecting them. Patients may interpret this difference in communication style as a reflection of women physicians' being more caring, nurturing, and humane.

Female physicians also spent more time providing preventive services for their patients than male physicians did, even when patient gender and health status were controlled for. Here, "preventive service" was defined as a physician's discussing, planning, or performing any screening task associated with disease prevention, or taking a history on disease prevention. This finding was both statistically and clinically significant and confirmed the conclusions of previous studies. As the public and the medical communities continue to focus on the importance of preventive care, the provision of these services is considered to be indicative of high-quality health care. And as health care organizations work to develop effective medical care delivery systems, they must consider the finding that physician gender influences the amount of preventive care given to patients.

Finally, even after controlling for patient gender and health status, as well as for the patient's general satisfaction prior to the visit, our study found patients to be significantly more satisfied with female physicians than with male physicians. In an effort to discover whether this could be explained by specific differences in practice style or was a consequence of patients' preconceived assumptions about male and female physicians, we felt it appropriate to control for certain behaviors in the statistical equation explaining patient satisfaction. These behaviors included preventive services, family information, and history taking. When this was done, the measured differences in patient satisfaction lost statistical significance. This means that a substantial portion of the patients' higher satisfaction with female physicians related not to the physicians' gender per se, but to measurable differences in practice style. Since patient satisfaction can be related to specific aspects of female physicians' practice styles, it follows that medical educators may be able to develop curricula designed to teach students physician behaviors that result in increased patient satisfaction.

CONCLUSION

In conclusion, male and female physicians do exhibit identifiable differences in the way they practice medicine, which in turn explain the differences in patient's satisfaction with them. Although there are no differences in the total time male and female physicians spend with their patients, female physicians engage in more preventive services, and their communication with patients places a greater emphasis on psychosocial issues and concerns. These differential practice styles lead to increased patient satisfaction and may lead to differences in other patient outcomes as well. It has been observed, however, that as women progress through medical school and residency training in a predominantly male-taught discipline (with only 26% of full-time faculty members being women), their attitudes and behaviors become less distinguishable from those of their male colleagues. Although female students tend to place a higher value on establishing a good interpersonal relationship with patients, on assessing the impact of disease on patients and their families, and on disease prevention and health promotion, the attitudinal differences between male and female students decrease as they advance in their medical training.

FURTHER READING

Arnold, R. M., Martin, S. C., & Parker, R. M. (1988). Taking care of patients: Does it matter whether the physician is a woman? *Western Journal of Medicine, 149,* 729–733.

This is an excellent review of studies examining practice style differences between male and female physicians.

Bertakis, K. D., Helms, L. J., Callahan, E. J., Azari, R., & Robbins, J. A. (1995). The influence of gender on physician practice style. *Medical Care, 33,* 407–416.

Female physicians spend significantly more time doing preventive services and discussing their patients' psychosocial issues, leading to significantly higher patient satisfaction with female physicians than with male physicians.

Franks, P., & Clancy, C. M. (1993). Physician gender bias in clinic decision making: Screening for cancer in primary care. *Medical Care, 31,* 213–218.

According to data from the 1987 National Medical Expenditure Survey, women reporting a female physician as their usual health care provider were less likely to be deficient for Pap tests, mammograms, and breast examinations than were patients identifying a male physician, but there was no gender bias evident for blood pressure checks.

Hall, J. A., Irish, J. T., Roter, D. L., Ehrlich, C. M., & Miller, L. H. (1994). Gender in medical encounters: An analysis of physician and patient communication in a primary care setting. *Health Psychology, 13,* 384–392.

This study of 100 routine medical visits found that female physicians had longer visits, made more positive and partnership statements, asked more questions, and gave more verbal and nonverbal indications of encouragement to their patients.

Linn, L. S., Cope, D. W., & Leake, B. (1984). The effect of gender and training of residents on satisfaction ratings by patients. *Journal of Medical Education, 59,* 964–966.

Both male and female patients seen by female physicians had significantly higher satisfaction scores than patients seen by male physicians.

Lurie, N., Slater, J., McGovern, P., Ekstrum, J., Quam, L., & Margolis, K. (1993). Preventive care for women: Does the sex of the physician matter? *New England Journal of Medicine, 329,* 478–482.

The medical claims for mammography and Pap tests for 97,962 women were reviewed, and it was demonstrated that women are more likely to undergo these tests if they see female rather than male physicians.

Roter, D., Lipkin, M., & Korsgaard, A. (1991). Sex differences in patients' and physicians' communication during primary care medical visits. *Medical Care, 29,* 1083–1093.

In this study of 537 adult visits, female physicians conducted medical visits differently than their male counterparts, spending more time with the patients and being more "patient-centered"; patients of women physicians talked more during the medical visit and were more actively involved in the medical dialogue.

Weisman, C. S., & Teitelbaum, M. A. (1985). Physician gender and the physician–patient relationship: Recent evidence and relevant questions. *Social Science and Medicine, 20,* 1119–1127.

This paper reviews the potential effects of physician gender on the physician–patient relationship and its outcomes.

141

What We Know about Women's Health

Elaine A. Blechman
Kelly D. Brownell
Amy W. Helstrom

*O*ur authors have presented an abundance of information about women's health. Each chapter contributes to a growing body of knowledge about what women and the practitioners who care for them can do to maximize women's physical and mental well-being. We leave you with some thought-provoking examples.

LIFE COURSE PERSPECTIVES

Sandra P. Thomas: "Women arrive at midlife with a stronger and more integrated sense of self than men, because women have dealt more actively with conflicting expectations, options, values, and role commitments throughout young adulthood." Evelyn B. Thoman: "Aspects of a mother's health are markedly affected by the synchrony achieved between her own psychological needs and biological rhythms and those of her baby." Susan G. Millstein and Bonnie L. Halpern-Felsher: "Data from the 1988 National Survey of Family Growth indicate that among 15- to 19-year-old females, 53% have experienced coitus at least once, with rates varying by race/ethnicity: 49% of Hispanic-American, 52% of European-American, and 61% of African-American girls are sexually active by the age of 19 years." Heather Carmichael Olson: "It is now recognized that the teratogenic effects of alcohol are a public health problem, as they can cause abnormal fetal development and a full spectrum of alcohol-related birth defects among women who drink while pregnant."

STRESS AND COPING

H. J. Eysenck: "Women's health is strongly affected by psychological factors such as stress and personality that determine in part the occurrence and outcome of cancer and coronary heart disease." K. Daniel O'Leary: " . . . there is no consistent evidence that helping an individual will increase marital satisfaction. On the other hand, there is evidence from over a dozen studies that conjoint marital therapy leads to increases in marital satisfaction." Thomas Ashby Wills: "People with more social support have lower levels of depression, a lower risk of mortality, and a greater likelihood of recovery from clinical illness." Frank D. Fincham: "Marital satisfaction is important in predicting the course and resolution of depressive episodes."

PREVENTION

Patricia M. Dubbert: "Women can achieve many physical and mental health benefits from at least 30 minutes of moderate-level physical activity each day." John W. Osborne: "Brushing one's teeth once a day for 3–5 minutes would be better than two to three times per day for 30 seconds each." Kathleen J. Sikkema: "The epidemiology of HIV infection among women is changing, with heterosexual transmission rather than a woman's own injection drug use now accounting for the majority of new infections." Joel D. Killen: "By age 18, about two-thirds of adolescents in the United States have tried smoking." Jalie A. Tucker: "The ratio of male to female problem drinkers is about 3:1, but women who drink heavily are more socially stigmatized and tend to develop problems more rapidly and at lower levels of alcohol consumption compared to men." Heidi D. Nelson: "Estrogen use in a large cohort of older women is associated with approximately a 50% decrease in risk for wrist fractures and all nonspinal fractures." Joni A. Mayer: "In the past decade, rates of mammographic screening among U.S. women age 50 and older have increased substantially."

HEALTH CARE POLICIES, PARADIGMS, SETTINGS, AND PRACTICES

Jacqueline Wallen: "Women who abuse alcohol or drugs, or who have partners who abuse alcohol or drugs, use more health care services than other women." Rona L. Levy: "Changes in the structure and financing of health care are likely to have a significant impact on behavioral medicine research for women and the delivery of health care services to women."

BODY IMAGE AND SUBSTANCE USE

Corinne G. Husten: "Cigarette smoking is the leading preventable cause of death among women in the United States." Janet Polivy and Traci L. McFarlane: "For many people, dieting may prove counterproductive and lead to weight gain and other problems rather than weight loss." Karen Heffernan: "The incidence of bulimia nervosa has increased markedly over the past three decades, affecting 1–3% of college women." Rena R. Wing: "Obesity affects over one-third of all U.S. women, with more than 50% of middle-aged

African-American and Mexican-American women affected." Sharon Hall: "Women drug treatment patients have different needs than men patients; both the history of drug use treatment and societal perception of women drug users complicate treatment."

SEXUALITY AND REPRODUCTION

Judith G. Rogers: "Women with disabilities are the forgotten minority. People cannot even imagine a woman with a disability as a parent." Ruth A. Lawrence: "Breast feeding has been rediscovered as the optimal source of infant nutrition because of a growing body of knowledge about the nutritional, immunological, psychological, and other health benefits to infants and mothers." Katherine A. O'Hanlan: "Although one alcoholic beverage daily may be beneficial in preventing cardiac disease, more than one beverage daily reduces bone density."

PHYSIOLOGICAL CONDITIONS WITH BEHAVIORAL/PSYCHOSOCIAL COMPONENTS

Catherine M. Stoney: "Coronary heart disease (CHD) is the leading cause of death among women, and the decline in mortality rates due to CHD has been slower among women than among men since 1979." C. David Jenkins: "Cardiovascular mortality—long the number one cause of death in older women—has been decreasing substantially in the last 25 years in the United States, because women and men have reduced their risk factors." Patricia A. Ganz: "Cancer is the second leading cause of death for women currently, and in the 21st century will likely surpass heart disease as the number one cause." Karen B. Schmaling: "Pregnancy is associated with the apparent worsening of asthma symptoms for some women and improvement in others." William E. Haley: "Alzheimer's disease takes its greatest toll on women, who are not only at higher risk than men for Alzheimer's disease, but most commonly take on the role of family caregiver for an impaired relative." Patricia A. Wisocki: "Preliminary reports indicate that behavioral treatments are effective interventions for pain and other problems associated with arthritis and osteoporosis for elderly women." Mark H. Hermanoff: "In 1987 lung cancer surpassed breast cancer for women and is now the leading cause of cancer death for women in the United States."

LINKAGES BETWEEN MENTAL AND PHYSICAL HEALTH PROBLEMS

William C. Sanderson: "Agoraphobia is diagnosed three times as often in women as in men." Richard R. J. Lewine: "As 50–60% of the pregnancies of schizophrenic women are unplanned, one of the first issues is that of family planning and the use of contraceptives." Lily D. McNair: "For every major health category, mortality rates for African-American women are higher than those for European-American women." Albert M. Woodward: "As a group, [Hispanic women] are more likely to face a barrier to entry [to health care] because of lack of insurance coverage." David R. Baines: "Most of the causes of mortality and morbidity [among Native American women] cam be significantly reduced by prevention programs and strategies and behavioral changes in the population."

Index

Mayer, Joni A., 212
Mayer, K., 446
Mayes, M., 704, 705
Mayeux, R., 550
Mayocchi, L., 74
McAlister, A., 232
McAnarney, E. R., 481
McArthur, J. W., 454, 455
McCabe, S. B., 112
McCrady, B. S., 405
McDonald, E., 787
McDonald-Haile, J., 474
McFarlane, Jessica Motherwell, 459, 462
McGarvey, S. T., 619, 622
McGinn, L. K., 740
McGinnis, J. M., 297
McGlashan, T. H., 773, 775, 776
McGlone, J., 16, 19
McGonagle, K. A., 736, 757, 762, 763
McGovern, P., 181, 853
McGrath, E., 752, 754, 756
McGrath, P. C., 593
McGrory, C. H., 686
McGuigan, S., 467
McKinlay, A., 253
McKinlay, J., 83, 86
McKinlay, S. M., 83, 86
McLanahan, S., 168
McLean, Peter D., 754, 756
McLeod, J. D., 174, 763
McLerran, D. F., 260
McNamara, G., 123
McNeilly, A., 505
Meadows, E. A., 746
Media, and gender role socialization, 42–44
Medical curricula and training, 303–307
  curricular initiatives, 305–306
  model training approaches, 306
  and morbidity/mortality, 304
  and gender bias, 304–305
Meilahn, E. N., 85, 401
Melin, B., 809
Mellits, E. D., 68
Melnick, S., 663, 838
Melton, L. J., 227, 396
Melzack, R., 467, 792
Mendelsohn, G., 638
Menopause
  and disease prevention, 521
  estrogen therapy for indications for, 521–524
    nutritional alternatives to, 524–525
  and progestogens, 525–526
  risk and safety issues, 524–525
Menstrual cycle, 450–451
  and gastrointestinal physiology, 644–645
  and immunity, 679–680
  and migraine headaches, 656–657

Mental health. *See also* well being
  optimism and, 146–147
  social support and, 119–120
Mentally retarded, parents of. *See* parents of mentally retarded adults
Mercer, M. B., 202
Mestman, J. H., 622
Metzger, D. A., 454, 455
Meyer, T. J., 591, 594
Meyerowitz, B. E., 590, 594
Micciolo, R., 112
Michelson, D., 694
Mickelson, O., 357
Midlife
  C. G. Jung on development during, 82
  coping during, 84
  psychosocial influences on health, 83
  stress during, 83–84
Midlife crisis, 82–83
Migaly, M., 705
Migraine headaches
  menstrual cycle and, 656–657
Miklowitz, David J., 749–751
Mikulincer, M., 104, 107, 154
Milburn, A. K., 468
Military
  Gulf War veteran readjustment, 327
  health care needs, 325–326
    of childbearing women, 326
  stressors of
    nontraditional roles and, 325
    in wartime duty, 324
    work environment and, 324–325
  work and family stress, 326–327
Miller, B., 217, 220, 244, 419, 552, 553
Miller, D. A., 746
Miller, L. H., 853
Miller, N. S., 312
Miller, R. H., 297
Miller, T. Q., 134, 138
Millman, R. B., 424
Millstein, Susan G., 49
Milne, K., 493
Minichiello, W. E., 736
Minkoff, H., 663
Mintz, J., 750
Miranda, J., 207
Mitchell, C. M., 474, 653
Mitchell, D., 558, 563, 565
Mitchell, J. T., 746
Mitton, J. E., 773, 776
Moffat, F. L., 589, 593
Moffat, F. L., Jr., 151
Moffitt, T. E., 55, 57
Mogil, J. S., 699
Molfese, V. J., 481

Monk, T. H., 749, 750
Montemayor, R., 63
Montgomery, L. M., 115, 117
Moore, M. E., 686
Moore, R., 207
Moore, R. E., 207
Moore, S., 63
Moorjani, S., 718
Moos, M. K., 332
Moos, R. H., 161
Moreland, K. L., 301
Morgan, S. P., 68, 161
Morganit, C., 565
Morokoff, Patricia J., 441, 442, 445
Morrill, A. C., 202
Morris, J., 273
Morris, N. M., 63
Morris, T., 151
Morrison, T. L., 365, 368
Morrissette, D., 534
Morrow, C., 30
Morrow, M., 603
Mortola, J. F., 454, 456
Morton, D., 151, 576, 591, 593, 804
Morton, D. L., 151, 591, 593
Moss, A. R., 207
Moten, J., 705
Mothers. *See* breastfeeding; childrearing; parents; pregnancy
Mount, J. H., 493
Mowbray, C. T., 782
Mozley, L. H., 18
Mozley, P. D., 18
Mrazek, D. A., 569
Mrazek, P. R., 237
Muff, A. M., 746
Mullan, J. T., 549
Mullen, P. D., 430
Muller, D. C., 718
Multiple sclerosis
  cognitive aspects, 690
  emotional aspects, 690
  interventions to enhance coping, 691–692
  psychotherapeutic approaches to, 692–693
  stress and, 689–690
Munroe-Blum, H., 775, 776
Murdock, T., 746
Murphy, D. A., 197, 202, 445
Myerson, J. C., 454, 456
Myrstren, A.-L., 809

Nachman, G., 474, 653
Nadeau, A., 718
Nakamura, C. Y., 832
Narcolepsy, 795
Narcotics Anonymous. *See* drug abuse, treatment; twelve-step programs